D. P. A

Drug Therapy in Infants

Pharmacologic Principles and Clinical Experience

Robert J. Roberts, M.D., Ph.D.

Professor, Departments of Pediatrics
   and Pharmacology
University of Iowa College of Medicine

1984

W. B. Saunders Company

Philadelphia • London • Toronto • Mexico City • Rio de Janeiro • Sydney • Tokyo

W. B. Saunders Company: West Washington Square
Philadelphia, PA 19105

1 St. Anne's Road
Eastbourne, East Sussex BN21 3UN, England

1 Goldthorne Avenue
Toronto, Ontario M8Z 5T9, Canada

Apartado 26370 — Cedro 512
Mexico 4, D.F., Mexico

Rua Coronel Cabrita, 8
Sao Cristovao Caixa Postal 21176
Rio de Janeiro, Brazil

9 Waltham Street
Artarmon, N.S.W. 2064, Australia

Ichibancho, Central Bldg., 22-1 Ichibancho
Chiyoda-Ku, Tokyo 102, Japan

Library of Congress Cataloging in Publication Data

Roberts, Robert J.
  Drug therapy in infants.

  Includes index.
  1. Infants — Diseases — Chemotherapy.   2. Pediatric
pharmacology.   I. Title.   [DNLM: 1. Drug therapy — In
infancy and childhood.   2. Pharmacology, Clinical — In
infancy and childhood.   WS 366 R646d]
RJ560.R63   1984   615.5'8'0880542   83-20033
ISBN 0-7216-7604-9

Drug Therapy in Infants:
Pharmacologic Principles and Clinical Experiences   ISBN   0-7216-7604-9

Last digit is the print number: 9   8   7   6   5   4   3   2   1

*Dedicated to my wife, Donna,
and children, Rob and CeAnn*

FOREWORD

Pediatricians, neonatologists, and other physicians caring for infants should not need to be reminded that therapeutic principles established for adults or even for older children are not applicable to the neonate. Indeed, some of the major therapeutic misadventures in the history of medicine have resulted from the assumption that newborns are no more than smaller versions of adults, and that principles of drug usage can be extrapolated to infants purely on the basis of size. Physicians who have seen infants devastated by sulfanilamide-associated kernicterus, the death of infants with the gray syndrome treated with "usual" doses of chloramphenicol, deafness resulting from streptomycin, and numerous other examples of drug-related problems should be aware that therapies applied to infants must be based on therapeutic principles established for infants. The appropriate use of pharmocologic agents in infants and children demands a critical knowledge and appreciation of the influences of normal and abnormal development on clinical pharmacology. It is exceedingly important to view drug administration to infants against the background of developmental changes in drug binding, distribution, and metabolism. Our therapeutic errors in the past have to a large extent resulted from a failure to recognize that infants are different from other age groups.

It is also important that we avoid ritualizing therapies provided to sick newborns and that therapies be carried out with a clear knowledge of developmental pathophysiology and of the risks and benefits of the agents given. For example, it is extremely difficult for any newborn admitted to an intensive care unit to escape the hospital without receiving methylxanthines, antibiotics, or furosemide, in addition to many other drugs. While these therapies may be indicated in some instances, it is essential that we maintain a critical approach to the administration of these and other agents and base drug use on the likelihood of therapeutic success rather than on ritual. In many cases drugs are used without strong evidence for efficacy, further emphasizing the need for carefully performed clinical trials.

Dr. Roberts has done an outstanding job of dealing with these important questions. He has utilized his excellent background as a neonatologist and a superb base of pharmacologic information to provide a text that is both critical in approach and rich in information concerning those drugs that are most frequently used in newborn nurseries and in infants. The unique aspects of drug therapy in the newborn are discussed within the context of the pathophysiology of the disorders for which drugs are being administered. The book also covers important practical issues of concern to the neonatologist. Special concerns involving the administration of drugs through intravenous lines in newborns and the effect of exchange transfusion on drug distribution are well described. Indeed, what comes across throughout the book is the need for drug therapy to be based on a sound understanding of developmental pathophysiology. For example, the chapter concerned with administration of anti-convulsants includes a discussion of the etiology and significance of seizures in the newborn. Similarly, the chapter on diuretics includes a description of developmental renal physiology as it relates to diuretic administration. This excellent blending of practical issues important to the neonatologist and pediatrician with a modern approach to developmental pharmacology is what will make this volume an essential resource for those caring for newborns. The book is written with clarity and authority and should be of immense help to those who wish to apply sound pharmacologic principles in neonatal therapeutics.

JOSEPH B. WARSHAW

PREFACE

The growing body of pediatric literature gives testimony to the interest and advances in the use of drugs for the treatment of neonates and older infants. Both a greater understanding of pathophysiology and the continued development and investigation of therapeutic agents have been major contributors to successful therapeutic manipulation. The early foundation for clinical pharmacology in infants rested largely on the superficial assumption that cursory extrapolation of adult drug experience to the infant was reasonable and appropriate; however, clinical studies prompted by experience suggesting age-related differences in drug disposition, and carried out with the aid of more sophisticated analytic techniques, have now amply demonstrated the unique complexity of pharmacology in infants.

The writing of this text was stimulated in part by the rapid growth of therapeutic knowledge in neonatal medicine; such knowledge is crucial in preventing therapeutic catastrophes such as the chloramphenicol-induced "gray baby syndrome." Another major inspiration was the intellectual enthusiasm of pediatric residents and neonatology fellows and staff at the University of Iowa College of Medicine as well as at other institutions. This enthusiasm served to reinforce my belief in the need for a comprehensive text on drug therapy in infants.

This book has been organized into two sections. The first section is a broad overview of general pharmacologic principles important to drug management of infant disease, including pharmacokinetics. (A portion of this information was previously published in a comprehensive text on neonatal disease.[a]) The second section is a comprehensive review of drugs that are currently utilized in the treatment of disease in infants. The chapters dealing with specific drugs include well-established and proven therapies along with recent developments in therapeutic manipulation of certain neonatal diseases. Owing to limitations of space, not every experience with drug therapy in infants can be presented, nor can every detail be provided for the drugs that are discussed; therefore, a comprehensive listing of relevant literature is provided, and the reader is encouraged to refer to this body of information for additional details. Whenever possible, a summary statement or conclusion has been offered regarding therapeutic approaches. Continued development of new drugs and therapies, however, may antiquate currently accepted treatment; perhaps definitive therapy for diseases not fully understood at present will be devised for inclusion in future editions of this book.

---

[a] Avery ME, Taeusch HW Jr (eds): Schaeffer's Diseases of the Newborn, 5th ed. Philadelphia, WB Saunders, 1983.

I wish to express my appreciation and gratitude to all my colleagues, especially Drs. Richard Andersen, James Bale, Edward Bell, William Bell, Edward Clark, Allen Erenberg, Herman Hein, Larry Mahoney, Jean Robillard, Gail McGuinness, Robert Thompson, Harold Williamson, Eckhard Zeigler, Kenneth Nakamura, Jon Wispe, and Richard Leff, for their unselfish assistance in the preparation of the book; to my two Department Chairmen, Drs. J. P. Long and Fred Smith, Jr., who have been exemplary inspirational role models; and to Denise Morrell, who has tirelessly deciphered and translated my handwriting and dictation into the contents of this text.

I hope the information contained in this text will be useful to both the student and the practicing physician in the care of their patients, and that the voids and controversies will prompt the academically inclined to carry out carefully designed, scientific investigations that will fill these voids and resolve the controversies.

ROBERT J. ROBERTS

CONTENTS

SECTION
ONE
PHARMACOLOGIC PRINCIPLES
AND PHARMACOKINETICS

ONE

Pharmacologic Principles in Therapeutics in Infants

For all physicians, including pediatricians and neonatologists, the major emphasis during educational training and subsequent clinical practice is on diagnosis and treatment of disease. To achieve maximal therapeutic advantage during the course of patient care, the appropriate "drug of choice" must be selected. This selection requires an accurate diagnosis of the disease, as well as a thorough understanding and knowledge of both the clinical status of the infant and the therapeutic agent chosen. Unfortunately, all too often the major concern resides in the selection of the therapeutic agent rather than in the details of its pharmacology and administration: dose, route, interval, and duration. Yet these aspects are likely to have a major impact on the potential for patient benefit.

The amount of drug given — the **dose** — determines whether its effect is therapeutic or toxic. Moreover, the **route** and **interval of administration** may have a sizable impact on the onset and duration of pharmacologic effect of each dose given. Any decision about **duration of therapy** must take into account the costs, both financial and toxicity-related, associated with the therapeutic program selected. The influence of the infant's **existing disease state** on these factors must also be considered. Without an awareness of the possible impact of these factors on therapeutic outcome, which can be considerable, unexpected or undesirable effects may be recognized only by the so-called "trial-and-error" approach or may even go unrecognized. If these factors are not fully appreciated, an excellent drug may be poorly used, so that optimal therapeutic benefits or potentially beneficial treatments are not realized.

Among the more important principles of pharmacology is the **site of action** of a drug.

Theoretically, if an adequate concentration of drug can be maintained at the site(s) of action for the duration of therapy, the ideal therapeutic objective can be achieved. However, since the site of action is generally far removed from the site of administration, the drug must undergo absorption from the site of administration and then transfer to the site of action. Additional intervening events, such as competitive distribution to tissue sites other than the site of action including sites of toxicity, metabolism, and excretion, can compromise achievement of the ideal response.

The term **drug disposition** refers to the absorption, distribution, storage, metabolism, and excretion of the drug in the body (see Fig. 1–1). As described more fully later in the chapter, drug disposition can be significantly altered by a variety of disease states affecting the respective organ systems involved in drug absorption, distribution, metabolism, or excretion. Altered drug disposition has been observed primarily in congestive heart, liver, or renal failure and in pathophysiologic states of hypoxemia and acidosis; these observations have been thoroughly reviewed by Rane.[24] (Details of the disposition of specific drugs are provided in later chapters.)

Compared with available data on adults, there is a paucity of information regarding drug disposition in infants. The disastrous experiences in earlier years, such as chloramphenicol-induced "gray baby syndrome," are dramatic illustrations of the importance of understanding and appreciating the fundamental principles involved in drug disposition in infants.

For optimal results with drug therapy, knowledge is needed not only of the mechanisms and details of disposition but also of the kinetics of the process. The term **pharmacokinetics** refers

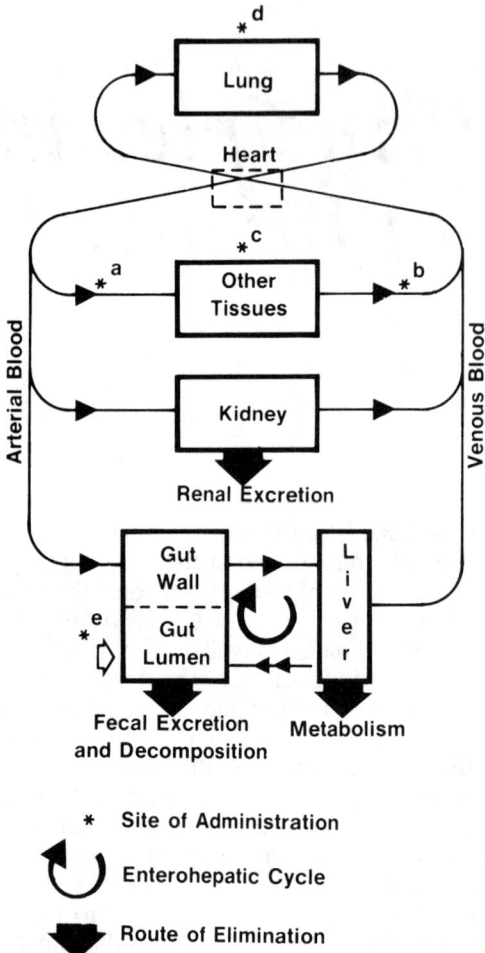

Figure 1–1. Once absorbed from any of the many possible sites of administration, a drug is distributed by blood to all sites within the body including the eliminating organs. Sites of administration are *a*, artery; *b*, peripheral vein; *c*, muscle and subcutaneous tissue; *d*, lung; and *e*, gastrointestinal tract. The lines with arrows refer to the mass movement of drug in blood (→) or bile (◂◂). The absorption and disposition of virtually any drug can be followed from site of administration to site of elimination. (From Rowland M, Tozer TN: Clinical Pharmacokinetics: Concepts and Application. Philadelphia, Lea and Febiger, 1980.)

to the mathematical (kinetic) expression of drug disposition. Numerical (quantitative) expressions characterizing one or more aspects of a drug's absorption, distribution, metabolism, or excretion have been devised; these are discussed in detail in Chapter 2. Pharmacokinetics is useful in clinical practice only if the dynamics of the clinical effects of the drug—its **pharmacodynamics**—can be temporally related to concentration of drug.

Absorption. The sites at which drugs can be administered are either **intravascular**—intravenous (IV), intra-arterial (IA)—or **extra-** vascular—oral (PO), sublingual, buccal, intramuscular (IM), subcutaneous (SQ), rectal. Intravascular administration routes deliver the drug directly to the bloodstream, but with extravascular routes of administration, the drug must be absorbed—that is, pass through tissue or cell membranes—in order to reach the blood. The movement of drugs through membranes from site of administration is by passive diffusion and therefore is largely determined by factors known to regulate rates of diffusion: the physicochemical properties of the drug molecule and of the membrane itself, pH of the drug's biological environment, and local blood flow.

Absorption of a drug from intramuscular injection sites depends largely on vascular perfusion surrounding the site of injection. Inflammation with vasoconstriction, avascular tissue, and shock can drastically modify both rate and extent of drug absorption. A recent study in adults has demonstrated that injections intended to be intramuscular were usually intralipomatous.[5] Although the therapeutic advantage of one over the other is unknown, clearly there is currently little control over where the drug bolus is actually delivered following intramuscular injection. Certain drugs are not suitable for intramuscular administration because of tissue insolubility problems (local precipitation), such as with phenytoin and diazepam, or because of significant pain on administration, such as with digoxin.

Absorption of drugs from the gastrointestinal tract in neonates should be expected to be under the same influences as those operating in older infants, children, and adults. Since the basic mechanism for drug absorption from the gastrointestinal tract is by diffusion, the major factors that can alter the rates and extent of drug absorption include gastrointestinal motility (surface area and contact time of the drug with the absorptive area), pH (degree of ionization of the drug), and gastrointestinal contents, including bacterial flora. Rane[24] points out the importance of considering the physiologic differences and developmental changes affecting these factors in the neonate; significant differences include the highly alkaline gastric contents until about 12 hours of life or beyond; a greater proportion of weight or surface area of gastrointestinal tract to the whole body; and the presence of β-glucuronidase in the gut.[28] β-Glucuronidase may have particular importance since it is capable of converting glucuronide-conjugated drug present in the gastrointestinal tract (e.g., subsequent to biliary excretion) to free drug, so that reabsorption into the systemic circulation is possible; such reabsorption may explain the prolonged or accentuated pharmacologic activity seen with the administration of certain drugs (e.g., see Indomethacin in Chap. 9). Despite frequent reference in the literature to differences in the neonatal gastrointestinal tract compared with that in the adult and the impact these differences may have on drug absorption, few controlled studies have actually examined questions of drug bioavailability and rate of absorption in neonates. One exception is the report by Bell and colleagues,[1] which dispels the notion that the premature infant absorbs vitamin E poorly from the intestinal tract. Other earlier studies reported reduced absorption of a triple sulfa suspension in low-birth-weight (premature) infants versus full-term infants; hypoglycemic effect of oral insulin observed when given within minutes after birth but not after several hours; and greater oral absorption of ampicillin and nafcillin in newborns compared with adults.[29] In a review of developmental differences in drug absorption, Hoffmann[11] concluded that drugs absorbed by passive diffusion from the gut are absorbed at higher rates in immature animals. However, these increased absorption rates do not always result in higher blood levels of drug because of greater volumes of distribution.

Oral drug absorption may be affected by other factors, including several possible mechanisms of drug loss. If drug decomposition or failure of dissolution of the pharmaceutical preparation occurs, the drug will not be available for absorption from the gastrointestinal tract. Metabolism during passage through the intestinal wall or liver can also occur. The loss of drug as a consequence of being absorbed from the gastrointestinal tract and subsequently extracted by hepatic elimination mechanisms before reaching the systemic circulation is known as the **first-pass effect.** Certain drugs show a significant first-pass effect in adult humans due to hepatic elimination;[27] these are listed in Table 1–1. Unfortunately, no similar data regarding first-pass effect exist for infants, although there may be notable differences between infants and adults in hepatic clearance phenomena (uptake, metabolism, and excretion), and in the amount of competing substrates such as endogenous hormones and bilirubin.[18]

It is important to realize that rates and extent of drug absorption from the site of administration cannot and should not be routinely equated with therapeutic efficacy. For example,

Table 1–1. DRUGS WITH RELATIVELY LOW ORAL AVAILABILITY DUE TO HIGH FIRST-PASS HEPATIC EXTRACTION

aspirin	methylphenidate
chlormethiazole	morphine
desipramine	nitroglycerin
hydralazine	nortriptyline
isoproterenol	pentazocine
lidocaine	propranolol
meperidine	salicylamide

Information largely from studies in adult humans.
Adapted from Williams RL, Mamelok RD[27] and Rowland M, Tozer TN: Clinical Pharmacokinetics: Concepts and Application. Philadelphia, Lea and Febiger, 1980.

to conclude drug A will be better than drug B simply on the basis of "percent" of dose available for absorption or "percent" of dose absorbed (bioavailability) ignores the importance of considering the "absolute" amount of drug absorbed. This amount may be sufficient to produce the desired effect but may represent a small percentage of the dose that was administered.

In summary, absorption of a drug from the site of administration can be a critical determinant of drug effect. Therefore, the site of administration must be selected on the basis of the patient's condition and knowledge of the drug. For example, in cardiac resuscitation of infants, epinephrine must be administered in such a way that it reaches the heart as rapidly as possible. Since vascular circulation may be nonexistent at the time of epinephrine administration, the intracardiac route has been employed. Intratracheal administration has also been shown to be effective because of the relatively short course of circulation to the heart and coronary circulation and the reduced morbidity compared with that associated with cardiac puncture.[8]

Distribution. Distribution refers to the reversible movement of drug from one location in the body to another. It is the process that leads to the partition of drugs among the various body organs and tissues (compartments). The distribution of a drug is determined by several factors, including blood flow, pH and composition of body fluids and tissues, physicochemical properties of the drug (lipid solubility, ionization constant), and extent of drug binding to plasma or other body proteins. The distribution of different drugs to body tissues will therefore vary in rate and amount. The influence of the route of administration on drug distribution must also be appreciated. Figure 1–1 vividly illustrates, for example, that the heart and lung are direct recipients of drugs administered intravenously, whereas the liver acts as a primary recipient for drugs given orally. Competition between organs for drugs can ultimately affect the amount of drug reaching the desired sites of effect (see Fig. 2–1). Persistence of fetal circulation can occur in neonates suffering from a variety of conditions (e.g., respiratory distress and postasphyxial syndromes). A right-to-left vascular shunt produces a hemodynamic abnormality that will markedly alter the distribution of blood, and of accompanying drug, away from the lung and to other tissues and organs. This is a major problem when the desired site of effect is the lung, such as with tolazoline treatment of pulmonary hypertension (see Chap. 7).

Of the controlling factors for drug distribution, the most important are (1) vascular perfusion of the tissue or organ, (2) drug diffusion, and (3) plasma protein binding. Generally, the greater the tendency for a drug to concentrate in a tissue, the longer the time required to deliver to that tissue the amount of drug required to reach distribution equilibrium. However, if diffusion, not perfusion, is the major rate-limiting factor, this principle may not hold. Varying penetration of different drugs into the cerebrospinal fluid illustrates this point.[3] If either perfusion or diffusion is rate-limiting to a given drug's distribution, then prediction of that drug's tissue distribution is possible. However, the large differences in perfusion and diffusion characteristics of different organs and tissues make it very difficult or impossible to predict reliably the rate and extent of distribution of drugs with both perfusion and diffusion rate factor considerations.

The third factor believed to be important as a modulator of drug distribution in the body is the **binding of drugs to plasma proteins.** In general, acidic drugs bind to albumin while basic drugs bind to alpha$_1$-acid glycoprotein and lipoproteins.[22] In drug–protein binding an equilibrium mechanism operates to produce a balance between two reversible processes: (1) dissociation of the drug–protein complex, resulting in free drug, and (2) a rebinding of the free drug to vacant sites on the protein. The rate of formation of free drug is proportional to the concentration of the complex, and the rate of drug–protein complex formation is proportional to the concentration of protein with available binding sites.[4] Factors affecting drug–protein binding other than the quantity of protein and drug and the intrinsic affinity properties of drug and protein include temperature, pH, and presence of competitive binding substances.

It is generally accepted that the binding of drug to plasma protein can be a modulating factor not only in the drug's distribution in the body but in dose–response relationships and the rate of elimination of drug from the body. The effects of intrinsic binding properties, of different amounts of plasma protein (newborn versus adult), or of number of available protein binding sites for a drug (competitive binding, such as by bilirubin or other drugs) on the distribution of drug between plasma and the remainder of the body are represented by the three theoretical curves in Figure 1–2. The changing slope of each curve means that there is not a fixed relationship between the concentration of drug in the plasma and the amount of total drug in the body. The major change in the

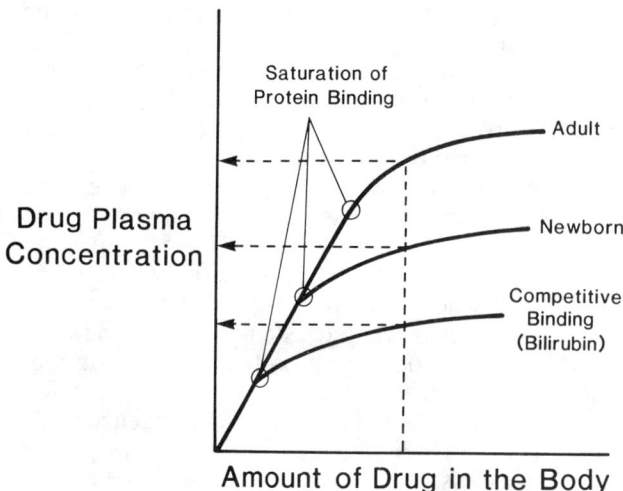

Figure 1–2. Graph showing differences in plasma protein binding of drugs resulting from intrinsic differences in or changes in the actual amount of plasma protein (*Newborn* vs. *Adult*) or from changes in available binding sites for drug (*Competitive Binding*). Note the changing relationship between the concentration of drug in the plasma and the amount of drug in the body. (From Roberts RJ: In Avery ME, Taeusch HW Jr (eds): Schaffer's Diseases of the Newborn, 5th ed. Philadelphia, WB Saunders, 1983.)

relationship occurs as a consequence of saturation of plasma protein binding sites (the point at which the rate of increase in plasma drug concentration diminishes with increasing body load of drug). If the changing equilibrium between plasma concentration and total body content of drug as depicted in this figure is not appreciated, serious problems can result. For example, the dashed lines illustrate how differences in protein binding between patients can result in a different plasma drug concentration for each curve despite equivalent amounts of total drug in the body (i.e., equal doses administered). If drug doses are increased in the newborn in an attempt to achieve the "effective" plasma drug concentration shown for the adult, the total amount of drug in the body of the newborn will be greater, possibly leading to toxicity or an cxaggerated response. Since plasma protein – bound drug is in equilibrium with free (unbound) drug in the plasma, this fraction (free drug) is typically increased under conditions of reduced quantity or decreased binding capacity of plasma protein. Because free drug is generally believed to be the pharmacologically active fraction in plasma or serum, an increase in the total plasma drug concentration may not be necessary to achieve equal pharmacologic effect in the case of reduced protein binding. For example, in adults with asthma, increasing bronchodilation is observed over the plasma concentration range for total (bound plus unbound) theophylline, 5 to 20 μg/ml, but toxicity becomes more likely above 20 μg/ml.[21] Let us assume tentatively the applicability to neonates with apnea of this upper limit or desired concentration, since it is set by toxicity, not efficacy. At the theophylline plasma concentration of 17 μg/ml, 56% of the drug is affixed to protein in adult plasma. The therapeutic plasma concentration range in adults of 10 to 20 μg/ml, therefore, corresponds to 4.4 to 8.8 μg/ml of unbound theophylline. If, as expected, only 36% of theophylline is bound to protein in full-term newborn cord plasma, the concentration limits for unbound drug of 4.4 to 8.8 μg/ml would correspond to an effective plasma concentration range for total theophylline of 6.9 to 13.8 μg/ml. This computed range for theophylline is remarkably similar to that (6.6 to 11.0 μg/ml) found appropriate by Shannon and colleagues[26] during treatment of premature infants with apnea. Therefore, because of differences in plasma protein binding, similar plasma drug concentrations may not result in similar pharmacologic effects. Thus, plasma protein binding differences may influence the translation of adult ideal therapeutic plasma concentration ranges to those for the newborn.

The possible influence of competitive protein binding by endogenous substrates such as bilirubin or by other drugs on drug distribution (drug plasma – tissue concentration relationships) is also illustrated in Figure 1 – 2. The presence in blood of two drugs that compete for protein binding sites results in a reduced binding capacity for one or both drugs. As a consequence, there are greater amounts of free (unbound) drug in plasma and a shift in equilibrium, driving drug into tissues. Thus, the result is the same as if the actual amount of plasma drug-binding protein were reduced. It is important to recognize that a changing relationship can also occur between the plasma concentration and amount of endogenous material (bilirubin) in tissue in such competitive binding situations. Binding of drug could result in fewer protein binding sites for bilirubin; this "released" bilirubin would redistribute to tissue. The less rapid rate of rise in the curve means that a large change in total body bilirubin content could be occurring in the face of smaller changes in plasma bilirubin concentration. This possibility may explain how a highly protein-bound drug could predispose the infant to the development of kernicterus. However, as demonstrated by the work of Brodersen,[4] the binding constant of bilirubin to albumin is much greater than that of any drug, meaning that no drug is capable of displacing bilirubin already bound to primary binding sites on albumin. On the contrary, bilirubin should be expected to prevent or to displace drugs from albumin binding sites. This, in fact, has been shown to occur with ampicillin, penicillin, phenobarbital, and phenytoin in neonates with hyperbilirubinemia.[6, 25] Some drugs, however, can bind to unoccupied sites, thereby inhibiting the subsequent binding of or changing the binding affinity for bilirubin (allosteric effects). Drugs with such potential are relatively few and include certain analgesic and anti-inflammatory agents (phenylbutazone and salicylate), ampicillin, sulfonamides, and x-ray contrast media.[4a, 4b] The majority of drugs have an insignificant competitive effect.

The actual quantity of drug present in the plasma must be considered in examinations of drug protein binding.[4a] It has been recognized for many years that the percent bound value is valid only for a specific drug concentration.[7] If a drug is 100% bound to plasma protein but present only in microgram quantities, its potential for competing for bilirubin binding sites on albumin is considerably less than that of a drug only 50% bound but present in milligram quantities, if their binding constants and molecular weights are approximately equal. The theoretical number of drug molecules bound to plasma protein can be computed from the following equation:

$$\text{number of drug molecules bound} = \frac{\text{plasma drug conc.}}{\text{molecular weight}} \times \text{percent protein bound}$$

Compare this number for drug A, 100% bound, with that for drug B, 50% bound, of similar molecular weight (m.w.), when a greater amount of drug B is present:

$$\text{number of drug A molecules bound} = \frac{1\ \mu g}{\text{m.w.}} \times 100\% = \frac{1}{\text{m.w.}}$$

$$\text{number of drug B molecules bound} = \frac{1000\ \mu g}{\text{m.w.}} \times 50\% = \frac{500}{\text{m.w.}}$$

Clearly, drug B at such concentrations would be likely to displace a much greater quantity of bilirubin—500 times more, as computed—even though it is only 50% bound. A recent finding that suggests another mechanism by which drugs may increase the risk of kernicterus is the fact that albumin-bound bilirubin can enter the brain following alteration of the blood–brain barrier.[16] However, considerable debate continues over the pathophysiology of kernicterus and the influence of competitive drug–protein binding.[16a]

Table 1–2 lists the plasma protein–binding percentages for several drugs in the neonate. The wide range of values for different drugs reflects not only the relative affinity of the drug for the available protein-binding sites but also the different concentrations of drug found in the plasma following therapeutic doses. From Table 1–3 it can be seen that only with drugs that are greater than 95% plasma protein–bound is the majority of the drug located within the plasma compartment.[2] Since at lower percent protein binding the majority of the drug is located outside the plasma compartment, there is little quantitative change in drug distribution with disturbances in drug–protein binding. Clinically important displacement of drug from protein binding sites probably is limited to drugs bound more than 80% to 90%.

The binding of many drugs (including digoxin, propranolol, lidocaine, diazoxide, theophylline, salicylate, nafcillin, phenytoin, pheno-

Table 1–2. PLASMA PROTEIN BINDING OF DRUGS IN THE NEONATE

Drug	Plasma Protein Binding (% Drug Bound)[a]
indomethacin	95
salicylate	95*
furosemide	95
diazepam	84–98
diazoxide	88*
phenytoin	70–90*
nafcillin	50–90*
cephalothin	72
propranolol	70*
sulfisoxazole	65–80
penicillin	65*
methicillin	65
dexamethasone	63
meperidine	60
phenobarbital	10–30*
lidocaine	10–50*
chloramphenicol	45*
gentamicin	45
theophylline	36*
morphine	30
digoxin	14–26
caffeine	25
atropine	20
procainamide	<20
ampicillin	7–12*
isoniazide	0

[a] Approximate values obtained from several different studies that utilized a variety of analytical techniques (the range of values in part reflect these variables), by Ehrenebo et al,[6] Hamar and Levy,[10] Kurz et al,[15] Krasner and Yaffe,[14] Morselli,[18] and Pruitt and Dayton.[23] See also sections on specific agents in later chapters for additional details and references.
* Plasma protein binding demonstrated in controlled study to be significantly less than in the adult.

barbital, chloramphenicol, and penicillins) to plasma protein has been reported to be diminished in newborns compared with that in adults other than pregnant women.[14, 15, 18, 22, 23] The cause of the deficient or diminished plasma protein binding of drugs at birth is not understood. Although decreased plasma protein concentration in the neonate has often been offered as an explanation, actual experimental testing of this hypothesis has provided contradictory evidence.[10,15] Competition by endogenous ligands, including allosteric effects, and qualitative differences in neonatal plasma protein are possible contributors. The postnatal age at which adult binding capacity is attained is unknown, since most studies have been restricted to cord plasma samples. With phenytoin, adult protein-binding equivalency has been observed before the age of 3 months. The complexity of drug–protein binding phenomena is exempli-

Table 1–3. TOTAL AMOUNT OF DRUG (BOUND + UNBOUND) IN PLASMA AND OUTSIDE PLASMA AT DIFFERENT DEGREES OF PLASMA PROTEIN BINDING IN ADULTS

Binding to Plasma Proteins (%)	Drug in Plasma (% Total Amount in Body)	Drug Outside Plasma (% Total Amount in Body)
0	6.7	93.3
50	12	88
60	15	85
70	19	81
80	26	74
90	42	58
95	59	41
98	78	22
99	88	12
100	100	0

From Boréus LO: Principles of Pediatric Pharmacology. In Monographs in Clinical Pharmacology. Vol 6, p 60. New York, Churchill Livingstone, 1982.

fied by the fact that there are a number of drugs that bind identically to neonatal and adult plasma protein.

Protein binding outside of the vascular compartment is known to occur with several drugs, including digoxin (myocardial, skeletal, and smooth muscle) and glucocorticoids (lung). The digoxin-binding proteins in the myocardium are considered to have a high degree of specificity for digoxin and are a major driving influence on the quantity of digoxin that passively diffuses into the myocardial tissue. Binding of digoxin as it enters the milieu of the myocardial cell maintains the effective concentration gradient between free drug in plasma and myocardial cell. This process is termed **facilitated diffusion.** Disease or developmental differences in drug-binding protein in extravascular loci can influence dose–response relationships. Tissue binding studies using various neurotransmitters (norepinephrine, dopamine) have become a valuable analytical tool for examining what are believed to be their true pharmacologic receptor sites. For the tissue studied, the number of receptors corresponds to the degree of response observed to either endogenously released or exogenously administered catecholamine.

Metabolism. Many drugs undergo metabolic conversion prior to elimination from the body. Biotransformation of a drug in general results in a more polar, less lipid-soluble molecule that can be expected to be more rapidly eliminated than the parent compound by renal excretion or other routes. Although biotransformation frequently provides a mechanism for more rapid clearance of the administered drug from the body, it can also result in production of active compounds that are either therapeutic or toxic

in their effects (see Table 2–4). Both the drug and its metabolite(s) may be pharmacologically active; for example, theophylline is partially metabolized to caffeine in neonates being treated for apnea (see Chap. 6). The intensity of effect and its duration will be dependent on the rate of elimination of each compound from the site(s) of action. Therefore, the disposition (metabolism, distribution, excretion) of the administered drug as well as the metabolite(s) can be a major therapeutic consideration, particularly with regard to interpretation of blood level values that reflect only one of the compounds.

There are two major categories of drug metabolic reactions: the **nonsynthetic** reactions, including oxidation, reduction, or hydrolysis, and the **synthetic** or **conjugation** reactions. For many drugs, metabolism occurs by several competing pathways, with the amount of each final metabolite being determined by the relative rate of the respective metabolism pathway. Although the liver is regarded as the major organ responsible for biotransformation of drugs, many other organs and tissues in the body possess considerable potential to metabolize drugs, including the blood, lung, gastrointestinal tract, and kidney.

Characteristic of any enzymatic reaction, including those associated with drug metabolism, is a limitation in the capacity of the process. The relative deficiency at birth in the capacity to oxidize a drug, as well as the rate of maturation of that capacity, varies with the drug. Both characteristics, the deficiency at birth and the rate of maturation, also exhibit marked individual variability. Most drugs, including phenytoin, phenobarbital, diazepam, amobarbital, tolbutamide, nortriptyline, mepivicaine, theophylline, and caffeine, exhibit prolonged plasma half-lives or low body clearance rates shortly after birth.[19] Even among those drugs poorly disposed of, there are quantitative differences. For example, elimination of the methylxanthines is substantially slower than that of phenytoin, relative to adult values. As the capacity to oxidize these drugs improves, there is a concomitant diminution in individual variation. The rate of maturation seems more rapid with phenytoin and phenobarbital than with the methylxanthines. Body clearance rate for phenytoin surpasses adult values by age 2 weeks, whereas that rate for theophylline is still deficient at age 2 months. There is little evidence to support the view that xenobiotic induction, midgestationally or perinatally, plays an important role in these processes.

The influence of gestational age and of birth per se on drug metabolism is not clearly defined. The capacity to oxidize antipyrine or diazepam is more deficient in premature infants than in their full-term counterparts. There is some evidence in humans that birth does initiate maturation of drug-oxidizing function, although the rate of maturation may be slower in very-low-birth-weight infants. The aspects of birth that trigger maturation are undefined. The deficiency in body clearance rates associated with most oxidized drugs at birth correlates well with fetal hepatic concentrations of cytochrome *P450* mono-oxygenase activity observed midgestationally. The differences in degree of deficiency and in rate of maturation of drug-oxidizing function can be attributed speculatively to different subclasses of cytochrome *P450,* each of which likely possesses distinctive substrate specificity.

Certain important conjugative processes, especially glucuronidation, have been found to be diminished in newborns compared with those in older neonates and infants. Chloramphenicol-induced "gray baby syndrome" has been explained by a reduced rate of glucuronide conjugation, resulting in an unexpected rate of accumulation of toxic amounts of the drug.

Most of the foregoing comments in reference to oxidation apply as well to the process of glucuronidation. One exception is the virtual absence of glucuronidative capacity in midgestational human fetal liver. Sulfation, as distinct from glucuronidation, is active in the neonate, as evidenced by metabolite patterns of acetaminophen.[17] Acetylation, glutathione conjugation, mercapturic acid formation, and conjugation with amino acids are processes likely to be somewhat deficient at birth. Maturational

characteristics of hepatic blood flow, transport of drugs into hepatocytes, intracellular binding of drugs, and biliary secretion, alone or in combination, are likely to influence the hepatic disposition of certain drugs and have been extensively reviewed in the literature.[24]

With respect to conjugation reactions it is now clear that some drugs, such as indomethacin, are subject to substantial enterohepatic recirculation, just as is bilirubin. Beta-glucuronidase activity in the newborn intestine may be seven-fold greater than adult values;[29] this finding strongly suggests that, although glucuronidation activity may appear low based on drug plasma levels, the drug is in fact being conjugated, excreted in the bile, deconjugated, and then reabsorbed into the systemic circulation.

Besides the fact that the mechanisms regulating drug metabolism from birth are poorly understood, the influences of specific illness, nutritional state, drug interactions (e.g., prenatal treatment with glucocorticoid), and other factors on drug metabolism in the neonate remain virtually unexplored. The oxygen dependence of many drug metabolism pathways has been demonstrated by extensive work both in vitro and, to a limited degree, in vivo.[12] Oxygen is required for drug-metabolizing systems directly as a substrate for oxidative reactions and as a participant in the electron transport–high-energy bond synthesis reactions. It would therefore be reasonable to anticipate an association between hypoxemic states and altered drug metabolism; yet no such clinical studies have been reported for any age group. It may be difficult to define or isolate the influence of hypoxemia on drug metabolism alone, since hypoxemia can cause altered biochemical or biophysical or even pathologic function, as well as alter other aspects of drug disposition. For example, Myers and coworkers[20] have established in animals and human neonates that hypoxemia significantly alters aminoglycoside serum half-life. Since metabolism of aminoglycosides is essentially nonexistent, other aspects of disposition, such as renal elimination, must be entertained to explain these findings.

Although the preceding discussion has emphasized the metabolic conversion of the parent drug to metabolite(s), considerable attention has recently focused on the activation processes required for conversion of some "pro" drugs to active forms. For example, several drugs are administered as salts or esters (chloramphenicol succinate, erythromycin estolate, alpha-tocopherol acetate), because the pro drugs are chemically more stable or soluble as pharmaceutical preparations. These salt or ester dosage forms of the drugs are assumed to be rapidly and completely hydrolyzed (enzymatically or nonenzymatically), thus releasing the active form of the drug. However, published evidence exists to demonstrate that for some drugs or patients this assumption is incorrect. Chloramphenicol is administered as an ester intravenously because chloramphenicol itself is poorly soluble in water. The ester has no direct antimicrobial activity and must be hydrolyzed following intravenous or intramuscular administration to release the active chloramphenicol base. Kauffman and colleagues[13] found that, in infants and children, rate of hydrolysis and degree of renal elimination of nonhydrolyzed chloramphenicol-3-monosuccinate were sufficiently variable to explain the wide range in half-life values and the poor correlation between dose and serum concentration of free chloramphenicol. Thus, dosage requirements may have to be increased not for reasons of increased metabolism of the administered drug but because of decreased conversion of the administered pro drug to its active constituent. With regard to the better-appreciated scenario of decreased metabolism requiring decreased dosage, this is a paradox. The conclusion that rapid hydrolysis would occur seems rather surprising in light of existing knowledge about blood esterase activity in neonates. Differences between infants and adults in procaine hydrolysis and in chlorinesterases, arylesterases, and acetylsalicylic acid esterases have been reported by a number of investigators since 1955.[18]

In contrast to the decreased rate of drug metabolism observed in the immediate newborn period, a dramatic increase in the metabolism of certain drugs has been reported to occur following the first 1 to 2 weeks of life and continuing for several months or years. Thus, the clearance rates for some drugs such as phenytoin, phenobarbital, and theophylline may pass from a fraction of adult rates to 2 to 6 times the adult rates.[19] Obviously, such a dramatic change could have a very significant therapeutic consequence, shifting the concern within a matter of days or few weeks of birth from that of risk of overdosing (toxicity) to that of underdosing (inefficacy). As has been pointed out by Morselli,[18] it is surprising how little attention has been paid to this period of transition in drug metabolism with respect to either its practical aspects or the mechanism(s) involved.

Excretion. The dominant pathway for drug elimination from the body is by renal excretion. The most important characteristics of neonatal renal function relative to drug elimination include a low glomerular filtration rate, glomerular preponderance, nephron heterogeneity, low effective renal blood flow, and low tubular function, compared with findings in the adult. The deficient glomerular filtration and renal tubular secretion in the neonate merit great concern since many drugs in clinical use are eliminated almost entirely by the kidney through these mechanisms. Neonatal glomerular filtration rate is about 30% of that of the adult expressed per unit of body surface area. The plasma disappearance rates of aminoglycosides, which are eliminated mainly by glomerular filtration, reflect these changes in glomerular filtration rate. The dosage schedules recommended for these drugs have taken this into account. Renal blood flow may influence the rate at which drugs reach and are eliminated by the kidney. The average effective renal plasma flow, as measured by the *para*-aminohippurate clearance rate (C_{PAH}), is 15% of that of the adult in the neonate less than 12 hours of age, assuming complete extraction of PAH. The rate at which renal clearance matures appears to vary, not only among infants but also with different drugs. Urinary pH also can influence the rate of renal excretion of drugs that are subject to non-ionic diffusion.

It is important to appreciate that the extent of urine output does not necessarily reflect the status of renal function and, correspondingly, the capacity for renal drug elimination. For example, in the neonate as in the adult, non-oliguric renal failure can occur.[9] In the very small premature (< 1200 g), an inappropriately high urine output state may exist owing to tubular dysfunction or immaturity. It would be inappropriate to anticipate that the normal or increased urine output in these neonates reflects the potential for normal plasma clearance of drugs dependent upon renal elimination, such as aminoglycosides (see Chap. 4).

References

1. Bell EF, Brown EJ, Milner R, et al: Vitamin E absorption in small premature infants. Pediatrics 63:830, 1979.
2. Boréus LO: Principles of Pediatric Pharmacology. In Monographs in Clinical Pharmacology. Vol 6, p 60. New York, Churchill Livingstone, 1982.
3. Bonati M, Kanto J, Tognoni G: Clinical pharmacokinetics of cerebrospinal fluid. Clin Pharmacokinet 7:312, 1982.
4. Brodersen R: The mechanism of drug-induced displacement of bilirubin from albumin. P 177. In Stern L, Hansen BF, Kilderberg P (eds): Intensive Care in the Newborn. New York, Masson Publishing, 1976.

4a. Brodersen R, Friis-Hansen B, Stern L: Drug-induced displacement of bilirubin from albumin in the newborn. Dev. Pharmacol. Ther. 6:217, 1983.

4b. Brodersen R, Ebbesen F: Bilirubin-displacing effect of ampicillin, indomethacin, chlorpromazine, gentamicin, and parabens in vitro and in newborn infants. J Pharm Sci 72:248, 1983.

5. Cockshott WP, Thompson GT, Howlett LJ, Seeley ET: Intramuscular or intralipomatous injections? N Engl J Med 306:356, 1982.

6. Ehrnebo M, Agurell S, Jalling B, Boréus LO: Age differences in drug binding by plasma proteins: Studies on human foetuses, neonates, and adults. Eur J Clin Pharmacol 3:189, 1971.

7. Goldstein A: The interactions of drugs and plasma proteins. Pharmacology 1:102, 1949.

8. Greenberg MI, Roberts JR, Baskin SI, Wagner DK: The use of endotracheal medication for cardiac arrest. Top Emerg Med 1(2):29, 1979.

9. Grylack L, Medani C, Hultzen C, et al: Nonoliguric acute renal failure in the newborn. Am J Dis Child 136:518, 1982.

10. Hamar C, Levy G: Serum protein binding of drugs and bilirubin in newborn infants and their mothers. Clin Pharmacol Ther 28:58, 1980.

11. Hoffmann H: Absorption of drugs and other xenobiotics during development in experimental animals. J Pharmacol Ther 16:247, 1982.

12. Jones DP: Hypoxia and drug metabolism. Biochem Pharmacol 30:1019, 1981.

13. Kauffman RE, Miceli JN, Strebel L, et al: Pharmacokinetics of chloramphenicol and chloramphenicol succinate in infants and children. J Pediatr 98:315, 1981.

14. Krasner J, Yaffe SJ: Drug–protein binding in the neonate. In Morselli PL, Garattini S, Sereni F (eds): Basic and Therapeutic Aspects of Perinatal Pharmacology. P 357. New York, Raven Press, 1975.

15. Kurz H, Mauser-Ganshorn A, Stickel HH: Differences in the binding of drugs to plasma proteins from newborn and adult man. I. Eur J Clin Pharmacol 11:463, 1977.

16. Levine RL, Fredericks WR, Rapoport SI: Entry of bilirubin into the brain due to opening of the blood–brain barrier. Pediatrics 69:255, 1982.

16a. Levine RL, Maisels MJ (eds): Hyperbilirubinemia in the newborn. Report of the Eighty-Fifth Ross Conference on Pediatric Research. Columbus, Ohio: Ross Laboratories, 1983.

17. Miller RP, Roberts RJ, Fischer LJ: Acetaminophen elimination kinetics in neonates, children, and adults. Clin Pharmacol Ther 19:284, 1976.

18. Morselli PL: Clinical pharmacokinetics in neonates. Clin Pharmacokinet 1:81, 1976.

19. Morselli PL, Franco-Morselli R, Bossi L: Clinical pharmacokinetics in newborns and infants. Age-related differences and therapeutic implications. Clin Pharmacokinet 5:485, 1980.

20. Myers MG, Roberts RJ, Mirhij NJ: Effects of gestational age, birth weight, and hypoxemia on pharmacokinetics of amikacin in serum of infants. Antimicrob Agents Chemother 11:1027, 1977.

21. Neims AH, Aranda JV, Loughnan PM: Principles of neonatal pharmacology. In Schaffer AJ, Avery ME (eds): Diseases of the Newborn. 4th ed., p. 1020. Philadelphia, WB Saunders, 1977.

22. Piafsky KM, Woolner EA, Sci M: The binding of basic drugs to alpha$_1$-acid glycoprotein in cord serum. J Pediatr 110:820, 1982.

23. Pruitt AW, Dayton PG: A comparison of the binding of drugs to adult and cord plasma. Eur J Clin Pharmacol 4:59, 1971.

24. Rane A: Basic principles of drug disposition and action in infants and children. In Yaffe SJ (ed): Pediatric Pharmacology: Therapeutic Principles in Practice. P 7. New York, Grune and Stratton, 1981.

25. Rane A, Lunde PKM, Jalling B, et al: Plasma protein binding of diphenylhydantoin in normal and hyperbilirubinemic infants. Pediatr Pharmacol Ther 78:877, 1971.

26. Shannon DC, Gotay F, Stein IM, et al: Prevention of apnea and bradycardia in low-birthweight infants. Pediatrics 55:589, 1975.

27. Williams RL, Mamelok RD: Hepatic disease and drug pharmacokinetics. Clin Pharmacol 5:528, 1980.

28. Yaffe SJ, Stern L: Clinical implications of perinatal pharmacology. In Mirkin BL (ed): Perinatal Pharmacology and Therapeutics. P 382. New York, Academic Press, 1976.

29. Yaffe SJ, Juchau MR: Perinatal pharmacology. Ann Rev Pharmacol 14:219, 1974.

TWO

Pharmacokinetics:
Basic Principles and Clinical Application

BASIC PHARMACOKINETICS

Designing an optimal therapeutic program for the infant requires not only a thorough understanding of the pharmacology of the drug under consideration but a rigorous and thoughtful examination of the infant's physiologic, biochemical, and clinical status. These requirements relate to the fact that the ultimate outcome of drug therapy represents a continual interplay among the intrinsic pharmacology of the drug; the organ, cellular, or subcellular responses to the drug; and the effect of the disease process on these events. The physician's ability to anticipate the therapeutic outcome is further compromised by the biologic variations among infants.

One of the more useful management tools for dealing with the complex interplay among the biochemical, physiologic, and clinical circumstances that can influence pharmacotherapeutic outcome is the use of quantitative measurements of drug concentrations in serum or plasma. The onset, intensity, and duration of drug effects — drug pharmacodynamics — are proportional to the concentration of the drug at the site of action. Thus, if the concentration of a drug at the site of action is in equilibrium with and relatable to the serum or plasma level, then drug concentrations measured in this compartment should correlate well with the drug's clinical effect. Recall that **pharmacokinetics** refers to the mathematical expression of the time course of drug movement in the body, useful only in relation to the **pharmacodynamics** — the resulting alterations in biochemical or physiologic events or processes that can be appreciated by clinical criteria.

The goal in pharmacotherapeutics is to achieve and to maintain a drug concentration at the site of action that will produce the maximum desired effect with a minimal risk of toxicity — the so-called **target concentration concept.** By understanding and appropriately applying pharmacokinetics, the physician should be able to predict and to adjust accurately the concentration of drug in the blood at any time after a dose or series of doses. For each infant, the ideal dosing requirements can be predetermined and subsequent doses adjusted to achieve a more ideal level of drug when an unusual drug dynamic or kinetic response is observed. Again, the critical assumption is that the intensity of action of the drug at the site of action is directly proportional to its concentration in the compartment being monitored (i.e., blood). The following discussion introduces some of the basic concepts and terms used in drug pharmacokinetics.

Body compartments. Blood plasma or serum is a practical and convenient resource material for drug measurements; plasma or serum levels of a drug typically are an accurate reflection of its amount and concentration in the body. Not only does the blood receive a drug from the site of administration, but it carries the drug to all other tissues — compartments — in the body, including those that represent the site of effect as well as those tissues that eliminate the drug from the body. The possible movements of a drug from site(s) of administration to site(s) of elimination is depicted schematically in Figure 2–1.

Single-compartment pharmacokinetics is considered the least complex situation in drug movements in the body. Presumably, after its introduction into the blood, the drug rapidly equilibrates with the tissues of the body so that the rate at which the blood concentration changes reflects the rate at which concentra-

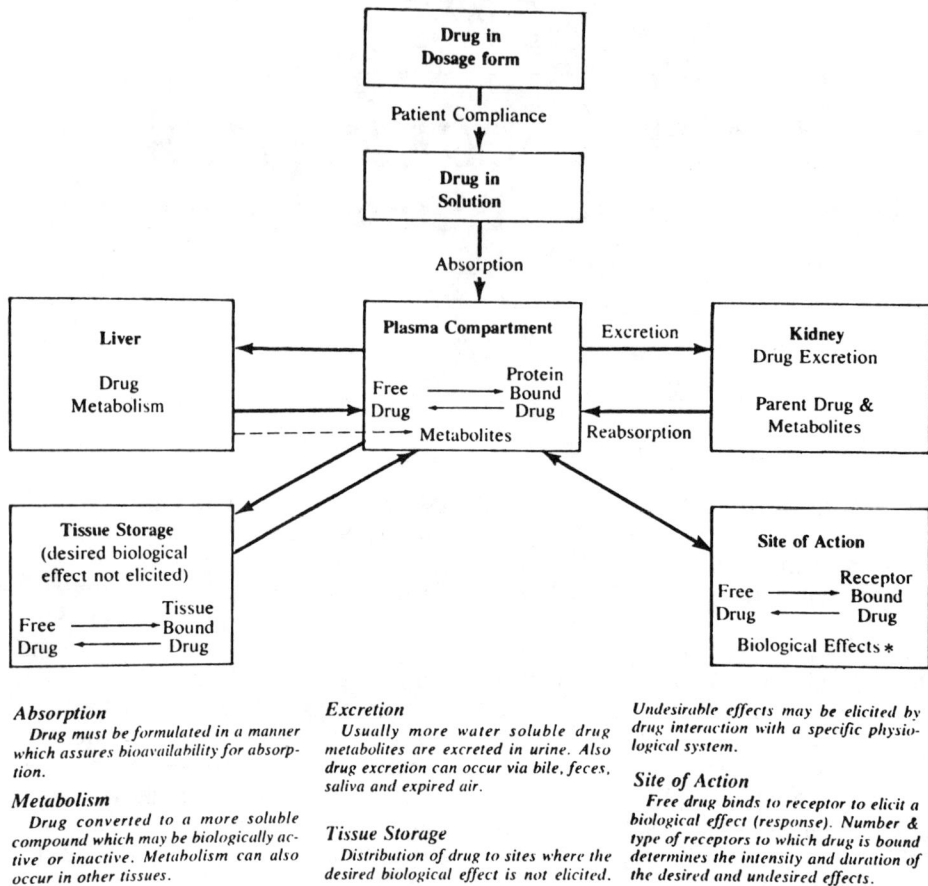

Figure 2-1. Possible movements of a drug from site(s) of administration to site(s) of elimination, showing the factors that affect drug concentration at the site of action. (From Pippenger CE: Pediatr Clin North Am 27:891, 1980.)

tions of drug change in most tissues of the body. Thus, measurement of drug concentration in blood and other tissues at various times after injection will reveal a parallel pattern of drug decline in all major tissues, as shown in Figure 2-2. Note also that even though the concentrations in various tissues are different at any one time, the rates at which the tissue and blood concentrations decline are equivalent. This similarity in drug flux in all major tissues indicates that the body may be considered as a single compartment. With single-compartment kinetics, the movement of drugs follows the laws of **first-order kinetics,** meaning that the instantaneous rate at which the amount of drug changes within the body depends upon the amount of drug present at that time.

Thus, with first-order kinetics of drug elimination, the greater the amount of drug in the body, the faster is its rate of removal. It is fortunate that many drugs follow first-order kinetics, because this means large potentially toxic doses are eliminated at a faster rate than smaller therapeutic doses. The other advantage of first-order pharmacokinetics is that knowledge of the dose of drug or plasma concentration of drug at any time can be used to calculate the amount of drug in the body or concentration of drug in the plasma at any time, provided the rate constant for elimination of that drug is known:

$$A_b = \text{dose } (e^{-kt})$$

where A_b = amount of drug in body at time t
e = natural log
k = elimination rate constant

or

$$C_p = C_p^0 \, e^{-kt}$$

where C_p = plasma concentration of drug at any time t
C_p^0 = plasma concentration of drug at time $t = 0$ (extrapolated graphically by going back to zero time on the log concentration versus time curve; see Fig. 2-2)

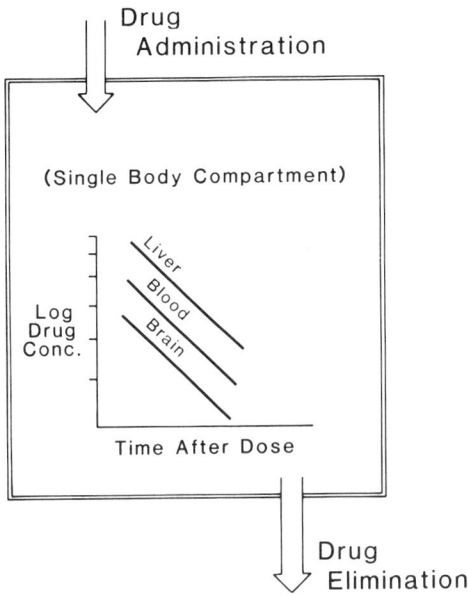

Figure 2-2. Representation of single-compartment drug disappearance curves. (From Roberts RJ: In Avery ME, Taeusch, HW Jr (eds): Schaffer's Diseases of the Newborn, 5th ed. Philadelphia, WB Saunders, 1983.)

The terms rate and rate constant must not be confused. A **rate** refers to an actual change in drug amount (or concentration) per unit of time (e.g., mg/min). A **rate constant** (k) is a non-changing value with reciprocal units of time (hr^{-1}) that describes a particular kinetic process and may be regarded as simply the fractional rate of drug removal; the value of k does not refer to the actual amount of drug eliminated per unit time. Thus, through the use of these equations, the amount of drug in the body or in plasma at any time after any selected dose can be predicted.

The fraction of the drug dose that would be remaining in the body is represented by the following:

$$\frac{\text{fraction of dose}}{\text{remaining in the body}} = \frac{A_b}{\text{dose}} = \frac{C}{C^0} = e^{-kt}$$

where A_b = amount of drug in the body
C = concentration of drug in plasma
C^0 = concentration of drug in plasma at zero time

Because $k = 0.693/(T\frac{1}{2}$ value) and $e^{-0.693} \approx \frac{1}{2}$, this equation for fraction of dose remaining in the body simplifies to $A_b/\text{dose} = (\frac{1}{2})^n$, where n is the number of half-lives involved since the time of dosing. As an example, about 25% of a bolus dose of a drug would remain after 2 half-lives

($\frac{1}{2} \times \frac{1}{2}$), and 6.25% after 4 half-lives ($\frac{1}{2} \times \frac{1}{2} \times \frac{1}{2} \times \frac{1}{2}$). To calculate the actual drug concentration (C_p) at these times,

$$C_p = C_p^0 \times (\tfrac{1}{2})^n$$

Volume of Distribution. The relationship between plasma concentration of the drug (C_p) and the total amount of drug in the body (A_b) is given by the following equation:

$$C_p = \frac{A_b}{V_d}$$

where V_d is the **volume of distribution** of the drug in the body. This calculation requires that distribution equilibrium be achieved between the drug in plasma and in tissues. V_d is a mathematical term relating A_b and C_p and has no physiologic identity. It is very useful, however, in predicting the plasma concentration of a drug resulting from a given dose. For example, for gentamicin,

A_b^0 = 2.5 mg/kg
V_d = 0.4 l/kg
$C_p^0 = \dfrac{2500\ \mu g/kg}{400\ ml/kg} = \dfrac{6.25\ \mu g/ml}{\text{after administration}}$ at zero time

Also note that if the dose is doubled, the plasma concentration will double. Thus, dosage adjustment with drugs that follow first-order single-compartment kinetics is straightforward with a predictable result if the plasma concentration resulting from a given dose is known.

Drug Half-life. The **half-life** of a drug in the blood or other compartment is the time required for any given concentration in the blood (or other compartment) to decline to one half of the initial value. For example, if it takes 1 hour for the plasma level of a drug to decline from 6 μg/ml to 3 μg/ml, the half-life is 1 hour. As noted earlier, half-life, $T\frac{1}{2}$, is related to the first-order rate constant for elimination, k, by the following equation:

$$T\tfrac{1}{2} = \frac{0.693}{k}$$

The values for elimination rate constant (k), half-life ($T\frac{1}{2}$), and the volume of distribution (V_d) are assumed to be constant in an individual after any given dose of any one drug. Therefore, for drugs with first-order single-compartment kinetics, these values are independent of the drug dose. However, for any given drug, these values may vary among individuals in the population. Disease states in particular can cause these values to change. It is important to appreciate these possible fluctuations when an unexpected intensity of drug response is observed. In addition, each drug has distinct physical properties and a specific method of disposition in the body. Pharmacokinetic parameters, therefore, vary widely among different drugs. Table 2–1 is a partial listing of drugs frequently employed in infants that can be usefully monitored; note that there is a wide variation in half-lives and, in some cases, a wide range of half-life values observed for a specific agent.

Clearance. Clearance represents the volume of blood or plasma which is completely cleared of drug per unit of time. Clearance, represented by Cl, is a direct index of drug elimination from the plasma compartment and takes into consideration changes in half-life as well as volume of distribution:

$$Cl = \frac{0.693 \times V_d}{T\frac{1}{2}\beta}$$

The clearance of a drug is, therefore, inversely proportional to its elimination half-life, $T\frac{1}{2}\beta$, and directly proportional to the apparent volume of distribution, V_d. Drug plasma half-life and elimination rate constant reflect rather than control volume of distribution. In situations of changing volume of distribution (see following section, Multicompartment Distribution) or elimination (see subsequent section, Dose-

dependent or Zero-order Kinetics), calculation of drug clearance is most appropriate because it normalizes the data:

$$Cl = \frac{\text{rate of elimination}}{\text{concentration}}$$

Multicompartment Distribution. Many drugs distribute in the body as if there were more than one compartment. The most realistic multicompartment model is the two-compartment open model depicted in Figure 2–3.[3] In this model there are two compartments: one a smaller central compartment composed of the plasma volume and richly perfused tissues, such as the brain, heart, liver, kidneys, and gastrointestinal tract, and a larger peripheral compartment corresponding to the rest of the body that is in equilibrium with the central compartment. Reversible transfer (diffusion) occurs between the central and peripheral compartments in proportion to the drug concentration in each compartment (i.e., first-order kinetics). The rate constants are represented by k_{12}, k_{21}, and k_{el}. Several independent processes operating simultaneously determine the concentration of a drug in the central compartment. After an intravenous dose the serum concentration curve would be observed to have the configuration shown in Figure 2–4 when plotted on semi-log paper. The accelerated portion of the disappearance curve at the earlier times following the dose administration—the alpha distribution phase, or α **phase**—represents the net distribu-

Table 2–1. SERUM HALF-LIFE AND THERAPEUTIC LEVELS OF SELECTED DRUGS USED IN THE TREATMENT OF DISEASE IN INFANTS

Drug	$T\frac{1}{2}$: Range (hr)	Serum Concentration Therapeutic Range (μg/ml)	Recommended Sampling Time After Dose (hr)
gentamicin	2–12 ⎫	⎧ Peak 5–8	1–2
tobramycin	2–12 ⎭	⎩ Trough 1–2	6–12
kanamycin	4–18	Peak 15–25	1–2
		Trough 2–4	6–12
chloramphenicol	10–24	Peak 15–20	1–2[a]
		Trough 5–10	4–8
digoxin	20–180	1–3	<8
phenobarbital	36–144	10–30	>6
phenytoin	15–105	10–20	>8
caffeine	37–231	7–20	>4[b]
theophylline	12–64	Peak 20	1
		Trough 10	>4[b]

[a] May have delayed hydrolysis of ester.
[b] Theophylline can be metabolized to caffeine in the neonate. See Chapter 6.
From Avery ME, and Taeusch HW Jr (eds): Schaffer's Diseases of the Newborn, 5th ed. Philadelphia, WB Saunders, 1983.

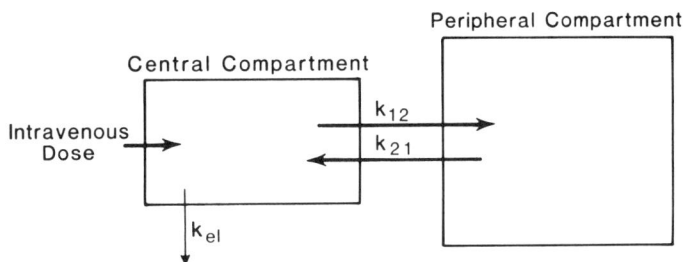

Figure 2-3. The two-compartment open model of drug distribution for agents having multicompartment distribution characteristics.

tion of a drug out of the plasma into tissues and simultaneous elimination of a drug from the body (k_{12} and k_{el} in Fig. 2-3). In other words, two or more processes are operating simultaneously to remove the drug from the blood or central compartment. During the linear phase — the beta elimination phase, or β **phase** — the peripheral compartment tissues are saturated, and the drug levels in the blood are declining through metabolism or excretion or both. During the β phase, there may be a reentrance of drug from the peripheral compartment to the central compartment (k_{21} in Fig. 2-3) because the reduced plasma drug levels will now favor diffusion of drug out of tissues as opposed to going into tissues (k_{12}) during the early (α phase), high-plasma-concentration period. Ordinarily the half-life of drugs following multicompartment pharmacokinetics is determined during the β phase. Pharmacokinetic equations used to make predictions of blood levels, volume of distribution, and so forth for drugs for which kinetics follow the two-compartment model are more complex than those shown previously for the one-compartment model.[3] Errors in pharmacokinetically derived predictions can occur when kinetics are assumed to follow the one-compartment model if in fact they follow a more complex multicompartment model.[2] Drugs having a multicompartment model of distribution include aspirin, ampicillin, digoxin, meperidine, and propranolol.

Dose-dependent or Zero-order Kinetics. The pharmacokinetics of a drug are described as

dose-dependent (or concentration-dependent) when the half-life of the drug changes with increasing doses (or levels of drug in the blood). This dependency of half-life on drug dose or drug concentration usually arises because elimination processes (e.g., metabolism or excretion) become saturated when sufficient amounts of the drug are present in the body. For some drugs, elimination processes appear to be saturated at low or therapeutic doses, so that dose-dependent kinetics prevail at the usual doses. Once saturation of elimination mechanisms occurs, the drug is eliminated at a constant rate (e.g., mg/hr), and the term **zero-order** or **saturation kinetics** is employed. Thus, the rate of decline of the drug in the body is constant and is not proportional to the amount of drug in the body, as is the case with first-order kinetics. Many drugs exhibit zero-order kinetics when high concentrations are present in the body, but after the drug levels fall owing to existing elimination processes, first-order kinetics prevail. As a result, progressively shorter half-lives are observed as the concentration of drug in the blood decreases. The plasma disappearance curve for such situations is shown in Figure 2-5. Some examples of drugs that show saturation-type kinetics are provided in Table 2-2.

Multiple Doses and the "Plateau Principle." During the typical course of drug therapy, many doses of a drug are ordinarily administered. Each additional dose is usually given before the previous dose (or doses) has been completely eliminated from the body, resulting in the addi-

Figure 2-4. Serum drug disappearance curve in multicompartment pharmacokinetics, showing the α and β phases. (From Roberts RJ: In Avery ME, Taeusch HW Jr (eds): Schaffer's Diseases of the Newborn, 5th ed. Philadelphia, WB Saunders, 1983.)

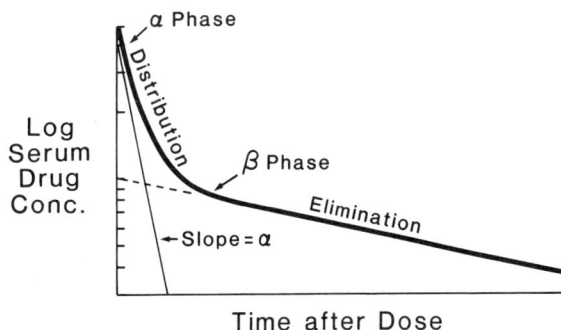

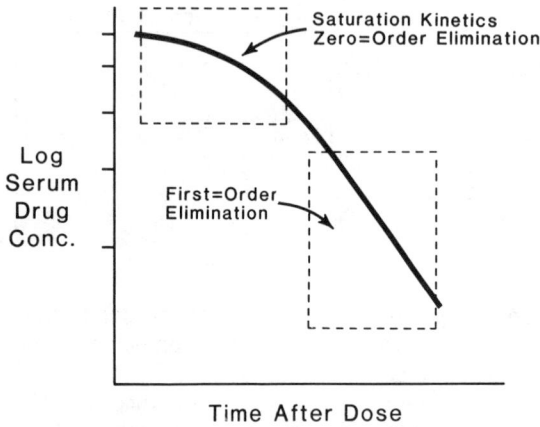

Figure 2-5. Graph depicting saturation or zero-order (serum concentration–dependent) and first-order (serum concentration–independent) pharmacokinetics. (From Roberts RJ: In Avery ME, Tacusch HW Jr (eds): Schaffer's Diseases of the Newborn, 5th ed. Philadelphia, WB Saunders, 1983.)

tion of more drug to that already present. Thus, with repeated administration the plasma level of the drug will increase until the rate of drug elimination (which is increasing with the increasing plasma drug level) equals the amount of drug administered at each dosing interval. Careful examination of the hypothetical serum level curve shown in Figure 2-6 reveals important principles that should be kept in mind when selecting a dosage regimen for therapy. The serum drug curve in the figure results from an oral dose given every 4 hours of a drug with a half-life of 4 hours. Note that (1) 4 half-lives (16 hours) are needed for the drug to reach what is essentially steady state or plateau level; (2) during the interval between doses, drug blood levels fluctuate owing to absorption and elimination; (3) once steady state has been reached (approximately 4 to 6 half-lives) the maximum and minimum drug blood levels are the same after each dose; and (4) after repeated administration using an interval of 1 half-life, a maximum (or minimum) drug blood level will be reached at steady state that is 1.4 times higher than that reached after the first dose.

Table 2-2. DRUGS DEMONSTRATING SATURATION KINETICS WITH THERAPEUTIC DOSES IN NEONATES

caffeine
chloramphenicol
diazepam
furosemide
indomethacin
phenytoin

The objective of any dosage regimen is to maintain the patient's drug blood level within a maximum safe concentration (below toxicity) and the minimum effective concentration. Figure 2-7 illustrates possible errors in dosage: The dose interval in *Curve 1* is too short, resulting in accumulation of a drug above a maximum safe concentration. The dose interval for *Curve 3* is too long, resulting in subtherapeutic levels. The optimal therapeutic regimen is represented in *Curve 2.*

Continuous Infusion of Drugs (First-order Kinetics). Elimination of the fluctuations in blood levels between doses can be achieved by continuous infusion of the drug. Upon infusion the drug will accumulate in the body to a plateau level, at which time the rate of elimination will equal the rate of infusion. The steady-state plasma concentration (C_{ss}) is determined by the rate of infusion (R_{inf}) and the clearance (Cl):

$$C_{ss} = \frac{R_{inf}}{Cl}$$

Any change in infusion rate will produce a proportional change in plasma concentration if clearance remains constant. Thus, if the plasma steady-state level at a given rate of constant infusion is known, any desired steady-state level can be easily accomplished.

The delay in time between the onset of infusion and attainment of steady state is determined by the half-life of the drug. Thus, in 1 half-life the plasma concentration will equal 50% of the steady-state concentration. For a drug with a half-life of 100 hours (phenobarbital, Table 2-1), over 300 hours (approximately 2 weeks) would be required to achieve over 90% of the expected plateau plasma level. When the drug infusion is discontinued, the plasma drug level will decline at a rate equal to the drug half-life. In general about 3 to 5 half-lives are required to achieve steady-state plateau levels or to rid the body of the drug once the infusion of the drug is stopped.

Loading Dose. In order to minimize the time required to achieve therapeutic levels of selected drugs, particularly those with a half-life of more than 12 hours, loading doses of the drug can be sometimes employed. The loading dose required for a drug will be determined by the volume and rate of distribution. Loading doses can be hazardous, particularly with drugs distributed slowly into extravascular tissues or those preferentially taken up by certain tissues, thereby producing toxic levels. Digoxin is an

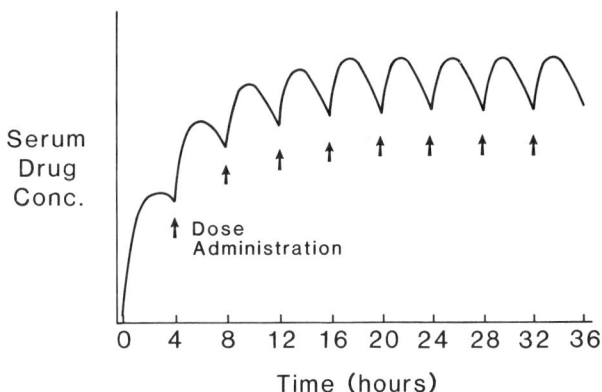

Figure 2-6. With multiple dosing, serum drug levels accumulate to steady-state or plateau concentrations. (From Roberts RJ: In Avery ME, Taeusch HW Jr (eds): Schaffer's Diseases of the Newborn, 5th ed. Philadelphia, WB Saunders, 1983.)

example of the latter type of agent; the total loading dose (digitalization) must be divided into two or three smaller doses in order to reduce the likelihood of toxicity. A summary of the effects of varying dose, dose interval, and loading dose is shown in Figure 2-8.[3]

Zero-order Kinetics in Drug Accumulation. When drug elimination follows zero-order kinetics and the drug is being administered at a rate greater than the rate of elimination, the drug will accumulate and blood levels will rise indefinitely. A plateau level will not occur since the drug is eliminated at a rate that does not increase as the blood drug level increases. This is obviously an undesirable situation likely to eventually result in drug toxicity. It is important to recognize that drugs may have first-order kinetics at low doses or blood levels, but that at high doses or blood levels, elimination mechanisms (metabolism and excretion) become saturated and zero-order kinetics prevail. For those drugs, blood level curves may appear as shown in Figure 2-9.

Drug Absorption, Elimination, and Bioavailability. The shape of a drug blood level versus time curve after dosing depends upon the rela-

tive rates of absorption and elimination of the drug. With each process (absorption and elimination) assumed to follow first-order kinetics, theoretical drug blood level curves can be constructed for various conditions (Fig. 2-10). At the initiation of drug administration, the rate of absorption will be maximal and the rate of elimination will be zero. As the drug is absorbed, the rate of absorption decreases while the rate of elimination increases. At the maximum or peak serum concentration the rates of absorption and elimination are equal. Subsequently the rate of elimination exceeds the rate of absorption. Peak blood levels are lower following extravascular administration compared with those for the intravenous route unless the rate of infusion is less than the rate of absorption from extravascular sites.

The effect of various rates of absorption of the same drug dose on the plasma concentration is shown in the first set of curves in Figure 2-10. Curve *a* results when the rate constant for absorption is far in excess of that for elimination. It is similar to the curve expected after an intravenous dose. Curve *b* represents an absorption rate constant less than in curve *a* but still in

Figure 2-7. Effects of multiple dosing at different time intervals between doses on serum drug concentration. *Curve 1* represents accumulation to toxic levels; *Curve 2*, optimal therapeutic levels; *Curve 3*, subtherapeutic levels.

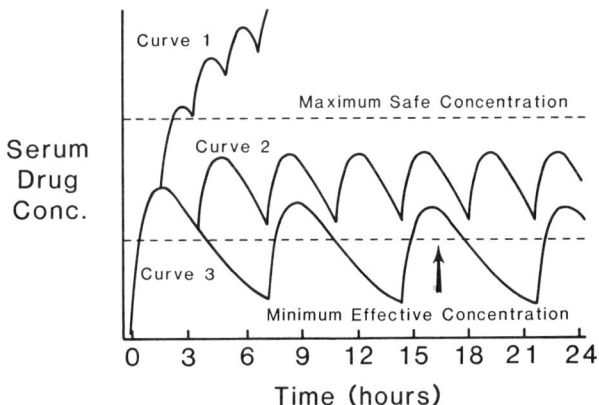

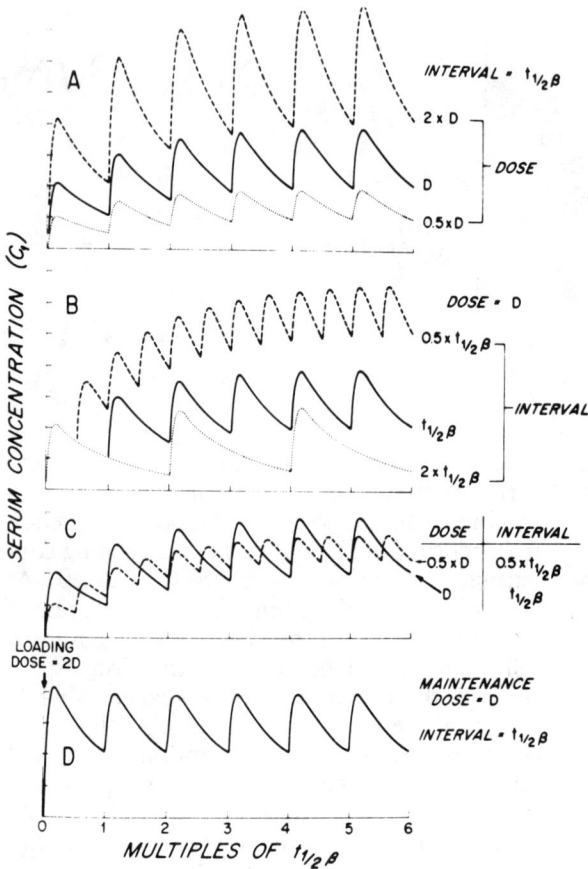

Figure 2-8. Effects of multiple dosing with different doses (*A*) dose intervals (*B*) and dose and interval (*C*) and loading doses (*D*) on serum drug levels. (From Greenblatt DJ, Koch-Weser J: N Engl J Med 293:264, 1975.)

Figure 2-9. Serum drug level–time curve showing rapid accumulation that results with too-frequent drug administration. Note change from first-order kinetics to saturation (zero-order) kinetics.

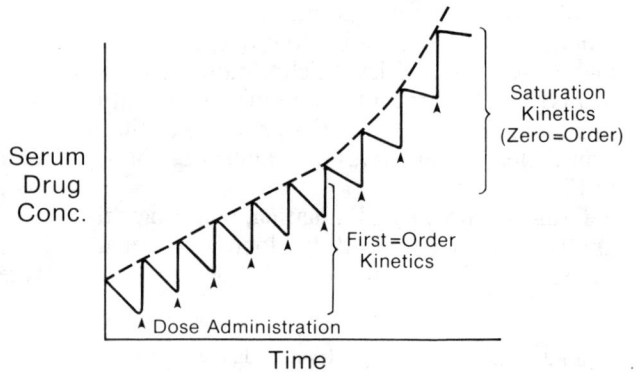

Figure 2-10. Effects of different rates of absorption, dosages, and rates of elimination on serum drug concentrations (based on first-order absorption and elimination kinetics). See text for details.

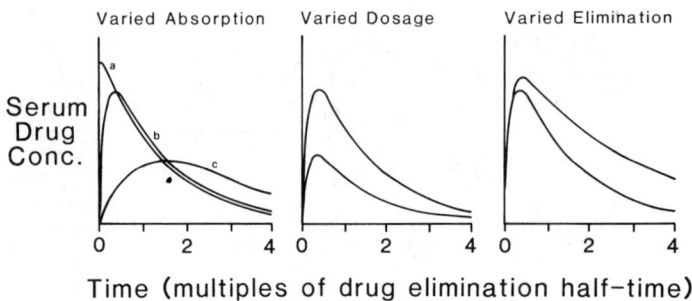

excess of the elimination rate constant. Curve *c* results from assuming equal rate constants for absorption and elimination. If 100% of the administered dose is absorbed, the area under the three example serum level curves (*a*, *b*, and *c*) would be equal no matter what relative rates of absorption and elimination were operating. The area under the curve (AUC) is a useful parameter because it is directly proportional to the amount of drug that is absorbed. Details regarding AUC calculations can be found in the literature.[5]

The middle set of curves in Figure 2–10 represents the effect of altering dosage but not changing the relative rate constants for absorption and elimination. Blood levels are lower for lower doses, but the shape of the curve is not altered. Note that the peak blood levels result at the same time regardless of the dose. The right-hand set of curves in the figure represents the effect of changing the elimination rate constant. The curves shown are for drugs with identical absorption rates but different half-lives; one has a lower elimination rate constant. Note that the blood levels are similar during the absorption phase, but that the peak is higher for the drug with the low elimination because of elimination of less drug during the absorptive phase. Since both desirable and undesirable effects of drugs can relate to blood level concentrations, inspection of Figure 2–10 will serve to emphasize that differences in drug responses can occur on the basis of altered drug absorption or elimination as well as dosage.

CLINICAL APPLICATION OF PHARMACOKINETICS

The previous discussions have centered on general pharmacologic principles and associated pharmacokinetic definitions. This section is devoted to pharmacokinetics-based techniques that can be meaningfully applied in most clinical settings to achieve an ideal dosage regimen. Rather than following only the clinical response to the drug (therapeutic or toxic) to establish the optimal dose and dosing interval, the pharmacokinetic approach utilizes measurements of the amount of drug present in the body or plasma.[5] For this kinetic approach to be valid, therapeutic and toxic responses must relate to a given concentration of drug in the plasma compartment (see Fig. 2–7). Ultimately, the validity of the kinetic approach must be confirmed in each infant by assessment of the therapeutic response.

A variety of factors have been identified that should prompt pharmacokinetic evaluation of a patient's therapeutic program.[1] Drugs having a narrow therapeutic window (i.e., toxic levels not greatly different from therapeutic levels), such as aminoglycosides, chloramphenicol, digoxin, and theophylline, can be more ideally managed with blood level monitoring. Clinical evidence of therapeutic failure or of toxicity is also a strong rationale for blood level monitoring. Monitoring of drug levels to improve patient motivation or compliance or to follow a change of the drug dosage form or dosage regimen is also acceptable. Certain drug–drug interactions can modify the pharmacologic effect of the involved medications, producing alteration of drug concentration. Impaired elimination of a drug because of hepatic or renal dysfunction frequently results in substantial or unpredictable alterations in drug elimination. Optimizing of drug dosing under any of these circumstances can be more readily accomplished with drug level monitoring. Finally, unfortunate accidents with overdose can be documented and followed by drug blood level measurements.

Design of a dosage regimen can be based on pharmacokinetic information to keep the plasma concentration of drug within certain maximum and minimum values. To establish the appropriate **dosing interval,**

$$\tau_{\max} = \frac{\ln(C_{\max}/C_{\min})}{k}$$

where $\tau_{\max}$ = maximum dosing interval that will keep plasma drug concentration at steady state within maximum and minimum units

$C_{\max}$ = maximum desired plasma concentration

$C_{\min}$ = minimum desired plasma concentration

Since $k = 0.693/T_{\frac{1}{2}}$,

$$\tau_{\max} = 1.44 \times T_{\frac{1}{2}} \times \ln(C_{\max}/C_{\min})$$

The maximum **maintenance dose** that can be given at the defined interval ($\tau_{\max}$) can be calculated from

$$D_{\max} = \frac{V_{\mathrm{d}}}{F}(C_{\max}/C_{\min})$$

where D_{max} = maximum maintenance dose
V_d = volume of distribution
F = availability of drug for route of administration chosen

The maintenance dose and the interval of administration τ can be adjusted to suit best the infant's overall care program from the following relationship:

$$\frac{\text{dose}}{\tau} = \frac{D_{max}}{\tau_{max}}$$

If the ratio of the dosing interval chosen to the drug's half-life $(\tau/T\frac{1}{2})$ is much less than one and if rapid establishment of therapeutic blood levels is desired, then a loading dose of the drug should be calculated from

$$D_L = \frac{V_d}{F} \times C_{max}$$

where D_L = loading dose
V_d = volume of distribution
F = availability
C_{max} = maximum desired plasma drug concentration

The **average plasma concentration** at steady state for any route of drug administration can also be calculated as long as the drug's availability and clearance remain constant with both time and dose:

$$C_{ave} = \frac{F \times D_{max}}{Cl \times \tau}$$

where F = availability
D_{max} = maximum maintenance dose
Cl = clearance
τ = dosing interval

Although single doses are the most commonly employed regimen for drug administration, in some cases a continuous infusion of drug is preferred. This is particularly true when it is possible to maximize the therapeutic effect and at the same time to minimize toxicity by minimizing fluctuations in drug plasma levels. Also, for drugs having very short durations of action (dopamine, tolazoline, prostaglandin E), a constant infusion is typically better. The only factors governing the amount of drug present at steady state (plateau) are the rate of infusion

and the elimination rate constant:

$$C_{ss} = \frac{R_{inf}}{Cl}$$

or

$$R_{inf} = C_{ss} \times Cl$$

where C_{ss} = steady state concentration of drug
R_{inf} = rate of infusion
Cl = clearance

If clearance remains constant, any change in infusion rate should produce a proportional change in plasma concentration. The time required to reach steady-state plasma levels is controlled by the half-life of the drug. For practical purposes, the plateau level is reached after approximately 4 to 6 half-lives. Administration of a bolus dose prior to constant infusion will virtually eliminate this time delay in reaching steady-state plasma levels:

$$\text{bolus dose} = \frac{R_{inf}}{k}$$

where R_{inf} = infusion rate
k = elimination rate constant

For most drugs existing drug pharmacokinetic data (V_d, $T\frac{1}{2}$, F, k, Cl) can be identified. Unfortunately, the vast majority of these data has been derived from human adults and not infants. Table 2–1 provides a summary of blood level values for drugs that have been monitored in a meaningful fashion in infants. Some useful relationships to assist in acquiring other drug values for infants can be realized from the following formula:

$$\frac{Cl}{F} = \frac{(\text{dose}/\tau)}{C_{ave}}$$

where Cl = clearance
F = availability
τ = dosing interval
C_{ave} = average plasma concentration

Since $F = 1$ with intravenous administration (i.e., 100% availability), this formula reduces to

$$Cl = \frac{(\text{dose}/\tau)}{C_{ave}}$$

Although measurements of plasma drug concentrations and employment of pharmacokine-

Table 2–3. FACTORS AFFECTING THE CLINICAL RESPONSE TO THE ADMINISTERED DRUG

Factors Affecting Response	Example(s)
Without Alteration of Drug Plasma Level	
presence of active metabolites	see Table 2–4
altered pharmacologic response (tolerance or resistance)	epinephrine, norepinephrine, isoproterenol
drug–drug interactions (altering drug effect but not drug levels)	
pharmacogenetic idiosyncrasy	see Table 2–5
sex	antenatal glucocorticoid; prevention of respiratory distress syndrome (RDS) in female fetus
With Alteration of Drug Plasma Level	
change in drug disposition	
hepatic dysfunction (metabolism)	chloramphenicol
renal dysfunction (excretion)	aminoglycoside
altered protein binding (measure free drug)	phenytoin
genetic origin	see Table 2–5
disease (thyroid, cardiac, gastrointestinal, pulmonary, burns, malignancy)	
drug–drug interactions	quinidine/digoxin (binding); phenobarbital/phenytoin (metabolism)
age	phenytoin, phenobarbital, diazepam, theophylline

tics may ordinarily facilitate optimal therapeutic management, they may correlate very poorly with clinical outcome for a variety of reasons. Table 2–3 summarizes some of the common factors that can influence a given drug's effects in the absence of appropriate or anticipated changes in the plasma level of the drug—for example, the presence of active metabolites (see Table 2–4). A change may occur in the anticipated therapeutic response resulting from an

Table 2–4. DRUGS WITH ACTIVE METABOLITES

Drug Administered	Active Metabolite(s)
acetohexamide	hydroxyhexamide
acetylsalicylic acid	salicylic acid
allopurinol	alloxanthine
amitriptyline	nortriptyline
chloral hydrate	trichloroethanol
chloramphenicol	glycolic acid metabolite
codeine	morphine
cortisone	cortisol
diazepam	desmethyldiazepam, oxazepam
digitoxin	digoxin
digoxin	digoxigenin derivatives
imipramine	desipramine
lidocaine	desethyllidocaine
meperidine	normeperidine
nortriptyline	desmethylnortriptyline
phenylbutazone	oxyphenylbutazone
prednisone	prednisolone
primidone	phenobarbital
procainamide	N-acetylprocainamide
propranolol	4-hydroxypropranolol
quinidine	3-hydroxyquinidine
theophylline	caffeine
verapamil	norverapamil

existing plasma concentration of the drug. As a consequence, there is a shift in the dose (plasma concentration)–response relationship for a given infant (see Fig. 2–11).

A difference in response to a given plasma concentration of a drug can be considered another expression of differences among persons analogous to genetic determinants of physical features, such as size or hair and eye color. Many genetic conditions have been demonstrated to affect pharmacokinetics or pharmacodynamics;[6] Table 2–5 lists some examples. Failure to appreciate the importance of individual differences in dose–response relationships can lead to therapeutic failure in some patients and toxicity in others. This realization should encourage continued pursuit of clinical evidence of drug effects even with circumstances of ideal target level concentrations of the drug in plasma. Figure 2–11 illustrates an expression of individual variation that can present significant difficulty in drug therapy: The slope of the dose–response curve for *Infant C* is different from that for *Infants A* or *B*. Therefore, careful monitoring will be particularly important, in this infant, both clinically and with drug plasma level measurements, because a given change in dose (or plasma concentration) is different from that for *Infant A* or *B*. In *Infant C* small changes in dose or plasma levels are associated with large changes in effect.

With certain drugs, on the other hand, serum concentration is irrelevant: The large doses commonly used in penicillin therapy, for example, are known to be essentially without toxicity. Other drugs such as antihypertensives can

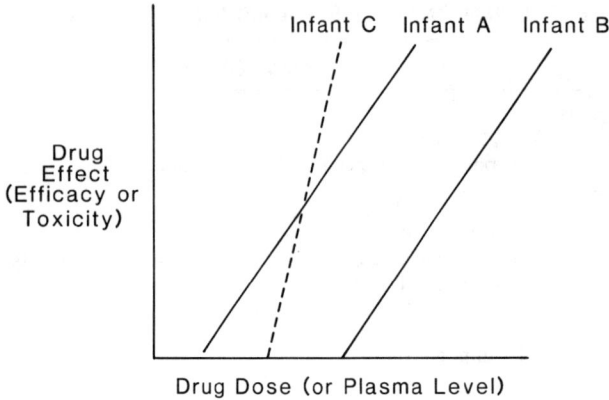

Figure 2–11. Dose–response relationships in three different infants. For *Infant A* and *Infant B*, there is a uniform shift to the right: The lines are parallel, indicating different potency of drug dose (or plasma level) but the same incremental change in response per change in dose (or plasma level). For *Infant C,* there is nonuniform or nonparallel shift relative to that for *Infant A* and *Infant B*, with a greater incremental change in effect occurring per change in dose (or plasma level).

Table 2–5. GENETIC FACTORS AFFECTING DRUG KINETICS OR DYNAMICS

Genetic Factor or Condition	Drug(s) Affected or Involved	Response
acetylation: fast or slow	isoniazid; hydralazine	increased toxicity (slow)
hydroxylation: slow	phenytoin	increased toxicity
hydrolysis: slow	succinylcholine; administered esters of chloramphenicol, and erythromycin	prolonged action; reduced efficacy
glucose 6-phosphate dehydrogenase (G6PD) deficiency, favism	various drugs: antimalarials, analgesics, sulfonamides, nitrofurantoin, chloramphenicol	RBC hemolysis
anticoagulant resistance	warfarin	resistance
glaucoma	corticosteroids	aggrevate glaucoma
malignant hyperthermia	various anesthetics	uncontrolled increase in body temperature
mongolism	atropine	increased heart rate beyond usual induced response

Adapted from Vesell ES: Advances in pharmacogenetics. In Progress in Medical Genetics. Steinberg AG and Bearn AG (eds), Vol IX. New York, Grune & Stratton, Inc, 1973, p. 291.

be more easily quantitated by clinical parameters than by blood level measurements. The effects of still other drugs, such as furosemide, simply do not correlate with blood levels, because the concentration at the locus of effect is not in constant equilibrium with the blood (see Chap. 8, Diuretics).

References

1. Aranda JV, Turmen T, Cote-Boileau T: Drug monitoring in the perinatal patient: Uses and abuses. Ther Drug Monit 2:39, 1980.
2. Dvorchik BH, Vesell ES: Significance of error associated with use of the one-compartment formula to calculate clearance of thirty-eight drugs. Clin Pharmacol Ther 23:617, 1978.
3. Greenblatt DJ, Koch-Weser J: Clinical Pharmacokinetics. N Engl J Med 293:702, 1975.
4. Pippenger CE: Rationale and clinical application of therapeutic drug monitoring. Pediatr Clin North Am 27:891, 1980.
5. Rowland M, Tozer TN: Clinical Pharmacokinetics: Concepts and Applications. Philadelphia, Lea and Febiger, 1980.
6. Vesell ES: Advances in pharmacogenetics. In Progress in Medical Genetics. Steinberg AG and Bearn AG (eds), Vol IX, New York, Grune & Stratton, 1973, p. 291.

THREE

Special Considerations in Drug Therapy in Infants

INTRAVENOUS DRUG ADMINISTRATION

Lack of awareness of or attention to critical aspects of clinical monitoring of drug concentrations in infants can lead to disasters even in the face of sophisticated pharmacokinetic and analytical methodology. Kauffman[13] has reviewed in detail the various factors that must be taken into consideration to ensure appropriate therapeutic drug monitoring technique. To summarize, the physician must recognize that drug concentrations in the blood are not static (except with constant infusion), as are levels of most endogenous substances such as electrolytes. Therefore, the timing relative to administration of samples for drug level monitoring must be accurate. In this regard, Roberts[20] has outlined methods for preventing the unique problems of intravenous (IV) drug delivery in the infant that can contribute to the difficulties in accurate timing of blood samples. Figures 3-1 and 3-2 demonstrate the problems associated with a delay in drug delivery as a result of the rate of IV flow or injection of drug via a distal site in the IV system. Lack of appreciation of time delay can obviously result in mis-timing of peak or trough blood level samples obtained for purposes of optimizing drug therapy. Adjustment of drug dosages based on such data could easily place the patient at risk either for toxicity on the basis of increased dosage (in response to low drug blood level) or for therapeutic failure owing to underdosing (in response to high drug blood level). Of additional concern is loss of drug as a consequence of routine changing of IV sets as a procedure for minimizing problems of bacterial contamination. It was determined by examining drug dosing times and IV set replacement times in the

neonatal unit at University of Iowa Hospitals and Clinics that approximately 36% of the total daily dose of various intravenous medications was unknowingly lost in the discarded intravenous sets.[12] Obviously, situations in which immediate discontinuation of IV medication administration is desired (e.g., toxic reactions) could also be compromised if the medication remaining in the IV system is not appreciated. If the IV is not completely flushed or replaced, a considerable length of time can be involved before the IV system is free of drug. For example, if continuous infusion of drug (e.g., dopamine, isoproterenol) is accomplished by infusion into another main IV line and is discontinued by simply clamping or disconnecting this secondary IV system, drug already in the main IV system may continue to be infused for a considerable length of time (see Fig. 3-1).

Benzing and Loggie[4] were first to present a method for IV administration of drugs to pediatric patients. Their technique utilized retrograde injection of a dosage volume that equals exactly one third of the IV fluid rate (ml/hr). Other studies using the retrograde technique[9,12] indicate that unexpected delivery times with the manual retrograde injection technique are probably the result of admixture of the dosage volume with the IV fluid, which prolongs the infusion of the dose to the patient.

Drug delivery systems have now been devised to minimize these problems. In studies by Leff and Roberts,[16] drug dosage volumes were calculated for theoretical patients weighing 1 and 5 kg to establish a data base for designing a uniform IV drug delivery protocol. Dosage volumes for 30 of the most frequently employed IV medications ranged from 0.06 to 5.0 ml; mean

A. Infusion Rate = 3 ml/hr

B. Infusion Rate = 25 ml/hr

Gentamicin
Injection Sites

●————● Butterfly
o————o Flashball
△·············△ Y Site
▲—·—·—▲ Metriset

Time from Injection into I.V. System (Hours)

% Remaining to be Infused

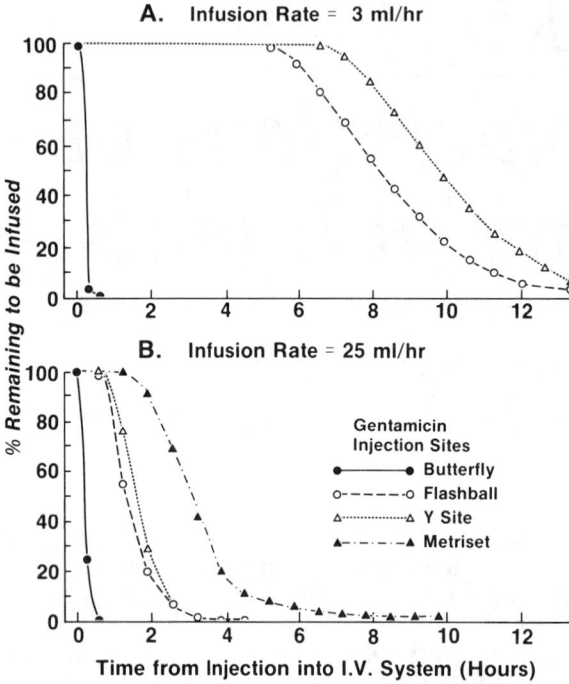

Figure 3–1. Effects of different IV infusion rates and different injection sites on time required for delivery of drug dose. For example, at 3 ml/hr *(A),* actual infusion of drug begins at 160 minutes after injection into the IV system (flashball site) and is completed 6 hours later (i.e., 400 minutes). At a more rapid IV infusion rate of 25 ml/hr *(B)* the delay in start of actual infusion is less, as is the duration required for delivery of the dose. Note the major difference between injection sites (butterfly vs. flashball site). (Adapted from Gould T, Roberts RJ: J Pediatr 95:465, 1979.)

drug dosage volumes were 0.4 and 1.3 ml for the 1-kg and 5-kg patients, respectively (Table 3–1). The calculated average maintenance IV fluid flow rates were 4 and 20 ml/hour for the respective patient weights.

A series of experiments examined the actual time required to deliver medications from the IV systems shown in Figure 3–3 to theoretical patients, utilizing the previously described dosage volumes and IV flow rates (Table 3–1). The time to deliver the drug was determined by retrograde injection of a marker dye (methylene blue) at the flashball site and visual observation of the clearance of the dye from the IV tubing. Drug delivery time was influenced by both dosage volume and IV flow rate (Fig. 3–4). The slower the IV flow rate and the larger the dosage volume, the longer the drug infusion time; the smaller the dosage volume and the faster the IV flow rate, the shorter the drug infusion time.

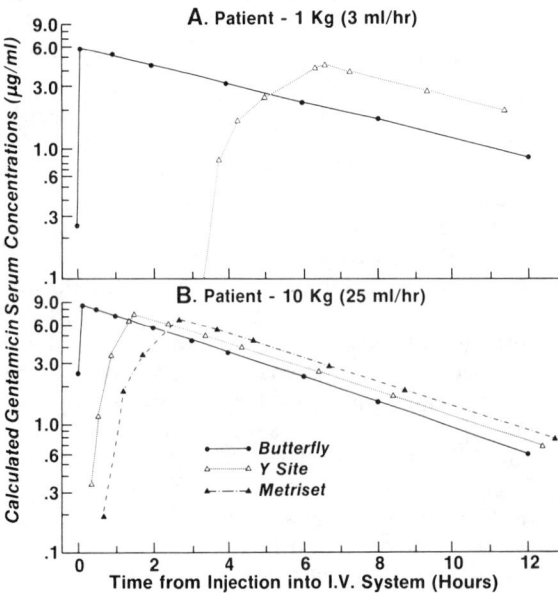

A. Patient - 1 Kg (3 ml/hr)

B. Patient - 10 Kg (25 ml/hr)

●———● *Butterfly*
△———△ *Y Site*
▲—·—·—▲ *Metriset*

Calculated Gentamicin Serum Concentrations (μg/ml)

Time from Injection into I.V. System (Hours)

Figure 3–2. Effects of IV injection site (butterfly, Y site, or Metriset) on serum gentamicin concentrations. Drug levels were calculated from infusion data shown in Figure 3–1 for a 1-kg patient at 3 ml/hr *(A)* and a 10-kg patient at 25 ml/hr *(B).* Note in *A* that with use of the Y site there is a three-hour delay before drug levels begin to rise in the serum. (Adapted from Roberts RJ: Pediatr Clin North Am 28:23, 1981.)

Table 3–1. REPRESENTATIVE DOSAGE
VOLUMES AND IV FLOW RATES CALCULATED
FOR INFANTS

Patient Wt (kg)	Calculated Dosage Volume (ml)[a]		Approximate IV Flow[b] (ml/hr)
	Mean	Range	
1	0.4	0.06–1.0	4
5	1.3	0.25–5.0	20

[a] Dosage volumes for 30 of the most frequently employed IV medications were identified using a computerized inventory system. Volume calculations were based on the drug concentration available from the manufacturer or the hospital pharmacy for IV administration.
[b] Intravenous flow rate calculations are based on 100 mg/kg/24 hr.
From Leff RD, Roberts RJ: J Pediatr 98:631, 1981.

Note that retrograde injection of a dosage volume much larger than one half the volume contained in the IV tubing between the injection site and overflow syringe (see Fig. 3–3B) will result in loss of medication into the overflow syringe.

On the basis of these studies it was concluded that an alternative method for introducing the drug into the IV system is needed when the manual retrograde injection technique results in either unacceptably prolonged or too-rapid delivery time.[16] An IV system employing a mechanical syringe infusion device was developed to allow absolute control over the rate of drug delivery to the patient (Fig. 3–5). Mechanical infusion of drug into the IV system produces an equal rate of drug infusion; the rate of flow of IV fluid and the drug dosage volume do not influence the rate of drug delivery from the IV system. Several syringe pumps compatible with the basic design and requirements of the infusion system are available. Each syringe infusion pump has features that may be more or less desirable, depending on the experience and preference of the hospital, medical, nursing, and pharmacy staff, or on requirements in the individual patient.

Thus, the rate of IV drug delivery to the patient has been shown to be subject to variation depending on the site chosen for drug injection into the IV system, the rate of flow of the IV solution, and the drug dosage volume. Variation in the rate of drug delivery among patients is common in the pediatric population because of the wide range of drug dosage volumes and maintenance IV fluid requirements. A uniform protocol to minimize these factors and to assure control of the rate of drug delivery to the patient is therefore essential. The mechanical infusion technique provides the opportunity for absolute control over the rate of drug delivery to the patient irrespective of the dosage volume and existing IV flow rate. The use of a distal injection site and low-volume tubing further assures that drug delivery time is neither delayed nor prolonged. Unfortunately, only general guidelines with regard to optimal rates of delivery can be found in the literature for most drugs.[19] Complicated multiple drug therapy and coadministration of drugs, blood products, venous nutritional preparations, and so forth, also require consideration in designing an optimal IV system.

Additional factors to consider in IV drug therapy include binding of drug to IV filter devices[22] and specific gravity of drug solution. These physicochemical variables can have a profound influence on drug delivery time, particularly when a reservoir of any kind (e.g., filter device) is incorporated into the IV system.[18]

Although not unique to IV drug therapy, errors in drug computations during newborn intensive care have been documented to occur with alarming frequency; Perlstein and coworkers reported approximately an 8% error.[17] The neonate is particularly vulnerable because individually calculated doses based on age, weight, or gestational age are typically involved.[17] The unfortunate similarity in appearance of dosage units (nanogram, ng; microgram, μg or mcg; milligram, mg or mgm; gram, g or gm), even when written legibly, certainly adds to the difficulty. Manufacturers of pharmaceutical preparations have traditionally failed to appreciate the advantages of a pediatric dosage form that would allow greater accuracy in preparing the small doses needed for neonates, although pediatric dosage forms are becoming more widely available. The technique involved in dilution of adult pharmaceutical preparations is of particular concern: If the dead space in syringes is not appreciated, the dose delivered may be substantially larger than intended, resulting in "dilution intoxication." Berman and colleagues[5] described such a situation with digoxin. They measured the amount of digoxin contained in the calibrated chamber and dead space of a tuberculin syringe filled to the 0.05-ml level and found that it averaged 14 μg (range 12–18 μg) compared with the 5 μg contained in the intended 0.05-ml dosage volume (digoxin is commercially available as a 100 μg/ml "pediatric" injection). If the 0.05-ml volume is subsequently diluted in the same syringe to increase the dosing delivery volume under the guise of improved accuracy, the di-

A.

(existing i.v. system)

occlude, i.v. line

or

low volume tubing

Pump

release pump tubing to
accommodate retrograde
drug injection

retrograde drug injection
site (flashball or 4-way
stopcock)

B.

(existing i.v. system)

open 4-way stopcock before
retrograde drug injection

P
u
m
p

occlude line during
retrograde injection

or

low volume tubing

close 4-way
stopcock after
drug injection

retrograde drug injection
site (flashball or 4-way
stopcock)

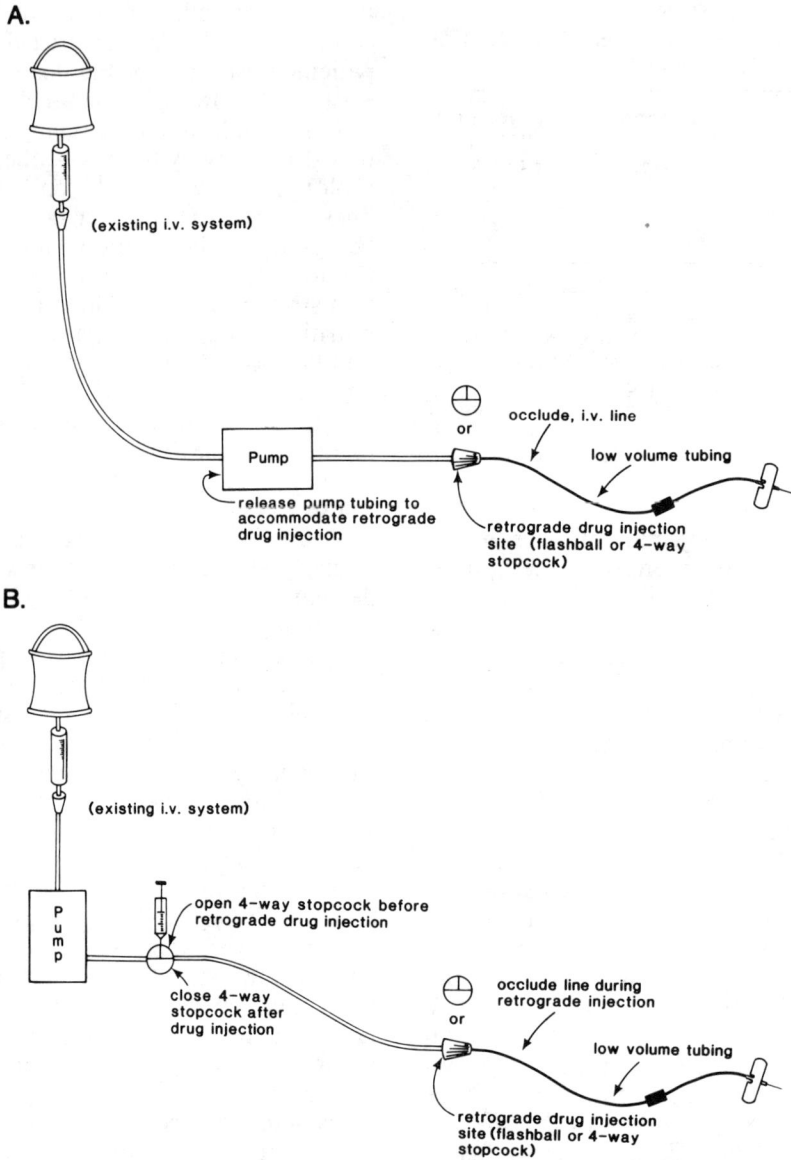

Figure 3 – 3. A, Construction of IV system for manual retrograde injection. An injection site (flashball or stopcock) and low-volume extension tubing are located at the distal end of the existing IV set-up. *B,* Construction of IV system for retrograde injection modified for a volume-infusion pump device unable to accept retrograde injections. To the existing IV system is attached an extension set with a proximal four-way stopcock and distal flashball injection site. A large-volume syringe is attached to the four-way stopcock and acts as an overflow reservoir for the IV fluid displaced by the dosage volume. (From Leff RD, Roberts RJ: J Pediatr 98:631, 1981.)

goxin contained in the dead space will be drawn into the actual delivery volume, resulting in inadvertent overdosing. An instance of morphine intoxication in a neonate following inappropriate dilution technique has also been reported.[27] Other potent medications with similar potential because of high concentrations in available products are listed in Table 3 – 2. It is obvious on inspection of the calculated dose volumes that, for some drugs, accurate administration is virtually impossible without prior dilution. A two-syringe technique must be employed to avoid dilution errors. A summary of the variety of special considerations important to accurate and precise drug therapy in infants is presented in Table 3 – 3.

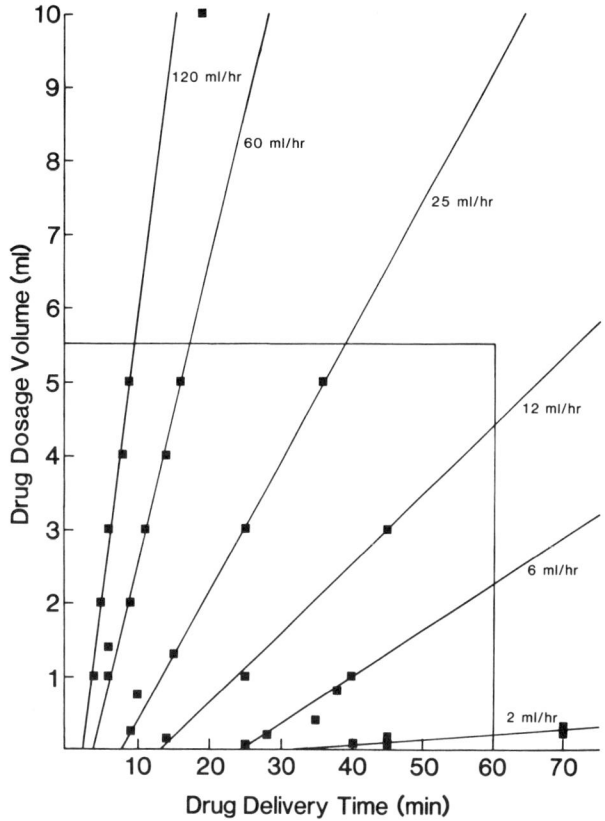

Figure 3-4. Influence of dosage volume (ordinate) or IV flow rate (individual data lines) on time required to complete drug delivery (abscissa) with use of a manual retrograde injection technique (see Fig. 3-3). (From Leff RD, Roberts RJ: J Pediatr 98:631, 1981.)

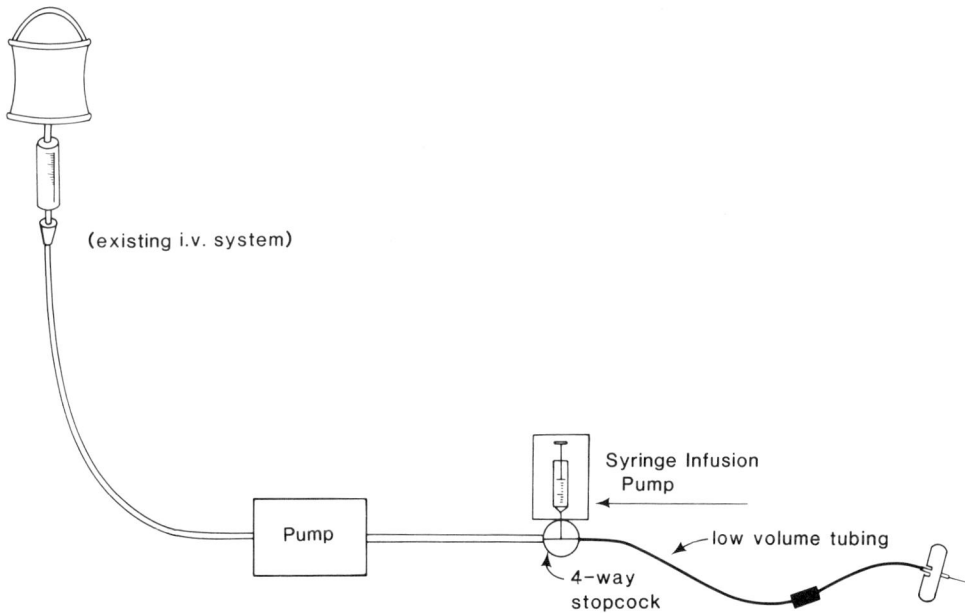

Figure 3-5. Construction of mechanical (syringe) infusion system. A four-way stopcock and low-volume extension tubing are attached distal to the existing IV system. The dosage syringe is attached directly to the four-way stopcock before placement on the syringe infusion device. (From Leff RD, Roberts RJ: J Pediatr 98:631, 1981.)

Table 3–2. POTENT MEDICATIONS WITH POTENTIAL FOR "DILUTION INTOXICATION" DUE TO CONCENTRATION IN AVAILABLE PHARMACEUTICAL PREPARATIONS

| Drug | Available Concentration[a] | Calculated Individual Dose[b] | | Dose Delivered with Flush[c] | Delivered Dose (% Calculated) |
		Volume (ml)	Amount		
atropine	0.4 mg/ml	0.0025	0.01 mg	0.016 mg	160
diazepam	5 mg/ml	0.05	0.1 mg	0.18 mg	180
digoxin	100 μg/ml	0.05	5 μg	6.5 μg	130
epinephrine	1 : 10,000	0.1	10 μg	11.5 μg	115
hydralazine	20 mg/ml	0.05	1 mg	1.3 mg	130
insulin	100 U/ml	0.001	0.1 U	0.115 U	115
morphine	8 mg/ml	0.013	0.1 mg	0.22 mg	220
phenytoin	50 mg/ml	0.08	4 mg	4.75 mg	120

[a] Preparation chosen for calculation represents lowest concentration in a commercially available form.
[b] Calculated dose based on recommended maintenance dose for 1-kg infant.
[c] Dose delivered by flush determined by combining the desired measured dosage contained in the calibrated chamber of the syringe with the drug in the dead space (0.015 ml) delivered by flushing a 1-ml tuberculin syringe.

DOSING REQUIREMENTS IN ORGAN FAILURE

The generalization that disease states or evidence of isolated organ failure (e.g., renal, hepatic, cardiac, lung) can be expected to alter the disposition of drugs is reasonable. But the assumption that organ failure is the major contributor (qualitatively and quantitatively) to variability in pharmacokinetics or pharmacodynamics compared with the contribution of individual variation cannot be supported by examination of the literature. Nevertheless, it is important to anticipate influences of organ failure on drug effects when the drugs used are known to have altered disposition with altered state(s) of organ(s) function.

Hepatic Dysfunction. Because the liver is the major site for drug metabolism, an impression prevails that particular care is necessary when administering drugs to infants with disease states expected to diminish hepatic metabolic function (e.g., drug metabolism, uptake, excretion). Although this is a fair presumption, actual studies of the influence of hepatic disease have produced conflicting results, prompting some investigators to conclude that it is often difficult to predict in a given patient with hepatic impairment whether the effect will be retarded, unchanged, or accelerated drug elimination.[25]

For drugs known to be subject to high hepatic extraction (first-pass effect; see Table 1–1), changes in hepatic blood flow may substantially change the clearance of the drug (increased bioavailability). In such cases, reduction of the initial and subsequent doses may be necessary; determination of serum drug levels would be particularly helpful. Table 3–4 summarizes drug kinetics reported to be influenced by liver disease; note that the data have been derived from studies in adults with a variety of liver diseases and thus may not necessarily be applicable in infant therapeutics.

The effect of liver disease can extend beyond modification of intrinsic drug clearance by the liver. Since the liver is the major organ for synthesis of circulating proteins involved in drug binding (albumin, alpha$_1$ globulin), alterations in unbound fraction of drug present in plasma can also be expected. Generally, only

Table 3–3. PHARMACOTHERAPEUTIC REQUIREMENTS IN THE INFANT PREDISPOSING TO ERRORS

I. Individual dosage calculation
   Increased likelihood of arithmetic errors in calculations based on weight, gestational age, and so forth, compared with use of "universal dose" in adult patient
II. Use of dosage units having similar appearance (e.g., μg or mcg, mg, ng)
III. Preparation of very small therapeutic dosages from concentrated formulations generally available commercially (see Table 3–2)
IV. Slow IV rates
   Predispose to delay in delivery or omission of dose due to inadvertent discarding, or to osmotic-related loss or delay in delivery with use of large-volume tubing or filtering device
V. Delivery of very small dosage volumes
   IV: loss in dead space of IV system, stopcock, Y site, or syringe
   PO: loss in delivery (nasogastric tube dead space) or from oral cavity
   IM: leak from injection site of significant portion of the very small volume injected

Table 3-4. EFFECTS OF HEPATIC DYSFUNCTION ON PLASMA CLEARANCE OF COMMONLY USED DRUGS

Drug	Cirrhosis	Acute Viral Hepatitis	Obstructive Jaundice
amobarbital	↓		
ampicillin	↓ or 0		
antipyrine	↓	↓	↓
chloramphenicol	↓ or 0		
clindamycin	↓		
diazepam	↓	↓	
digoxin	0	↑	
heparin	↓		
hexobarbital		↓	
isoniazid	↓		
lidocaine	↓	0	
meperidine	↓	↓	
pentobarbital	↓		
phenobarbital	↓	↓ or 0	
phenytoin		0	
prednisolone	0		
propranolol	0		
theophylline	↓		
tolbutamide		↑	
warfarin		0	

Plasma clearance: ↑ = increased; ↓ = decreased; 0 = no change.

[a] Hepatic dysfunction includes a diverse group of clinical conditions such as hepatitis (acute) and cirrhosis (chronic). Because these data have been derived from adult studies, it is inappropriate to assume that they would also apply in infants with or without similar causes of hepatic dysfunction.

Adapted from Rowland M et al: In Benet LZ (ed): Effect of Disease States on Drug Pharmacokinetics. Washington DC, American Pharmaceutical Association, 1976; and from Williams RL, Mamelock RD: Clin Pharmacokinet 5:528, 1980.

drugs greater than 90% protein-bound demonstrate significant changes in pharmacokinetics as a result of changes in protein binding.[6] Changes in pharmacodynamics may also occur secondary to liver disease: In adults with chronic liver disease, an increased sensitivity to drugs active in the central nervous system has been observed.[7]

General guidelines for drug use in hepatic disease are difficult to formulate, because liver disease itself is complex in etiology and pathophysiology, and because it can affect not only metabolism and excretion but also protein binding, tissue distribution, and receptor responsiveness. In general, even with severe hepatic dysfunction, alterations in drug disposition beyond two- to threefold are unlikely.[24] Even so, in a patient with serious liver dysfunction an attempt should be made to utilize drugs that are eliminated by extrahepatic mechanisms with therapeutic activity unaffected by liver disease and not known to produce hepatotoxicity themselves. In the absence of information on the use of a specific drug in hepatic failure, cautious and individualized therapy based on the known pharmacologic features of the drug and careful clinical observations of parameters of therapeutic effect is a reasonable guideline.

Renal Dysfunction. The period of time a drug and any metabolites remain in the body, and therefore the duration and intensity of pharmacologic effect, is often determined by the status of kidney function because of the major role of kidneys in elimination of a large number of drugs and metabolites from the body (see Chap. 1). In contrast to the liver, a number of very sensitive indicators are available for identification, characterization, and quantitation of renal dysfunction. For drugs such as digoxin and the aminoglycosides, elimination depends almost entirely upon the kidneys; therefore, an estimation of the glomerular filtration rate (GFR) can reflect accurately the dosing requirements for these drugs under conditions of renal dysfunction. It should be appreciated that in acute tubular necrosis or other situations of rapidly changing glomerular filtration, the onset of changes in creatinine clearance (indicator of GFR) may be significantly delayed. Serum urea nitrogen concentration as determined by BUN levels should not be considered an accurate guide to drug dose adjustment in renal disease.[8] Other drugs depend not at all on renal function for elimination; still others depend both on renal and nonrenal routes (Table 3-5). The great majority of work reported in the literature deals with antimicrobial drugs in adults; relatively little work has been done with other drugs or drugs in infants.

As is the case with hepatic dysfunction, renal failure can have a variety of influences on drug kinetics and dynamics. Alteration in nonrenal elimination, protein binding, and volume of distribution of drugs has been reported with renal failure.[11] Renal failure can also lead to the accumulation of pharmacologically active or toxic metabolites of drugs. Drugs with this potential (e.g., procainamide) are best avoided in renal failure because of the complexity surrounding dosing considerations. Welling and Craig[23] have recently reviewed in detail the known influences of renal dysfunction on drug disposition.

Whether or not dosage adjustment will be necessary for any given drug depends primarily on the degree of renal dysfunction, the percent-

Table 3-5. CLASSIFICATION OF DRUGS BASED ON PRIMARY ROUTE OF ELIMINATION

Renal Elimination Mechanism

amikacin	cephalothin	lithium
cefazolin	gentamicin	tobramycin
cephalexin	kanamycin	vancomycin
cephaloridine		

Nonrenal Elimination Mechanisms

acetaminophen	isoniazid	prazosin
amphotericin	meperidine	propranolol
chloramphenicol	minoxidil	quinidine
clindamycin	morphine	reserpine
clonidine	naloxone	rifampin
codeine	nitroprusside	steroids
diazepam	pentobarbital	theophylline
heparin	phenothiazine	
hydralazine	phenytoin	

Renal and Nonrenal Elimination Mechanisms

ampicillin	digoxin	penicillin G
carbenicillin	lincomycin	phenobarbital
cephalothin	methicillin	procainamide
diazoxide	nafcillin	
dicloxacillin	oxacillin	

Data derived largely from studies in adults.
Adapted from Gibson TP: In Evans WE et al (eds): Applied Pharmacokinetics: Principles of Therapeutic Drug Monitoring. San Francisco, Applied Therapeutics, Inc., 1980.

age of drug cleared via the kidney (Table 3-5), and the therapeutic index of the particular drug, particularly under conditions of renal dysfunction. For example, most penicillins and some cephalosporins have wide therapeutic indices, and no dosage adjustment is necessary in cases of mild or moderate renal dysfunction. Although a large number of techniques based on nomograms, tables, or computer programs have been produced in an attempt to deal with the problem of dosage adjustment in renal failure, none is uniformly successful. Therefore, a rigid approach to determining drug dosage in infants with renal dysfunction should be discouraged.

Basically, three adjustments in dosage are possible: (1) prolongation of the dosing interval, (2) reduction in the maintenance dose, or (3) both prolongation in dosing interval and reduction in maintenance dose. In the third method, originally proposed by Kunin,[14] some proportion of the usual maintenance dose (typically one half) is administered at a dosing interval equal to the drug half-life in the patient. Determining which of the three possibilities is best requires an appreciation of the likely drug plasma disappearance versus time curve resulting from each method and a knowledge of the ideal peak and trough levels (therapeutic window) for the drug being given. The factor of time must be considered in this decision because diffusion of drug from one site or compartment to another is dependent not only on concentration but on time or duration of that concentration.

In order to establish a dosage regimen for a patient with renal failure, the following information is required: (1) the normal dosage regimen, (2) estimate of the existing renal function (fraction of normal), and (3) fraction of the unchanged drug normally eliminated by renal excretion. Figure 3-6 shows the plasma disappearance curves possible with the three different dosage adjustments: Curve 1 represents a change only in interval; curve 2 represents a change only in dose; and curve 3 represents a change in both dose and interval. The resulting plasma levels obviously will depend on the magnitude of the changes made in dose or interval of administration. The majority of published methods for dosage adjustment have as the major objective an average plasma drug level equal to that observed with normal renal function.[1-3, 11, 14, 23] In Figure 3-6, a hypothetical drug is administered to an infant with sufficient renal dysfunction to cause a significant prolongation of the $T\frac{1}{2}$. In general, the initial or loading dose of drug should not be altered with renal dysfunction. It is the compromise in elimination of this initial dose and subsequent doses that demands adjustment of the

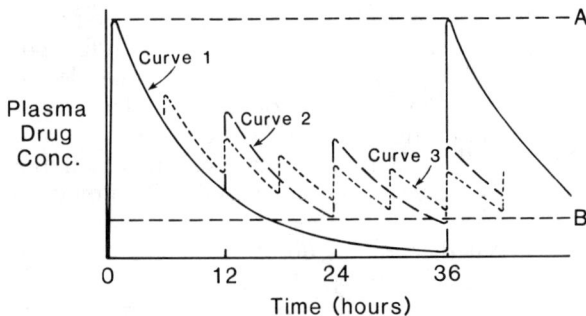

Figure 3-6. Theoretical plasma concentration profiles for three possible dosage modifications in a neonate with renal dysfunction. *Curve 1* represents change only in dosage interval (increased from every 12 hours to every 36 hours); *Curve 2*, a change only in dose; *Curve 3*, a change in both dose and interval (reduced). The horizontal lines represent the therapeutic window: Line *A*, the toxic threshold; line *B*, the minimum effective concentration.

maintenance dosage. Although the total area under the three individual plasma disappearance curves and average plasma drug concentration figured on a per-day basis is equal in the figure, the peak and trough plasma levels and the associated period of time spent at high or low plasma drug levels are obviously different. This may have a significant influence on toxicity (time at high plasma levels) or efficacy (time at low plasma levels). It could be argued, therefore, that a change in both dose and interval will produce the most ideal situation. Unfortunately there is still considerable debate regarding this concept, because little in the way of scientific investigation has been accomplished. Table 3–6 presents a guide to rational drug dosage in patients with significant renal dysfunction. More complete information is provided with discussions of specific agents in later chapters.

The use of Table 3–6 or published nomograms or programs in situations involving renal dysfunction should never take the place of monitoring plasma or serum drug levels or the clinical response for evidence of toxicity. This is especially important for drugs with high percentage of renal clearance ($>90\%$) and patients who have profound and sudden changes in renal function. Another note of caution is in order regarding the fact that most existing nomograms and programs have not been prepared for use in the infant. The use of these techniques in cases of renal failure also requires the following assumptions: no change in drug availability, no active or toxic metabolites formed, no change in ability to metabolize the drug, no concentration-dependent kinetics, and no change in other aspects of drug disposition or dynamics.

Table 3–6. MAINTENANCE DOSE INTERVALS FOR SELECTED DRUGS USED IN INFANTS WITH RENAL DYSFUNCTION[a]

Drug	Major Route of Elimination	Increase in Dose Interval (renal function <10% normal)
Analgesics (Antagonists)		
meperidine	hepatic	unchanged
morphine	hepatic	unchanged
naloxone	hepatic	unchanged
Cardiovascular Agents		
diazoxide	renal	unchanged
digoxin	renal	×2–?
hydralazine	hepatic	×1–2
lidocaine	hepatic	unchanged
procainamide	renal	×2–3
propranolol	hepatic	unchanged
Diuretics		
furosemide	renal	unchanged
spironolactone	hepatic	avoid use
thiazides	renal	avoid use
Sedatives and Hypnotics		
amobarbital	hepatic	unchanged
diazepam	hepatic	unchanged
phenobarbital	hepatic/renal	×1–2
phenothiazines	hepatic/renal	×2–3
secobarbital	hepatic	unchanged
Other Agents		
atropine	nonrenal	unchanged
caffeine	renal	×2–?
corticosteroids	renal	unchanged
heparin	nonrenal	unchanged
indomethacin	hepatic/renal	unchanged
phenytoin	hepatic	unchanged
theophylline	hepatic	unchanged
tubocurarine	renal	unchanged

[a] For drugs not listed see discussions under specific agents. Antibiotic recommendations are given in Table 4–4.
Adapted from Bennett WM et al: JAMA 230:1544, 1974; Ann Intern Med 93:62, 1980; and Ann Intern Med 93:286, 1980.

A Warning. The use of any pharmacokinetics-based dosing program or scheme for all infants, irrespective of the type of evidence for organ failure, will undoubtedly result in widely different drug dosages. Important and serious questions must be considered regarding the balance between efficacy and toxicity resulting from rigid employment of any dosage adjustment protocol. Until the necessary well-controlled clinical studies are accomplished, the decision process to determine the appropriate dosage regimen for individual infants must include consideration of the clinical status of the patient together with pharmacokinetic models to individualize drug therapy.

EXCHANGE TRANSFUSION

Other aspects of function in infants undergoing drug therapy may be so compromised that exchange transfusion may be required (e.g., in hyperbilirubinemia or severe sepsis). It is, therefore, appropriate to consider the effect of exchange transfusion on drug clearance. There have been few studies, and little information is available on drug loss resulting from exchange transfusion in neonates. In an attempt to fill this void, methods for pedicting or calculating drug loss have been published.[15, 26] The hypothetical loss of a variety of drugs due to exchange transfusion is shown in Table 3–7.

In general, the extent of drug loss due to exchange transfusion is related to the drug's volume and rate of distribution, the drug blood level at the time of exchange (peak vs. trough), the number of blood volumes exchanged, and the rate at which the exchange is conducted.[10, 15, 26] Whether any resulting increase in drug loss is associated with adverse therapeutic consequences must be considered on an individual basis. In most cases, antibiotic therapy will not be compromised, particularly if the exchange is conducted during a trough level period. Replacement of antibiotic may be required with repeated exchange transfusions. One possible remedy is the addition of a therapeutic concentration of drug to the exchange blood prior to the procedure. This technique may be particularly efficient when the multiple exchange procedures interfere with or postpone the routine antibiotic administration. Replacement of anticonvulsant drugs and digoxin is usually unnecessary because the quantity of drug lost is quite small. In contrast, considerable loss of theophylline is possible. The use of blood level determinations following exchange

Table 3–7. THEORETICAL DRUG LOSS FROM THE BODY SUBSEQUENT TO EXCHANGE TRANSFUSION

Drug	% Loss One Volume Exchange	% Loss Two Volume Exchange
amikacin	7.1	13.8
ampicillin	7.7	14.7
carbamazepine	3.7	7.2
carbenicillin	5.6	10.9
colistin	18.7	33.9
diazepam	2.3	4.5
digoxin	1.2	2.4
furosemide	4.9	9.5
gentamicin	5.2	10.1
kanamycin	5.6	10.9
methicillin	10.1	19.1
oxacillin	19.6	35.4
penicillin G (crystalline)	6.0	11.6
penicillin G (procaine)	2.4	4.8
phenobarbital	6.4	12.3
phenytoin	3.1	6.2
theophylline	17.8	32.4
tobramycin	10.3	19.6
vancomycin	5.7	11.0

Adapted from Lackner TE: J Pediatr 100:811, 1982.

will be extremely helpful in documenting the need for any drug replacement due to loss with exchange transfusion.

References

1. Bennett WM, Singer I, Coggins CJ: A guide to drug therapy in renal failure. JAMA 230:1544, 1974.
2. Bennett WM, Muther RS, Parker RA, et al: Drug therapy in renal failure: Dosing guidelines for adults. Part I: Antimicrobial agents, analgesics. Ann Intern Med 93:62, 1980.
3. Bennett WM, Muther RS, Parker RA, et al: Drug therapy in renal failure: Dosing guidelines for adults. Part II. Sedatives, hypnotics, and tranquilizers; cardiovascular, antihypertensive and diuretic agents; miscellaneous agents. Ann Intern Med 93:286, 1980.
4. Benzing G III, Loggie J: A new retrograde method for administering drugs intravenously. Pediatrics 52:420, 1973.
5. Berman W Jr, Whitman V, Marks KH, et al: Inadvertent overadministration of digoxin to low-birth-weight infants. J Pediatr 92:1024, 1978.
6. Blaschke TF: Protein binding and kinetics of drugs in liver diseases. Clin Pharmacokinet 2:32, 1977.
7. Branch RA, Morgan MH, James J, Read AE: Intravenous administration of diazepam in patients with chronic liver disease. Gut 17:975, 1976.
8. Dossetor JB: Creatininemia versus uremia. The relative significance of blood urea nitrogen and serum creatinine concentrations in azotemia. Ann Intern Med 65:1287, 1966.
9. Eling R, Brissie EO: Intravenous infusion of drugs by a retrograde technique. Am J Hosp Pharm 31:740, 1974.
10. Fuquay D, Koup J, Epstein MF, Smith AL: Effect of

exchange transfusion on serum gentamicin concentration. Dev Pharmacol Ther 3:214, 1981.

11. Gibson TP: Influence of renal disease on pharmacokinetics. In Evans WE, Schentag JJ, Jusko WJ (eds): Applied Pharmacokinetics: Principles of Therapeutic Drug Monitoring. Chapter 3, p 32. San Francisco, Applied Therapeutics, Inc, 1980.

12. Gould T, Roberts RJ: Therapeutic problems arising from the use of the intravenous route for drug administration. J Pediatr 95:465, 1979.

13. Kauffman RE: The clinical interpretation and application of drug concentration data. Pediatr Clin North Am 28:35, 1981.

14. Kunin CM: A guide to use of antibiotics in patients with renal disease. Ann Intern Med 67:151, 1967.

15. Lackner TE: Drug replacement following exchange transfusion. J Pediatr 100:811, 1982.

16. Leff RD, Roberts RJ: Methods for intravenous drug administration in the pediatric patient. J Pediatr 98:631, 1981.

17. Perlstein PH, Callison C, White M, et al: Errors in drug computations during newborn intensive care. Am J Dis Child 133:376, 1979.

18. Rajchgot P, Radde IC, MacLeod SM: Influence of specific gravity on intravenous drug delivery. J Pediatr 99:658, 1981.

19. Rapp RP, Elgert JF, Piecoro JJ: Guidelines for the administration of commonly used intravenous drugs. Drug Intell Clin Pharm 14:193, 1980.

20. Roberts RP: Intravenous administration of medication in pediatric patients: Problems and solutions. Pediatr Clin North Am 28:23, 1981.

21. Rowland M, Blaschke TF, Meffin PJ, Williams RL: Pharmacokinetics in disease states modifying hepatic and metabolic function, In Benet LZ (ed): The Effect of Disease States on Drug Pharmacokinetics. Chapter 4, p 53. Washington DC, American Pharmaceutical Association, 1976.

22. Wagman GH, Bailey JV, Weinstein MJ: Binding of aminoglycoside antibiotics to filtration materials. Antimicrob Agents Chemother 7:316, 1975.

23. Welling PG, Craig WA: Pharmacokinetics in disease states modifying renal function. In Benet LZ (ed): The Effect of Disease States on Drug Pharmacokinetics. Chap 10, p 155. Washington DC, American Pharmaceutical Association, 1976.

24. Wilkinson GR: Influences of liver disease on pharmacokinetics. In Evans WE, Schentag JJ, Jusko WJ (eds): Applied Pharmacokinetics: Principles of Therapeutic Drug Monitoring. Chapter 4, p 57. San Francisco, Applied Therapeutics, Inc., 1980.

25. Williams RL, Mamelock RD: Hepatic disease and drug pharmacokinetics. Clin Pharmacokinet 5:528, 1980.

26. Yakatan GJ, Smith RB, Leff RD, Kay JL: Pharmacokinetic considerations in exchange transfusion in neonates. Clin Pharmacol Ther 24:90, 1978.

27. Zenk KE, Anderson S: Improving the accuracy of mini-volume injections. Infusion, 7, Jan/Feb 1982.

SECTION TWO
DRUGS

FOUR

Antimicrobial Agents

The utilization of antimicrobial agents in neonates has increased tremendously because of accumulated investigative experience in neonates for a greater number of drugs and an improved clinical sophistication in diagnosis of neonatal infection. An estimated 5% of all newborn infants receive antimicrobial agents in the first few days of life; of these, almost all receive two drugs, a penicillin and an aminoglycoside.[88] In newborn intensive care units the frequency of antimicrobial drug exposure is much higher, approaching 50%.[4] There is, however, an element of frustration in neonatal infectious disease management resulting from the constant state of change in organism sensitivity and the inherent difficulties in critically evaluating drug therapy in neonates for both efficacy and toxicity. This chapter presents basic and clinical information on the more commonly employed antimicrobial drugs for the treatment of neonatal infection.

CONSIDERATIONS IN SELECTING THE THERAPEUTIC REGIMEN

Antimicrobial agents are drugs that kill microorganisms or inhibit their growth; this group of drugs includes the antibacterial agents, antifungal agents, and antiviral agents. Antibacterial agents may be **bacteriostatic** (inhibiting), **bactericidal** (destroying), or both (likewise, antifungal agents may be fungistatic or fungicidal, and so on). An important class of antibacterials is the **antibiotics** (e.g., penicillin), which are biochemical substances produced by various species of microorganisms; all other antimicrobials are chemicals not derived from microorganisms (e.g., sulfa drugs, isoniazid).

Classification schemes for the antimicrobial agents are based either on mechanism of action or on chemical structure. The mechanisms of action for antimicrobials that have been identi-

fied are listed in Table 4–1. A more detailed description of mechanisms of action is presented in the discussions of specific agents.

The determining factor in successful employment of any antimicrobial agent is the achievement of sufficient concentration of drug to inhibit or kill the pathogenic organism. Obviously, this concentration must be below that toxic to human cells. If host defense mechanisms (e.g., white blood cells or immune mechanisms) are intact, then the concentration of antimicrobial required may be substantially less (bacteriostatic) than that required in a compromised host, where bactericidal concentrations may be required. If the concentration of drug required to inhibit or kill the organism is greater than the concentration of drug that can be safely achieved with respect to the host, the microorganism must be considered resistant to this drug.

There are a number of factors that have an impact upon the susceptibility of any given organism to a drug. First, the antimicrobial agent must reach the locus of the microorganism. Many microorganisms involved in neonatal infections are able to survive or even replicate in phagocytic cells of the reticuloendothelial system. Because of the decreased microbicidal activity of phagocytes in the newborn, intracellular activity of antimicrobial agents may be of great importance. Rifampin, chloramphenicol, and trimethoprim are the most active drugs intracellularly. Other antimicrobial drugs either are taken up by cells but appear to be inactive intracellularly (lincomycin) or are excluded from cells (penicillins, cephalosporins, aminoglycosides). This aspect of tissue distribution has been reviewed in detail by Wilson and colleagues.[232] Local factors such as pus and other binding substances like hemoglobin, which can bind penicillins and tetracyclines,[43] can reduce the effective concentration of antimicrobials. The pH of the local environment can signifi-

Table 4–1. MECHANISMS OF ACTION FOR
ANTIMICROBIAL AGENTS

Effect on Microbial Cells	Representative Drug(s)
inhibition of cell wall synthesis or activation of host enzymes that disrupt cell walls to cause loss of viability	penicillins, cephalosporins, vancomycin
increase in cell membrane permeability, resulting in loss of intracellular constituents	amphotericin B
altered function of ribosomes, causing disruption of protein synthesis (reversible inhibition)	chloramphenicol, tetracyclines, erythromycin, lincomycin, clindamycin
binding of drug to ribosomes, causing misreading of mRNA code and production of abnormal polypeptides	aminoglycosides
disruption of nucleic acid metabolism	rifampin, metronidazole
blocking of essential metabolism events critical to microorganism (antimetabolites)	trimethoprim, sulfonamides, metronidazole

cantly affect antimicrobial activity: In low (acid) pH, a marked loss in activity occurs with the aminoglycosides, macrolides, and lincomycin, while the activity of other drugs may be enhanced. The anaerobic conditions found in the relatively avascular anaerobic environment of abscesses may impede the activity of the aminoglycosides.[224]

As previously mentioned, the contribution of host defense mechanisms to the outcome of any antimicrobial regimen can be immense. The rate of bacterial killing with many antimicrobial agents is further dependent on the number of bacteria present versus the concentration of drug in tissue — that is, **tissue concentration.** Major factors influencing the antimicrobial tissue concentration that have been identified include drug serum protein binding; binding of drug at the tissue site; delays in drug penetration due to membranes; transport systems that control drug tissue penetration; blood flow to the tissue site; and the effects of disease on penetration both to site of action and to local binding sites.

Tissue concentration is particularly important in treatment of infections of the central nervous system (CNS). In order for a drug to be effective in such infections, it must be able to penetrate the blood–brain barrier. The integ-

rity of the blood–brain barrier is diminished during the more acute active phase of the illness, but as the infection is eradicated and the inflammatory reaction subsides, drug penetration reverts toward normal (lessens). Therefore, drug dosage should not be reduced as the patient improves, and the drug should certainly not be discontinued until the cerebrospinal fluid (CSF) is proved to be sterile. The ratio of plasma to CSF drug concentration or percentage of plasma drug concentration in the CSF is often considered indicative of the potential value of the drug in treating CNS infections. Such ratios or percentages can be very misleading, however, since the major determinant of effect is the actual drug concentration values, not percentage or ratio. A drug with low percentage in the CSF (i.e., low ratio of CSF to plasma values) may in fact be more effective than a second drug with a high percentage in the CSF (i.e., high ratio of CSF to plasma values), because the actual CSF concentration reached with the former drug may in fact be higher. Attempts to circumvent the blood–brain barrier by intrathecal or intraventricular administration have drawn mixed reactions and results.[121,141,144] There are technical difficulties in entering the lateral ventricles, which may be very small in the early stages of CNS infection subsequent to cerebral swelling. Other problems include poor diffusion of drug throughout the CNS from the site of intrathecal injection due to undirectional flow of CSF; density of the injected solution; and presence of purulent and sometimes loculated exudate characteristic of neonatal meningitis.

Even with ideal tissue concentrations there may be therapeutic failures because of the presence or development of **resistance** on the part of the microorganism. Antibacterial resistance may exist because the drug cannot reach the site of action on or within the bacteria for any of several reasons. For example, some microorganisms possess enzymes at or within the cell surface that inactivate the drug before it ever reaches its site of action. The influx of drug into the microorganism can also be impeded by a lack of a transport system(s) required for entrance, by lack of optimal pH for passage of the drug through the cell membrane, or because of a structural (membrane)-based impermeability to the drug.

Bacteria can develop resistance to antimicrobial drugs by chromosomal mutation, recombination, or acquisition of plasmids.[82] Mutation-based antimicrobial resistance is not directly induced by the drug; it occurs spontaneously.

The antimicrobial agent inhibits the nonmutants, permitting (selecting for) growth of the surviving mutants. The mechanisms responsible for mutational resistance are shown in Table 4–2. Plasmids are extrachromosomal DNA elements of bacteria and include R factors. The mechanisms for plasmid-mediated resistance, which are the most common determinants of drug resistance in bacteria, are also listed in Table 4–2.

The process of selecting the ideal or optimal antimicrobial therapeutic regimen is a complex procedure that requires sound clinical judgment and detailed knowledge of pharmacologic and microbiologic factors. The goal should always be to choose the drug that is most effective and selective for the infecting microorganism. At the same time, consideration must be given to those clinical and pharmacologic factors that relate to the potential for adverse reactions. Antimicrobial agents all have the potential to produce toxicity either directly or secondarily (e.g., by selecting for highly resistant bacteria). The identification of the involved pathogens on the basis of clinical experience or microbiologic techniques is a critical step in the selection process, allowing a rational choice of one or more antimicrobials for possible use.[47] Table 4–3 is a general summary of the antimicrobial spectrum of drugs with neonatal experience. It is imperative that such tabulated information *not* be used as the definitive and final selection step; invariably there are other factors worthy of consideration that must not be ignored.

Subsequent testing of microbial sensitivity by the Kirby-Bauer or disk diffusion technique[13] or by serial dilutions of antimicrobials in solid agar or broth media containing appropriate microorganisms can be very helpful. From these procedures the lowest concentration of antimicrobial that prevents visible growth after 18 to 24 hours of incubation, known as the **minimum inhibitory concentration (MIC),** can be determined. The lowest antimicrobial concentration that results in a 99.9% or greater decline in bacterial number is known as the **minimum bactericidal concentration (MBC).** The MIC and MBC values can be very useful when employed in conjunction with information on drug concentration in serum or plasma. Favorable consideration can be given to a drug with actual or anticipated serum levels that are significantly greater than the MIC; conversely, a drug with an MIC that approaches a blood level concentration associated with toxicity should be avoided.

Among the final criteria for selection of the ideal antimicrobial agent are the clinical findings and complications that might affect the pharmacokinetics and pharmacodynamics of the drugs under consideration. Variability in pharmacokinetic parameters associated with the disposition of antibiotics in neonates is as great as with any drug category. Among the factors contributing to this variability are gestational and postnatal age, weight, and disease state. Dysfunction of virtually any major organ, particularly the kidneys[20,97] but also the liver,[124] can affect antibiotic disposition, and multiple organ failure may further increase the range of the variability. Table 4–4 summarizes the literature with respect to the potential influence of renal or hepatic failure on antibiotic dosage requirements. (See Chap. 3 for details of managing dosage programs in patients with evi-

Table 4–2. MECHANISMS RESPONSIBLE FOR RESISTANCE TO ANTIMICROBIAL DRUGS

Mechanism	Antimicrobial
Mutational Resistance	
increased production of antimicrobial-inactivating enzyme otherwise present in low concentrations (beta-lactamases)	ampicillin, cefamandole
permeability alteration	penicillin, chloramphenicol, tetracycline, streptomycin, aminoglycosides
target site alteration: block of attachment to ribosomal unit	streptomycin, erythromycin
Plasmid-mediated Resistance	
increased production of beta-lactamase	penicillins, cephalosporins, methicillin
intrinsic; possibly altered drug transport	methicillin
O-nucleotidylation, O-phosphorylation, O-acetylation	aminoglycosides
alteration of cell membrane transport	tetracycline
increased production of acetyltransferase	chloramphenicol
production of resistant dehydropteroate synthetase	sulfonamide
production of resistant dihydrofolate reductase	trimethoprim
enzymatic methylation of ribosomal RNA: blocks binding	erythromycin, lincomycin

Adapted from Grieco MH: Med Clin North Am 66:25, 1981.

Table 4-3. ANTIMICROBIAL SPECTRUM OF DRUGS EMPLOYED IN NEONATES[a]

Drug	Cocci (+)	Cocci (−)	Microorganisms Bacilli (+)	Bacilli (−)	Other Organisms (+)
aminoglycosides				E. coli; Enterobacteriaceae, Proteus, spp., Serratia, Acinetobacter, Pseudomonas spp.	
cephalosporins	S. aureus, streptococci	Neisseria spp.	L. monocytogenes	Enterobacteriaceae, Klebsiella spp., E. coli, Proteus spp., H. influenzae, Acinetobacter	
penicillin	S. aureus, streptococci	Neisseria spp.	Clostridium spp., Corynebacterium diphtheriae		Treponema, Actinomyces, Leptospira
ampicillin	streptococci	Neisseria spp.	L. monocytogenes	E. coli, Proteus mirabilis, Salmonella, Shigella, H. influenzae, Bordetella spp.	
carbenicillin, ticarcillin, piperacillin				Pseudomonas and Proteus spp., Enterobacteriaceae	
methicillin and nafcillin	S. aureus				
chloramphenicol	streptococci (CNS)	N. meningitidis	L. monocytogenes, Clostridium	H. influenzae, Bacteroides spp., Salmonella, Campylobacter fetus	Rickettsia
clindamycin				Bacteroides spp., Fusobacterium fusiforme	
erythromycin	S. aureus	N. gonorrhoeae	C. diphtheriae, L. monocytogenes	Flavobacterium, Bordetella spp.	Mycoplasma pneumoniae, Chlamydia spp.
isoniazid					M. tuberculosis
metronidazole				Bacteroides spp.	Trichomonas vaginalis
rifampin	S. aureus	N. meningitidis (carrier)	Flavobacterium	M. tuberculosis	
tetracyclines		N. gonorrhoeae	Clostridium spp.	Hemophilus ducreyi, Brucella, Pseudomonas spp., Vibrio cholerae	Treponema spp., M. pneumoniae, Rickettsia, Chlamydia spp.
vancomycin	S. aureus	Clostridium difficile			
nystatin, amphotericin, flucytosine, ketoconazole, miconazole					Candida albicans, Cryptococcus, Aspergillus, Histoplasma

[a] Data compiled from numerous sources in the literature (see References at end of chapter). This table is meant only as a general outline of the spectrum of microorganisms potentially susceptible to the various drugs listed; the drug of choice cannot be ascertained solely from these data as the order of choice must be based on additional considerations as discussed in the text.

Table 4-4. ANTIMICROBIALS THAT MAY REQUIRE DOSAGE ADJUSTMENT IN NEONATES WITH SIGNIFICANT KIDNEY OR LIVER DYSFUNCTION

Drugs	Metabolized	Major Route of Excretion: Kidney (K) or Liver (L)	Recommended Dosage Change: Dose (D) or Interval (I)	Normal Dosing Interval or Dose	Dosage Adjustment Recommendation[a]		Organ Failure[b]
					50-10% Normal Function	<10% Normal Function	
Aminoglyco-sides			(monitor serum levels)				
amikacin	no	K	I	8-12 hr	24 hr	24-48 hr	kidney
gentamicin	no	K	I	8-12 hr	12-24 hr	24-48 hr	kidney
kanamycin	no	K	I	8-12 hr	24-48 hr	>48 hr	kidney
tobramycin	no	K	I	8-12 hr	12-24 hr	24-48 hr	kidney
Cephalosporins[c]							
cefazolin	no	K	I	8-12 hr	16-24 hr	24-96 hr	kidney
cephalothin	yes (small %)	K	I	6-8 hr	none	12-24 hr	kidney
cefotaxime	yes	K	I	8-12 hr	16-24 hr	24-36 hr	kidney
moxalactam	no	K	I	12 hr	12-24 hr	24-48 hr	kidney
cefoperazone	no	L (K)	none	12 hr	none	none	kidney
Penicillins[d]							
ampicillin	yes (small %)	K (L)	I	6-8 hr	8-12 hr	12-16 hr	kidney
carbenicillin	yes (small %)	K (L)	I	6-8 hr	12-18 hr	18-24 hr	kidney
methicillin	yes (small %)	K (L)	I	8-12 hr	12-16 hr	16-24 hr	kidney
nafcillin	yes	L (K)	I	12 hr	12-18 hr	24 hr	liver
penicillin	yes (small %)	K (L)	I	8-12 hr	none	12-18 hr	kidney
piperacillin	yes (<10 %)	K (L)	I	4-6 hr	none	8-12 hr	kidney/liver
ticarcillin	yes (small %)	K	I	6-8 hr	12-18 hr	18-24 hr	kidney
Other Agents							
chloramphenicol	yes (large %)	L (K)	(monitor serum levels D (I))	5 mg/kg	½-¾ dose	<½ dose	liver
clindamycin	yes (large %)	L (K)	D	10 mg/kg	none	½ dose	liver
erythromycin	yes •	L (K)	D	20 mg/kg	none	½ dose	liver
isoniazid	yes (large %)	L (K)	D	10 mg/kg	none	½ dose	liver
metronidazole	yes	L (K)	I	12 hr	none	23 hr	liver
rifampin	yes (large %)	L	D	10 mg/kg	none	½ dose	liver
tetracycline	yes	K	avoid	—	—	—	kidney
vancomycin	no	K	I	8-12 hr	40-120 hr	120-240 hr	kidney

[a] The extent of liver or kidney dysfunction necessary before dosage adjustment is required varies with the different drugs and will likely be influenced by other considerations such as extent of clinical illness (host factors) and infecting organism (MIC, MBC). The maintenance dosage adjustment for 50-100% or <10% normal organ function represents the need to increase the interval of administration (reduced frequency) or decrease the dose, although both may be necessary. The initial (loading) dose usually is the same regardless of the status of liver or kidney function. Serum drug levels should be monitored whenever possible for optimal therapy.

[b] Kidney = dosage alteration necessary with kidney dysfunction; liver = dosage alteration necessary with liver dysfunction.

[c] The only cephalosporin not requiring dosage adjustment with renal dysfunction is cefoperazone. Cefotaxime is only moderately affected compared with moxalactam.

[d] Penicillins not requiring dosage adjustment with renal dysfunction include nafcillin and oxacillin. In patients with combined hepatic and renal failure, dosage adjustment may be necessary with many penicillins, although there is a wide margin of safety with most.

Adapted from Bennett WM et al: Ann Intern Med 93:62, 1980; Jackson EA, McLeod DC: Am J Hosp Pharm 31:137, 1974; Kunin CM: Ann Intern Med 67:151, 1967; Lesar TS, Zaske DE: Med Clin North Am 66:257, 1982; and Whelton A: Med Clin North Am 66:267, 1982.

dence of organ failure.) In general, the major impact of renal or hepatic failure, besides that on drug selection, is on maintenance dosage rather than modification of the initial dose.

Usual dosages of antimicrobial agents are shown in Table 4-5. (Special dosing considerations are discussed under specific agents.) Although shortening of dosing interval in infants older than 1 week of age is recommended for drugs eliminated by renal mechanisms, it is critical to appreciate that the time of renal maturation is not absolute in all neonates. Further-

Table 4-5. RECOMMENDED ANTIBACTERIAL DOSAGE SCHEDULES FOR NEONATES[a]

Drug	Dosage	Serum Drug Level Monitoring: Essential = E Recommended = R)
amikacin	7.5 mg/kg q 12 hr, IV or IM (need to increase interval to q 18–24 hr if $T\frac{1}{2} > 8$ hr or decrease interval to q 8 hr if $T\frac{1}{2} < 4$ hr	E
ampicillin		
meningitis	50 mg/kg q 8–12 hr, IV (q 6 hr > 1 week of age)	R
other indications	25 mg/kg q 8–12 hr, IV or IM (q 6–8 hr > 1 wk of age)	
carbenicillin	100 mg/kg IV initially, then 75 mg/kg q 6–8 hr (100 mg/kg IV q 6 hr > 1 week of age)	R
cephalosporins		
cephalothin	20 mg/kg q 6–8 hr IV or IM	
cefazoline	20 mg/kg q 8–12 hr IV or IM	
cefoperazone	50 mg/kg q 12 hr IV	
cefotaxime	50 mg/kg q 12 hr IV (q 8 hr > 1 week of age)	
moxalactam	100 mg/kg IV loading dose, then 50 mg/kg q 12 hr IV (q 8 hr > 2 months of age)	
chloramphenicol	20 mg/kg PO or IV initially, then 5 mg/kg PO or IV q 6 hr (start maintenance dose 12 hr after loading dose). Maintenance dose requirements may vary from 2.5 up to 12.5 mg/kg PO or IV q 6 hr	E
clindamycin	10 mg/kg IV q 8 hr	
erythromycin	20 mg/kg q 12 hr PO	
gentamicin	2.5 mg/kg q 12 hr IV or IM (need to increase interval to q 18–24 hr if $T\frac{1}{2} > 8$ hr or decrease interval to q 8 hr if $T\frac{1}{2} < 4$ hr)	E
isoniazid	10 mg/kg PO q day	R
kanamycin	7.5 mg/kg q 12 hr IV or IM (need to increase interval to q 18–24 hr if $T\frac{1}{2} > 8$ hr or decrease interval to q 8 hr if $T\frac{1}{2} < 4$ hr)	E
methicillin		
meningitis	50 mg/kg q 8 hr IV	R
other indications	25 mg/kg q 8–12 hr IV or IM (q 6–8 hr > 1 week of age)	
metronidazole	15 mg/kg IV loading dose, then 7.5 mg/kg IV q 12 hr	R (meningitis)
nafcillin		
meningitis	50 mg/kg q 8 hr IV	R
other indications	20 mg/kg q 8 hr IV or IM	
netilmicin	2–3 mg/kg IV q 12 hr	
oxacillin	25 mg/kg q 12 hr IV or IM (q 6–8 hr > 1 week of age)	
penicillins		
penicillin G		
meningitis	75,000 U/kg q 8 hr IV (q 6 hr > 1 week of age)	R
sepsis	25,000–50,000 U/kg q 12 hr IV or IM (q 8 hr > 1 week of age)	
benzathine	50,000 U/kg one dose	
procaine	50,000 U/kg q 24 hr	
piperacillin	50 mg/kg IV q 4–6 hr	R
rifampin	10 mg/kg PO q 12 hr	
ticarcillin	100 mg/kg IV initially, then 75 mg/kg q 6–8 hr (100 mg/kg q 6 hr > 1 week of age)	R
tobramycin	2.5 mg/kg q 12 hr IV or IM (need to increase interval to q 18–24 hr if $T\frac{1}{2} > 8$ hr or decrease interval to q 8 hr if $T\frac{1}{2} < 4$ hr)	E
trimethoprim-sulfamethoxazole	loading dose: trimethoprim 3 mg/kg IV sulfamethoxazole 10 mg/kg IV maintenance dose trimethoprim 1 mg/kg IV q 12 hr sulfamethoxazole 3 mg/kg IV q 12 hr	R
vancomycin	15 mg/kg q 12 hr IV (q 8 hr > 1 week of age)	

[a] These data represent usual starting and maintenance doses for full-term infants. With seriously compromised infants or low-birth-weight premature infants (<2 kg), reduction in dosage may be necessary. Usually an increase in *interval* of administration is warranted rather than lowering of individual dose, although both may be necessary in some neonates (see under specific agents and Chap. 3). Monitoring of serum drug levels will assist in optimizing dosage adjustments, particularly with changing organ function as the newborn matures or recovers from the initial illness.

more, preceding or coexisting serious illness can have a significant impact on intrinsic maturational events as well as on drug disposition. *Thus, in seriously ill neonates, clinical status may be of greater importance than chronologic age in ascertaining optimal dosage requirements.*

The recommended dose and interval of administration for the various antimicrobials (Table 4–5) have frequently been derived by combining in vitro activity of a drug against a variety of microorganisms with the achievable concentrations of drug in blood (or urine). The major dose-limiting factors include frequency of administration necessary to maintain drug concentration above MIC, risk of toxicity, and cost of the drug. Despite the atmosphere of legitimacy surrounding published dosage recommendations for antimicrobial agents, the ideal dosage regimen has probably not been sufficiently examined for most antimicrobial drugs. For example, the major determinant of effectiveness (for a particular microorganism) could be high concentrations achieved briefly one or more times daily for one drug but sustained lower levels attained with constant infusion for another. Kunin[117] has thoroughly reviewed many of the issues involved in dosage schedule determinations. Basically, intermittent dosage schedules are routinely employed primarily because of the belief that there is greater penetration of drug into target tissues, convenience of administration, and better compliance. The magnitude of the intermittent dose is determined by toxicity and expense. The duration of antimicrobial therapy necessary for optimal response is another therapeutic topic for debate.

It is critical to appreciate that each individual dose will largely determine the peak tissue concentrations developed, and that interval of administration will determine how many times throughout the course of treatment this peak concentration occurs. Unfortunately, antimicrobial dosages can be found in the literature as total daily dosage with the indication that this dose should be divided 2, 3, or 4 times. Obviously, if the same total dose is divided by 2 versus 4, there will be large differences in the resulting individual dose, and consequently in the resulting peak concentration. Even more confusing is the recommendation of a range of daily doses along with a range of dosing intervals. It is, therefore, advantageous and prudent to list dosages on an individual dose basis along with the recommended interval of administration; this also eliminates confusion and possible errors in calculations since the division step is eliminated.[175] If toxic peak levels develop, the dose should be reduced (assuming that the toxic peak level was not due to accumulation of drug as a consequence of too short a dosing interval). If the serum drug clearance is diminished (prolonged $T\frac{1}{2}$), then the interval of administration should be increased to preclude accumulation of toxic amounts of drug (see Chaps. 1 through 3 for further discussion of these pharmacokinetic principles).

ANTIBACTERIAL AGENTS

PENICILLINS AND THEIR DERIVATIVES

Pharmacology. Penicillins have been the most widely employed and useful antibiotics since the fortuitous discovery of penicillin in 1928. The basic structures of the various penicillins are shown in Table 4–6. The penicillin nucleus itself is the chief structural requirement for biologic activity. The side chain (R) determines the major pharmacologic and antibacterial features of the various penicillins. The basic mechanism of action of the penicillins involves interruption of certain of the complex enzymatic events associated with bacterial cell wall synthesis, although all the details remain incomplete.[174] Resistance to the penicillins can exist because of structural differences in the enzymes involved in bacterial cell wall synthesis that make them immune to the penicillins, or because the penicillin is unable to penetrate the bacterial cell wall sufficiently to reach the otherwise vulnerable enzyme system (e.g., gram-negative bacteria have a relatively complex cell wall with an outer protective membrane, lipopolysaccharide, and capsule). Resistance can also exist because of enzymatic destruction of the beta-lactam ring by penicillinases (see Table 4–6). The penicillins differ in their susceptibil-

Table 4-6. STRUCTURAL AND PHARMACOLOGIC PROPERTIES OF THE PENICILLINS

basic structure

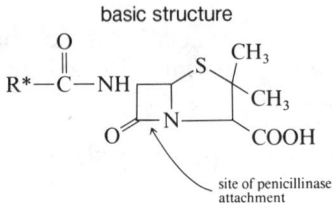

site of penicillinase attachment

Drug	R*—Group	Resistance to Penicillinase
penicillin G	—CH$_2$—	no
penicillin V	—OCH$_2$—	no
ampicillin	—CH— NH$_2$	no
amoxicillin	HO— —CH— NH$_2$	no
methicillin	(OCH$_3$, OCH$_3$)	yes
oxacillin	N—O—CH$_3$	yes
nafcillin	OC$_2$H$_5$	yes
carbenicillin	—CH— COOH	no
ticarcillin	—CH— COO— —CH$_3$	no
piperacillin	—CH— NHCO NHCO	no

ity to the beta-lactamases (penicillinases), depending on the capability of the molecular side chain to interfere with the penicillinase enzyme activity. The density of bacteria and the duration of an infection can also influence the activity of the penicillins. Rapidly multiplying bacteria (in a recently developed infection) are generally more susceptible to penicillin antimicrobial action than are older, less rapidly multiplying bacteria. Protein and pus do not appreciably decrease the bactericidal activity of penicillins, and they are active with low pH and oxygen tension. However, penetration of penicillins into areas of purulent exudate is generally poor; higher-than-normal tissue and plasma drug concentrations are required in order to maintain therapeutic effectiveness.

Clinical Toxicology. Penicillins are very well tolerated by infants, although as a group penicillins account for a significant percentage of all drug-induced allergic reactions reported in children and adults. There is no good evidence that any one of the penicillin derivatives possesses a greater or lesser potential for causing an allergic reaction. Clinical manifestations of penicillin allergy include (in order of decreasing frequency) maculopapular rash, urticarial rash, fever, bronchospasm, vasculitis, serum sickness, exfoliative dermatitis, Stevens-Johnson syndrome, and anaphylaxis.[194] No data have been reported on the overall incidence of these reactions in infants, but for adults it ranges from 0.7% to 10%.[66] Hypersensitivity reactions can occur with any dose or dosage form of penicillin. Cross-sensitivity between penicillins is to be expected. On the other hand, untoward reactions may not necessarily occur with subsequent courses of penicillin therapy.

The most important contributor to the allergic reaction is the breakdown product of penicillin resulting from cleavage of the beta-lactam ring. This moiety acts as a hapten along with penicillin and other penicillin breakdown products by combining with proteins, with subsequent initiation of antibody formation.

Other toxic reactions associated with the penicillins are rare but include bone-marrow depression, granulocytopenia, and hepatitis. Local reactions at the site of administration are not uncommon. Tragic demise of the sciatic nerve has been associated with accidental injection of penicillins into the nerve. Significant CNS toxicity (lethargy, twitching, multifocal myoclonus, or localized or generalized seizure activity) has been associated with levels of penicillin in the CSF greater than 10 μg/ml in adults.

Penicillin G

Clinical Pharmacology. The absorption of an oral dose of penicillin G is better in newborn infants than in older infants and children, in whom gastric juice at pH 2 or less destroys the antibiotic. Absorption is mainly in the duodenum and is complete within 30 to 60 minutes. Studies in premature and full-term neonates revealed serum penicillin concentrations of $1-2$ µg/ml 1/2 to 1 hour after administration of approximately 20,000 IU/kg PO of penicillin G.[94,125] Because only about one third of the oral dose is actually absorbed, this route should be reserved for older infants and children where clinical experience has shown it to be effective in specific infections. Penicillin V has as its sole virtue greater stability than penicillin G in acid environments (greater absorption after oral administration). With parenteral administration of penicillin G (IM, SQ, or IV), the magnitude and duration of drug concentrations in plasma will be determined by many factors, including dose, rate of infusion (IV) or absorption from injection site (IM or SQ), and renal function. The serum half-life ($T\frac{1}{2}$) for penicillin in neonates is inversely related to creatinine clearance rate[137] and ranges between 1 and 2.5 hours (Fig. 4–1). The peak serum levels range between 10 and 25 µg/ml with doses around 20,000 IU/kg IM and 35–40 µg/ml with doses of 50,000 IU/kg. Using an average dose of 330,000 IU/kg of penicillin G, Grossman and Ticknor observed mean serum levels of 140 µg/ml 2 to 4 hours after IM injection in neonates.[84]

Procaine and benzathine penicillin G are repository preparations that release penicillin G slowly from the area injected (IM) and thereby produce relatively low but persistent concentrations of antibiotic in the serum. Procaine penicillin G 50,000 IU/kg IM produces a mean serum level of 7 to 8 µg/ml for 12 hours and 1.5 µg/ml at 24 hours in neonates less than 1 week of age.[137] In older neonates the 24-hour level is less (0.4 µg/ml). Benzathine penicillin G, 50,000 IU/kg IM, results in serum values of between 0.4 and 2.6 µg/ml 12 to 24 hours following administration to newborn infants; after 12 days serum levels range between 0.07 and 0.09 µg/ml.

Penicillin G is widely distributed throughout the body, although there are large differences in the concentrations developed in various fluids and tissues. Significant concentrations can be found in liver, bile, joint fluid, lymph, kidney, and urine. Levels of penicillin in CSF are considerably lower than in plasma because of poor

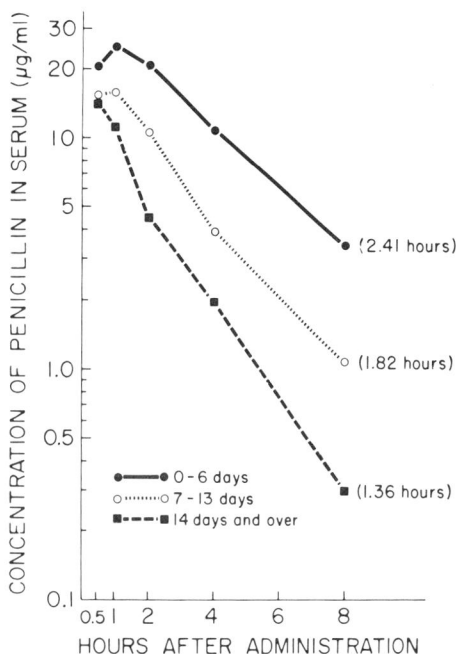

Figure 4 – 1. Serum dose–response curves in neonates given 16,650 IU/kg IM of penicillin G at various ages. Serum half-life values are given in parentheses. (From McCracken GH Jr et al: J Pediatr 82:692, 1973.)

penetration of the blood–brain barrier, and because penicillin is rapidly secreted from the CSF into the blood by an active transport process.[209] With severe renal failure, other organic acids can accumulate in the CSF and compete with penicillin for these same transport systems, causing greatly elevated CSF concentrations of penicillin and leading to toxic concentrations in the brain and possibly convulsions.[210] In neonates with meningitis, peak CSF levels of penicillin range between 0.5 and 2 µg/ml with doses of 50,000 IU/kg.[140]

Excretion of 60% to 90% of an IM dose of penicillin G occurs via the urine within a few hours of administration. Approximately 10% is eliminated by glomerular filtration and 90% by tubular secretion. When renal function is impaired sufficiently to cause a significant prolongation in the half-life, some of the penicillin may be metabolized by the liver (< 10%). This, along with biliary excretion, can explain why excessive accumulation of penicillin does not generally occur with renal failure. If hepatic and renal dysfunction coexist, some adjustment in dosage interval will be necessary (Table 4–4).

Therapeutic Indications. Penicillin G is highly effective against many but not all gram-positive and gram-negative cocci. It is considered satisfactory therapy for susceptible pneumococci, streptococci, and staphylococci. Infants with group B streptococcal infections should receive greater than standard doses (meningitis: 100,000 IU/kg IV every 8 hours; sepsis: 50,000 IU/kg IV every 8 hr) to prevent relapse and to encourage rapid eradication of the organisms from the CSF. Pencillin prophylaxis for early-onset group B streptococcal disease in newborns has not been shown to be efficacious.[279]

Benzathine penicillin G (50,000 IU/kg IM once) or procaine penicillin G (50,000 IU/kg/day IM for 10 days) is effective for asymptomatic (no CNS involvement) congenital syphilis. In syphilis with CNS involvement, procaine penicillin G (50,000 IU/kg/day IM for 14 to 21 days) or penicillin G (25,000 IU/kg IM q 12 hr for 14 to 21 days) is recommended. Other infectious conditions for which standard doses of penicillin G are recommended (Table 4–5) are listed in Table 4–7.

Ampicillin

Clinical Pharmacology. Ampicillin is considered to have a broader spectrum of antimicrobial activity than that of penicillin. It is bactericidal for both gram-positive and gram-negative bacteria. It is acid-stable and well absorbed after oral administration. Doses of 5 to 25 mg/kg IM produce peak serum levels of 16 to 60 μg/ml.[9,25,51] In studies conducted by Kaplan and colleagues,[102] doses of 50 to 100 mg/kg IM produced a wide range of peak serum levels in premature and full-term neonates, with the levels in prematures being higher than those in the full-term infants given equivalent doses (Fig. 4–2 and Table 4–8). The mean peak serum ampicillin concentrations in premature infants after single or multiple doses of 50, 75, or 100 mg/kg IM were 104, 166, and 204 μg/ml, respectively. For full-term neonates the mean peak serum concentrations of ampicillin were 75, 130, and 180 μg/ml for doses of 50, 75, and 100 mg/kg IM. Peak serum levels occur between 1/2 and 2 hours after IM administration.

The half-life of ampicillin in serum is inversely related to postnatal age, probably because renal clearance is a major contributor to ampicillin clearance. In low-dose ampicillin studies by Axline and coworkers,[9] the half-life was 4 hours in infants 2 to 7 days old, 2 to 8 hours in infants 8 to 14 days old and 1.7 hours in infants 15 to 30 days of age. In the higher-dose studies of Kaplan,[102] the mean serum half-life values were 3.1 to 4.7 hours and 4.7 to 6.2

Table 4–7. RECOMMENDED PENICILLINS FOR SELECTED CLINICAL ILLNESSES

Clinical Illness	Recommended Penicillin or Derivative
congenital syphilis tetanus neonatorum gonococcal infection: conjunctivitis, osteomyelitis, septic arthritis sepsis and meningitis: group A or nonenterococcal D streptococcis pulmonary infection: group B streptococcis skin infection: group A streptococcis abscess: group B streptococcis	penicillin G
gastrointestinal infection: *Salmonella* (complicated), necrotizing enterocolitis sepsis and meningitis:[a] initial therapy, group B streptococci, *L. monocytogenes,* and enterococci urinary tract infection: enterococcis	ampicillin
Staphylococcus aureus infection: conjunctivitis, sepsis and meningitis, osteomyelitis, septic arthritis, pulmonary infections, skin infections, abscess (alternative drug: see Vancomycin)	methicillin or nafcillin
Pseudomonas aeruginosa infection: conjunctivitis, peritonitis, sepsis and meningitis, pulmonary infections, urinary tract infections	carbenicillin,[a] ticarcillin,[a] piperacillin[a]

[a] Combined with aminoglycosides.

hours in full-term and premature infants, respectively, at the initiation of therapy; by the end of the 8 days of treatment, the half-life values were shorter: 1.1 to 2.9 and 1.4 to 5.3 hours in full-term and prematures, respectively. The mean serum levels at 12 hours after dosing with 50 to 100 mg/kg ranged from 18 to 57 μg/ml and were significantly less than these values at 7 to 10 days of age.

The peak concentration of ampicillin in CSF appears to occur 3 to 7 hours after IV administration. The CSF concentrations resulting from doses of 40 to 70 mg/kg IV increase from 2.5 μg/ml at 1 hour to 15.2 μg/ml 7 hours after IV administration.[102] The CSF concentrations are

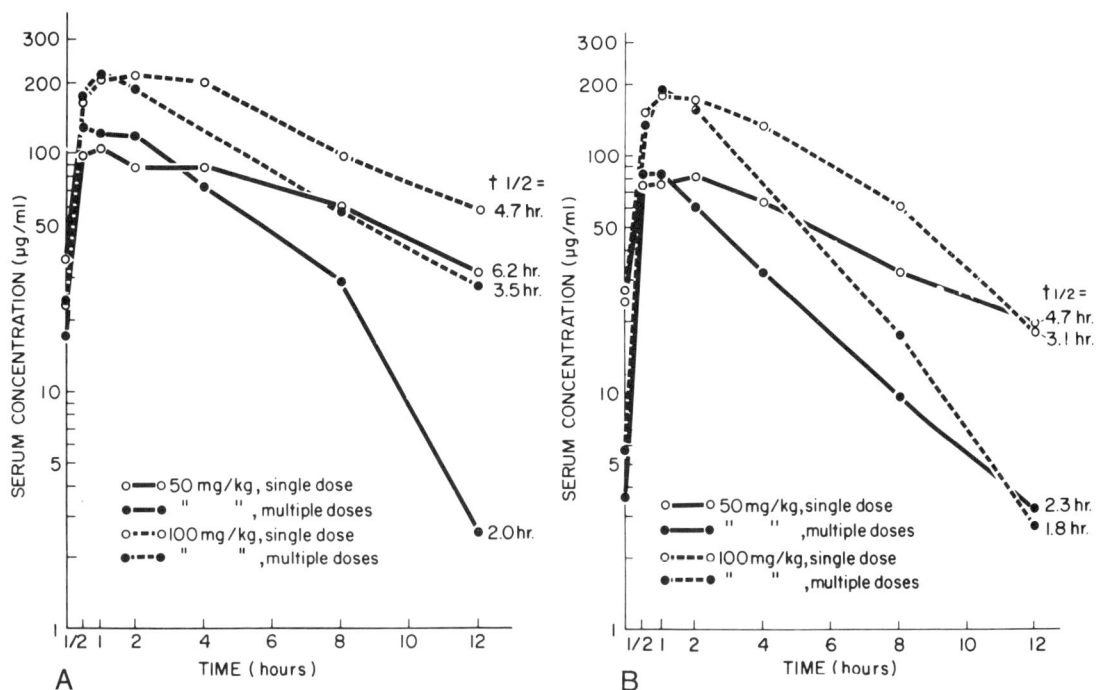

Figure 4-2. Ampicillin serum disappearance curves in full-term (*A*) and premature (*B*) neonates given single or multiple doses of 50 or 100 mg/kg IM. The numbers at the end of each curve represent the *T*½ for that infant. (From Kaplan JM et al: J Pediatr 84:571, 1974.)

tenfold greater than the MIC values for group B streptococci and *Listeria* and are equal to or several-fold greater than the MIC values for most susceptible *Escherichia coli* strains.

Excretion of ampicillin is primarily by renal mechanisms. Anywhere from 20% to 80% of the drug can be found in the urine within 12 hours of administration.[102] The percentage of ampicillin excreted in the urine appears independent of age and dosage but does increase with postnatal age. Severe renal impairment markedly prolongs the persistence of ampicillin in the serum. Because of increased incidence of adverse effects associated with continuing regular doses of ampicillin in adult patients with severe renal insufficiency, some dosage adjustment is indicated in these situations; increasing the interval of administration to once daily with anuria and monitoring serum levels (vs. MIC) is a reasonable approach. Ampicillin is also excreted in the bile and subsequently undergoes enterohepatic circulation.

Therapeutic Indications. The broad-spectrum coverage of ampicillin accounts for its usefulness against group B streptococcis, *Listeria monocytogenes,* and susceptible *E. coli* strains (see Table 4-3). Ampicillin is most often given in combination with an aminogly-

coside, in part because of in vitro evidence for a synergistic effect (see later section, Antimicrobial Combinations). In the treatment of certain infectious processes with ampicillin, particularly meningitis, optimal dose and interval of administration can be assessed by obtaining peak and trough serum and CSF ampicillin levels, which can be compared to the MIC for the involved organism. Peak serum levels of ampicillin of 40 to 80 µg/ml are 600 to 1000 times greater than the highest MIC values for group B streptococci and *Listeria* and 5 to 8 times higher than the MIC values for 90% of *E. coli* strains.[102] Trough serum levels of 2 to 20 µg/ml are 50 to 250 times higher than the MIC values for the gram-positive pathogens and equal to or slightly higher than those for *E coli.* The concentration of ampicillin in urine will typically exceed 1000 µg/ml, which negates any need to monitor urine ampicillin levels. See Table 4-5 for dosage recommendations.

Penicillinase-Resistant Penicillins

The major differentiating feature of the penicillinase-resistant penicillins, that is, methicillin, oxacillin, nafcillin, cloxacillin, and dicloxa-

Table 4–8. SUMMARY OF CLINICAL PHARMACOLOGY STUDIES OF AMPICILLIN, METHICILLIN, OXACILLIN, NAFCILLIN, CARBENICILLIN, AND TICARCILLIN IN NEONATES

Authors of Published Study[a]	Study Group[b]	Dose	Peak Serum Concentration[c] (μg/ml)	Serum Half-life[d] ($T_{\frac{1}{2}}$: hr)
Ampicillin				
Grossman and Ticknor[84]	24 full-term infants 68 full-term infants	5–20 mg/kg IM 5–20 mg/kg PO	16–54 2–32	
Axline et al[9]	35 prematures	10 mg/kg IM	13–19	4.0 (2–7 days old) 2.8 (8–14 days old) 1.7 (15–30 days old)
Boe et al[25]	9 full-term infants	25 mg/kg IM	47–57	2.2–3.4
Silverio and Poole[204]	10 full-term infants	10 mg/kg PO	3–5 (range)	
Kaplan et al[102]	39 neonates: premature and full-term	50–100 mg/kg IM q 8–12 hr, 40–70 mg/kg IV q 8 hr	104–204 (premature) 75–180 (full-term)	4.7–6.2 (premature, day 1) 1.4–5.3 (premature, day 8) 3.1–4.7 (full-term, day 1) 1.1–2.9 (full-term, day 8) 1.6 (1–5 wk old)
Driessen et al[51]	34 neonates: premature and full-term	12.5 mg/kg IM q 6 hr	17–55	1.0–4.1 (3–13 days old)
Methicillin				
Axline et al[9]	24 prematures	20 mg/kg IM	36–42	1.4–2.4 (4–33 days old)
Boe et al[25]	23 prematures 44 full-term infants	25 mg/kg IM	38–52 28–60	1.4–3.3 0.8–3.3
Sarff et al[196]	17 prematures 30 full-term infants	25–50 mg/kg IM	45–80	1.1–3.1 ($V_d = 0.36–0.53$ l/kg)
Oxacillin				
Burns et al[34]	10 prematures	20 mg/kg IM	47–42	1.2–1.6
Axline et al[9]	65 prematures	25–50 mg/kg IM	18–106	(<3)
Nafcillin				
O'Connor et al[166]	27 full-term infants	5–15 mg/kg IM	10–30	
Grossman and Ticknor[84]	17 full-term infants 24 full-term infants	5–20 mg/kg IM 5–20 mg/kg PO	12–37 4–21	
Banner et al[11]	13 prematures	50 mg/kg IV q 12 hr, or 33 mg/kg IV q 8 hr	90–160	1.2–5.5 (mean 3.2) ($V_d = 0.28–0.53$ l/kg; $Cl = 2.2 \pm 0.4$ ml/min/kg)
Yogev et al[237]	14 children: 2 neonates	50 mg/kg IV q 6 hr	13–308 (CSF: 0–10)	2.8–3.5 (neonates)
Carbenicillin				
Nelson and McCracken[162]	55 neonates: premature and full-term	75–100 mg/kg IM q 6–8 hr	117–217	3.4–5.7 (<2 wk old) 1.5–2.2 (2–6 wk old)
Ticarcillin				
Nelson et al[163]	36 neonates: premature and full-term	75–100 mg/kg IM or IV q 4–8 hr	125–189	4.9–5.6 (<1 wk old) 2.2 (1–5 wk old) ($V_d = 0.66–0.76$ l/kg; $Cl = 31–118$ ml/min/1.73 m²)

[a] Listed in order of publication. See References at end of chapter.
[b] Gestational age at birth is given if available.
[c] Peak serum concentration values represent mean values for each of the study groups unless otherwise noted.
[d] The half-life values represent mean values or ranges for each of the study groups unless otherwise noted; V_d = volume of distribution; Cl = clearance.

cillin, is that they are not hydrolyzed by penicillinase-producing strains of *Staphylococcus aureus*. The mechanism for the resistance to penicillinase resides in the molecular hindrance created by the side chains on the moiety attached to the beta-lactam ring (see Table 4–6). Methicillin differs from others in this group in that it is acid-unstable and therefore poorly absorbed from the gastrointestinal tract. There are very few other significant differences in the pharmacology of the various agents or from that discussed for the penicillins. The clinical usefulness of this group of drugs is limited to treatment of staphylococcal disease.

Methicillin

Clinical Pharmacology. Methicillin is not well absorbed by the oral route and is sufficiently destroyed by the acid environment to render oral therapy ineffective. Peak concentrations can be anticipated in serum within 1 to 2 hours after IM administration. The distribution and excretion of methicillin and penicillin G are essentially identical. Methicillin is primarily excreted by the kidney, with approximately 30% to 40% of the dose excreted in the urine during the first 6 hours after administration.[9]

The pharmacokinetic properties of methicillin determined from studies in neonates are shown in Table 4–8. Peak serum levels range from about 25 to 60 μg/ml after an IM dose of 20 to 25 mg/kg in infants including prematures, full-term newborns, and those of up to 1 month postnatal age.[9,25] Peak serum levels of 80 to 120 μg/ml result from a 50-mg/kg IM dose.[140] The serum levels of methicillin do not appear to be greatly different in premature versus full-term infants given equivalent doses. The half-life of methicillin ranges from 0.8 to 3.3 hours in infants from newborns to those 4 weeks of age and is generally prolonged in newborns, particularly prematures (Table 4–8). Sarff and colleagues[196] found the serum half-life of methicillin to range from 2.8 to 3.1 hours in premature infants less than 2 weeks of age and to be 1.1 hours in term infants 3 to 6 weeks of age.

There is very little known about the CSF levels of methicillin in neonates, although concentrations achieved are believed to be below or equal to the MIC of penicillinase-producing staphylococci.[100a,168] In a study by McCullough and coworkers[146] of CSF methicillin levels in 17 infants and children with a ventricular shunt, the drug (25 mg/kg IV or IM q 6 hr) was found in the CSF in only 1 patient (1.2 μg/ml). The mechanism for the development of resistance to

methicillin is not fully understood (see Table 4–2).

Therapeutic Indications. Methicillin has been considered the drug of choice for treatment of infections due to penicillinase-producing (penicillin-resistant) staphylococci in neonates. However, nafcillin has recently been proposed as an alternative drug of choice because of purported lower incidence of renal toxicity and better CSF drug levels (see under Nafcillin). See Table 4–5 for dosage recommendations.

Clinical Toxicology. A number of reports of methicillin-induced interstitial nephritis in adults and children have appeared in the literature, most often associated with larger doses of methicillin (>200 mg/kg per day). The onset generally is after the first week of therapy and is associated with hematuria, albuminuria, and renal cell and other casts in the urine. The reaction is typically reversible.[75] Yow and colleagues[241] reviewed methicillin-associated side-effects in children and found an 8% incidence of hematuria; other side-effects noted were hematologic, rash, and fever. Of all patients receiving the drug, 31.5% had signs of toxicity, although the true incidence rate was estimated to be 1.5% for all side-effects. Sarff and coworkers[196] found hematuria in 3.4% of patients treated with methicillin. A prospective study of adverse effects of methicillin, nafcillin, and oxacillin in pediatric patients (doses ranged from 100 to 150 mg/kg per day) revealed no significant differences in toxicity among the drugs, although the number of patients treated with methicillin showing toxicity was lower (11%) compared to nafcillin (19%) and oxacillin (25%).[158]

Nafcillin

Clinical Pharmacology. Nafcillin is inactivated to a variable degree by the acidic medium of the gastric contents. Its absorption from the gastrointestinal tract is also irregular. Nafcillin differs from the other penicillins in that a smaller percentage of the administered dose is eliminated by renal excretion (8–25%). The major fraction of the administered dose is excreted via hepatic clearance mechanisms; therefore, renal dysfunction does not significantly affect the serum clearance.[49] Infants with hepatic dysfunction obviously require consideration of dosage adjustment or use of an alternative drug (Table 4–4). Widely differing values for percentage of nafcillin bound to serum protein can be found in the literature (50–90%). There is no question regarding the effect of protein on in vitro antimicrobial activity of nafcillin (see Therapeutic Indications further on).[115] In clinical studies in infants and children, a mean serum concentration of nafcillin of 48 μg/ml was observed a half hour after a dose of 37.5 mg/kg IV.[64] Pharmacokinetic studies in premature infants indicated a dose of 20 mg/kg IV given every 8 hours would achieve a mean peak serum concentration of 80 μg/ml and a steady-state nadir of 17 μg/ml.[11] After 5 or 6 doses of 50 mg/kg IV given every 6 hours, peak serum nafcillin levels have been observed to range from 13 to 308 μg/ml.[237] Peak CSF nafcillin levels exceeded 1 μg/ml in patients with CSF glucose levels greater than 40 mg/dl. Patients with ventriculitis appear to attain greater CSF levels of nafcillin, although detectable levels have been found in patients without ventriculitis.[100a] McCullough and colleagues[146] administered nafcillin (25 mg/kg IV or IM q 6 hr) to 20 infants and children with ventricular shunts without infections or ventriculitis; CSF levels of nafcillin ranged from 0 (in 9 patients) to 0.166 μg/ml (in 11 patients). The sampling time ranged from 1/2 to 3 hours after dosing.

Therapeutic Indications. Nafcillin may be considered a drug of choice in neonates who require a penicillinase-resistant penicillin, particularly if there is evidence of renal dysfunction. Controversy over the choice of nafcillin versus methicillin has evolved in part because of the marked effect of proteins on the antimicrobial activity of nafcillin in contrast to methicillin. Kunin[116] compared the MICs of nafcillin and methicillin against staphylococcis in trypticase soy broth and 100% pooled human serum. The MIC for nafcillin was 0.3 ± 0.05 μg/ml in broth but 2.5 ± 0.25 μg/ml in serum, a tenfold difference. Methicillin MIC was no different in broth versus serum (1.5 ± 0.25 μg/ml). Since proteins are present particularly in CSF infections, protein binding is a necessary consideration in evaluating and interpreting the clinical significance of differences in chemically determined levels of methicillin and nafcillin. In one controlled clinical trial in pediatric patients,[109] there was no significant difference in clinical efficacy between nafcillin and methicillin. However, another study demonstrated greater penetration of nafcillin into the CSF compared with methicillin.[146] Ventricular fluid levels of nafcillin exceeded the MIC (median 0.2–0.6 μg/ml) for staphylococcal organisms obtained from a group of hydrocephalic infants and children with meningitis, indicating a potential usefulness for nafcillin in neonates with this illness.[237] See Table 4–5 for dosage recommendations.

Clinical Toxicology. In a prospective, controlled, comparative study of methicillin and nafcillin in 75 infants and children, Kitzing and coworkers[109] found evidence of urologic toxic effects in 5.3% of infants and children receiving methicillin (50 mg/kg IV q 6 hr) but none in those patients treated with nafcillin (37.5 mg/kg IV q 6 hr). These authors concluded that nafcillin is preferable to methicillin for treatment of susceptible gram-positive coccal infections. A number of cases of agranulocytosis or granulocytopenia have been reported with nafcillin use.[80,242]

Oxacillin

Clinical Pharmacology. The basic difference of oxacillin from methicillin resides in its stability in acidic medium and its rapid but incomplete absorption (30–80%) after oral administration. The remainder of its pharmacology, except for significantly greater protein binding, is similar to that of methicillin. Despite good oral bioavailability of the drug, PO administration is not recommended.

Mean peak serum level of oxacillin after 20 mg/kg IM is approximately 50 μg/ml, or 100 μg/ml after a dose of 50 mg/kg IM.[9,34] The mean serum oxacillin half-life values are 1.6 hours in premature infants 1 to 2 weeks of age and 1.2 hours in infants 3 weeks of age. Approximately 15% to 30% of the dose is excreted in the urine within 6 hours of administration.[9] No alteration in dosage is required with renal dysfunction. The incidence of hepatotoxicity appears to be greater with oxacillin than with methicillin or nafcillin.[158]

Therapeutic Indications. There is no therapeutic rationale for using oxacillin rather than nafcillin or methicillin. The oral bioavailability of oxacillin is not sufficient to justify use of this drug or the oral route for treatment of penicillin-resistant staphylococcal disease.

Carbenicillin and Ticarcillin

Pharmacology. Carbenicillin and ticarcillin are penicillinase-susceptible penicillin derivatives (see structure in Table 4–6) useful in serious infections caused by ampicillin-resistant *Pseudomonas* species, *Proteus* strains, and certain other gram-negative microorganisms. The activity of carbenicillin and ticarcillin, like that of the other penicillins, is dependent upon entering the bacterial cell wall, avoiding destruction by beta-lactamases, and binding to penicillin-binding proteins involved in septum formation. Carbenicillin and ticarcillin must be administered parenterally, since they are not absorbed from the gastrointestinal tract. Peak concentrations in serum are reached within 1/2 to 2 hours after IM administration. Maximal serum concentrations are about fourfold greater with the IV route than those with IM administration. The volume of distribution and serum half-life of carbenicillin is essentially identical to ticarcillin and similar to that of the other penicillin derivatives.[300] Tissue concentrations are also similar for the two drugs. Greater than 80% of the dose of carbenicillin or ticarcillin is cleared by the kidneys; the small remaining percentage of the dose, slightly more with ticarcillin, undergoes hepatic metabolism.

Clinical Pharmacology. Peak serum carbenicillin concentrations of 150 to 175 μg/ml result from doses of 100 mg/kg IV.[162] The serum half-life of carbenicillin correlates significantly with postnatal age and creatinine clearance, indicative of excretion of the drug primarily by renal mechanisms. The mean half-life for low-birth-weight neonates ($<$ 2 kg) is 5 to 6 hours, as it is during the first 3 days of life in full-term neonates. By 3 to 4 weeks of age the half-life is betwen 2 to 3 hours in all infants. Levels of carbenicillin in urine are 10- to 50-fold greater than the MIC for *Pseudomonas* and *Proteus* species after a dose of 25 to 50 mg/kg. Studies by Nelson and colleagues[163] with ticarcillin in neonates indicate peak serum levels of 125 to 189 μg/ml after IM doses of 75 to 100 mg/kg. Information published on CSF levels attained with carbenicillin and ticarcillin in adults with meningitis indicates levels of 26 to 172 μg/ml (30–50% of serum level).[165]

Therapeutic Indications. If bacterial infection with ampicillin-resistant *Pseudomonas* or *Proteus* species is proved or strongly suspected, the use of carbenicillin or ticarcillin can be considered.[56] Combination therapy with an aminoglycoside has been frequently employed (see later section, Antimicrobial Combinations). To date, there has not been adequate evidence to indicate that one drug is superior to the other in the treatment of susceptible organisms. Bacterial resistance may appear in vitro during therapy with suboptimal doses. Peak concentrations of 150 to 175 μg/ml should be maintained throughout the duration of therapy. Loading doses of 100 mg/kg IV will establish these therapeutic levels, which can be maintained with 75 mg/kg given every 6 to 8 hours, depending on renal function (i.e., postnatal age). The optimal interval between doses is not known. There should be no difference in dosage between carbenicillin and ticarcillin, because there is no difference in their pharmacokinetics and antibacterial properties. Dosage reductions are indicated with renal dysfunction. With less than 10% renal function, the dosage should be reduced by one third, by increasing the dosage interval to every 18 to 24 hours (Table 4–4). Severe liver dysfunction may also require a reduction in dosage. Monitoring of serum drug levels is indicated in these circumstances.

Clinical Toxicology. Carbenicillin and ticarcillin are capable of producing all of the various side-effects associated with the penicillins. In addition, congestive heart failure may be aggravated by the excessive sodium found in these preparations: Both carbenicillin and ticarcillin are disodium salts containing 4.7 and 5.2 mEq of sodium per gram of drug, respectively. Hypokalemia may also occur because of the obligatory excretion of cation with the large amount of nonreabsorbable anion (carbenicillin or ticarcillin) presented to the distal renal tubule.[38] Carbenicillin and ticarcillin also interfere with platelet function; bleeding may develop secondary to abnormal platelet aggregation,[201] which is a dose-related phenomenon. Carbenicillin and ticarcillin can react chemically with aminoglycosides in IV solutions, resulting in inactivation of their antibacterial activity (see later section, Antimicrobial Combinations). For this reason, these drugs should never be physically combined during infusion.[178] Formation of chemical complexes also occurs in vivo after administration of both aminoglycosides and penicillins to patients with severe renal failure.[221] The penicillin–aminoglycoside complex is known to be microbiologically inactive, but the possible adverse effects of the combination remain unknown.

Piperacillin

Pharmacology. A new group of extended-spectrum penicillins has recently been added to the large family of penicillin antimicrobial agents. Piperacillin, meclocillin, and azlocillin compose the so-called ureidopenicillin or ureidopenicillin-like agents. These drugs are monosodium salts and have a much lower sodium content (1.85 to 2.17 mEq/gm drug) than the disodium salts carbenicillin and ticarcillin. The ureidopenicillins are generally bactericidal except for certain *Pseudomonas, Escherichia coli,* and *Klebsiella* strains. Piperacillin is more active than carbenicillin or ticarcillin against *Pseudomonas aeruginosa* and against many Enterobacteriaceae (*Klebsiella pneumoniae, Serratia marcescens, E. coli, Enterobacter, Citrobacter,* and *Proteus*).[255,300]

Piperacillin is effective with intramuscular or intravenous administration but is not absorbed from the gastrointestinal tract. The volume of distribution approximates the extracellular fluid compartment. Therapeutic concentrations are reached in a number of tissues and fluids including wound fluid; subcutaneous, skeletal muscle, tonsillar, renal and liver tissues; and CSF, bile, bronchial, and urine fluids.[255,286,294] Piperacillin and the other ureidopenicillins are only minimally metabolized (10%); the majority of the dose (60–80%) is excreted primarily as active drug by glomerular filtration and tubular secretion. Unlike carbenicillin and ticarcillin, between 20 and 30% of the dose of the ureidopenicillins is excreted as active drug in the bile.[300]

Clinical Pharmacology. There is very limited information on the pharmacokinetics of piperacillin in infants. Neonates less than 30 days old have been reported to have a serum half-life of the drug of between 3 and 3.5 hours.[255] These values are substantially different from those reported for infants 1 to 6 months old (47 ± 7 minutes).[294] Older infants and children are reported to have serum half-lives of about 30 minutes.[294,299] Peak serum concentrations of piperacillin following IV infusions of 50-mg/kg doses ranged from between 91.6 and 268.3 μg/ml. (Approximately 60%—range 39–88% —of the dose was recovered in the urine within 4 hours of administration).[294] Most Enterobacteriaceae and *Pseudomonas aeruginosa* are inhibited by a dose of 25 μg/ml or less of piperacillin.

Therapeutic Indications. The ureidopenicillins should be considered second-line antimicrobials to be used in combination with an aminoglycoside. When there is no direct evidence for superior clinical efficacy, their use should be restricted to clinical situations in which carbenicillin or ticarcillin have expected disadvantages, such as when there is a need for a lower sodium load, when there are problems with hypokalemia or platelet dysfunction or renal failure, and when the infecting organism is known to be sensitive to the ureidopenicillins. The ureidopenicillins should not be used in infections involving gram-positive organisms.

In adults, piperacillin can achieve sufficient concentrations in the CSF to exceed the MIC of susceptible strains, including that of gram-negative enteric organisms.[255]

Existing information is consistent, with a recommended dosage of piperacillin for infants of 50 mg/kg IV every 4 to 6 hours.[294] The appropriate dose and dosing interval for neonates have not been established. Modification of dosage appears necessary only in patients with severe renal and hepatic dysfunction (Table 4–4). The fact that these drugs exhibit nonlinear dose-dependent pharmacokinetic properties requires extreme caution in employing dosages higher than those currently recommended.

Clinical Toxicology. Piperacillin has a low frequency of toxicity associated with its use in adults and older infants and children. There are scattered reports of fever, allergic reactions, (rash, pruritus, serum sickness), gastrointestinal problems (diarrhea, nausea, vomiting), local intolerance at the site of the IM administration, headache, dizziness, fatigue, leukopenia, neutropenia, eosinophilia, and elevated alkaline phosphatase, SGOT, and creatinine levels.[255] Patients allergic to pencillins are at risk for developing allergic reactions to the ureidopenicillins as well.

Compared with carbenicillin and ticarcillin, the sodium load of the ureidopenicillins is less than half, and there is less frequent development of hypokalemia and platelet dysfunction.[300]

CEPHALOSPORINS

The cephalosporin antibiotics that have reached the stage of clinical use are all derivatives of cephalosporin C, which has a strong structural similarity to penicillins (see Table 4–9). A whole family of cephalosporin antibiotics has evolved by the addition of various chemical side chains to the cephalosporin C nucleus. Modifications at position 7 of the beta-lactam ring are believed to alter antibacterial activity, while modification of position 3 of the dehydrothiazine ring alters metabolism, pharmacokinetic properties, and toxicity. Like the penicillins, the cephalosporins inhibit the third stage of bacterial cell wall synthesis. Resistance to the cephalosporins may be related to an inability of the antibiotic to penetrate to or interact with its normal site of action; in addition, some bacteria produce beta-lactamases that cleave the beta-lactam ring of the cephalosporins, thereby inactivating them. The susceptibility of the various cephalosporins to beta-lactamases varies according to the different side chain groups (Table 4–9).

The cephalosporins differ significantly in various aspects of disposition, including extent of absorption following oral administration and plasma protein binding, concentrations reached in various tissues and fluids (including CSF), percentage metabolized, and major route(s) of excretion.[45,164,182] The antibacterial spectrum also differs for the various cephalosporins; relevant details for each drug are presented in the following sections.

Cephalothin

Pharmacology. Cephalothin should be given by the IV route because it is not well absorbed orally and produces considerable pain upon IM injection. Although cephalothin may localize in many tissues and fluids, it does not enter the CSF to a significant extent and should not be used for treatment of CNS infections. About half of the administered dose is eliminated unchanged in the urine, and up to 20% to 30% is metabolized and subsequently excreted in the urine. Excretion can be delayed with renal dysfunction, requiring an increase in the interval of administration to prevent drug accumulation.

Clinical Pharmacology. In one study, neonates given 12.5 mg/kg IM had serum cephalothin levels of 22, 2.4, and 0.5 μg/ml at 1/2, 6, and 12 hours after administration, respectively.[202] These values are slightly lower than serum levels observed in full-term infants given an identical dose. In another study, a dose of 20 mg/kg in healthy full-term infants produced serum cephalothin levels of between 14 and 93 μg/ml (mean 47 μg/ml) at 1/2 hour and a mean of 1.9 μg/ml 8 hours after the dose. Continuous IV infusion studies (40 mg/kg/day) yielded serum levels of 24 to 35 μg/ml in premature infants and 7 to 22 μg/ml in full term infants; a larger continuous-infusion dose of 80 mg/kg/day IV produced serum levels of 50 to 150 μg/ml in prematures and 30 to 50 μg/ml in full-term infants. There were no adverse effects noted.[86]

Therapeutic Indications. There is currently very little therapeutic indication for the use of this drug in neonates. See Table 4–10 for in vitro antimicrobial activity.

Cefazolin

Pharmacology. Because of a smaller volume of distribution, the serum concentrations of cefazolin are higher than those of cephalothin when equivalent doses are used. The half-life for cefazolin is about twice as long as that for cephalothin. It is not metabolized, and nearly the entire dose can be recovered from the urine within 24 hours of administration. The drug is highly bound to serum proteins.

Clinical Pharmacology. Peak serum concentrations of cefazolin are in the range of 55 to 65 μg/ml 1 hour after a 25-mg/kg IM dose; trough levels of 13 to 18 μg/ml occur at 12 hours. The serum half-life values are between 3 and 4 1/2 hours.[40]

Therapeutic Indications. There is very little therapeutic indication for the use of cefazolin in neonates at the present time. See Table 4–10 for in vitro antimicrobial activity.

Cefamandole

Pharmacology. Cefamandole is a **second-generation** cephalosporin that is active against a wide spectrum of gram-negative enteric organisms and against ampicillin-resistant strains of *Hemophilus influenzae* and methicillin-resistant strains of *S. aureus*. Half-life and serum protein binding are similar to those seen with cephalothin, but higher serum levels are attained with cefamandole. The drug is excreted unchanged in the urine.

Clinical Pharmacology. Cefamandole has had only limited clinical use in neonates. In one study, serum concentrations attained with IM and IV doses of 17 and 33 mg/kg were similar, ranging from 35 to 84 μg/ml (peak); the mean half-life in neonates was approximately 1 hour, and the volume of distribution calculated to be between 0.26 and 0.48 l/kg.[2] These pharmacokinetic values are similar to those reported in older infants and children.[36] The ability of cefamandole to cross the blood-brain barrier is insufficient for its use in meningitis.

Therapeutic Indications. There is no therapeutic indication for the use of this drug in neonates at the present time.

Cefoxitin

Pharmacology. Cefoxitin is a second-generation cephalosporin with antimicrobial activity

Table 4-9. STRUCTURE AND PHARMACOLOGIC PROPERTIES OF THE CEPHALOSPORINS

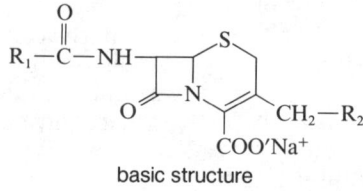

basic structure

Cephalosporin	Structure R_1	R_2	Resistance to Beta-Lactamases	Metabolized	Excretion	CSF Penetration
First-generation						
cephalothin			yes	yes (<30%)	urine > bile	no
cefazolin			poor	no	urine > bile	no
Second-generation						
cefamandole			yes	no	urine > bile	poor
cefoxitin			yes	no	urine > bile	poor
Third-generation						
cefotaxime			yes	yes	urine (65%) > bile	yes
moxalactam*			yes	no	urine (90%)	yes
cefoperazone			yes	no (<1%)	bile > urine (20–30%)	yes
ceftriaxone			yes	no	urine (60%), bile (30%)	yes

*(Also, oxygen is substituted for sulfur in basic structure.)

Table 4 – 10. COMPARATIVE IN VITRO ANTIMICROBIAL SPECTRA OF THE CEPHALOSPORINS[a]

Microorganism	Cephalothin or Cephapirin	Cefazolin	Cefamandole	Cefoxitin	Cefotaxime	Moxalactam	Cefoperazone
Gram-positive							
S. aureus	++++	+++	++++	+++	+++	++	++
S. pneumoniae	+++	+++	++++	+++	+++	++	+++
S. pyogenes	+++	+++	++++	+++	+++	++	++
S. faecalis	–	–	–	–	–	–	–
Gram-negative							
E. coli	+++	+++	++++	++++	++++	++++	+++
Klebsiella	++	+++	++++	++++	++++	++++	++++
Enterobacteriaceae	–	–	++	–	+++	+++	++
Serratia	–	–	–	+	+	+++	++
Proteus (indole-positive)	–	–	++	++	++++	++++	+++
H. influenzae	–	+	++	++	++++	++++	++++
N. gonorrhoeae	+++	+++	++++	+++	++++	++++	++++
Acinetobacter	–	–	–	–	++	–	+
P. aeruginosa	–	–	–	–	+	+	+++
Bacteroides fragilis	–	–	–	+++	++	+++	++

[a] In vitro activity expressed as relative potency of drug against the specific organism, with + = lowest and ++++ = highest; – = no activity.

similar to that of cefamandole except for the Enterobacterioceae, against which it is ineffective. Unlike cefamandole, cefoxitin is reliably active against *Bacteroides fragilis*. The drug is poorly absorbed from the gastrointestinal tract, but IV or IM administration produces peak serum levels within 2 hours. The drug penetrates poorly into the CSF. About 70% to 80% of the drug in serum is protein-bound. Very little metabolism of the drug occurs (< 5%); over 75% of the dose is excreted unchanged in the urine.[29]

Clinical Pharmacology. In studies with cefoxitin in prematures and full-term neonates, doses of 30 to 35 mg/kg IV given every 8 hours produced mean serum concentrations (at steady state) of 60 μg/ml (range 42 – 143 μg/ml).[189] The peak serum levels were 43 to 177 μg/ml; the trough levels were between 6.5 and 37 μg/ml. The elimination half-life was 3.8 hours (range 2 – 6.9 hr), and the volume of distribution 0.58 l/kg (range 0.23 – 1.26 l/kg). Although some conflicting data exist, the majority of studies with cefoxitin indicate the drug does not reach adequate therapeutic concentrations in the CSF after IV administration. Feldman and co-workers, employing doses of 75 mg/kg IV given every 6 hours in infants (mean age 14 mo), found a mean peak CSF concentration of between 4 and 6 μg/ml. They concluded that cefoxitin is inadequate used alone in pediatric patients with meningitis. No significant adverse effects were observed in these studies.

Therapeutic Indications. The use of this drug as a single therapeutic agent in neonatal infections is not indicated.

Clinical Toxicity. A retrospective review of clinical studies of cefoxitin indicates the drug is well tolerated.[223] Drug-related reactions include rash (observed in 2.2% of patients), thrombophlebitis (in 5.3%), positive direct Coombs' test (in 2.4%), eosinophilia (in 2.9%), and increase in liver enzymes (in 3%).

Cefotaxime

Pharmacology. Cefotaxime is one of the new **third-generation** cephalosporins, which can be generally characterized as being very resistant to beta-lactamases and having an increased spectrum of activity and potency against gram-negative organisms.[45,52] Cefotaxime distributes widely into most body fluids and tissues. Plasma protein binding is estimated to range between 25% and 50%. The ability of cefotaxime and the other third-generation cephalosporins to reach therapeutic levels in the CSF may prove to be of great use in the treatment of neonatal meningitis. Cefotaxime is the only current third-generation cephalosporin that is metabolized to inactive metabolites (Table 4 – 9).

Clinical Pharmacology. The IV route should be used for cefotaxime administration to achieve optimal therapeutic concentrations in the serum. The drug penetrates into bile, bronchial secretions, lung tissue, CSF, ascitic fluid, and middle ear fluid. Doses of 25 mg/kg IV result in peak serum drug levels of greater than 50 μg/ml, which decrease to 5 to 20 μg/ml by 6 hours after administration.[100] Doses of 50 mg/kg IV produce peak serum levels of 116 to 133 μg/ml.[145] Pre-term neonates have significantly lower clearance rates for cefotaxime than those found in full-term neonates (23 vs. 44 ml/min/1.73 m^2, respectively).[145] In addition, the elimination half-life decreases during the course of treatment. Studies of cefotaxime pharmacokinetics in 17 preterm low-birth-weight neonates given 50 mg/kg IV or IM every 12 hours revealed mean peak serum levels of 87 $\pm$ 36 μg/ml and mean body clearances of 1.7 $\pm$ 0.9 ml/min/kg.[253] The volume of distribution is 0.4 to 0.5 l/kg in infants. Additional pharmacokinetic details are outlined in Table 4–11. Adjustment of dosage according to the degree of renal dysfunction has been recommended by some investigators (Table 4–4),[45] although others indicate no dosage adjustment is necessary even in patients with renal function

Table 4–11. SUMMARY OF PEDIATRIC CLINICAL PHARMACOLOGY STUDIES OF THE THIRD-GENERATION CEPHALOSPORINS

Authors of Published Study[a]	Study Group	Dose	Peak Serum Concentration (μg/ml)	Serum Half-life[c] ($T_{\frac{1}{2}}$: hr)	CSF Concentration[d] (μg/ml)
Cefotaxime					
Kafetzis et al[100]	18 prematures 14 full-term infants	25 mg/kg IV (50 mg/kg for meningitis)	60–80	5.7 2–3.5	7–30
McCracken et al[145]	30 neonates	50 mg/kg IV	116–130	4.6 (premature) 3.4 (full-term)	
deLouvois et al[253]	17 neonates (33 $\pm$ 4 wks)	50 mg/kg IV or IM q 12 hr	87 $\pm$ 36	3.1 + 0.8 $V_d = 0.56 \pm 0.4$ l/kg	
Moxalactam					
Schaad et al[198]	62 neonates	25–100 mg/kg IV or 50 mg/kg IM	56–234	5.4–7.6 (<1 wk old); 4.4 (1–4 wk old)	2–34 (mean 14.3; 50-mg/kg dose)
Kaplan et al[103]	39 children (2–90 mo)	20–50 mg/kg IV	30–113	1.8–2.0	5.7 (50-mg/kg dose)
Thirumoorthi et al[220]	16 children (1–54 mo)	15–50 mg/kg IV	4.5–86.5 (range at 2 hr)		0–42
Latif et al[118]	37 children (9 mo–14 yr)	25 mg/kg IV	41.1	1.5	
Nahata et al[158]	12 children (8–45 mo)	50 mg/kg IV	25–100	2	
Keyserling et al[108]	34 children (2–15 yr)	50 mg/kg IV q 8 hr	106	1.5 (range 71–141 min)	
Reed et al[282]	30 patients (7 days–26.3 yrs)	50 mg/kg IV q 8 hr	<1 yr ($N = 10$) 148 $\pm$ 30	2.5 $\pm$ 1.1 hr $V_d = 0.39 \pm 0.1$ l/kg	
Ceftriaxone					
Schaad and Stoeckel[199]	5 infants (7–15 mo)	50 mg/kg IV, single dose	219	6.5 (range 4.1–7.7; $V_d = 0.39$ l/kg)	
Del Rio et al[48]	32 children (2–42 mo)	50 mg/kg IV q 8–12 hr	205–263	4	0.9–2.2
Chadwick et al[37]	17 children (0.6–52 mo)	50–75 mg/kg IV, single dose	184–267	4.2	4.5–6.0
McCracken et al[270]	40 neonates (1–45 days)	50 mg/kg IV ×1	136–173	5.2–8.4 $V_d = 0.5$ to 0.6 l/kg	
Steele et al[291]	30 neonates and children (8 days–2 yr)	50 or 75 mg/kg IV ×1	230–295	5.4–5.8 $V_d = 0.4$ l/kg	5.4–6.4

[a] Listed in order of publication. See References at end of chapter.
[b] Peak serum concentration values represent mean values or ranges for each study group unless otherwise noted.
[c] The half-life values represent mean values or ranges for the study group indicated.
[d] CSF concentrations are ranges unless otherwise indicated; V_d = volume of distribution.

less than 10% of normal.[229] No information in this regard has been obtained in neonates.

Therapeutic Indications. The effectiveness of third-generation cephalosporins against gram-negative bacilli, their apparent safety, and the adequate CSF concentrations attained upon systemic administration of these agents provide considerable optimism for their use in treating neonatal meningitis. The use of cefotaxime probably should be avoided in CNS infections with *Streptococcus faecalis, Pseudomonas aeruginosa,* and *Bacteroides fragilis.* The main spectrum includes *E. coli, Proteus, Klebsiella, H. influenzae,* and *S. aureus* (see Table 4–10). A significant rate of relapse following cefotaxime therapy for gram-negative bacillary meningitis[26] and group A streptococcal meningitis[95] in adults emphasizes the need for careful assessment of this newer antimicrobial agent in neonates.

The recommended dose of cefotaxime is 50 mg/kg IV or IM given every 12 hours in infants less than 1 week old and every 8 hours in infants 7 to 28 days of age.[145,253]

Clinical Toxicity. Very few significant side-effects have been reported. There is no evidence of unfavorable effects on renal or hepatic function.[239,253] Side-effects reported include rashes, phlebitis, diarrhea, leukopenia or granulocytopenia, and eosinophilia.

Moxalactam

Pharmacology. Moxalactam is a third-generation cephalosporin with structural features characteristic of neither a true penicillin nor a cephalosporin.[185] Moxalactam is a mixture of R and S epimers, which possess different in vitro antibacterial activity and different pharmacokinetics.[159] The pharmacologic features of moxalactam are similar to those of cefotaxime, with the following exceptions: Moxalactam is not metabolized and is eliminated almost entirely by renal mechanisms, and it has greater susceptibility to beta-lactamases as well as decreased protein binding.[164] Dosage adjustment is recommended in patients with renal dysfunction (see Table 4–4), although some sources indicate no adjustment is necessary because of the drug's wide therapeutic index of safety.

Clinical Pharmacology. The disappearance of moxalactam from serum following IM or IV administration is diphasic in character, with the elimination phase half-life correlating with chronologic and gestational ages of the neonate. The average half-life in neonates less than 1 week of age is 6.2 hours versus 4.4 hours in

neonates 1 to 4 weeks old.[198] The peak concentrations of moxalactam range from 100 to 130 μg/ml in serum and 0 to 34 μg/ml in CSF after a 50-mg/kg IV dose. These levels exceed by many times the MIC for most gram-negative bacilli isolated from the CSF of neonates with meningitis.[198] Studies in older infants and children (Table 4–11) have yielded some conflicting data, especially with respect to drug CSF levels.[50] As pointed out by Dillon,[50] variation in analytic technique may account for some of these different clinical observations, especially with respect to the drug's R and S epimers.[159] Moxalactam also appears to be chemically unstable, raising concern regarding administration technique. The rapid rate of clearance ($T\frac{1}{2} = 2$ hr) and multiple-compartment distribution of the drug also mandate attention to experimental details such as exact serum or CSF sampling times relative to time of dosing.

Therapeutic Indications. Studies by Schaad and colleagues[198] indicate that moxalactam may provide a therapeutic advantage in neonates with gram-negative bacillary meningitis (excluding that caused by *Pseudomonas aeruginosa*). The in vitro sensitivities for moxalactam[71] are very similar to those of cefotaxime (Table 4–10). Dosage recommendations for moxalactam in neonatal meningitis include a loading dose of 100 mg/kg IV and a maintenance dose of 50 mg/kg IV every 12 hours in infants less than 1 week old or every 8 hours in those older than 2 months.[282]

Clinical Toxicity. Adverse effects in general have been few and minor, although some serious effects have been reported with moxalactam use in adults.[164,276] Coagulopathy has been associated with the use of this agent in 2.5% of adult patients.[171] Moxalactam has been shown to produce hypoprothrombinemia, which can be prevented by the use of vitamin K. Dose-dependent increased bleeding time and thrombocytopenia are also listed by the manufacturer as possible contributing complications to the coagulopathy.[228] The limited studies of moxalactam in neonates have shown it to be well tolerated.

Cefoperazone

Pharmacology. Cefoperazone is a new third-generation cephalosporin with little reported experience in pediatric patients, especially neonates. It is considered to have a broad spectrum of antimicrobial activity against aerobic and anaerobic gram-positive and gram-negative organisms (see Table 4–10) and is proposed to be the most active third-generation cephalosporin against *Pseudomonas*.[45,259] The drug has been shown to be effective with both IV and IM administration. Excretion occurs primarily by biliary elimination (70–80%), with the remaining dose excreted unchanged in the urine. Patients with biliary obstruction excrete the majority of the drug in the urine.[212] In adults, only about 1% of the dose is believed metabolized.[203] The drug is highly protein-bound (65–90%) at usual serum concentrations. No significant accumulation of drug occurs with severe renal failure.[259]

Clinical Pharmacology. Peak serum levels in preterm infants (32–36 weeks) receiving a single 50 mg/kg IV dose have been reported to be 136 ± 28 μg/ml and 720 ± 264 μg/ml after a single 250 mg/kg IV dose.[246] The plasma half-life values ranged between 2.7 and 7.7 hours. Rosenfeld and coworkers[285] evaluated cefoperazone pharmacokinetics in 28 newborn infants ranging in gestational age from 27 weeks to full-term. The mean peak serum concentration of cefoperazone following a dose of 50 mg/kg IV was 159 ± 22 μg/ml in those <33 weeks, 110 ± 41 μg/ml in those 33–36 weeks, and 109 ± 29 μg/ml in those >37 weeks. The drug serum half-life ranged from 5 to 9 hours. CSF levels of cefoperazone ranged from 1 to 9.5 μg/ml. Peak serum concentrations in adults reach 250 μg/ml after recommended doses (1–2 g); the half-life is about 2 hours. Therapeutic concentrations may remain up to 12 hours following a single dose.[44] By in vitro testing of antimicrobial activity (agar and broth dilution techniques), MIC standards have been set as follows: ≤ 16 μg/ml, susceptible; 16–63 μg/ml, moderately susceptible; ≥ 64 μg/ml, resistant. The apparent volume of distribution of cefoperazone, 0.1 to 0.4 l/kg, is similar to that of the other third-generation cephalosporins. Therapeutic levels of cefoperazone have been measured in a variety of body fluids and tissues in adults. Bile and urine concentrations are many-fold greater than concurrent serum concentrations.[45]

Therapeutic Indications. There is insufficient experience with cefoperazone in neonates to justify its routine use in this age group at this time. However, the therapeutic indications for cefotaxime apply to cefoperazone as well, except that cefoperazone is more effective for treatment of *Pseudomonas* infections. The recommended dose for infants is 50 mg/kg, given IV every 12 hours.[246,285]

Clinical Toxicology. Side-effects reported with cefoperazone are similar to those for the other cephalosporins. Fever, rash, diarrhea, and pain at the injection site are the most common reactions.[259] Intestinal side-effects of cefoperazone may occur in up to 20% of patients receiving the drug and may be sufficiently severe to require discontinuation of the therapy.[249] Disulfiram-like reactions[146a] and antiprothrombin effects[68] also have been reported.

Ceftriaxone

Pharmacology. Ceftriaxone is another third-generation cephalosporin with broad in vitro activity against the major etiologic agents in infant and childhood bacterial meningitis. In both in vitro and animal model testing, ceftriaxone appears to have lower MICs and superior efficacy compared with other third-generation cephalosporins.[37]

Clinical Pharmacology. Several clinical studies have been conducted with ceftriaxone in neonates and infants. After IV administration of 50 mg/kg, peak plasma concentrations range from 136 to 295 μg/ml.[37,48,199,270,290] The serum half-life values reported range from 4 to 8.4 hours, with no major differences between infants and children; these values are considerably longer than those reported in full-term infants for moxalactam (2–4 hr), cefotaxime (2–3.4 hr), and cefoperazone (1.4 hr). Calculated plasma clearance values range from 27.9 to 52.6 ml/hr/kg. The reported volume of distribution ranges from 0.3 to 0.6 l/kg. Serum protein binding studies indicate that about 85% of ceftriaxone is bound at therapeutic serum concentrations, which is less than for adults.[199]

CSF levels of 2 to 11 μg/ml have been reported with doses of 50 to 75 mg/kg. The CSF levels of ceftriaxone attained are sufficient to consider the drug useful in the treatment of meningitis.[119,291] The elimination of ceftriaxone is believed to be primarily by the renal route (two thirds), with the remainder excreted via hepatic mechanisms. Based on these pharmacokinetic observations, the recommended dosage for infants is 50 mg/kg IV given every 12 hours.

Therapeutic Indications. The drug is not currently available in the United States.

A Warning

Further investigations of the newer third-generation cephalosporins in neonates are warranted before they assume the status of first-line drugs of choice, particularly since basic questions of disposition and pharmacokinetics remain. Moreover, concern exists with respect to clinical efficacy (CSF penetration) and reports of resistance and relapse.[30]

AMINOGLYCOSIDES

Pharmacology. The aminoglycoside antibiotics include neomycin, kanamycin, gentamicin, tobramycin, amikacin, and netilmicin. All of these drugs contain amino sugars in glycosidic linkage to a hexose nucleus (Fig. 4–3); despite some differences in chemical structure, they are nearly identical in their absorption, distribution, and excretion.[187]

Aminoglycoside molecules contain multiple

cationic sites; the polarity conferred by this arrangement plays an important role in the poor oral absorption, poor penetration into CSF, and rapid renal excretion of these agents. A very small percentage of dose (<5%) is absorbed following oral administration.[85] However, significant absorption of neomycin and gentamicin has been found in neonates with necrotizing enterocolitis,[160,266] although neomycin appears not to be absorbed in patients with ulcers or other types of inflammatory bowel disease.[27] Instillation of aminoglycoside antibiotics into body cavities (peritoneal, pleural) or topical application to large wounds, burns, or cutaneous ulcers can result in toxic accumulation systemically, particularly if the patient also has renal dysfunction.[107]

All aminoglycosides are absorbed rapidly from IM and SQ injection sites. However, repeated IM administration, particularly in very

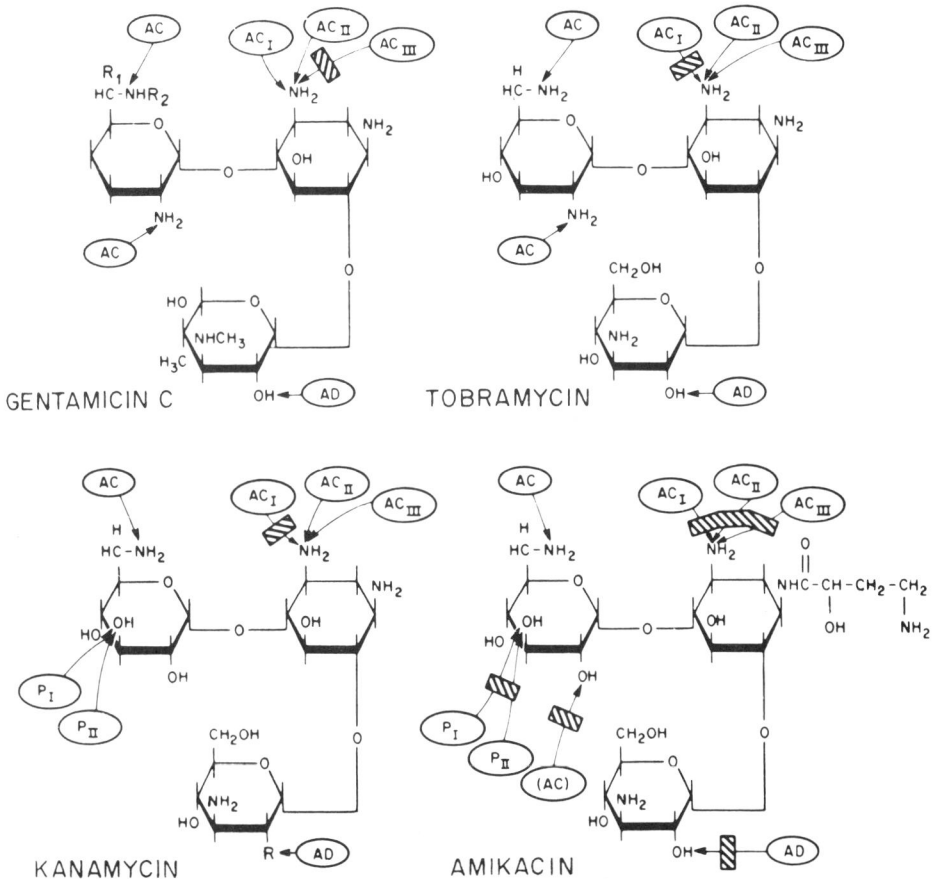

Figure 4–3. Aminoglycosides: Structures and sites of inactivation resulting from plasmid-mediated enzyme activity. In gentamicin C, R_1 and $R_2 = CH_3$; in gentamicin C_2, $R_1 = CH_3$, $R_2 = H$; in gentamicin C_{1a}, R_1 and $R_2 = H$. In kanamycin A, $R = OH$; in kanamycin B, $R = NH_2$. ▨ = regions of the molecule protected from enzyme activity; *AC*, acetylase; *AD*, adenylylase; *P*, phosphorylase. (From Sande MA, Mandell, GL: In Gilman, Goodman, Gilman (eds): The Pharmacologic Basis of Therapeutics, 6th ed. New York, Macmillan, 1980.)

small prematures, may be associated with tissue scarring and very variable rates of absorption, which will result in erratic serum drug concentrations. To provide absolute control over rate and quantity of delivery, particularly in seriously ill neonates, the IV route with a 30-minute infusion should be employed.

Because of the polar character of the aminoglycoside molecule, most of the absorbed drug remains outside of cells and the CNS. Only a small percentage (<20%) is bound to plasma proteins. The volume of distribution of the aminoglycosides has been reported to range from 0.4 to 0.9 l/kg (mean 0.6 l/kg) in neonates,[187] which is larger than the values of 0.2–0.3 reported for children and adults. The renal cortex develops high concentrations of aminoglycoside, which is a major factor in the nephrotoxic potential of these agents. Other highly perfused organs such as the liver and lung usually also have aminoglycoside concentrations exceeding those in serum. Concentrations in muscle, fat, and bone are less than those found in serum; concentrations in bile may reach 30% of serum concentrations, a consequence of minor hepatic clearance of these drugs. Penetration of respiratory tissue and secretions is also poor; concentrations attained are less than serum concentrations.[288] CNS inflammation does increase penetration by the aminoglycosides, but the clinical impact of the resulting increased drug concentrations is uncertain. In experimental studies, CSF penetration by aminoglycoside increased from 10% of serum levels to 20% in meningitis.[213] In general, the concentrations of aminoglycoside reached in the CNS following parenteral administration (IV or IM) are less than ideal for treatment of meningitis.[35] The elimination of aminoglycosides is almost entirely by glomerular filtration; concentrations of unchanged aminoglycoside in the urine are generally greater than 50 μg/ml. Urinary recovery is less than the administered dose because of sequestration of drug in various tissues. There is no evidence that the aminoglycosides are metabolized. Liver disease has no apparent effect on aminoglycoside pharmacokinetics. There is a good correlation between aminoglycoside elimination from the body and renal function (i.e., creatinine clearance).

Bertino and colleagues[22] have determined that double-volume exchange transfusions in neonates decrease serum gentamicin concentrations by 18.5 ± 4.2%. Rebound serum concentrations were inversely related to the number of doses received by the patient prior to the exchange. The authors concluded that addi-

tional doses of drug are not indicated, particularly if exchange is conducted late in the dosing interval.

The aminoglycosides are bactericidal, probably as a result of their known ability to inhibit protein synthesis (initiation) by causing misreading of the RNA template at the level of the ribosome. To produce this effect on protein synthesis the drug must be transported to the site of effect; this may possibly occur via two active transport processes linked to electron transport, oxidative phosphorylation, and the respiratory quinones in the cell membrane.[31] The rate of drug reaching the site of action is believed to account for the variation in sensitivity seen in vitro of different microbial strains. Since the transport process to the site of action can be influenced by pH, divalent cations, osmolality, and oxygen tension, the antimicrobial activity of the aminoglycosides may be markedly reduced in the anaerobic environment of an abscess and in acidic urine. In meningitis, pH may be a factor because of the known decline in CSF pH secondary in part to the increase in lactic acid content.[18]

Inactivation of aminoglycosides by microbial enzymes is the major mechanism of resistance, although alteration in the ribosomal binding site or failure of transport of the antibiotic to the site of effect may also contribute (Table 4–2).[82] The multiple enzymes involved in metabolism of the aminoglycosides are in the bacterial membrane located in or near the site of drug transport.

The antimicrobial activity of several aminoglycosides is shown in Table 4–12. These agents are effective primarily against aerobic, gram-negative bacilli; they have little effectiveness against anaerobic microorganisms or gram-positive bacteria.[70,110] It is imperative to appreciate that considerable difference in microorganism sensitivity can exist from one hospital to the next because of alterations in susceptibility to the aminoglycosides induced by the nature of their use.

Clinical Pharmacology. The pharmacokinetics of aminoglycosides in neonates have been studied by a number of investigators (Table 4–13). Reported peak serum levels after IM or IV administration have varied widely, depending on the dose, rate of infusion (IV) or absorption (IM), timing of serum sample, number of doses (accumulation), gestational or postnatal age, and clinical status of the patients (problems known to affect serum levels include renal dysfunction and hypoxemia).[96,157,257] The numerous factors that can influence aminoglycoside

Table 4-12. ANTIMICROBIAL ACTIVITY (MIC) OF SEVERAL AMINOGLYCOSIDES

	Kanamycin	Gentamicin	Tobramycin	Amikacin
		Serum Concentration Range[a] ($\mu g/ml$)		
	<16 to 4.8	<10 to 1-2	<10 to 1-2	<16 to 4-8
Bacterium		Aminoglycoside MIC[b] ($\mu g/ml$)		
Staphylococcus aureus	1 (90%)	0.25 (95%)	0.25 (95%)	1 (95%)
Escherichia coli	3 (95%)	1 (95%)	1.6 (80%)	2 (98%)
Proteus mirabilis	3 (90%)	1.6 (8%)	0.8 (90%)	6.3 (90%)
Pseudomonas aeruginosa	25 (5%)	3 (40%)	1.6 (85%)	4 (95%)
Klebsiella pneumoniae	12 (60%)	0.8 (95%)	0.8 (90%)	3 (95%)
Enterobacteriaceae	6 (90%)	1.6 (90%)	1.6 (85%)	6 (95%)
Serratia marcescens	6 (30%)	1.6 (50%)	3.2 (40%)	6 (90%)

[a] Theoretical ideal range of serum drug values (peak to trough, respectively) attained during each dosing interval.

[b] MIC (minimum inhibitory concentration) is determined in vitro and may not relate to clinical circumstance. In addition, host factors and sensitivity of the microorganism can vary substantially, limiting the utility of this compiled information. Values in parentheses are the cumulative percentage of isolated strains considered sensitive to the drug.

Data from Finland M et al: J Infect Dis 134:S57, 1976.

serum levels, coupled with the narrow "therapeutic window" for safe, effective, and nontoxic serum drug levels, necessitate the monitoring of aminoglycoside serum levels in every sick neonate.

The pharmacokinetics of the various aminoglycosides are presented in the following sections. Basically, dosage adjustments can be readily and simply accomplished because of the linear (nonsaturation) pharmacokinetics of the aminoglycosides. Assessment of serum drug levels at several time points (preferably peak, mid-interval and pre-dose) and plotting these values on semilog graph paper allows visual determination of ideal dose or dose interval to achieve the desired peak and trough serum levels. Correction of excessive peak serum drug levels can generally be best achieved by dose adjustment; however, decrease in dose is rarely necessary because accumulation of aminoglycoside typically accounts for excessive serum levels. Instead, the dosing interval should be increased sufficiently to allow the serum aminoglycoside levels to decrease to an appropriate (trough) level (see Table 4-12) before administration of the next dose. Szefler and co-workers[217] recommend a dosing interval of 18 hours in neonates of less than 35 weeks' gestation who demonstrate prolonged clearance rates ($T\frac{1}{2} = 8 \pm 2$ hr) of gentamicin or tobramycin. If inadequate peak levels are observed (see Table 4-12), the dose calculation should be checked and possible errors in sampling time should be ruled out (see Chap. 3) before the dose is increased. See Chapter 2 or reviews on aminoglycosides for additional practical discussion of aminoglycoside dosage adjustments.[187,301]

Clinical Toxicology. All the aminoglycosides have demonstrated the potential to produce ototoxicity (vestibular and auditory) and renal toxicity. Although there is little argument that the toxicity of aminoglycosides relate to the amount of drug at the site of toxicity, controversy exists over whether peak or trough serum levels reflect the most useful assessment of toxicity. Some investigators have proposed using area-under-the-curve (AUC) values—that is, area under the curve described by aminoglycoside serum concentration versus time—or total aminoglycoside dose to predict toxicity.[200] Studies have demonstrated that ototoxicity results from progressive destruction of vestibular and cochlear sensory cells. Although early changes induced by the aminoglycosides may be reversible, cellular regeneration does not occur after sensory cells are lost. Many studies have unfortunately not measured vestibular function in neonates, probably because of the technical difficulty involved. However, Eviatar and Eviatar[57] found a higher incidence of vestibular dysfunction than that of sensorineural hearing loss in neonates exposed to aminoglycosides; this finding emphasizes the importance of this expression of aminoglycoside ototoxicity. It is also important to realize that increased risk of ototoxicity is to be expected with prolonged use, high dosage, and preexisting renal dysfunction, or when other ototoxic drugs such as furosemide or noise coexist in the environment of the neonate.[58,59] The true incidence of ototoxicity of the aminoglycosides is uncertain because of the limited number of studies in neonates and the technical difficulties associated with such studies.[57,69]

Table 4–13. SUMMARY OF CLINICAL PHARMACOLOGY STUDIES OF AMINOGLYCOSIDES IN NEONATES

Author(s) of Published Study[a]	Study Group[b]	Dose	Peak Serum Concentration[c] (μg/ml)	Serum Half-life[d] ($T_{\frac{1}{2}}$: hr)	Peak CSF Concentration[c] (μg/ml)
Kanamycin					
Simon and Axline[205]	11 prematures (0.8–2.5 kg)	6.3–8.5 mg/kg IM	17.5	8.9	8–10
Eichenwald[55]	12 neonates: premature and full-term	7.5–10 mg/kg	16–28		10
McCracken[138]	120 neonates: premature and full-term	7.5 mg/kg IM	12.6 / 15.4 / 7.8		6.5
Chang et al[35]	49 neonates (28–40 wk)	5 mg/kg IM q 8 hr			undetectable levels in 6 patients
Howard and McCracken[92]	65 neonates (30–38 wk)	7.5 mg/kg IM / 10 mg/kg IM	17–22 / 22–26	3.8–8.6 ($V_{d} = 0.7$ l/kg) / 4.3–4.5	5.6 (7.5-mg/kg dose)
McCracken et al[142]	17 neonates (32–42 wk)	7.5 mg/kg IM or IV / 10 mg/kg IM or IV	21 / 27–29	4.5–5.1	
Driessen et al[51]	27 neonates: premature and full-term	7.5 mg/kg IM q 12 hr	25.2	1.8–5.5 ($V_{d} = 0.9$ l/kg)	
Beachler et al[14]	41 neonates: premature and full-term	7.5 mg/kg Im q 12 hr	15–20	2.8–7.3 ($V_{d} = 0.6$–0.8 l/kg)	
Gentamicin					
McCracken and Jones[135]	42 neonates: premature and full-term	1.0 mg/kg IM / 1.5 mg/kg IM q 8–12 hr	1.4–2.5 / 2.2–4.4	6 / 4.5 (3 > 1 wk of age)	1.5 (average)
Howard et al[91]	45 neonates (low-birth-weight)	1.5–2.5 mg/kg IM q 12 hr	3.3–4.3		
McCracken et al[136]	77 neonates: premature and full-term	1.5–2.5 mg/kg IM or IV q 12 hr	2.6–4.1	3.5–5.5	1.2 (average)
Nelson and McCracken[162]	28 neonates: premature and full-term	2.5 mg/kg IM q 8–12 hr	3.9–5.3	2.3–5.9	

Study	Patients	Dosage			
Paisley et al[169]	18 neonates (28–42 wk)	0.75–2.4 mg/kg IV or IM q 6–12 hr	2.2–2.6	2.7–4.6	
Chang et al[35]	23 neonates (28–40 wk)	2.5 mg/kg IV q 8 hr	5.3		<1.0 in 4 patients
Assael et al[7]	82 neonates (25–42 wk)	2–2.5 mg/kg IM q 12 hr	2.5–5.7		0.2–1.0 (IM)
Lee et al[12]	16 neonates: premature and full-term	2.5 mg/kg IM q 8 hr; 2 mg intraventricularly q 24 hr	0.3–3.4		3.4–21 (intraventricular dose)
McCracken et al[142]	9 neonates (32–42 wk)	2.5 mg/kg IM or IV q 12 hr	5.2–6.3	3.7–4.3	
McCracken et al[144]	32 neonates	2.5 mg/kg IM or IV q 8–12 hr; 2.5 mg/kg intraventricularly			0.1–3.7 (IM or IV) 48 in ventricular fluid, 32 in lumbar fluid (intraventricular dose)
Szefler et al[217]	84 neonates (26–>38 wk)	2.5 mg/kg IM q 12–18 hr	6.2–7.4	8 (26–34 wk) 6.7 (35–37 wk) 5 (full-term)	
Leff and Roberts[122]	23 neonates (26–40 wk)	2.5 mg/kg IM or IV q 8 hr	8.7–2.2	5.9	
Friedman et al[257]	80 neonates (<36 wk)	2.5 mg/kg IV q 8–12 hr	5.0–6.2	14.6 hrs (asphyxia) 8.2 hrs (control) 11.3 to 16.1 hrs	
Hindmarsh et al[268]	18 neonates (<32 wk, <1.5 kg)	2.5 mg/kg q 18 hr or 3.0 mg/kg q 24 hr IM	6.4–7.5		
Tobramycin Kaplan et al[101]	19 neonates: premature and full-term	2.0 mg/kg IM q 12 hr	4.5–5.2	8.7 (<1.5 kg) 4.6 (>2.5 kg) 6 (>1 wk of age)	
Itsarayoungyuen[96]	30 neonates	2.5 mg/kg IM q 12 hr	5.2–7.5		
Arbeter et al[243]	25 neonates (27–40 wk)	2.5 mg/kg IV q 8–12 hr	5–10	12.2 hrs (<1 kg) 8.9 hrs (1–1.5 kg) 10.8 hrs (1.5–2 kg) 6.4 hrs (2–2.9 kg) 5.9 hrs (>3 kg)	
Nahata et al[275]	18 neonates	2.5 mg/kg IV	6.5 ± 1.8 (1–1.5 kg) 7.8 ± 1.8 (1.5–2 kg) 7.1 ± 1.9 (>2 kg)	9.5 ± 3.7 hrs (1–1.5 kg) 7.5 ± 1.6 hrs (1.5–2 kg) 5.6 ± 1.2 hrs (>2 kg)	

Table continued on following page

Table 4-13. SUMMARY OF CLINICAL PHARMACOLOGY STUDIES OF AMINOGLYCOSIDES IN NEONATES (Continued)

Author(s) of Published Study[a]	Study Group[b]	Dose	Peak Serum Concentration[c] (μg/ml)	Serum Half-life[d] ($T_{\frac{1}{2}}$: hr)	Peak CSF Concentration[c] (μg/ml)
Amikacin					
Howard et al[93]	45 neonates	7.5 mg/kg IM or IV	17–20 (IM)	4.9–7.1 (V_d = 0.6 l/kg)	4.4 (7.3 in ventricular fluid)
Sardemann et al[195]	37 neonates: premature and full-term	7.5 mg/kg IM or IV	18.5 ± 4.9	3–6	
Myers et al[156]	36 neonates (30–42 wk)	7.5 mg/kg IM or IV q 12 hr	17.7 ± 5.4	5.4 ± 2.0	
Cookson et al[42]	35 neonates (24–37 wk)	7.5–10 mg/kg IM q 12 hr	9–21	4.4–7.2	
Prober et al[181]	40 neonates (30 wk)	7.5 mg/kg IV q 12 hr	20–22	6–7 (est.)	
Philips et al[177]	18 neonates (24–40 wk)	7.5 mg/kg IV q 12 hr (loading dose = 10 mg/kg)	trough levels 16.6 ± 11.9 (<1 kg) 6.4 ± 4.3 (>1 kg)		
Assael et al[8]	29 neonates (28–42 wk)	7.2 mg/kg IV q 12 hr	Cl = 0.86 ± 0.29 ml/min/kg V_d = 0.8 ± 0.21 l/kg	6.8 ± 2.9	

[a] Listed in order of publication. See References at end of chapter.
[b] Gestational age at birth is given if available.
[c] Peak serum concentration values and CSF values represent mean values unless otherwise noted.
[d] The half-life values represent mean values or ranges unless otherwise noted; V_d = volume of distribution; Cl = clearance.

The mechanism of the renal toxicity associated with the aminoglycosides is more complex than simple dose-related renal damage. The primary site of damage is the proximal tubule, where concentrations of drug may reach 10 to 20 times those found in serum. Studies of cellular transport mechanisms have provided evidence for a link between normal renal proximal tubular reabsorption of basic amino acids and the damage caused by aminoglycosides: Transmembrane transport of the drug may occur by the same transport system responsible for reabsorption of basic amino acids. Once the drug is inside the cell, initial damage occurs in the lysosome, followed by release of aminoglycoside molecules into the intracellular environment, where they act to uncouple oxidative phosphorylation and inhibit mitochondrial ATP formation. Direct injury to transport functions of the tubular cells can also occur.[200] Usually, the onset of nephrotoxicity is seen after 5 to 7 days of therapy.[5] Signs of renal tubular injury include urinary excretion of granular casts and protein followed by increasing serum creatinine levels. The acute renal failure is often nonoliguric or may be polyuric. Measurement of certain enzyme activity in urine (alanine aminopeptidase — AAP, N-acetyl-β-glucosamidase — NAG, β-glucuronidase, muramidase) to detect aminoglycoside-induced renal injury has recently been accomplished but the clinical importance of these observations is unknown.[1,293] Fortunately, the tubular damage is reversible.

Since renal dysfunction is commonly associated with very ill neonates, particularly those with sepsis or meningitis, differentiation between drug-induced versus disease-induced renal dysfunction is important. Aminoglycoside therapy should not be summarily discontinued in any neonate with increasing serum creatinine levels, particularly if the infection is caused by aminoglycoside-susceptible microorganisms. The patient with oliguric renal failure is not necessarily at greater risk for nephrotoxicity so long as serum levels are maintained in the therapeutic range. The fact that aminoglycosides accumulate only in the renal cortex subsequent to glomerular filtration may be an important protective mechanism. Experimental evidence exists showing that immature and partially functional proximal tubular cells are resistant to the development of further aminoglycoside-induced damage.[131] This observation may explain in part the observation of recovery of renal function despite continued aminoglycoside therapy. Extreme care should be exercised if aminoglycoside therapy is to be contin-

ued in any neonate with progressive renal dysfunction (see under Tobramycin). Utilizing a variety of indices of renal status, Itsarayoungyuen and colleagues[96] concluded from a double-blind comparison of gentamicin and tobramycin that there was no difference in renal status in the two treatment groups; overt renal abnormalities were noted in about 15% of the neonates. The authors appropriately point out the difficulty of determining to what extent the changes in renal status were dependent on the patient's underlying disease or drug therapy. The fact that the neonatal kidney appears to acquire lower aminoglycoside tissue concentrations than those attained in adults[8] may be associated with a decreased risk of nephrotoxicity in neonates.

Another toxicity associated with the use of aminoglycosides is neuromuscular blockade. Reports of this adverse effect have largely been confined to adults who undergo general anesthesia or who are also receiving other neuromuscular blocking agents.[180] Potentiation of neuromuscular weakness and precipitation of respiratory failure have been associated with the use of aminoglycosides in infants with botulism.[269] Certain aminoglycosides are more likely than others to produce neuromuscular blockade; the order of potency for the various agents has been assigned as follows:

neomycin > kanamycin > amikacin > gentamicin > tobramycin

Since this side-effect can occur in neonates, such a possibility should be considered in the differential diagnosis of neuromuscular abnormalities in neonates.

Kanamycin

Clinical Pharmacology. Kanamycin was the most frequently employed aminoglycoside in the 1960s, but increasing resistance and the appearance of other aminoglycosides led to diminished use. Simon and Axline[205] found peak mean serum concentrations of 17.5 μg/ml at 1 hour following IM doses of 6.3 to 8.5 mg/kg in premature infants. The serum half-life of kanamycin was found to be inversely related to postnatal age. Studies by McCracken and colleagues[138] showed considerable variation in peak serum kanamycin concentrations, which ranged from 6.7 to 29 μg/ml (mean 15.4 μg/ml) in full-term neonates and from 4.7 to 27.8 μg/ml (mean 12.6 μg/ml) in premature neonates following an IM dose of 7.5 mg/kg. Using a more specific radioisotope assay, Chang and coworkers[35] also documented marked variability in kanamycin serum concentrations; doses of 5 mg/kg IV produced an average serum concentration of 7.8 μg/ml at 1 hour in neonates. More recently, in a well-designed study, Beachler and colleagues[14] examined the pharmacokinetics of kanamycin in three groups of neonates selected according to birth weight and chronologic age. They found mean peak serum levels between 15.6 and 19.6 μg/ml after a dose of 7.5 mg/kg IM given evey 12 hours. The mean peak concentrations varied inversely with chronologic age but were not influenced by birth weight; mean serum half-life did vary inversely with birth weight, gestational age, and chronologic age. The general consensus is that variation in serum concentration of kanamycin, as well as of the other aminoglycosides, is to be expected, and monitoring of serum levels should be done to establish the ideal dosage for each neonate.

CSF concentrations of kanamycin are approximately one fifth to one half the serum levels in neonates with meningitis. Howard and McCracken[92] found peak CSF kanamycin levels of 2.4 to 12 μg/ml (mean 5.6 μg/ml) 4 hours after a dose of 7.5 mg/kg IM. Other studies observed mean peak CSF levels of kanamycin of 10 μg/ml.[55]

Therapeutic Indications. Kanamycin has been frequently employed in the past, but resistant organisms have become commonplace. Kanamycin has little activity against *Pseudomonas aeruginosa* (Table 4 – 12). Since its toxicity potential is the same as the other aminoglycosides, sensitivity studies of the involved microorganism(s) should be a major determining factor in its employment. Initial therapy with kanamycin can be considered appropriate in situations where resistant microorganisms have previously not been a problem (e.g., non-nosocomial source of infection or low frequency of gentamicin, tobramycin or amikacin use). The initial dosage regimen, pending alteration on the basis of serum concentration measurements, should be 7.5 mg/kg IV or IM given every 12 hours (in infants < 1 wk of age) or 8 hours (in infants > 1 wk of age). The optimal peak serum concentration is believed to be 15 to 25 μg/ml; levels exceeding 30 μg/ml should be avoided because of increasing risk of ototoxicity or renal toxicity (see Clinical Toxicology under Aminoglycosides). In general, infants with $T\frac{1}{2} > 8$ hours require a dosing interval of 18 to 24 hours while those with a $T\frac{1}{2} < 4$ hours require a dosing interval of 8 hours (Table 4 – 5).

Measurement of kanamycin serum levels is necessary to confirm the appropriateness of any dosing change.

Gentamicin

Clinical Pharmacology. The clinical pharmacokinetics of gentamicin in neonates have been examined by a number of investigators (Table 4 – 13). Peak serum levels occurring 30 minutes to 2 hours after administration (IV or IM) generally range between 4 and 8 μg/ml with doses of 2.5 mg/kg. The average serum half-life is 3 to 6 hours in neonates and correlates with creatinine clearance. Generally, premature infants have significantly longer aminoglycoside serum half-life values than those found in full-term infants, resulting in the need for a more prolonged dosing interval. Hindmarsh et al. observed mean $T\frac{1}{2}$ values between 11.3 and 16.1 hours for premature infants of less than 32 weeks gestational age and 1.5 kg birth weight.[268] Very sick, hypoxemic neonates are also likely to have prolonged gentamicin clearance rates.[156] Friedman et al. found a prolonged $T\frac{1}{2}$ (14.6 ± 4.8 hr) and clearance (0.66 ± 0.43 ml/min) in asphyxiated premature neonates compared with nonasphyxiated controls ($T\frac{1}{2} = 8.2 ± 2.0$ hr; clearance = 1.17 ± 0.44 ml/min).[257]

The CSF concentration of gentamicin in infants with meningitis ranges from 0 to 3.7 μg/ml with doses of 2.5 mg/kg,[144] which are less than ideal. Chang and colleagues[35] reported that CSF gentamicin levels were undetectable in most instances in neonates with therapeutic peak serum concentrations. Because of these observations, direct injection of gentamicin into the lumbar subarachnoid or ventricular space has been used in order to achieve therapeutic levels of drug in the CSF. The lumbar approach has not resulted in improved clinical outcome for a variety of reasons, including inadequate access to the ventricles because of the unidirectional flow of CSF.[18] On the other hand, direct intraventricular administration (1 – 2 mg) raises the CSF gentamicin levels well above MIC values.[121] However, there are problems with this approach, including technical difficulties (such as in reentering the lateral ventricles) and concern regarding toxicity.[18,144] Eradication of gram-negative bacilli has been reported following initiation of intraventricular therapy with gentamicin after systemic or intrathecal therapy had failed.[121,302]

Therapeutic Indications. The emergence of kanamycin-resistant microorganisms requires consideration of the use of gentamicin and other newer aminoglycosides. It must be recognized that liberal use in confined hospital populations encourages the emergence of bacteria resistant to the aminoglycosides involved. The in vitro sensitivities of various bacteria to gentamicin are shown in Table 4–12. Orally administered gentamicin has been shown to be of no value in the treatment of necrotizing enterocolitis.[266]

The recommended dose of gentamicin is 2.5 mg/kg IM or IV given every 12 hours. A longer dosing interval (18–24 hrs) should be employed in neonates with prolonged aminoglycoside plasma clearance ($T\frac{1}{2} > 8$ hr for gentamicin) and a shorter dosing interval (8 hr) for infants with shorter plasma aminoglycoside clearance ($T\frac{1}{2} < 4$ hr) (Table 4–5). All infants receiving gentamicin should have serum drug level determinations done within the first 2 days of therapy, or after the first dose in cases of known renal dysfunction, to ensure the attainment of serum drug levels associated with optimal efficacy and minimal risk of toxicity. With proven gram-negative bacillary meningitis, consideration has been given in the past to intraventricular administration of gentamicin (1–3 mg) because of its poor penetration into the CSF when given parenterally. Whether this is actually beneficial to the patient remains controversial.

Tobramycin

Clinical Pharmacology. The clinical pharmacology of tobramycin is identical with that of gentamicin (Table 4–13), although less information is available regarding CSF penetration by tobramycin. One study in neonates without meningitis found levels of 0.6 to 1.5 μg/ml of tobramycin in CSF 4 hours after a 1.3-mg/kg IM dose in one half of the neonates, while the remainder of the study group had undetectable CSF levels.[140] Ototoxic and nephrotoxic effects have been reported for tobramycin, but there is experimental and clinical evidence that tobramycin may be less nephrotoxic than gentamicin in adults, particularly those with preexisting renal dysfunction.[114,207]

Therapeutic Indications. Tobramycin has been shown to have greater in vitro activity against *Pseudomonas aeruginosa* compared with gentamicin.[139] This use should be guided by bacterial sensitivity studies. In one study involving a double-blind, randomized evaluation of neonates treated with either gentamicin or tobramycin, no significant differences in toxicity could be identified.[96] However, in situa-

tions of preexisting renal dysfunction, employment of tobramycin, the more expensive drug, may be justified because of evidence for less nephrotoxicity.[114,207] The dosage recommendations for tobramycin are identical with those for gentamicin (Table 4–5).

Amikacin

Clinical Pharmacology. Amikacin is inactivated by only one of the several known aminoglycoside-inactivating enzymes associated with resistance. Thus, amikacin may be effective in treating gram-negative organisms resistant to other aminoglycosides.[240] Peak serum concentrations of 10 to 30 μg/ml are achieved 20 to 60 minutes after IM administration. The amikacin serum half-life in neonates ranges from 3 to 9 hours and appears to correlate with postnatal age (Table 4–13). Although there are reports to the contrary,[42] CSF levels range from 0.8 to 9.2 μg/ml 1 to 12 hours after a 7.5-mg/kg IM dose of amikacin.[93] There are no known differences in ototoxic or nephrotoxic characteristics of amikacin compared with the other aminoglycosides. Philips and Cassady[176] have reviewed the pharmacology and use of amikacin in neonates.

Therapeutic Indications. Use of amikacin should be restricted to gram-negative bacilli known to be resistant to the other aminoglycosides and sensitive to amikacin (Table 4–12). The recommended dose for neonates is 7.5 mg/kg IM or IV every 12 hours (Table 4–5). Cookson and colleagues[42] recommended a dose of 10 mg/kg IM every 12 hours, based on observations in low- and very-low-birth-weight newborns. A shorter dosing interval or larger dose is generally reserved for neonates who demonstrate more rapid serum clearance of the drug. The optimal therapeutic peak serum level is considered to be 15 to 20 μg/ml, although some investigators regard levels of 20 to 40 μg/ml as therapeutic.[206] The ideal trough levels are between 3 and 5 μg/ml, which should be above the in vitro MIC values for the involved microorganisms. Doses employed for direct administration into ventricular or intrathecal space have been between 2 and 5 mg.

Netilmicin

Netilmicin is a recent addition to the aminoglycoside group of antimicrobials that is claimed to have less nephrotoxic and ototoxic potential than gentamicin. The drug does appear to be effective in vitro against organisms resistant to gentamicin and tobramycin, particularly *Staphylococcus aureus*.[261] Doses of netilmicin of 2.5 to 4 mg/kg given IM every 12 hours resulted in an average peak serum concentration of 5.4 ± 2.3 μg/ml in neonates and older infants.[267] The serum half-life values ranged between 3.8 and 5.5 hours. Phillips and Milner[277] have reported peak netilmicin serum levels of 5.2 to 12 μg/ml with doses of 3.0 or 2.5 mg/kg given IV every 12 hours but excessive trough levels (> 3 μg/ml). The recommended dose is 2.0 to 3.0 mg/kg IV given every 12 hours. In older infants (4 to 7 weeks old) 3.0 mg/kg should be given IV every 8 hours.[277] The use of netilmicin in neonates should be considered experimental.

OTHER ANTIBACTERIAL AGENTS

Chloramphenicol

Pharmacology. Chloramphenicol was discovered in 1948, synthesized successfully in 1949, and marketed for general use by 1949—a remarkable but perhaps too-expedient history, as viewed retrospectively. The chemical structure of chloramphenicol and related compounds is shown in Figure 4–4. The drug is available as the lipid-soluble base or water-soluble esters of succinate (for IV use) or palmitate (the oral preparation). Both esters are biologically inactive "prodrugs" and must be hydrolyzed following administration to release the active moiety

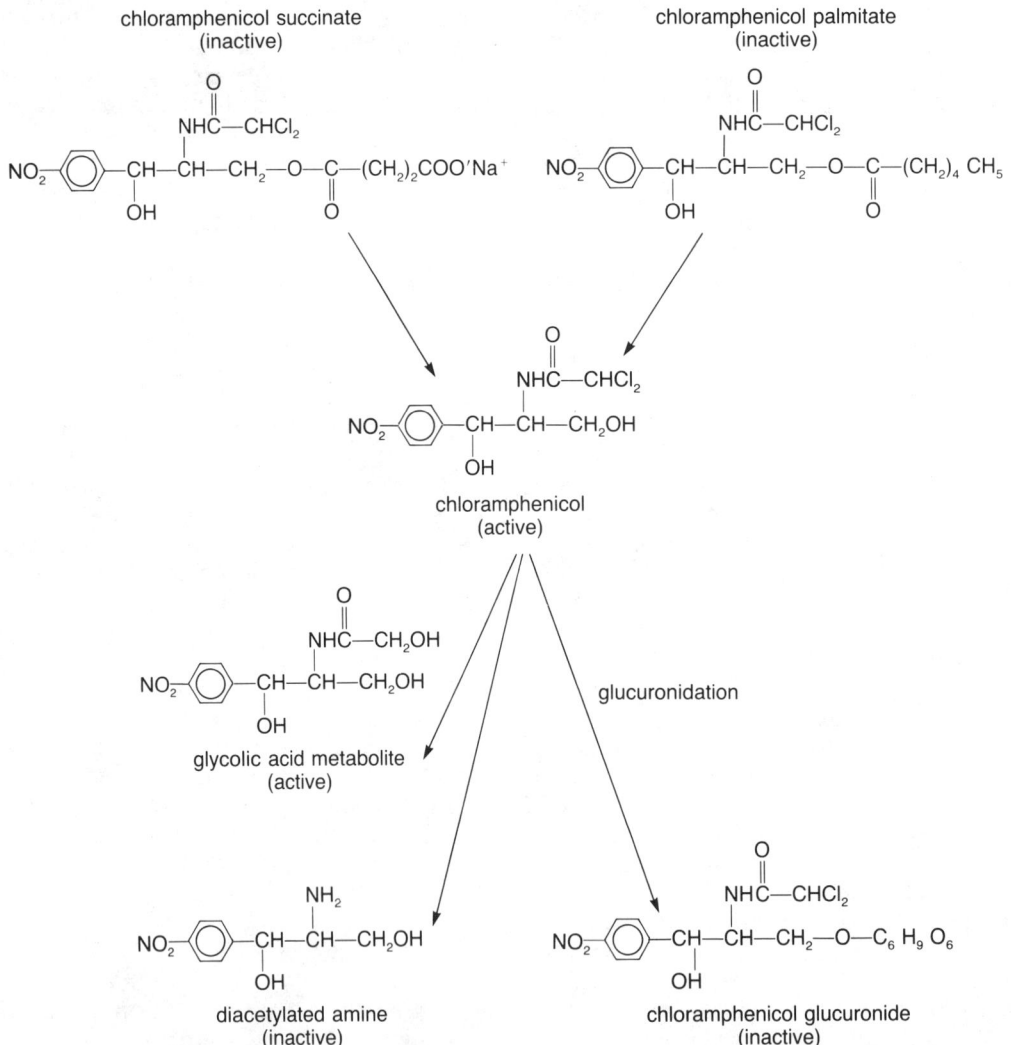

Figure 4–4. Structural formulas of chloramphenicol and its esters and metabolites. The antibacterial effect of chloramphenicol is dependent on the integrity of the propanol moiety. (Adapted from Meissner HC, Smith AL: Pediatrics 64:348, 1979.)

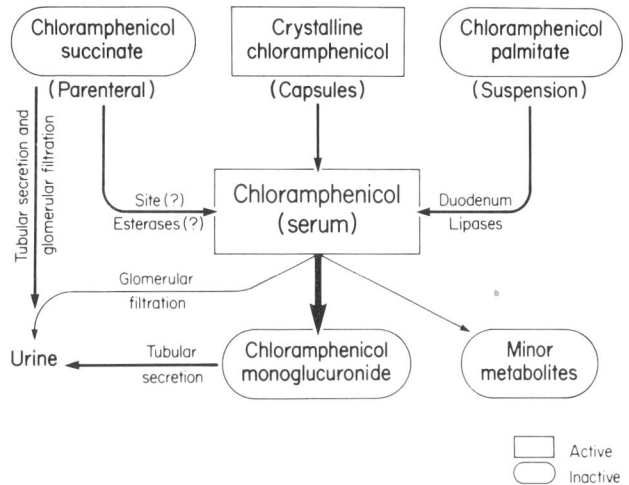

Figure 4–5. Disposition of chloramphenicol esters, base, and metabolites. (From Dajani AS, Kauffman RE: Pediatr Clin North Am 28:195, 1981.)

(Fig. 4–5). Chloramphenicol palmitate is believed to be hydrolyzed in the proximal small bowel, and the free base is subsequently rapidly and completely absorbed. Serum levels of chloramphenicol lower than expected have been reported after oral administration of chloramphenicol palmitate to neonates. This result has been ascribed to reduced hydrolysis of the prodrug ester owing to limited gastrointestinal lipase activity.[149] Chloramphenicol succinate administered IV must also be hydrolyzed for release of the active free base; the site of hydrolysis is unknown. The degree of hydrolysis can be unpredictable and variable from patient to patient, with significant clinical consequences.[103,193] Infants during the first month of life appear to hydrolyze the succinate ester less readily than do older infants and children. An average of 9% to 40% (range 0–80%) of the administered dose of chloramphenicol succinate ester can be recovered unchanged in the urine.[106,193,274] Free chloramphenicol is metabolized by hepatic glucuronyl transferases. The hepatic glucuronyl transferase system is highly vulnerable to influence by a wide variety of agents, including drugs (e.g., phenobarbital, phenytoin) that can alter the rate of conjugation of chloramphenicol.[24,112,238]

There is an apparent dichotomy with respect to the interactions between chloramphenicol and phenytoin and phenobarbital. In a report by Koup and coworkers,[111] an adult patient demonstrated a 60% and 30% decrease in clearance of phenytoin and phenobarbital, respectively, after the administration of chloramphenicol. Krasinski and colleagues[112] reported only subtherapeutic levels of chloramphenicol coadministered with phenobarbital but elevated levels of chloramphenicol given concur-

rently with phenytoin. The apparent differences in the consequences of concurrent administration of chloramphenicol with phenytoin or phenobarbital are difficult to resolve. Chloramphenicol is known to inhibit the metabolism of phenytoin and phenobarbital, which would explain the elevation of their serum levels as reported by Koup and coworkers.[111] Phenobarbital is known to stimulate the glucuronidation of chloramphenicol, which would explain the reduction in chloramphenicol serum levels reported by Krasinski's group.[112] In the neonate, whether chloramphenicol will cause an elevation of phenytoin serum levels, or phenytoin an elevation of chloramphenicol serum levels, or both, is not clear. Nahata and Powell[274] did not observe any consistent effect of phenobarbital or phenytoin on the kinetic parameters of chloramphenicol succinate or chloramphenicol in premature infants. A significant reduction in chloramphenicol serum levels has been reported in older infants also receiving phenobarbital therapy.[248] Although data in neonates are lacking, saturation of conjugation capacity may likely occur within the dose ranges of chloramphenicol commonly employed. The glucuronide conjugate of chloramphenicol is believed to be nontoxic and is inactive as an antimicrobial.

Sack and coworkers[193] have speculated that the liver may be the anatomic site of hydrolysis of the prodrug succinate ester as well as the locus for conjugation of the active chloramphenicol. Liver dysfunction may thus diminish the rate of formation of both chloramphenicol and its conjugate after administration of the prodrug (chloramphenicol succinate). Therefore, variation in hydrolysis of the administered ester, variation in rate of renal elimination of administered (unhydrolyzed) ester prodrug or chloramphenicol base, and variation in hepatic conjugation of chloramphenicol base can all significantly influence the serum-chloramphenicol-concentration-versus-time curve and easily explains the widely varying serum chloramphenicol concentrations observed in ill neonates, in whom renal or hepatic immaturity is expected.

The lipid solubility of chloramphenicol undoubtedly contributes to its ability to distribute widely in body fluids and tissue. Levels in CSF are usually about one half of the serum concentration, although considerable variation is to be expected among patients. Unlike the free base, the succinate ester diffuses very poorly if at all into the CSF. Of administered or available free chloramphenicol, 85% to 90% is excreted as the glucuronide in the urine.

Chloramphenicol is considered a wide-spectrum antimicrobial agent, classified as bacteriostatic, although it may be bactericidal to certain species such as *H. influenzae* and *Neisseria meningitidis.* The susceptibility of various bacteria to chloramphenicol is shown in Table 4–14. The mechanisms for antimicrobial activity reside in the ability of chloramphenicol to inhibit peptide bond formation on bacterial ribosomal units by suppressing peptidyl transferase activity.[12] The binding of chloramphenicol takes place at a single ribosomal protein receptor, which is competitively inhibited by lincomycin, clindamycin, and macrolide antimicrobials. The major mechanism for resistance to chloramphenicol is by enzymatic acetylation, which is R-factor mediated (Table 4–2).

Clinical Pharmacology. Much of the existing data relative to pharmacokinetics and concentrations of chloramphenicol have been cast in doubt by the revelations of recent studies utiliz-

ing highly specific analytical assay techniques. Older colorimetric methods measured not only free chloramphenicol but esters and metabolites. Although the data are incomplete, MICs for most microorganisms susceptible to chloramphenicol are below 12 μg/ml (Table 4–14), and the risk of dose-dependent toxicity is minimal below 25 μg/ml, indicating that the ideal therapeutic "window" should be between 10 and 25 μg/ml. Generally, peak serum levels develop within 2 to 4 hours of PO or IV administration. In studies in low-birth-weight neonates, Glazer and colleagues[78] employed doses between 12 and 25 mg/kg given IV every 8 to 24 hours. Peak serum levels ranged from 10 to 36 μg/ml, reflecting variability from patient to patient as well as the different doses used. The serum half-life values ranged from 10 to 20 hours for most of the infants, but 4 of the 13 neonates studied had $T\frac{1}{2}$ greater than 48 hours. Black and coworkers[24] monitored serum chloramphenicol levels in a neonate who, over a three-week period, received individual doses of between 10 and 50 mg/kg IV; serum levels of 5 to 25 μg/ml were maintained. Nahata and Powell[274] observed steady state peak serum concentrations of chloramphenicol succinate ranging from 2.6 to 41.0 μg/ml and of chloramphenicol ranging from 10.1 to 59.8 μg/ml in premature infants (gestational age 28 to 37 weeks, chronological age 5 to 13 weeks) given chloramphenicol succinate 36 to 75 mg/kg/day by continuous intravenous infusion. The estimated half-life was 0.9 ± 0.3 hours (range 0.5 to 1.3 hours) for chloramphenicol succinate and 10 ± 6.9 hours (range 2.9 to 21.4 hours) for chloramphenicol. The renal clearance of chloramphenicol succinate was markedly lower in the prematurely born infants, which resulted in a greater fraction of the

Table 4–14. SUSCEPTIBILITY OF VARIOUS BACTERIA TO CHLORAMPHENICOL

Very Susceptible (MIC < 4.0 μg/ml)	Susceptible (MIC 4.0–12.5 μg/ml)	Relatively Resistant (MIC 12.5–25.0 μg/ml)	Resistant (MIC > 25.0 μg/ml)
groups A and B streptococci	*S. aureus* streptococci	group D streptococci Enterobacteriaceae *Serratia marcescens*	*Pseudomonas* spp. *Proteus* (indole-positive) spp.
Clostridium spp.	*L. monocytogenes*		
N. meningitidis *N. gonorrhoeae* *H. influenzae* *Bordetella pertussis*	*E. coli* *Klebsiella* spp. *Proteus* spp. *Salmonella* spp.		
Shigella spp.	*Vibrio cholerae*		
peptococci and peptostreptococci	*Clostridium* spp.		
Fusobacterium fusiforme	*Bacteroides fragilis*		

dose being hydrolyzed to chloramphenicol compared to the fraction in older infants and children. Rajchgot and colleagues[280] observed a total body clearance of chloramphenicol in 9 neonates (31 ± 2 weeks gestation; 10 ± 3 days postnatal age) of 1.1 ± 0.2 mg/min per kg and a $T\frac{1}{2}$ of 16.1 ± 2.9 hours (range 6 to 35 hours). Studies of CSF levels of chloramphenicol in neonates reveal concentrations between 4 and 20 μg/ml, which are equal to 20% to 80% of serum levels (Table 4–15).

The value of loading doses of chloramphenicol to rapidly achieve therapeutically ideal serum levels has been studied by Rajchgot and coworkers.[184] Loading doses of 12.5 mg/kg IV produced mean levels (±S.E.) of 7.9 ± 0.6, 8.8 ± 1.2, and 7.6 ± 1.1 μg/ml at 2, 4, and 12 hours after infusion, respectively. After a 20-mg/kg IV loading dose the mean serum chloramphenicol concentrations (±S.E.) were consistently between 10 and 20 μg/ml (15.5 ± 1.2, 15.9 ± 0.7, and 11.3 ± 0.9 μg/ml at 2, 4, and 12 hours after infusion). The actual peak serum concentrations of chloramphenicol

achieved after loading doses of 20 mg/kg IV were no different in neonates less than 2 days of age from those for infants averaging 17 ± 3 days of age (17.1 ± 1 μg/ml vs. 17.6 ± 1.9 μg/ml). The time at which the peak concentration was reached, however, was 2 hours following dosing in the older neonates and 4 hours in the neonates less-than-2-days old. The $T\frac{1}{2}$ estimated from the 4- and 12-hour serum levels measured in these infants was 12 hours in the older neonates (17 ± 3 days) and 22 hours in neonates less than 2 days of age. Rajchgot and coworkers[184] concluded that a loading dose of 20 mg/kg IV is appropriate for chloramphenicol therapy in neonates. Employing a frequency of administration of every 6 hours, the dose required to maintain therapeutic levels will vary, ranging from 2.5 to 5 mg/kg in the newborn and up to 12.5 mg/kg (IV or PO) in infants 1 week of age or older (Table 4–5). Serum chloramphenicol levels must be monitored to establish the optimal maintenance dose.

Therapeutic Indications. Chloramphenicol is most frequently employed for selected neonatal

Table 4–15. SUMMARY OF RECENT CLINICAL PHARMACOLOGY STUDIES ON CHLORAMPHENICOL IN PEDIATRIC PATIENTS

Author(s) of Published Study[a]	Study Group[b]	Dose	Peak Serum Concentration (μg/ml)	Serum Half-life[c] ($T\frac{1}{2}$: hr)	Peak CSF Concentration[c] (μg/ml)
Dunkle[53]	4 prematures (<1500 g)	12.5–17.5 mg/kg IV q 12 hr	20–40		16–20
Yogev and Williams[236]	2 neonates (1 mo)	20–30 mg/kg IV q 6 hr	16.5–23.5		4–10
Friedman et al[72]	40 infants: 8 neonates	12.5 mg/kg IV q 6–24 hr		8 (range 2.5–15)	5–20 (range)
Glazer et al[78]	13 infants (low-birth-weight, 25–36 wk)	12.5–25 mg/kg IV q 8–24 hr	10–36	5.5–>48 (range in 8 infants 5–15)	
Leitman[126]	107 neonates	6–12.5 mg/kg IV q 6 hr	<10–68		
Kauffman[105]	14 neonates	6–12.5 mg/kg IV q 6 hr	5–45		
Sack et al[193]	24 children (2 wk–7 yr)	12–25 mg/kg IV q 6–12 hr	28	4.6	
Rajchgot[184]	39 neonates (<2–55 days)	Loading: 12.5 mg/kg IV 20 mg/kg IV	8.8 ± 1.2 15.9 ± 0.7	Estimate: 22 (<2 days old) 12 (17 days old)	
Burckart et al[248]	10 infants (3–18 mo old)	25 mg/kg IV	20.9–94.0		
Nahata and Powell[274]	5 prematures (5–13 wk old)	36–75 mg/kg/ day by continuous IV infusion	10.1–59.8	10 + 6.9 (3–21)	
Rajchgot[280]	9 neonates (10 days old)	12.5 or 20 mg/kg IV	15–50	16.1 + 2.9 (6–35)	

[a] Listed in order of publication. See References at end of chapter.
[b] Gestational age at birth or age at time of study is given if available.
[c] Peak serum concentration and half-life and peak CSF concentration values represent mean values or ranges.

infections including those caused by aminoglycoside-resistant Enterobacteriaceae, anaerobes, or ampicillin-resistant *H. influenzae* and gram-negative bacillary meningitis. Based on available data (see Table 4–15), the recommended initial loading dose is 20 mg/kg, followed by a maintenance program of 5 mg/kg IV or PO given every 6 hours.[126] The first maintenance dose should be given 12 hours after the loading dose based on the pharmacokinetic data of Rajchgot et al.[184] A maintenance dose of 2.5 mg/kg may be necesary in very small premature infants who are very ill (Table 4–5). Doses usually are increased to 12.5 mg/kg PO or IV given every 6 hours after 1 week of age in full-term infants. *Serum drug level measurements are mandatory because of the unpredictability of the pharmacokinetics of chloramphenicol in neonates.* If the succinate ester is employed, consideration must be given to inadequate hydrolysis if lower-than-expected serum levels are observed (peak <15 μg/ml). A prolonged half-life (greater than the dose interval) as determined by peak, midpoint, and pre-dose serum levels will require increasing the interval to at least equal the half-life.[192] Because of the possibility of saturation kinetics associated with the glucuronide conjugation of chloramphenicol, any changes in dose or dose interval could result in disproportionate changes in serum drug levels (see Chaps. 1 and 2). Therefore, small incremental changes in dosages should ordinarily be made ($<30\%$) at one time. As previously discussed, liver and renal dysfunction can play varying roles in chloramphenicol dosage requirements; therefore, monitoring chloramphenicol serum levels is essential.

Clinical Toxicology. The principal toxicities of chloramphenicol involve two distinctive forms of bone marrow suppression and the classical entity known as the "gray baby syndrome."[149]

One form of bone marrow suppression manifests as anemia, increased serum iron, and maturation arrest of erythroid and myeloid precursors. These effects are dose-related and reversible and generally occur during the course of therapy. Keeping serum chloramphenicol levels to less than 25 μg/ml minimizes the occurrence of these manifestations, which are thought to represent the ability of chloramphenicol to inhibit mitochondrial protein synthesis. Early signs of toxicity include increased serum iron and free erythrocyte protoporphyrin, reticulocytopenia, and eventually decreased erythrocyte count.

The more serious toxicity of chloramphenicol is a non–dose-related aplastic anemia,

which is typically irreversible and often appears after the drug has been discontinued.[23] The mechanism for this toxicity is unknown, although toxic intermediate metabolites of chloramphenicol may be responsible via damage to DNA or inhibition of DNA synthesis.[83,155] All blood cell lines are affected. No valid scientific data are available to support the commonly held belief that the occurrence of aplastic anemia is related to the oral administration of chloramphenicol.[278]

The gray baby syndrome was observed in infants who were receiving very large doses of chloramphenicol (100 to 200 mg/kg/day) and had serum concentrations in excess of 70 μg/ml.[129,216] This toxic effect, resulting from excessive doses of chloramphenicol, is believed to be related to a disturbance of mitochondrial electron transport.[258] Symptoms in affected neonates usually include abdominal distension, pallid cyanosis, and vasomotor collapse, with progression to death within a matter of hours of the onset. Avoiding chloramphenicol serum levels of greater than 50 μg/ml eliminates this toxic problem. Treatment of serious chloramphenicol overdose (>50 μg/ml serum levels) has included exchange transfusions and charcoal hemoperfusion.[256]

For details of toxic interaction with other drugs, see later sections, Antimicrobial Combinations, and under Phenobarbital and Phenytoin in Chap. 5.

Clindamycin

Pharmacology. The early enthusiasm for clindamycin because of its effectiveness against many aerobic and anaerobic gram-positive bacteria and anaerobic gram-negative bacteria has dissipated because of the emergence of treatment failure, the occurrence of serious side-effects, and the development of newer drugs with a similar spectrum of activity. Clindamycin inhibits bacterial protein synthesis by binding to a specific ribosomal subunit of bacteria;[123] lincomycin also competes for this particular binding site. Clindamycin is primarily bacteriostatic at therapeutically attainable concentrations.

Clindamycin is rapidly and completely absorbed from the gastrointestinal tract. It distributes widely and penetrates well into respiratory tissues, pleural fluid, soft tissues, bones, and joints. There are very few data with respect to CSF drug levels, but clindamycin is believed to poorly penetrate the blood–brain barrier and has not been commonly used to treat CNS infections. The greater portion of an adminis tered dose is metabolized by the liver, with only about 10% excreted unaltered in the urine. Because the majority of drug is metabolized, renal dysfunction has little influence on dose requirements. Specific recommendations for dosage adjustment in hepatic dysfunction are not available, but serum concentrations should be monitored in patients with severe liver disease.

Clinical Pharmacology. There is little published work on the use of clindamycin in infants. In one study, infants under 6 months of age who received oral doses of clindamycin palmitate (3 mg/kg q 6 hr) had peak serum concentrations of between 1 and 3 μg/ml.[132]

Therapeutic Indications. The absolute indications for the treatment with clindamycin are few, particularly in neonates. Its major use in adults has been in the treatment of anaerobic infections including bacteremia and pulmonary, intra-abdominal and pelvic infections, but chloramphenicol and metronidazole appear to be preferred drugs in such situations. Feigin and colleagues[61] employed clindamycin successfully in the treatment of osteomyelitis and septic arthritis in children, including several less than 1 month of age; the dosage in infants was 10 mg/kg IV or PO every 8 hours. (Table 4–5).

Clinical Toxicology. The most serious side-effect of clindamycin, which has limited its use, is pseudomembranous colitis, characterized by diarrhea, abdominal pain, fever, and mucus and blood in the stools. This syndrome, which may be lethal, is apparently due to the production of an exotoxin by clindamycin-resistant strains of *Clostridum difficile*;[123] if symptoms appear, clindamycin should be discontinued immediately. Agents that inhibit peristalsis, such as opiates, may prolong or worsen the condition and should not be employed. Vancomycin and metronidazole have been used successfully to treat clindamycin-associated colitis. The reported incidence of diarrhea associated with clindamycin use ranges between 2% and 20%.[218]

Erythromycin

Pharmacology. Erythromycin is one of the macrolide antibiotics, so named because they contain a many-membered lactone ring to which are attached one or more deoxy sugars. Erythromycin is considered both bactericidal and bacteriostatic, depending upon the concentration of drug and the microorganism. Several preparations of erythromycin have been marketed: a free base form and estolate or ethylsuc-

cinate esters, all well absorbed from the gastrointestinal tract, and gluceptate or lactobionate for IV administration. The hydrolysis of the erythromycin esters may be less predictable than was previously believed[81,234] and presents problems similar to those seen with the chloramphenicol esters (see under Chloramphenicol). Erythromycin diffuses into intracellular fluids, and antibacterial levels are achievable in all tissues except brain and CSF. A very small percentage of administered dose is excreted in active form in the urine; the drug does concentrate in the liver and is excreted in active form in the bile. Erythromycin inhibits microbial protein synthesis by binding to the ribosomes of sensitive microorganisms. Erythromycin can interfere with the binding of chloramphenicol because of their similar ribosomal binding characteristics.[81]

Clinical Pharmacology. In one report, erythromycin estolate given to prematures (10 mg/kg PO q 6 hr) produced levels of 1 to 2 μg/ml 3 to 4 hours after administration.[33] These blood levels are similar to those observed by Fujii and colleagues[74] in full-term neonates. Serum levels appear to be independent of gestational or postnatal age.

Therapeutic Indications. The use of erythromycin in neonates other than as a substitute for penicillin in situations of significant allergic intolerance has been limited to the systemic treatment of chlamydial infections[17,191] and for prophylaxis against pertussis.[3] The recommended dose is 20 mg/kg PO given every 12 hours. (Table 4–5).

Clinical Toxicology. The most significant side-effect reported for erythromycin is intrahepatic cholestasis, seen primarily with use of the estolate ester, although other preparations of erythromycin have also been involved.[214] Manifestations usually start after 10 to 20 days of treatment and subside upon withdrawal of erythromycin. Kuder[113] reported a 2.5% incidence of loose stools as the only side-effect in over 10,000 neonates treated with erythromycin.

Isoniazid

Pharmacology. Isoniazid is well absorbed when administered either PO or IM, with peak concentrations developing within 2 hours. It diffuses readily into whole body fluids and tissues and penetrates well into the caseous material associated with tuberculosis infection as well as CSF. The majority of the dose of isoniazid is metabolized and subsequently excreted in the urine. Patients can be divided into distinct groups on the basis of the rate at which they metabolize isoniazid (rapid acetylators and slow acetylators).[226] The incidence of some side-effects of isoniazid has been associated with its rate of metabolism, although controversy exists over the exact mechanism.

Clinical Pharmacology and Therapeutic Indications. Isoniazid is both tuberculostatic and tuberculocidal, although one or two cell divisions of *Mycobacterium tuberculosis* must occur before inhibition of growth develops. Miceli and coworkers[150] recently presented results of isoniazid therapy in two newborn infants who were recipients of the drug transplacentally; the serum half-life values observed were 7.8 and 19.8 hours, respectively (serum levels ranged between 0.2 and 4 µg/ml). In children ranging in age from 1 1/2 to 15 years, half-life values have been reported to range from 2.3 to 4.9 hours.[167] The recommended dose for infants is 10 mg/kg given once daily (Table 4–5). Serum level measurements of isoniazid should be done to minimize the development of toxicity problems (usual serum peak concentrations are 3 to 5 µg/ml).

Clinical Toxicology. The incidence of untoward effects associated with isoniazid is dose-related; about a 15% incidence is observed with doses exceeding 10 mg/kg per day. Peripheral neuritis is the most common adverse reaction. Prophylactic administration of pyridoxine has been shown to prevent the development of peripheral neuritis, which is believed to reflect pyridoxine deficiency: Isoniazid reduces tissue levels and increases the excretion of pyridoxine, which leads to the deficiency state.[284] Other side-effects associated with isoniazid therapy include rash, fever, and hepatotoxicity.[292] Because all these side-effects can be very serious in nature, careful monitoring of serum drug levels during isoniazid therapy is necessary.

Metronidazole

Pharmacology. Metronidazole is a nitroimidazole compound that is directly microbicidal for many anaerobic organisms, including *Bacteroides* species. Metronidazole is thought to act as an electron "sink," depriving the microorganism of required reducing equivalents that are critical in the metabolism of these anaerobic cells. The reduction of metronidazole not only creates a gradient that favors further uptake of the drug into the microorganism but, more importantly, results in the formation of reactive intermediate compounds (free radicals) that are

toxic to the cell.[154] Available evidence indicates that these toxic intermediate compounds bind to DNA, thereby interfering with its function as a template for protein synthesis.[39,54]

After oral administration metronidazole is almost completely absorbed; peak serum concentrations are attained within 1 to 3 hours.[152] The drug distributes throughout the body, reaching therapeutic levels in tissues, secretions, CSF, and abscesses. The drug is poorly bound to plasma proteins (<20%). In adults less than 20% of the administered dose is excreted unchanged in the urine, most being hydroxylated and conjugated by the liver, then excreted by renal mechanisms.[286] The major metabolite (1-[2 hydroxyethyl]-2 hydroxymethyl-5-nitroimidazole) also possesses some antianaerobic activity.[265] In neonates metabolism of metronidazole appears to be substantially less than in adults.[98]

Clinical Pharmacology. In a study of metronidazole pharmacokinetics in neonates, Jager-Roman and colleagues[98] gave 11 neonates 7.5 or 15 mg/kg IV of metronidazole. Plasma and CSF drug concentrations were respectively 11 and 18, 15 and 14, and 12 and 11.5 µg/ml at 2, 6, and 12 hours after dosing. The elimination half-life ranged from 25 to 75 hours, the longer half-life being associated with 28- to 30-week-gestation infants. The apparent volume of distribution (0.54 to 0.8 l/kg) did not correlate with gestational age. On the basis of their observations, these authors recommended an initial loading dose of 15 mg/kg IV in both term and pre-term infants, followed by a maintenance dose of 7.5 mg/kg given every 12 hours.

Hall and colleagues[265] examined the blood levels of metronidazole and its major metabolite in 24 neonates treated intravenously. The dosing regimen consisted of 7.5 mg/kg given as a 30-minute infusion every 8 hours. The duration of therapy ranged from 1.5 to 10 days. The mean peak blood level was 9.6 µg/ml (range 4.3 to 24.1 µg/ml) from 1 to 5 hours after the first dose and 19.3 µg/ml (range 8.8 to 28.9 µg/ml) from 10 to 15 hours after the final dose. The mean elimination half-life of metronidazole was 23 ± 13 hours. Measurement of metronidazole in the CSF of neonates with meningitis has revealed concentrations of between 7 and 80 µg/ml with doses of 30 to 80 mg/kg/day PO or IV.[281] Hepatic dysfunction and extreme prematurity may necessitate a longer dosing interval. No modification of dose appears necessary for renal dysfunction.

Therapeutic Indications. Anaerobes have been isolated from as many as 26% of all cases of neonatal bacteremia, although the true significance of these isolates remains unclear, except in the case of perforation of the gastrointestinal tract. Metronidazole has been successfully employed in neonates with *Bacteroides fragilis* meningitis[21] and is clearly the drug of choice for treatment of meningitis caused by *Bacteroides* species as well as other susceptible anaerobes. Metronidazole is an alternative to clindamycin and chloramphenicol for the treatment of non-meningitis anaerobic infections of various types. Since there is no antagonism between metronidazole and other antimicrobials against *Bacteroides* species or aerobic bacteria, combination therapy with a suitable antimicrobial agent is possible. The recommended dose is 15 mg/kg IV initially, followed by 7.5 mg/kg IV every 12 hours (Table 4–5). Although higher doses have been employed, this dosing recommendation should be expected to achieve plasma concentrations of metronidazole that exceed the reported MIC for anaerobic isolates (2–8 μg/ml).[247,265]

Clinical Toxicology. Metronidazole appears to have a very low incidence of toxicity. Neutropenia and sensory polyneuropathy have been reported in a few adult patients receiving high doses over a prolonged period.[152] During metronidazole therapy the urine may be colored a deep red-brown owing to the presence of metabolites of the drug. Although only experimental evidence in animals exists, concern has been expressed regarding the carcinogenicity potential of this agent. Two retrospective studies in adults have shown no increase in the incidence of cancer following exposure to metronidazole.[16,73]

Rifampin

Pharmacology. Rifampin inhibits and kills a wide variety of microorganisms and is considered the most active antibiotic known against staphylococci. Rifampin is approximately 1000-fold more active than methicillin on a weight basis against coagulase-negative staphylococci.[188] The antibacterial effect is exerted through inhibition of DNA-dependent RNA polymerase, thus preventing normal synthesis of RNA.[60] Rifampin is well absorbed from the gastrointestinal tract, with plasma concentrations greater than 5 μg/ml developing within 4 hours of oral dosing with 10 mg/kg. Rifampin appears to penetrate effectively almost all body tissues and fluids. It has been successfully employed for CNS infections as well as for osteomyelitis. Plasma clearance is chiefly through hepatic uptake, metabolism, and biliary excre-

tion. There is significant enterohepatic circulation. Because only a very small percentage of the dose is excreted in the urine, there is no necessity for dosage adjustment with renal failure; hepatic dysfunction, however, does require a decrease in dose (see Table 4–4).

Clinical Pharmacology and Therapeutic Indications. Rifampin remains a valuable therapeutic agent in treatment of tuberculosis as a part of a multiple-drug regimen. The use of rifampin against other pathogens has been of a more recent vintage. Almost all bacteria may rapidly develop resistance to rifampin; therefore, except for short-term use in prophylactic treatment of meningitis contacts, this drug should not be used alone, particularly in staphylococcal infections. Rifampin should be employed along with another drug active against the effective organism.[133] Rifampin has been used successfully in cases of infected CSF shunts[188] and for unusual cases of neonatal meningitis due to *Flavobacterium meningosepticum* that were resistant to aminoglycosides, ampicillin, and chloramphenicol.[120] It has also been used successfully to treat infants with serious gram-negative infections resistant to most other antibiotics.[161]In a study by Naveh and Friedman,[161] both intraventricular and parenteral doses of rifampin were employed. CSF concentrations following a 20-mg/kg IM dose were 0.8 to 1.1 μg/ml (peak) versus 10 to 100 μg/ml after a 2- to 5-mg dose given intraventricularly. Rifampin also appears to be the drug of choice for meningococcal prophylaxis. More recently, preliminary studies suggest similar efficacy for prophylactic use in contacts of children with *H. influenzae* disease.[79] Although pharmacokinetic studies in neonates are insufficient, the recommended dose is 10 mg/kg given every 12 hours PO (Table 4–5).

Clinical Toxicology. A variety of toxic effects have been reported for rifampin, including rashes, renal failure, and various CNS disturbances. Because rifampin is a very potent inducer of microsomal enzyme metabolism, it can adversely affect therapy with other drugs. Most patients receiving rifampin, besides developing a red urine from the drug itself, show evidence of proteinuria without apparent ill effect.[60]

Tetracyclines

Pharmacology. Tetracyclines have a broad spectrum of action against many bacteria, actinomycetes, rickettsiae, mycoplasmas, and chlamydia. These agents are all adequately but irregularly and incompletely absorbed from the gastrointestinal tract. Divalent and trivalent cations (i.e., calcium, magnesium, iron) are chelated by the tetracyclines, significantly impairing their absorption. The volume of distribution exceeds that of body water, indicating sequestration in certain tissues (liver). Biliary levels are five times greater than plasma levels, in keeping with the fact that some of the administered tetracycline is excreted via the bile and subsequently undergoes enterohepatic circulation; this also results in apparent prolonged tetracycline serum clearance. The tetracyclines are stored in bone, dentin, and enamel of teeth prior to eruption, explaining their toxic potential in these tissues.[225,263] All the tetracyclines are excreted in the urine and feces. The mechanism of action of the tetracyclines involves inhibition of protein synthesis by binding of drug to ribosomes, as with the aminoglycosides.

Clinical Pharmacology. Tetracycline and oxytetracycline pharmacokinetics have been studied in neonates given IM or IV doses of 10 mg/kg.[77] Peak tetracycline serum levels were 4 μg/ml after IM administration and slightly higher after IV administration. Oxytetracycline levels reached 3 to 5 μg/ml at 2 hours after IM administration (10 mg/kg). Demethyl chlortetracycline administered to premature and full-term neonates produced serum levels in the range of 0.4 to 2.2 μg/ml after 1.5 mg/kg was given orally every 6 hours.[76]

Therapeutic Indications. The only indication for use of the tetracyclines in neonates is for *Chlamydia* infections (e.g., inclusion blennorrhea). Topical application (ophthalmic ointment or drops) is effective for this condition, although recent recommendations call for the coadministration for at least 2 weeks of erythromycin, 10 mg/kg every 8 hours, with the topical tetracycline.[186,191]

Clinical Toxicology. Tetracyclines may affect developing bones and teeth by forming chelates with calcium and related cations, thus concentrating in areas of new bone growth and dentition (see Chapter 11). Wallman and Hilton[225] evaluated 50 infants exposed to tetracyclines as neonates and found 46 to have discoloration of teeth with or without enamel hypoplasia. Significant inhibition of bone growth has been reported in premature infants exposed to tetracyclines;[41] this effect subsided with discontinuation of the drug. Other reported side-effects of the tetracyclines include hypersensitivity reactions (cutaneous), local reactive effects (e.g., thrombophlebitis), blood dyscrasia, and manifestations of increased intracranial pressure and hepatotoxicity.[67,153]

Vancomycin

Pharmacology. Vancomycin was originally introduced for its effectiveness against penicillin-resistant staphylococci. Newer antibiotics such as methicillin and nafcillin have relegated vancomycin to the role of alternative therapy for infections due to these microorganisms. However, recently it has been employed effectively in infections by methicillin-resistant staphylococci, including *S. aureus* and *S. epidermidis,* and for colitis due to *Clostridium difficile* that may develop following the use of certain antibiotics such as clindamycin.[62] Vancomycin exerts its bactericidal effect by interfering with the phospholipid cycle of cell wall synthesis in sensitive bacteria by binding with high affinity to precursors of this structure.[173] The drug also alters plasma membrane function and inhibits RNA synthesis. The drug is rapidly bactericidal for multiplying microorganisms. Vancomycin is poorly absorbed after oral administration, a property that makes it useful for the treatment of colitis. Its highly irritating properties require intravenous administration for parenteral therapy. Approximately 50% to 60% of the drug in plasma is bound to protein, and it diffuses readily into body fluid compartments, including the CSF in infants with inflamed meninges.[298] A large percentage of the drug is eliminated by the kidneys. In anuria, the half-life of vancomycin may be prolonged to greater than a week;[251] serum drug level monitoring is therefore imperative in these situations. In the presence of CNS infection, vancomycin has been detectable in CSF.[264]

Clinical Pharmacology. Following parenteral administration, vancomycin plasma disappearance is consistent with a two-compartment open-system pharmacokinetic model. In newborns a dose of 10 mg/kg IV produces serum concentrations of 11 to 20.5 μg/ml; 15 mg/kg IV produces peak levels of 17.1 to 34 μg/ml.[197] Serum half-life ranges from 5.9 to 9.8 hours in newborn infants but is only 4.1 hours in older infants. The volume of distribution ranges from 0.5 to 0.96 l/kg, and the plasma clearance rates are 15 to 30 ml/min/1.73 m^2 in neonates versus 50 and 81 ml/min/1.73 m^2 in older infants. The concentration of vancomycin found in CSF ranges from 1.2 to 4.8 μg/ml (mean 3.1 μg/ml), which represents from 7% to 21% of the concurrent serum concentration. The therapeutic serum concentration is believed to be between 40 and 25 μg/ml.[197]

Therapeutic Indications. Vancomycin should be considered only in very serious infections where the treatment of choice is unacceptable or failing, such as with methicillin-resistant *S. aureus* and *S. epidermidis*. As an oral agent vancomycin has been shown to be beneficial in patients with colitis caused by toxin-producing bacteria (see under Clindamycin). The recommended IV dosage schedule for newborns less than 1 week old is 15 mg/kg every 12 hours and every 8 hours in older neonates (Table 4–5); infusion should be accomplished over a 30- to 60-minute period.

Clinical Toxicology. The most serious adverse reaction to vancomycin is ototoxicity, which is manifested by auditory nerve damage and hearing loss. This effect is infrequent with serum concentrations of drug maintained below 30 µg/ml. Problems with nephrotoxicity have been largely eliminated with newer preparations of vancomycin and lower dosages. Vancomycin is thus not as nephrotoxic as was once thought, but administration by the parenteral route should be employed cautiously, and the drug avoided altogether when other nephrotoxic agents are being utilized. The drug has been well tolerated by infants and children.[197]

Trimethoprim – Sulfamethoxazole

Pharmacology. The combination of trimethoprim–sulfamethoxazole has been used clinically for the treatment of a variety of infections due to gram-positive and gram-negative organisms, although its use in neonates has been limited. The mechanism of action involves inhibition of sequential steps in the synthesis of tetrahydrofolic acid, an essential metabolic cofactor in bacterial synthesis of DNA. The drugs are extremely well absorbed from the upper intestinal tract, with peak serum levels developing within 4 hours of oral administration. Therapeutic drug levels have been demonstrated in the CSF. The majority of administered dose is excreted in the urine as either metabolites or unchanged drug. In patients with severe renal dysfunction (< 10% of normal function), one half the usual dose should be administered at the regular interval following a full loading dose; careful monitoring of blood levels should be performed.

Clinical Pharmacology. The serum half-life values for trimethoprim and sulfamethoxazole are much longer in neonates than those observed in adults and children. More importantly, in the newborn infant there is a poor correlation between the half-life value and creatinine clearance, which emphasizes the importance of serum drug level monitoring with their use, particularly in seriously ill infants. Peak

serum levels of trimethoprim after oral administration range from between 1 and 1.2 µg/ml versus 10 to 20 µg/ml for sulfamethoxazole after IV administration of 2.5 mg/kg of trimethoprim and 12.5 mg/kg of sulfamethoxazole every 6 hours. Identical IV doses resulted in peak serum levels of between 2.4 and 3.2 µg/ml of trimethoprim and 11.1 and 18.2 µg/ml of sulfamethoxazole.[244] In these same studies the serum half-life after repeated injections for sulfamethoxazole was reported to be about 8 to 9 hours compared with 5 to 6 hours for trimethoprim. In studies in 12 newborn infants, Springer and coworkers[211] observed peak serum levels between 3 and 6.4 µg/ml for trimethoprim and between 120 and 200 µg/ml for sulfamethoxazole following single daily intravenous doses of 5 mg/kg and 25 mg/kg of trimethoprim and sulfamethoxazole, respectively. The mean volume of distribution was 2.7 l/kg for trimethoprim and 0.48 l/kg for sulfamethoxazole. The half-lives of trimethoprim and sulfamethoxazole were significantly longer after repeated injections (14.7 to 40.8 hours and 14.7 to 36.5 hours, respectively) than after the first injection (10.8 to 27.2 hours and 10.2 to 27.7 hours, respectively).

Therapeutic Indications. The therapeutic indications for combination trimethoprim–sulfamethoxazole therapy in the neonate are unclear, except in very unusual situations documented by culture and sensitivity studies. Successful therapy of *Citrobacter* ventriculitis has been reported in a neonate who had failed to improve with other antimicrobial therapy.[262] The recommended dosage based on pharmacokinetic studies in neonates[211] is as follows: loading doses, 10 mg/kg IV sulfamethoxazole, 3 mg/kg IV trimethoprim; maintenance doses, 3 mg/kg IV sulfamethoxazole, 1 mg/kg IV trimethoprim, given every 12 hours. The fixed-combination preparation cannot be used to deliver these doses, since its ratio of sulfamethoxazole to trimethoprim is 5:1.

Clinical Toxicology. A major deterrent to therapy with trimethoprim–sulfamethoxazole is risk of kernicterus associated with the use of sulfonamides. However, sulfamethoxazole compared with the other sulfonamides is a weak displacer of bilirubin from albumin.[28] Other reported side-effects include serious skin reactions, such as toxic epidermal necrolysis, erythema multiforme, and exfoliative dermatitis; hepatotoxicity, including inflammation, necrosis, and cholestasis; bone marrow depression, including neutropenia (very common) and thrombocytopenia; and interstitial nephritis.[6,208,244] All of these toxic effects are considered reversible, although death has occurred in cases where therapy was continued despite clinical evidence of drug toxicity.

ANTIBACTERIAL COMBINATIONS

The simultaneous use of two or more antibacterial agents has evolved from the necessity for early intervention in suspicious or high-risk situations involving neonates and from the development of improved antibacterial agents. A better understanding of the pharmacokinetics of the drugs, in turn, has helped to define the clinical situations where the use of combination antibacterial therapy is definitely advantageous to patients.[219] Reasons for use of combined antibacterial therapy include the following: (1) treatment of mixed bacterial infections, (2) treatment of severe infection due to unknown microorganisms, (3) enhancement of antimicrobial activity, and (4) prevention of emergence of resistant microorganisms (such as to rifampin). Similarly, combinations of antibacterial agents may have detrimental consequences. For example, nephrotoxicity or ototoxicity may be greatly enhanced when two drugs with this toxic potential are simultaneously employed in the same patient. Lindberg and colleagues[128] reported an increase in incidence of sequelae associated with *H. influenzae* meningitis in neonates and children receiving both ampicillin and chloramphenicol compared with that found in patients receiving only one of these drugs. Chemical inactivation has been shown to occur with aminoglycosides and carbenicillin or ticarcillin; this finding must be appreciated in designing the dosing routine, particularly in patients with renal failure.[178] In addition to antagonism of activity and increased risk of toxicity, the financial cost associated with unnecessary multiple drug therapy can be considerable.

Various attempts have been made to predict synergism and antagonism by means of various pharmacologic parameters. A useful scheme originally devised by Jawetz and Gunnison[99] employs the concept that bacteriostatic drugs commonly antagonize the action of bactericidal drugs; in addition, two bactericidal drugs may exhibit synergism or have additive effects.[183] Table 4–16 lists the various antibacterial agents according to their primary mode of activity, along with the possible consequences of combined therapy.

SPECIFIC REGIMENS FOR USE IN NEONATES

Ampicillin and Gentamicin

The clinical rationale for use of the ampicillin–gentamicin combination resides primarily in the need for adequate coverage of unknown but suspected microorganisms responsible for an infection in a neonate. The clinical significance of the synergism between ampicillin and gentamicin against group B streptococci remains unclear.[187] Aminoglycosides also show synergism with methicillin or nafcillin against *Staphylococcus aureus* in vitro. Enterococcal group D streptococci often exhibit multiple antibiotic resistance. Because of the synergism between ampicillin and gentamicin against these organisms, this combined therapy is recommended. Although ampicillin alone is effective against *Listeria monocytogenes,* it is often combined with gentamicin because of in vitro demonstration of synergism. Mixed infections (e.g., in bowel perforation) involving susceptible organisms have also been successfully managed with combined ampicillin and gentamicin therapy.

Carbenicillin (or Ticarcillin) and Gentamicin (or Tobramycin)

Combined therapy with carbenicillin (or ticarcillin) and gentamicin (or tobramycin) is recommended for infections due to gram-negative bacilli (Enterobacteriaceae, including *E. coli,* and *Pseudomonas aeruginosa*) because of demonstrated synergistic activity in vitro and clinical studies in adults suggesting improved outcome.[172] The combination therapy also appears to prevent the rapid development of resistance to carbenicillin or ticarcillin. Mixed bacterial

Table 4–16. GROUPING OF ANTIMICROBIAL AGENTS ACCORDING TO PRIMARY BACTERICIDAL VERSUS BACTERIOSTATIC ACTION AND THE CONSEQUENCES OF COMBINATIONS

Bactericidal (Group 1)	Bacteriostatic (Group 2)
aminoglycosides	chloramphenicol
cephalosporins	erythromycin
penicillins	clindamycin
trimethoprim–sulfamethoxazole	lincomycin
	tetracyclines

Consequence of Combination
Group 1 + Group 1 = synergistic or indifferent
Group 1 + Group 2 = synergistic, additive, or antagonistic

From Rahal JJ Jr: Medicine 57:179, 1978.

infections involving anaerobes and aerobic gram-negative bacilli (e.g., intra-abdominal sepsis from intestinal perforation) are best treated with combination therapy, including semisynthetic penicillins (carbenicillin or ticarcillin) combined with an aminoglycoside. The important chemical interactions that can occur between these drugs may possibly compromise their antimicrobial activities. The clinical significance of such interactions remains unclear; nevertheless, the drugs should be administered separately. This combination regimen should be used with caution in neonates known to have significant renal dysfunction.[179]

Ampicillin and Chloramphenicol

The combination of ampicillin and chloramphenicol has been shown to be synergistic against *H. influenzae*,[63] although the rationale for use of this combination as initial therapy of suspected *H. influenzae* meningitis is based on the known frequency of resistance of the organism to ampicillin. Recently Kaplan and Mason[104] reported that ampicillin and chloramphenicol were synergistic against many unrelated gram-negative enteric organisms isolated from neonates with meningitis. The clinical significance of these in vitro observations is not known.

Recent studies suggest that chloramphenicol can inhibit the bactericidal activity of ampicillin against group B streptococci.[227] Such inhibition is consistent with the possibility, suggested by other studies, that chloramphenicol in combination with a penicillin is antagonistic for some bacterial species. Lindberg and colleagues[128] found an increase in complications in children with *H. influenzae* meningitis treated with both ampicillin and chloramphenicol. Mathies and coworkers[134] treated bacterial meningitis in children with either ampicillin alone or with combination of ampicillin, chloramphenicol, and streptomycin; a significantly greater mortality was observed in those receiving the combination compared with those receiving ampicillin alone. The clinical significance of the demonstration in vitro of chloramphenicol impairment of the bactericidal activity of gentamicin or gentamicin plus ampicillin remains unclear.[170] These observations clearly point out the importance of identification of the infecting organism rather than arbitrary use of chloramphenicol with ampicillin or gentamicin.

CONSIDERATIONS IN CHOOSING A COMBINATION REGIMEN

These few examples of clinically documented beneficial antimicrobial drug combinations stand in contrast to the actual employment of a variety of antimicrobial combinations seen in the clinical setting. Combination antimicrobial therapy often evolves from the addition of one or more agents to an existing regimen when the clinical condition of the neonate continues to deteriorate. Because of the potential for antagonistic interaction and increased risk of toxicity associated with two or more drugs given simultaneously, the prescribing physician must carefully reexamine the total therapeutic regimen in an attempt to substitute a more appropriate drug rather than add another agent to the antimicrobial regimen in use. Enthusiasm for antimicrobial combinations should also be limited by the realization that potential deleterious effects include suppression of normal flora, greater risk of secondary infection, and development of resistant microorganisms. Antimicrobial agents should not be routinely used in combination for the purpose of synergy unless the combination has been proved effective or unless one of the drugs is known to be unsatisfactory when used alone.

ANTIFUNGAL AGENTS

Nystatin

Pharmacology. Nystatin is a polyene antifungal agent with a chemical structure very similar to that of amphotericin B. Nystatin is both fungicidal and fungistatic but is without effect on bacteria, protozoa, or viruses. The mechanism of action is dependent upon the binding of nystatin to a sterol moiety, ergosterol, present in the membrane of sensitive fungi.[87] Increased permeability of the membrane to small molecules results, allowing leakage of cellular constituents and eventually producing cell lysis and death.[148]

Very little nystatin is absorbed from the gastrointestinal tract, skin, or mucous membranes. Patients with severe renal dysfunction may acquire measurable serum levels of the drug.

Therapeutic Indications. Nystatin is used primarily to treat *Candida* infections of skin, mucous membranes, and intestinal tract. In a double-blind placebo-controlled study, Munz and colleagues[273] determined that candidal diaper dermatitis responded equally well to topical nystatin cream (100,000 U/gm) and to combined therapy with nystatin cream and oral nystatin suspension (1 ml of 100,000 U/ml given by mouth 4 times per day). Eradication of *C. albicans* from either the skin or the gastrointestinal tract was similiar in the two groups, as was the incidence of recurrence of a rash. The oral dose for infants is 1 to 2 ml (100,000 U/ml suspension) given every 6 to 8 hours.

Amphotericin B

Pharmacology. Amphotericin B, like nystatin, is a polyene antifungal. Amphotericin B is either fungicidal or fungistatic, depending on the concentration of drug and the sensitivity of the fungus. The mechanism of action of amphotericin B is the same as for nystatin.

Amphotericin is poorly absorbed from the gastrointestinal tract.[252] After IV administration only a small percentage of the drug remains in the plasma compartment. More than 90% of the drug in serum is bound to protein. Details of tissue distribution and metabolism of amphotericin B are not known. In humans, CSF concentrations of amphotericin B are only about 2% to 4% of the serum concentrations. Impaired renal function is associated with increased plasma clearance of total plasma amphotericin but not of unbound drug. Therefore, the dosage does not need to be adjusted for renal failure unless it is very severe (< 10% of normal renal function) and attributable to amphotericin B itself.[272]

Clinical Pharmacology. No comprehensive studies of pharmacokinetics have been reported for infants, although Ward and coworkers[295] measured serum concentrations of amphotericin in an 800-gm infant with disseminated candidiasis. Doses of 0.5 mg/kg IV daily or 0.75 to 1 mg/kg IV every other day resulted in serum concentrations of amphotericin between 0.2 and 0.65 μg/ml. Serum concentrations decreased only slightly by 4 and 17 days after stopping therapy (0.16 and 0.19 μg/ml, respectively). In adults, peak serum concentrations of 1.9 μg/ml were observed, with levels falling to 0.6 μg/ml by 24 hours.[147] The half-life of elimination is estimated to be about 15 days. There is a very poor correlation between serum or CSF levels of amphotericin B and clinical response. Poor correlation between in vitro susceptibility and the clinical response is also often observed; lack of penetration by amphotericin to the site of infection or organisms and the clinical condition of the patient are felt to be contributing factors. There are also major problems with the in vitro testing, including the influence of inoculum size, temperature, duration of incubation, and medium composition on the results of MIC studies.[148]

Therapeutic Indications. Parenteral amphotericin B has been used successfully to treat both systemic fungal infections and severe superficial mycoses.[231] Dosage schedules for amphotericin B have largely been devised following observations of toxicity with large doses and other clinical experiences. The initial dose is given over a period of 2 to 6 hours IV; on each subsequent day the dose can be doubled until the desired dosage is achieved. Starting doses have ranged from 0.1 to 0.3 mg/kg given IV over a period of 2 to 6 hours. The usual maintenance dose is 0.5 to 1.0 mg/kg IV given once daily or every other day over 2 to 6 hours.[148,295] Recommended therapeutic serum concentrations of amphotericin B range between 0.2 and 0.5 μg/ml. Dosage need not be reduced in patients with preexisting renal failure. Unfortunately, no objective data exist regarding the appropriate length of therapy required, although most infants have been treated for an average of 40 days (range 14 to 70 days).[295] Amphotericin is frequently employed in combination with flucytosine.

Clinical Toxicology. Renal dysfunction resulting from a reduction in renal blood flow and GFR is the most important toxic effect of amphotericin B.[151] Impairment of distal nephron function has been attributed to a direct effect of amphotericin on the tubular mucosa resulting in increased permeability to sodium, potassium, hydrogen ion, water, and low-molecular-weight solutes. The result is a loss of potassium, hyposthenuria, renal tubular acidosis, and decreased tubular sodium reabsorption. Other toxicities associated with amphotericin B include anemia (common), thrombocytopenia and granulocytopenia (rare), hypokalemia, fever, nausea, and vomiting.[233] Opinions vary as to the value of antihistamines or steroids in counteracting the side-effects. Steroids can aggravate amphotericin-induced hypokalemia. After repeated doses renal dysfunction should be anticipated (20–60% of normal). Only when renal function deteriorates to less than 20% of normal should amphotericin B therapy be interrupted for a 2- to 5-day period.[148]

Ketoconazole

Pharmacology. Ketoconazole is a member of a newer group of imidazole antifungals that includes miconazole. The drug is orally effective against a broad spectrum of fungi, yeast, and dermatophytes. The mechanism of action is believed to involve impairment of the synthesis of ergosterol, the main sterol in fungal cell membranes.[289] There is limited information on the distribution of the drug in body tissues. Ketoconazole levels in CSF vary directly with those in the serum and with CSF fluid protein content.[250] In whole blood, 84% of ketoconazole is bound to plasma protein, 15% to blood cells, and 1% is present as free drug.[252] The drug is extensively metabolized by the liver to a number of oxidative metabolites, none of which appear to possess antifungal activity. The major route of excretion is the gut via the bile, with an insignificant percentage of the administered dose recovered in the urine.

Clinical Pharmacology. In adults therapeutic doses of ketoconazole (200 to 400 mg/day) produce peak serum concentrations of between 1 and 6.5 μg/ml.[252] Plasma elimination of ketoconazole is biphasic. Within the first 10 hours after dosing, the half-life appears to be dose-dependent, ranging between 1.5 to 4 hours with doses in adults of 200 mg, and 2.2 to 2.7 hours with doses of 400 mg. After this early distribution phase there is a slower terminal elimination phase that is also dose-dependent, with a half-life in adults from 6.5 to 9.6 hours after doses of 100 to 400 mg.[260] Renal or hepatic dysfunction appears to have little or no impact on ketoconazole pharmacokinetics.

Therapeutic Indications. Ketoconazole has several attributes that may prove significant, including oral efficacy, once daily dosing requirements, and relatively low toxicity. Its approved clinical uses include in oral candidiasis (1 ml of 20 mg/ml suspension given three times daily), chronic mucocutaneous candidiasis, candiduria, coccidioidomycosis, paracoccidioidomycosis, histoplasmosis, candidiasis, and chromomycosis.[289] Except for treatment of oral candidiasis, there is no reported experience of use in neonates. Its use in neonates must be considered experimental.

Clinical Toxicology. In general, ketoconazole is well tolerated. Nausea and vomiting are the most frequently reported adverse effects, followed by pruritus, abdominal pain, rash, dizziness, constipation, diarrhea, fever, chills, and headache. Transient elevations in liver enzymes in serum have been observed, but very few patients develop symptomatic liver dysfunction while taking ketoconazole.[289]

Miconazole

Pharmacology. Miconazole is a member of a newer group of imidazole antifungals. These agents have activity against a broad range of microorganisms including bacteria (S. aureus, Bacteroides fragilis), fungi, yeast, and dermatophytes (Aspergillus species, Blastomyces species including B. dermatitidis and B. brasiliensis, Cryptococcus neoformans, Candida species). The mechanism of action is not fully understood but appears to involve increases in membrane permeability (see under Nystatin). The drug is poorly absorbed from the gastrointestinal tract. Following IV administration miconazole distributes widely in body tissues, but relatively low concentrations (<50% of serum levels) are reached in the CSF. About 90% of the drug in serum is protein-bound. Less than 1% of the dose is excreted unchanged in the urine, the majority being metabolized by the liver and excreted via the GI tract.[89] None of the metabolites of miconazole possess antifungal properties.

Clinical Pharmacology. Miconazole has been employed in the treatment of neonates with systemic candidiasis.[215] The doses employed ranged from 3 to 15 mg/kg given every 8 to 12 hours IV infused over 1 hour. Peak serum concentrations ranged from 0.7 to 1.3 μg/ml for doses of 3.8 to 6.9 mg/kg IV. In adults the half-life of miconazole is about 20 to 25 hours.[89]

Therapeutic Indications. There are currently no specific therapeutic indications for miconazole, but this agent should be considered a second-line drug for use in cases where other antifungal therapy is ineffective. McDougall and colleagues[271] were unsuccessful in treating systemic candidiasis with IV miconazole in two neonates. The drug must be given intravenously in patients with systemic fungal infections and intrathecally in patients with meningitis to produce therapeutic levels in the CSF.[222] It is not clear, however, whether response rate is improved with intrathecal administration. The relationship between miconazole concentrations in serum and other body fluids and therapeutic effects and toxicity remains undefined. Therefore, therapeutic monitoring of miconazole concentrations in tissues does not appear to be useful at this time. The dosages employed in neonates have been between 3 and 15 mg/kg given intravenously every 8 to 12 hours.

Clinical Toxicology. Hyponatremia has been reported in half the patients receiving miconazole. Phlebitis, fever, chills, rash, vomiting, pruritus, hyperlipidemia, and hematological abnormalities have also been observed.[89]

Flucytosine

Pharmacology. Flucytosine (5-fluorocytosine, 5-FC) is a fluorinated pyrimidine that is metabolized by fungi to fluorouracil. Further metabolism then ensues, resulting in the formation of 5-fluorodeoxyuridylic acid, which leads to poorly or nonfunctioning RNA or inhibition of DNA synthesis. The end result is interference with vital cellular activities. Cells of the host fortunately convert very little flucytosine to fluorouracil in contrast to the fungi.

Flucytosine is well absorbed from the gastrointestinal tract and is therefore effective when given orally. The drug distributes into body water with only about 4% in serum bound to protein. There is essentially no metabolism of flucytosine. Peak serum levels develop within a few hours of administration, and 80% to 90% of the dose is excreted in the urine. There is a linear relationship between flucytosine serum clearance and creatinine clearance levels. Thus, dosage adjustments are important with renal failure. The drug does reach therapeutic levels in the CSF with the reported CSF-to-plasma ratios averaging greater than 60%.[222,252]

Clinical Pharmacology. Ward and colleagues[295] observed peak serum concentrations of flucytosine between 25 and 37 μg/ml and trough levels between 8 and 27μg/ml in premature neonates given 10 to 25 mg/kg IV or PO every 6 hours. These serum values are similar to those reported in adults receiving similar equivalent doses.[252] The half-life of flucytosine is between 3 and 6 hours in adults with normal renal function, which is slightly shorter than values reported for premature neonates.[254] Renal disease and dysfunction markedly influence flucytosine pharmacokinetics. The effects, if any, of severe hepatic disease on flucytosine pharmacokinetics have not been determined.

Therapeutic Indications. Flucytosine has been used in a variety of fungal infections with mixed success. It has a narrow spectrum of activity limited to *Cryptococcus neoformans, Candida* species, and *Cladosporium* species. There is significant variability in sensitivity of different isolates, particularly *Candida* species, up to 50% of which may be resistant. Resistance can also develop during therapy for cryptococcosis and candidiasis.[252] Because of the narrow spectrum of activity and the problem of resistance, flucytosine is frequently used in combination with amphotericin B, particularly with serious infections (cryptococcal meningitis).[19]

The recommended dose for neonates is 20–40 mg/kg given intravenously or orally every 6 hours. The mean steady state serum concentration of flucytosine recommended for effective antifungal chemotherapy is 35 to 70 μg/ml.[287] Serum flucytosine levels should be monitored, particularly when the drug is used in combination with amphotericin B, because of the anticipated development of renal dysfunction leading to reduced clearance of flucytosine. Renal dysfunction one half of expected normal will require increasing the dosing interval of flucytosine to every 12 hours, and less than 10% of normal renal function requires dosing every 24 hours. No change in individual doses should be made, since the drug is not metabolized.

Clinical Toxicology. Bone marrow function can be depressed by flucytosine, particularly if serum flucytosine concentrations exceed 100 to 124 μg/ml. Other side-effects reported include enterocolitis, nausea, vomiting, diarrhea, and hepatic injury. As suggested above, renal dysfunction may cause significant accumulation of the drug.

ANTIVIRAL AGENTS

Viruses and obligatory intracellular parasites have a replicative cycle so integrated into the cellular activities of the host mammalian cell that it has been difficult to identify chemotherapeutic agents that selectively attack the virus without producing toxicity to the host cell. **In-**

terferons, the first substances tested as antiviral agents, are proteins produced by human cells that exert nonspecific antiviral activity through cellular metabolic processes involving synthesis of both RNA and protein.[130] The status of interferons as antiviral agents is experimental. Several other compounds, including vidarabine (adenine arabinoside) and acyclovir, are also under investigation.

Because of the high morbidity and mortality rates associated with neonatal herpes simplex viral infections, all neonates with any clinical herpes simplex infection warrant systemic antiviral therapy.[230] Neonates with varicella–zoster infection who have evidence of pulmonary and CNS disease are also candidates for antiviral therapy. Vidarabine is the only antiviral agent of proven value in the treatment of neonatal herpes infection.[230]

Vidarabine

Pharmacology. Vidarabine (adenine arabinoside, Ara-A) is a purine nucleotide approved for topical therapy of herpetic keratoconjunctivitis and for systemic therapy of herpes simplex. It appears capable of inhibiting primarily the viral DNA polymerase but also the host cellular DNA polymerase.[130] Vidarabine distributes widely in tissues (kidney, liver, spleen, skeletal muscle, brain) and fluids.[297] The drug is metabolized and excreted primarily in the urine, and 60% of the dose is excreted over the first 24 hours after administration.

Clinical Pharmacology. Vidarabine was evaluated in a randomized controlled study for treatment of neonatal herpes simplex virus infections.[230] Morbidity and mortality were significantly affected, particularly in neonates with CNS and disseminated disease. Vidarabine was administered by the IV route at a dose of 15 mg/kg over a 12-hour period.

Vidarabine is rapidly metabolized in adults to an inactive metabolite. Plasma levels of active drug are about 0.2 μg/ml with doses of 10 to 15 mg/kg per day in adults or 30 to 35 mg/kg per day in neonates.[32] The drug and metabolite are cleared primarily by the kidney (60% of dose) with a half-life value of 3.5 to 6.0 hours in adults. Patients with renal dysfunction may accumulate toxic levels, requiring dosage adjustment.

The current recommended dose for neonates is 30 mg/kg per day IV infused over an 18- to 24-hour period for 10 consecutive days.[297] For infants over 1 month of age, the dose is reduced to 15 mg/kg per day IV infused over a 12-hour period. Because of the very poor solubility of the drug (1 mg soluble in minimum of 2.2 ml of IV fluid) the administered concentration must not exceed 0.7 mg/ml of standard IV fluid.

Clinical Toxicology. Side-effects associated with vidarabine use in adults include nausea, vomiting, diarrhea, rash, ataxia, dizziness, tremors, myoclonus, and bone marrow suppression.[130,230,297] These side-effects are minimal with doses of 15 mg/kg per day and have not been observed in neonates, although some of these toxicities would be difficult to appreciate in neonates with herpes simplex infection.

Acyclovir

Pharmacology. Acyclovir is an acyclic nucleoside with selective antiviral activity against herpes simplex and varicella–zoster virus by inhibition of viral DNA synthesis.[190] Acyclovir is preferentially taken up by herpes virus–infected cells and therefore has potentially less toxicity for normal, uninfected host cells. In vitro studies with Type I herpex simplex virus showed acyclovir to be 170 times more active than vidarabine.[130]

Acyclovir distributes in the body following a two-compartment open-system pharmacokinetic model, with the volume of distribution equaling about two thirds of the body weight (range 50–80%). Thus, dividing the administered dose by this distribution volume will provide an estimate of achievable plasma concentration of acyclovir. The drug is about 15% protein bound, with no major potential for significant interaction with other substances bound to protein (e.g., biliribin). Acyclovir is excreted largely unchanged into the urine by glomerular filtration (major mechanism) and tubular secretion. Only about 15% of the dose is metabolized.[127]

Clinical Pharmacology. Multidose intravenous pharmacokinetic studies in neonates[90,235] revealed dose-dependent proportional increases in plasma levels peaking at 20 to 163 μM with IV doses of 5 to 15 mg/kg. These plasma levels are well over 100 times the 50% inhibitory dose. Trough levels ranged between 1 and 129 μM with dosing intervals of every 8 hours. The average half-life was 3.2 $\pm$ 1.2 hours; total body clearance, 109 $\pm$ 39 ml/min/1.73 m^2; and volume of distribution, 27.5 $\pm$ 7 l/1.73 m^2. Of the administered dose, 60% to 70% was recovered in the urine.

The recommended dose for treatment of clinical herpes simplex infection in neonates is 10 mg/kg IV given every 8 hours for 10 days.[90] The dosing interval should be increased to every 24 hours if renal function is less than 25% of expected normal.[245] Studies in adults have demonstrated efficacy of acyclovir against herpes zoster with IV doses of 5 to 7.5 mg/kg every 8 hours.[15] Studies comparing the effectiveness of acyclovir and vidarabine against neonatal herpes simplex virus infections are in progress.

Clinical Toxicology. Toxicities associated with acyclovir are minor. Local irritation at the site of administration and transient renal dysfunction have been reported, although studies by Yeager[235] in neonates did not demonstrate any renal or other toxicities due to administration of acyclovir.

References

1. Adelman RD, Zakauddin S: Urinary enzyme activities in children and neonates receiving gentamicin therapy. Dev Pharmacol Ther 1:325, 1980.
2. Agbayani MM, Khan AJ, Kemawikasit P, et al: Pharmacokinetics and safety of cefamandole in newborn infants. Antimicrob Agents Chemother 15:674, 1979.
3. Altemeier WA III, Ayoub EM: Erythromycin prophylaxis for pertussis. Pediatrics 59:623, 1977.
4. Aranda JV, Collinge JM, Clarkson S: Epidemiologic aspects of drug utilization in a newborn intensive care unit. Semin Perinatol 6:148, 1982.
5. Appel, GB, Neu HC: The nephrotoxicity of antimicrobial agents (second of three parts). N Engl J Med 293:722, 1977.
6. Asmar BI, Maqbool S, Dajani AS: Hematologic abnormalities after oral trimethoprim–sulfamethoxazole therapy in children. Am J Dis Child 135:1100, 1981.
7. Assael BM, Gianni, V, Marini A, et al: Gentamicin dosage in preterm and term neonates. Arch Dis Child 52:883, 1977.
8. Assael BM, Parini R, Rusconi F, Cavanna G: Influence of intrauterine maturation on the pharmacokinetics of amikacin in the neonatal period. Pediatr Red 16:810, 1982.
9. Axline SG, Yaffe SJ, Simon HJ: Clinical pharmacology of antimicrobials in premature infants: II. Ampicillin, methicillin, oxacillin, neomycin, and colistin. Pediatrics 39:97, 1967.
10. Baker CJ: Group B streptococcal infections in neonates. Pediatr Rev 1:5, 1979.
11. Banner W, Gooch WM, Burckart G, Korones SB: Pharmacokinetics of nafcillin in infants with low birth weights. Antimicrob Agents Chemother 17:691, 1980.
12. Bartlett JG: Chloramphenicol. Med Clin North Am 66:91, 1982.
13. Bauer AW, Kirby WMM, Sherris JC, Turck M: Antibiotic susceptibility testing by a standardized single disk method. Am J Clin Pathol 45:493, 1966.
14. Beachler CW, Speer ME, Mason EO Jr, Yow MD: Pharmacology of kanamycin in the newborn. South Med J 75:301, 1982.
15. Bean B, Braun C, Balfour HH: Acyclovir therapy for acute herpes zoster. Lancet 2:118, 1982.
16. Beard CM, Noller KL, O'Fallon WM, et al: Lack of evidence for cancer due to use of metronidazole. N Engl J Med 301:519, 1979.
17. Beem MO, Saxon E, Tipple MA: Treatment of chlamydial pneumonia of infancy. Pediatrics 63:198, 1979.
18. Bell, WE, McGuinness GA: Suppurative central nervous system infections in the neonate. Semin Perinatol 6:1, 1982.
19. Bennett JE, Dismukes WE, Duma RJ, et al: A comparison of amphotericin B alone and combined with flucytosine in the treatment of cryptococcal meningitis. N Engl J Med 301:126, 1979.
20. Bennett WM, Muther RS, Parker RA, et al: Drug therapy in renal failure: Dosing guidelines for adults. Ann Intern Med 93:62, 1980.
21. Berman BW, King FH Jr, Rubenstein DS, Long SS: *Bacteroides fragilis* meningitis in a neonate successfully treated with metronidazole. J Pediatr 93:793, 1978.
22. Bertino JS, Kliegman RM, Myers CM, Blumer JL: Alteration in gentamicin pharmacokinetics during neonatal exchange transfusion. Dev Pharmacol Ther 4:205, 1982.
23. Best WR: Chloramphenicol-associated blood dyscrasias. JAMA 201:99, 1967.
24. Black SB, Levine F, Shinefield HR: The necessity for monitoring chloramphenicol levels when treating neonatal meningitis. J Pediatr 92:235, 1978.
25. Boe RW, Williams CPS, Bennett JV, Oliver TK Jr: Serum levels of methicillin and ampicillin in newborn and premature infants in relation to postnatal age. Pediatrics 39:194, 1967.
26. Bradsher RW: Relapse of gram-negative bacillary meningitis after cefotaxime therapy. JAMA 248:1214, 1982.
27. Breen KJ, Bryant RE, Levinson JD, Schenker S: Neomycin absorption in man: Studies of oral and enema administration and effect of intestinal ulceration. Ann Intern Med 76:211, 1972.
28. Brodersen R: The mechanism of drug-induced displacement of bilirubin from albumin. In Stern L, Hansen BF, Kilderberg P (eds): Intensive Care in the Newborn. Pp 17–84. New York, Masson Publishing, USA, 1976.
29. Brogden RN, Heel RC, Speight TM, Avery GS: Cefoxitin: A review of its antibacterial activity, pharmacological properties and therapeutic use. Drugs 17:1, 1979.
30. Broughton RA, Mason EO, Baker CJ: Relapse of *Escherichia coli* meningitis following therapy with moxalactam. Pediatr Infect Dis 1:24, 1982.
31. Bryan LE, Van Den Elzen HM: Effects of membrane-energy mutations and cations on streptomycin and gentamicin accumulation by bacteria: A model for entry of streptomycin and gentamicin in susceptible and resistant bacteria. Antimicrob Agents Chemother 12:163, 1977.
32. Bryson Y, Connor JD: Pharmacology and efficacy of Ara-A in neonates and adults. Abstract 974, Nineteenth Interscience Conference on Antimicrobial Agents and Chemotherapy, 1979.
33. Burns L, Hodgman J: Studies of prematures given erythromycin estolate. Am J Dis Child 106:280, 1963.
34. Burns L, Hodgman JE, Wehrle PF: Treatment of premature infants with oxacillin. Antimicrob Agents Chemother, 4:192, 1964.

35. Chang MJ, Escobedo M, Anderson DC, et al: Kanamycin and gentamicin treatment of neonatal sepsis and meningitis. Pediatrics 56:695, 1975.
36. Chang CT, Khan AJ, Agbayani MM, et al: Pharmacokinetics and safety of cefamandole in infants and children. Antimicrob Agents Chemother 14:838, 1978.
37. Chadwick EG, Yogev R, Shulman ST, et al: Single-dose ceftriaxone pharmacokinetics in pediatric patients with central nervous system infections. J Pediatr 102:134, 1983.
38. Chesney RW: Drug-induced hypokalemia. Am J Dis Child 130:1055, 1976.
39. Chien YW, Mizuba SS: Activity–electroreduction relationship of antimicrobial metronidazole analogues. J Med Chem 21:374, 1978.
40. Cho (Chang) N, Ito T, Saito T, Fukada M: Studies on cefazolin in obstetrics and gynecology with special reference to its clinical pharmacology in the neonate. Adv Microb Antineoplast Chemother: I(2), 1187, 1972.
41. Cohlan SQ, Bevelander G, Tiamsic T: Growth inhibition of prematures receiving tetracycline. Am J Dis Child 105:453, 1963.
42. Cookson B, Tripp J, Leung T, Williams JD: Evaluation of amikacin dosage regimes in the low and very low birth weight newborn. Infection 8(Suppl 3): S239, 1980.
43. Craig WA, Kunin CM: Significance of serum protein and tissue binding of antimicrobial agents. Ann Rev Med 27:287, 1976.
44. Craig WA, Gerber AU: Pharmacokinetics of cefoperazone: A review. Drugs 22(Suppl 1):34, 1981.
45. Cunha BA, Ristuccia AM: Third generation cephalosporins. Med Clin North Am 66:283, 1982.
46. Dajani AS, Kauffman RE: The renaissance of chloramphenicol. Pediatr Clin North Am 28:195, 1981.
47. Dashefsky B, Klein JO: The treatment of bacterial infections in the newborn infant. Clin Perinatol 8:559, 1981.
48. Del Rio M, McCracken Jr GH, Nelson JD, et al: Pharmacokinetics and cerebrospinal fluid bactericidal activity of ceftriaxone in the treatment of pediatric patients with bacterial meningitis. Antimicrob Agents Chemother 22:622, 1982.
49. Diaz CR, Kane JG, Parker RH, Pelsor FR: Pharmacokinetics of nafcillin in patients with renal failure. Antimicrob Agents Chemother 12:98, 1977.
50. Dillon HC Jr: Studies of moxalactam for gram-negative and *Haemophilus influenzae* meningitis: An appraisal. J Pediatr 99:907, 1981.
51. Driessen OMJ, Sorgedrager N, Michel MF, et al: Pharmacokinetic aspects of therapy with ampicillin and kanamycin in newborn infants. Eur J Clin Pharmacol 13:449, 1978.
52. Dudley MN, Barriere SL: Cefotaxime: Microbiology, pharmacology, and clinical use. Clin Pharmacy 1:114, 1982.
53. Dunkle LM: Central nervous system chloramphenicol concentration in premature infants. Antimicrob Agents Chemother 13:427, 1978.
54. Edwards DI: The action of metronidazole on DNA: J Antimicrob Chemother 3:43, 1977.
55. Eichenwald HF: Some observations on dosage and toxicity of kanamycin in premature and full-term infants. Ann NY Acad Sci 132:984, 1966.
56. Eichenwald HF, McCracken GH Jr: Antimicrobial therapy in infants and children. J Pediatr 93:337, 1978.
57. Eviatar L, Eviatar A: Aminoglycoside ototoxicity in the neonatal period: Possible etiologic factor in delayed postural control. Otolaryngol Head Neck Surg 89:818, 1981.
58. Falk SA: Combined effects of noise and ototoxic drugs. Environ Health Perspect 2:5, 1972.
59. Falk SA, Woods NF: Hospital noise—levels and potential health hazards. N Engl J Med 289:774, 1973.
60. Farr B, Mandell GL: Rifampin. Med Clin North Am 66:157, 1982.
61. Feigin RD, Pickering LK, Anderson D, et al: Clindamycin treatment of osteomyelitis and septic arthritis in children. Pediatrics 55:213, 1975.
62. Fekety R: Vancomycin. Med Clin North Am 66:175, 1982.
63. Feldman WE: Effects of ampicillin and chloramphenicol against *Haemophilus influenzae.* Pediatrics 61:406, 1978.
64. Feldman WE, Nelson JD, Stanberry LR: Clinical and pharmacokinetic evaluation of nafcillin in infants and children. J Pediatr 93:1029, 1978.
65. Feldman WE, Moffitt S, Manning NS: Penetration of cefoxitin into cerebrospinal fluid of infants and children with bacterial meningitis. Antimicrob Agents Chemother 21:468, 1982.
66. Fellner MJ: Penicillin allergy 1976: A review of reactions, detection and current management. Int J Dermatol 15:497, 1976.
67. Fields JP: Bulging fontanel: A complication of tetracycline therapy in infants. J Pediatr 58:74, 1961.
68. File TM Jr, Tan JS, Gardner WG, Baird I: Cefoperazone versus cefamandole in the treatment of acute bacterial lower respiratory tract infections. J Antimicrob Chemother 11:75, 1983.
69. Finitzo-Hieber T, McCracken GH Jr, Roeser RJ, et al: Ototoxicity in neonates treated with gentamicin and kanamycin: Results of a four-year controlled follow-up study. Pediatrics 63:443, 1979.
70. Finland M, Garner C, Wilcox C, Sabath LD: Susceptibility of "enterobacteria" to aminoglycoside antibiotics: Comparisons with tetracyclines, polymyxins, chloramphenicol, and spectinomycin. J Infect Dis 134(Suppl):S57, 1976.
71. Fitzpatrick BJ, Standiford HC: A comparative evaluation of moxalactam: Antimicrobial activity, pharmacokinetics, adverse reactions, and clinical efficacy. Pharmacotherapy 2:197, 1982.
72. Friedman CA, Lovejoy FC, Smith AL: Chloramphenicol disposition in infants and children. J Pediatr 95:1071, 1979.
73. Friedman GD: Cancer after metronidazole. N Engl J Med 302:519, 1980.
74. Fujii R, Grossman M, Ticknor W: Micromethod for determination of concentration of antibiotics in serum for application in clinical pediatrics. Pediatrics 28:662, 1961.
75. Galpin JE, Shinaberger JH, Stanley TM, et al: Acute interstitial nephritis due to methicillin. Am J Med 65:756, 1978.
76. Gibbons RJ, Reichelderfer TE: Transplacental transmission of demethylchloretracycline and toxicity studies in premature and full-term, newly born infants. Antibiot Med Clin Ther 7:618, 1960.
77. Gidion R, Marget W: Zur Frage der dosierung injizierbarer Tetracycline im sauglingsalter. Munchn Med Wochensch 103:967, 1961.
78. Glazer JP, Danish MA, Plotkin SA, Yaffe SJ: Disposition of chloramphenicol in low-birth-weight infants. Pediatrics 66:573, 1980.
79. Granoff DM, Daum RS: Spread of *Haemophilus in-*

fluenzae type b: Recent epidemiologic and therapeutic considerations. J Pediatr 97:854, 1980.

80. Greene GR, Cohen E: Nafcillin-induced neutropenia in children. Pediatrics 61:94, 1978.
81. Gribble MJ, Chow AW: Erythromycin. Med Clin North Am 66:79, 1982.
82. Grieco MH: Antibiotic resistance. Med Clin North Am 66:25, 1981.
83. Gross BJ, Branchflower RV, Burke TR, et al: Bone marrow toxicity in vitro of chloramphenicol and its metabolites. Toxicol Appl Pharmacol 64:557, 1982.
84. Grossman M, Ticknor W: Serum levels of ampicillin, cephalothin, cloxacillin, and nafcillin in the newborn infant. Antimicrob Agents Chemother, 5:214, 1965.
85. Grylack L, Boehnert J, Scanlon J: Serum concentration of gentamicin following oral administration to preterm newborns. Dev Pharmacol Ther 5:47, 1982.
86. Hallberg T, Svenningsen NW: Cephalothin in neonatal infections. Acta Paediatr Scand 206:110, 1970.
87. Hamilton-Miller JMT: Fungal sterols and the mode of action of the polyene antibiotics. Adv Appl Microbiol 17:109, 1974.
88. Hammerschlag MR, Klein JO, Herschel M, et al: Patterns of use of antibiotics in two newborn nurseries. N Engl J Med 296:1268, 1977.
89. Heel RC, Brogden RN, Pakes GE, et al: Miconazole: A preliminary review of its therapeutic efficacy in systemic fungal infections. Drugs 19:7, 1980.
90. Hintz M, Connor JD, Spector SA, et al: Neonatal acyclovir pharmacokinetics in patients with herpes virus infections. Am J Med 73:210, 1982.
91. Howard JE, Donoso E, Mimica I, Zilleruelo G: Gentamicin in infections in infants with low birth weights. J Infect Dis 124(Suppl):S232, 1971.
92. Howard JB, McCracken GH Jr: Reappraisal of kanamycin usage in neonates. J Pediatr 86:949, 1975.
93. Howard JB, McCracken GH Jr, Trujillo H, Mohs E: Amikacin in newborn infants: Comparative pharmacology with kanamycin and clinical efficacy in 45 neonates with bacterial diseases. Antimicrob Agents Chemother 10:205, 1976.
94. Huang NN, High RH: Effectiveness of penicillin administered orally at intervals of twelve hours. J Pediatr 42:532, 1953.
95. Iannini PB, Kinkel MJ: Cefotaxime failure in group A streptococcal meningitis. JAMA 248:1878, 1982.
96. Itsarayoungyuen S, Riff L, Schauf V, et al: Tobramycin and gentamicin are equally safe for neonates: Results of a double-blind randomized trial with quantitative assessment of renal function. Pediatr Pharmacol 2:143, 1982.
97. Jackson EA, McLeod DC: Pharmacokinetics and dosing of antimicrobial agents in renal impairment, part II. Am J Hosp Pharm 31:137, 1974.
98. Jager-Roman E, Doyle PE, Baird-Lambert J, et al: Pharmacokinetics and tissue distribution of metronidazole in the newborn infant. J Pediatr 100:651, 1982.
99. Jawetz E, Gunnison JB: Experimental basis of combined antibiotic action. JAMA 150:693, 1952.
100. Kafetzis DA, Brater DC, Kapiki AN, et al: Treatment of severe neonatal infections with cefotaxime. Efficacy and pharmacokinetics. J Pediatr 100:483, 1982.
100a. Kane JG, Parker RH, Jordan GW, et al: Nafcillin concentration in cerebrospinal fluid during treatment of staphylococcal infections. Ann Intern Med 87:309, 1977.
101. Kaplan JM, McCracken GH Jr, Thomas ML, et al: Clinical pharmacology of tobramycin in newborns. Am J Dis Child 125:656, 1973.
102. Kaplan JM, McCracken GH Jr, Horton LJ, et al: Pharmacologic studies in neonates given large dosages of ampicillin. J Pediatr 84:571, 1974.
103. Kaplan SL, Mason EO Jr, Garcia H, et al: Pharmacokinetics and cerebrospinal fluid penetration of moxalactam in children with bacterial meningitis. J Pediatr 98:152, 1981.
104. Kaplan SL, Mason EO Jr: *In vitro* synergy of ampicillin and chloramphenicol against gram-negative bacteria. Pediatr Pharmacol 1:305, 1981.
105. Kauffman RE, Miceli JN, Strebel L, et al: Pharmacokinetics of chloramphenicol and chloramphenicol succinate in infants and children. J Pediatr 98:315, 1981.
106. Kauffman RE, Thirumoorthi MC, Buckley JA, et al: Relative bioavailability of intravenous chloramphenicol succinate and oral chloramphenicol palmitate in infants and children. J Pediatr 99:963, 1981.
107. Kelly DR, Nilo ER, Berggren RB: Deafness after topical neomycin wound irrigation. N Engl J Med 280:1338, 1969.
108. Keyserling H, Feldman WE, Moffitt S, et al: Clinical pharmacokinetic evaluation of parenteral moxalactam in infants and children. Antimicrob Agents Chemother 21:898, 1982.
109. Kitzing W, Nelson JD, Mohs E: Comparative toxicities of methicillin and nafcillin. Am J Dis Child 135:52, 1981.
110. Korzeniowski DM, Hook EW: Aminocyclitols: Aminoglycosides and spectinomycin. In Mandell GL, Douglas RG Jr, Benett JE (eds): Principles and Practices of Infectious Diseases. Pp 249–273. New York, John Wiley & Sons, 1979.
111. Koup JR, Gibaldi M, McNamara P, et al: Interaction of chloramphenicol with phenytoin and phenobarbital. J Clin Pharmacol Ther 24:571, 1978.
112. Krasinski K, Kusmiesz H, Nelson JD: Pharmacologic interactions among chloramphenicol, phenytoin, and phenobarbital. Pediatr Infect Dis 1:232, 1982.
113. Kuder HV: Propionyl erythromycin: A review of 20,525 case reports for side effect data. Clin Pharmacol Ther 1:604, 1960.
114. Kumin GD: Clinical nephrotoxicity of tobramycin and gentamicin. JAMA 244:1808, 1980.
115. Kunin CM: Clinical pharmacology of the new penicillins. I. Importance of serum protein binding in determining antimicrobial activity and concentration in serum. Clin Pharmacol Ther 7:166, 1966.
116. Kunin CM: A guide to use of antibiotics in patients with renal disease. A table of recommended doses and factors governing serum levels. Ann Intern Med 67:151, 1967.
117. Kunin CM: Dosage schedules of antimicrobial agents: A historical review. Rev Infect Dis 3:4, 1981.
118. Latif R, Thirumoorthi MC, Buckley JA, et al: Pharmacokinetic and clinical evaluation of moxalactam in infants and children. Dev Pharmacol Ther 3:222, 1981.
119. Latif R, Dajani AS: Ceftriaxone diffusion into cerebrospinal fluid of children with meningitis. Antimicrob Agents Chemother 23:46, 1983.
120. Lee EL, Robinson MJ, Thong ML, Puthucheary DS: Rifamycin in neonatal flavobacteria meningitis. Arch Dis Child 51:209, 1976.

121. Lee EL, Robinson MJ, Thong ML, et al: Intraventricular chemotherapy in neonatal meningitis. J Pediatr 91:991, 1977.

122. Leff RD, Roberts RJ: Aminoglycoside dosage in pediatric patients: Considerations regarding pharmacokinetic-based dose adjustment in patients requiring high versus low dose therapy. Dev Pharmacol Ther 3:242, 1981.

123. LeFrock JL, Molavi A, Prince RA: Clindamycin. Med Clin North Am 66:103, 1982.

124. Lesar TS, Zaske DE: Antibiotics and hepatic disease. Med Clin North Am 66:257, 1982.

125. Levin B, Neill CA: Oral penicillin in the newborn. Arch Dis Child 24:171, 1949.

126. Lietman PS: Chloramphenicol and the neonate—1979 view. Clin Pharmacol 6:151, 1979.

127. Lietman PS: Acyclovir clinical pharmacology. Am J Med 73(Suppl):193, 1982.

128. Lindberg J, Rosenhall U, Nylen O, Ringner A: Long-term outcome of *Haemophilus influenzae* meningitis related to antibiotic treatment. Pediatrics 60:1, 1977.

129. Lischner H, Seligman SJ, Krammer A, Parmelee AH Jr: An outbreak of neonatal deaths among term infants associated with administration of chloramphenicol. J Pediatr 59:21, 1961.

130. Liu C: Antiviral drugs. Med Clin North Am 66:235, 1982.

131. Luft FC, Rankin LI, Sloan RS, Yum MN: Recovery from aminoglycoside nephrotoxicity with continued drug administration. Antimicrob Agents Chemother 3:284, 1978.

132. Lwin N, Collipp PJ: Absorption and tolerance of clindamycin-2-palmitate in infants below 6 months of age. Curr Ther Res 12:648, 1970.

133. Mandell GL, Moorman DR: Treatment of experimental staphylococcal infections: Effect of rifampin alone and in combination on development of rifampin resistance. Antimicrob Agents Chemother 17:658, 1980.

134. Mathies AW Jr, Leedom JM, Ivler D, et al: Antibiotic antagonism in bacterial meningitis. Antimicrob Agents Chemother, 7:218, 1967.

135. McCracken GH Jr, Jones LG: Gentamicin in neonatal period. Am J Dis Child 120:524, 1970.

136. McCracken GH Jr, Chrane DF, Thomas ML: Pharmacologic evaluation of gentamicin in newborn infants. J Infect Dis 124(Suppl):S214, 1971.

137. McCracken GH Jr, Ginsberg C, Chrane DF, et al: Clinical pharmacology of penicillin in newborn infants. J Pediatr 82:692, 1973.

138. McCracken GH Jr: Pharmacologic basis for antimicrobial therapy in newborn infants. Am J Dis Child 128:407, 1974.

139. McCracken GH Jr, Nelson JD: Commentary: An appraisal of tobramycin usage in pediatrics. J Pediatr 88:315, 1976.

140. McCracken GH Jr: Clinical pharmacology of antibacterial agents. In Remington JS, Klein JO (eds): Infectious Diseases of the Fetus and Newborn Infant. Pp 1020–1067. Philadelphia, WB Saunders, 1976.

141. McCracken GH Jr: Intraventricular treatment of neonatal meningitis due to gram-negative bacilli. J Pediatr 91:1037, 1977.

142. McCracken GH Jr, Threlkeld N, Thomas ML: Intravenous administration of kanamycin and gentamicin in newborn infants. Pediatrics 60:463, 1977.

143. McCracken GH Jr, Eichenwald HF: Part II. Therapy of infectious conditions. J Pediatr 93:357, 1978.

144. McCracken GH Jr, Mize SG, Threlkeld N: Intraventricular gentamicin therapy in gram-negative bacillary meningitis in infancy. Lancet 1:787, 1980.

145. McCracken GH Jr, Threlkeld NE, Thomas ML: Pharmacokinetics of cefotaxime in newborn infants. Antimicrob Agents Chemother 21:683, 1982.

146. McCullough DC, Kane JG, Harleman G, Wells M: Antibiotic prophylaxis in ventricular shunt surgery. II. Antibiotic concentrations in cerebrospinal fluid. Child's Brain 7:190, 1980.

146a. McMahon FG: Disulfiram-like reaction to a cephalosporin. JAMA 243:2397, 1980.

147. Meade RH III: Drug therapy reviews: Clinical pharmacology and therapeutic use of antimycotic drugs. Am J Hosp Pharm 36:1326, 1979.

148. Medoff G, Kobayashi GS: Strategies in the treatment of systemic fungal infections. N Engl J Med 302:145, 1980.

149. Meissner HC, Smith AL: The current status of chloramphenicol. Pediatrics 64:348, 1979.

150. Miceli JN, Olson WA, Cohen SN: Elimination kinetics of isoniazid in the newborn infant. Dev Pharmacol Ther 2:235, 1981.

151. Miller RP, Bates JH: Amphotericin B toxicity: A follow-up report of 53 patients. Ann Intern Med 71:1089, 1969.

152. Molavi A, LeFrock JL, Prince RA: Metronidazole. Med Clin North Am 66:121, 1982.

153. Mull MM: The tetracyclines. Am J Dis Child 112:483, 1966.

154. Müller M: Mode of action of metronidazole on anaerobic microorganisms. In Phillips I, Collier J (eds): Metronidazole P 223. London, Royal Society of Medicine and Academic Press, London, Grune & Stratton, New York, 1979.

155. Murray T, Downey KM, Yunis AA: Degradation of isolated deoxyribonucleic acid mediated by nitroso-chloramphenicol. Biochem Pharmacol 31:2291, 1982.

156. Myers MG, Roberts RJ, Mirhij NJ: Effects of gestational age, birth weight, and hypoxemia on pharmacokinetics of amikacin in serum of infants. Antimicrob Agents Chemother 11:1027, 1977.

157. Myers MG, Roberts RJ, Mirhij NJ: Effects of hypoxemia upon aminoglycoside serum pharmacokinetics. Curr Chemother 2:994, 1978.

158. Nahata MC, Debolt SL, Powell DA: Adverse effects of methicillin, nafcillin, and oxacillin in pediatric patients. Dev Pharmacol Ther 4:117, 1982.

159. Nahata MC, Durrell DE, Barson WJ: Moxalactam epimer kinetics in children. Clin Pharmacol Ther 31:528, 1982.

160. Nation RL, Huang S, Vidyasagar D, et al: Absorption of oral neomycin in premature infants with suspected necrotizing enterocolitis. Dev Pharmacol Ther 5:53, 1982.

161. Naveh Y, Friedman A: Rifampicin therapy in gram-negative bacteraemia in infancy. Arch Dis Child 48:967, 1973.

162. Nelson JD, McCracken GH Jr: Clinical pharmacology of carbenicillin and gentamicin in the neonate and comparative efficacy with ampicillin and gentamicin. Pediatrics 52:801, 1973.

163. Nelson JD, Kusmiesz H, Shelton S, Woodman E: Clinical pharmacology and efficacy of ticarcillin in infants and children. Pediatrics 61:858, 1978.

164. Neu HC: The *in vitro* activity, human pharmacology, and clinical effectiveness of new beta-lactam antibiotics. Ann Rev Pharmacol Toxicol 22:599, 1982.

165. Neu HC: Carbenicillin and ticarcillin. Med Clin North Am 66:61, 1982.

166. O'Connor WJ: Warren GH, Mandala PS, et al: Serum concentrations of nafcillin in newborn infants and children. Antimicrob Agents Chemother, 4:188, 1964.

167. Olson WA, Dayton PG, Israili ZH, Pruitt AW: Spectrophotofluorometric assay for isoniazid and acetyl isoniazid in plasma adapted to pediatric studies. Clin Chem 23:745, 1977.

168. Oppenheimer S, Beaty HN, Petersdorf RG: Pathogenesis of meningitis. VIII. Cerebrospinal fluid and blood concentrations of methicillin, cephalothin, and cephaloridine in experimental pneumococcal meningitis. J Lab Clin Med 73:535, 1969.

169. Paisley JW, Smith AL, Smith DH: Gentamicin in newborn infants: Comparison of intramuscular and intravenous administration. Am J Dis Child 126:473, 1973.

170. Paisley JW, Washington JA: Susceptibility of *Escherichia coli* K1 to four combinations of antimicrobial agents potentially useful for treatment of neonatal meningitis. J Infect Dis 140:183, 1979.

171. Pakter RL, Russell TR, Mielke H, West D: Coagulopathy associated with the use of moxalactam. JAMA 248:1100, 1982.

172. Parry MF, Neu HC: A comparative study of ticarcillin plus tobramycin versus carbenicillin plus gentamicin for the treatment of serious infections due to gram-negative bacili. Am J Med 64:961, 1978.

173. Perkins HR, Nieto M: Part IV. Inhibitors of the synthesis of peptidoglycans and other wall components. The chemical basis for the action of the vancomycin group of antibiotics. Ann NY Acad Sci 235:348, 1974.

174. Perlman D (ed): Structure–Activity Relationship Among the Semi-synthetic Antibiotics. New York, Academic Press, 1977.

175. Perlstein PH, Callison C, White M, et al: Errors in drug computations during newborn intensive care. Am J Dis Child 133:376, 1979.

176. Philips JB, Cassady G: Amikacin: Pharmacology, indications, and cautions for use, and dose recommendations. Semin Perinatol 6:166, 1982.

177. Philips JB, Satterwhite C, Dworsky ME, Cassady G: Recommended amikacin doses in newborns often produce excessive serum levels. Pediatr Pharmacol 2:121, 1982.

178. Pickering LK, Gearhart P: Effect of time and concentration upon interaction between gentamicin, tobramycin, netilmicin, or amikacin and carbenicillin or ticarcillin. Antimicrob Agents Chemother 15:592, 1979.

179. Pieper JA, Vidal RA, Schentag JJ: Animal model distinguishing *in vitro* from *in vivo* carbenicillin–aminoglycoside interactions. Antimicrob Agents Chemother 18:604, 1980.

180. Pittinger CB, Eryasa Y, Adamson R: Antibiotic-induced paralysis. Anesth Analg (Cleve) 49:487, 1970.

181. Prober CG, Yeager AS, Arvin AM: The effect of chronological age on the serum concentrations of amikacin in sick term and premature infants. J Pediatr 98:636, 1981.

182. Quintiliani R, French M, Nightingale CH: First and second generation cephalosporins. Med Clin North Am 66:183, 1982.

183. Rahal JJ Jr: Antibiotic combinations: The clinical relevance of synergy and antagonism. Medicine 57:179, 1978.

184. Rajchgot P, Prober CG, Soldin S, et al: Initiation of chloramphenicol therapy in the newborn infant. J Pediatr 101:1018, 1982.

185. Reed MD, Bertino JS Jr, Aronoff SC, et al: Evaluation of moxalactam. Clin Pharmacy 1:124, 1982.

186. Rees E, Tait A, Hobson D, et al: Persistence of chlamydial infection after treatment for neonatal conjuctivitis. Arch Dis Child 56:193, 1981.

187. Riff L, Schauf V: Use of aminoglycosides in the neonate. Semin Perinatol 6:155, 1982.

188. Ring JC, Cates KL, Belani KK, et al: Rifampin for CSF shunt infections caused by coagulase-negative staphylocci. J Pediatr 95:317, 1979.

189. Roos R, von Hattingberg HM, Belohradsky BH, Marget W: Pharmacokinetics of cefoxitin in premature and newborn infants studied by continuous serum level monitoring during combination therapy with penicillin and amikacin. Infection 8:301, 1980.

190. Rosenberry KR, Bryan CK, Sohn CA: Acyclovir: Evaluation of a new antiviral agent. Clin Pharmacy 1:399, 1982.

191. Rowe DS, Aicardi EZ, Dawson CR, Schachter J: Purulent ocular discharge in neonates: Significance of *Chlamydia trachomatis.* Pediatrics 63:628, 1979.

192. Sack CM, Koup JR, Smith AL: Chloramphenicol pharmacokinetics in infants and young children. Pediatrics 66:579, 1980.

193. Sack CM, Koup JR, Opheim KE, et al: Chloramphenicol succinate kinetics in infants and young children. Pediatr Pharmacol 2:93, 1982.

194. Sande MA, Mandell GL: Miscellaneous antibacterial agents; antifungal and antiviral agents. In Gilman AG, Goodman LS, Gilman A (eds): The Pharmacological Basis of Therapeutics, 6th ed. Chap 54, P. 1222. New York, Macmillan, 1980.

195. Sardeman H, Colding H, Hendel J, et al: Kinetics and dose calculations of amikacin in the newborn. Clin Pharmacol Ther 20:59, 1976.

196. Sarff LD, McCracken GH Jr, Thomas ML, et al: Clinical pharmacology of methicillin in neonates. J Pediatr 90:1005, 1977.

197. Schaad UB, McCracken GH, Nelson JD: Clinical pharmacology and efficacy of vancomycin in pediatric patients. J Pediatr 96:119, 1980.

198. Schaad UB, McCracken GH Jr, Threlkeld N, Thomas ML: Clinical evaluation of a new broad-spectrum oxa-beta-lactam antibiotic, moxalactam, in neonates and infants. J Pediatr 98:129, 1981.

199. Schaad UB, Stoeckel K: Single-dose pharmacokinetics of ceftriaxone in infants and young children. Antimicrob Agents Chemother 21:248, 1982.

200. Schentag JJ: Aminoglycosides. In Evans WE, Schentag JJ (eds): Applied Pharmacokinetics: Principles of Therapeutic Drug Monitoring. P. 174. San Francisco, Applied Therapeutics, Inc, 1980.

201. Shattil SJ, Bennett JS, McDonough M, Turnbull J: Carbenicillin and penicillin G inhibit platelet function *in vitro* by impairing the interaction of agonists with the platelet surface. J Clin Invest 65:329, 1980.

202. Sheng KT, Huang NN, Promadhattavedi V: Serum concentrations of cephalothin in infants and children and placental transmission of the antibiotic. Antimicrob Agents Chemother, 4:200, 1964.

203. Shimizu K: Cefoperazone: Absorption, excretion, distribution, and metabolism. Clin Ther 3(Suppl):60, 1980.

204. Silverio J, Poole JW: Serum concentrations of ampicillin in newborn infants after oral administration. Pediatrics 51:578, 1973.

205. Simon HJ, Axline SG: Clinical pharmacology of kan-

amycin in premature infants. Ann NY Acad Sci 132:1020, 1966.

206. Smith, CR, Baughman KL, Edwards CQ, et al: Controlled comparison of amikacin and gentamicin. N Engl J Med 296:349, 1977.

207. Smith CR, Lipsky JJ, Laskin OL, et al: Double-blind comparison of the nephrotoxicity and auditory toxicity of gentamicin and tobramycin. N Engl J Med 302:1106, 1980.

208. Smith LG, Sensakovic J: Trimethoprim–sulfamethoxazole. Med Clin North Am 66:143, 1982.

209. Spector R, Lorenzo AV: Inhibition of penicillin transport from the cerebrospinal fluid after intracisternal inoculation of bacteria. J Clin Invest 545:316, 1974.

210. Spector R, Snodgrass SR: The effect of uremia on penicillin flux between blood and cerebrospinal fluid. J Lab Clin Med 87:749, 1976.

211. Springer C, Eyal F, Michel J: Pharmacology of trimethoprim–sulfamethoxazole in newborn infants. J Pediatr 100:647, 1982.

212. Srinivasan S, Francke EL, Neu HC: Comparative pharmacokinetics of cefoperazone and cefamendole. Antimicrob Agents Chemother 19:298, 1981.

213. Strausbaugh LJ, Sande MA: Factors influencing the therapy of experimental *Proteus mirabilis* meningitis in rabbits. J Infect Dis 137:251, 1978.

214. Sullivan D, Csuka ME, Blanchard B: Erythromycin ethylsuccinate hepatotoxicity. JAMA 243:1074, 1980.

215. Sung JP, Rajani K, Chopra DR, et al: Miconazole therapy for systemic candidiasis in a cojoined (Siamese) twin and a premature newborn. Am J Surg 138:688, 1979.

216. Sutherland JM: Fatal cardiovascular collapse of infants receiving large amounts of chloramphenicol. Am J Dis Child 97:761, 1959.

217. Szefler SJ, Wynn RJ, Clarke DF, et al: Relationship of gentamicin serum concentrations to gestational age in preterm and term neonates. J Pediatr 97:312, 1980.

218. Tedesco FJ, Barton RW, Alpers DH: Clindamycin-associated colitis: A prospective study. Ann Intern Med 81:429, 1974.

219. Tenenbaum MJ, Kaplan MH: Antibiotic combinations. Med Clin North Am 66:17, 1982.

220. Thirumoorthi MC, Buckley JA, Aravind MK, et al: Diffusion of moxalactam into the cerebrospinal fluid in children with bacterial meningitis. J Pediatr 99:975, 1981.

221. Thompson MIB, Russo ME, Saxon BJ, et al: Gentamicin inactivation by piperacillin or carbinicillin in patients with end-stage renal disease. Antimicrob Agents Chemother 21:268, 1982.

222. Utz JP: Chemotherapy of systemic mycoses. Med Clin North Am 66:221, 1982.

223. van Winzum C: Clinical safety and tolerance of cefoxitin sodium: An overview. J Antimicrob Chemother 4(Suppl B):91, 1978.

224. Verklin RM Jr, Mandell GL: Alteration of effectiveness of antibiotics by anaerobiosis. J Lab Clin Med 89:65, 1977.

225. Wallman IS, Hilton HB: Teeth pigmented by tetracycline. Lancet 1:827, 1962.

226. Weber WW, Hein DW: Clinical pharmacokinetics of isoniazid. Clin Pharmacol 4:401, 1979.

227. Weeks JL, Mason EO Jr, Baker CJ: Antagonism of ampicillin and chloramphenicol for meningeal isolates of group B streptococci. Antimicrob Agents Chemother 20:281, 1981.

228. Weitekamp MR, Aber RC: Prolonged bleeding times

and bleeding diathesis associated with moxalactam administration. JAMA 249:69, 1983.

229. Whelton A: Antibiotic pharmacokinetics and clinical application in renal insufficiency. Med Clin North Am 66:267, 1982.

230. Whitley RJ, Nahmias AJ, Soong S, et al: Vidarabine therapy of neonatal herpes simplex virus infection. Pediatrics 66:495, 1980.

231. Whyte, RK, Hussain Z, deSa D: Antenatal infections with *Candida* species. Arch Dis Child 57:528, 1982.

232. Wilson CB, Jacobs RF, Smith AL: Cellular antibiotic pharmacology. Semin Perinatol 6:205, 1982.

233. Wilson R, Feldman S: Toxicity of amphotericin B in children with cancer. Am J Dis Child 133:731, 1979.

234. Yakatan GJ, Poynor WJ, Breeding SA, et al: Single- and multiple-dose bioequivalence of erythromycin pharmaceutical alternatives. J Clin Pharmacol 20:625, 1980.

235. Yeager AS: Use of acyclovir in premature and term neonates. Am J Med 73(Suppl):205, 1982.

236. Yogev R, Williams T: Ventricular fluid levels of chloramphenicol in infants. Antimicrob Agents Chemother 16:7, 1979.

237. Yogev R, Schultz WE, Rosenman SB: Penetrance of nafcillin into human ventricular fluid: Correlation with ventricular pleocytosis and glucose levels. Antimicrob Agents Chemother 19:545, 1981.

238. Young WS III, Lietman PS: Chloramphenicol glucuronyl transferase: Assay, ontogeny and inducibility. J Pharmacol Exp Ther 204:203, 1978.

239. Young JPW, Husson JM, Bruch K, et al: The evaluation of efficacy and safety of cefotaxime: A review of 2,500 cases. J Antimicrob Chemother 6(Suppl A):293, 1980.

240. Yow MD: An overview of pediatric experience with amikacin. Am J Med 62:954, 1977.

241. Yow MD, Taber LH, Barrett FF, et al: A ten-year assessment of methicillin-associated side effects. Pediatrics 58:329, 1976.

242. Zakhireh B, Root RK: Unusually high occurrence of drug reactions with nafcillin. Yale J Biol Med 51:449, 1978.

243. Arbeter AM, Saccar CL, Eisner S, et al: Tobramycin sulfate elimination in premature infants. J Pediatr 103:131, 1983.

244. Ardati KO, Thirumoorthi MC, Dajani AS: Intravenous trimethoprim-sulfamethoxazole in the treatment of serious infections in children. J Pediatr 95:801, 1979.

245. Blum MR, Liao SHT, De Miranda P: Overview of acyclovir pharmacokinetic disposition in adults and children. Am J Med 73:186, 1982.

246. Bosso JA, Chan GM, Matsen JM: Cefoperazone pharmacokinetics in preterm infants. Antimicrob Agents Chemother 23:413, 1983.

247. Brook I: Treatment of anaerobic infections in children with metronidazole. Dev Pharmacol Ther 6:187, 1983.

248. Burckart GJ, Barrett FF, Straughn AB, et al: Chloramphenicol clearance in infants. J Clin Pharmacol 22:49, 1982.

249. Carlberg H, Alestig K, Nord CE, et al: Intestinal side effects of cefoperazone. J Antimicrob Chemother 10:483, 1982.

250. Craven PC, Graybill JR, Jorgensen JH, et al: High-dose ketoconazole for treatment of fungal infections of the central nervous system. Ann Intern Med 98:160, 1983.

251. Cunha BA, Quintiliani R, Deglin JM, et al: Pharma-

cokinetics of vancomycin in anuria. Rev Infect Dis 3:S269, 1981.

252. Daneshmend TK, Warnock DW: Clinical pharmacokinetics of systemic antifungal drugs. Clin Pharmacokin 8:17, 1983.

253. de Louvois J, Mulhall A, Hurley R: The safety and pharmacokinetics of cefotaxime in the treatment of neonates. Pediatr Pharmacol 2:275, 1982.

254. Drouhet E, Borderon JC, Borderon E, et al: Evolution des concentrations serique de 5-fluorocytosine chez les prématures. Bull Soc Franc Mycol Med 3:37, 1974.

255. Fortner CL, Finley RS, Schimpff SC: Piperacillin sodium: Antibacterial spectrum, pharmacokinetics, clinical efficacy, and adverse reactions. Pharmacotherapy 2:287, 1982.

256. Freundlick M, Cynamon H, Tamer A, et al: Clinical and laboratory observations: Management of chloramphenicol intoxication in infancy by charcoal hemoperfusion. J Pediatr 103:485, 1983.

257. Friedman CA, Parks BR, Rawson JE: Gentamicin disposition in asphyxiated newborns: Relationship to mean arterial blood pressure and urine output. Pediatr Pharmacol 2:189, 1982.

258. Fripp RR, Carter MC, Werner JC, et al: Cardiac function and acute chloramphenicol toxicity. J Pediatr 103:487, 1983.

259. Funk EA, Strausbaugh LJ: Antimicrobial activity, pharmacokinetics, adverse reactions, and therapeutic indications of cefoperazone. Pharmacotherapy 2:185, 1982.

260. Gascoigne EW, Barton GJ, Michaels M, et al: The kinetics of ketoconazole in animals and man. Clin Res Rev 1:177, 1981.

261. Graninger W, Haubenstock A, Rameis H, et al: Netilmicin: A new aminoglycoside active against gentamicin-resistant *Staphylococcus aureus.* Drug Exp Clin Res 9:263, 1983.

262. Greene GR, Heitlinger L, Madden JD: *Citrobacter* ventriculitis in a neonate responsive to trimethoprim-sulfamethoxazole. Clin Pediatr 22:515, 1983.

263. Grossman ER, Walchek A, Freedman H, et al: Tetracyclines and permanent teeth: The relation between dose and tooth color. Pediatrics 47:567, 1971.

264. Gump DW: Vancomycin for treatment of bacterial meningitis. Rev Infect Dis 3:S289, 1981.

265. Hall P, Kaye CM, McIntosh N, et al: Intravenous metronidazole in the newborn. Arch Dis Child 58:529, 1983.

266. Hansen TN, Ritter DA, Speer ME, et al: A randomized, controlled study of oral gentamicin in the treatment of neonatal necrotizing enterocolitis. J Pediatr 97:836, 1980.

267. Henriksson P, Svenningsen N, Juhlin I, et al: Netilmicin in moderate to severe infections in neonates and infants: A study of efficacy, tolerance and pharmacokinetics. Curr Ther Res 24:108, 1978.

268. Hindmarsh KW, Nation RL, Williams GL, et al: Pharmacokinetics of gentamicin in very low birth weight preterm infants. Eur J Clin Pharmacol 24:649, 1983.

269. L'Hommedieu C, Stough R, Brown L, et al: Potentiation of neuromuscular weakness in infant botulism by aminoglycosides. J Pediatr 95:1065, 1979.

270. McCracken GH Jr, Siegel JD, Threlkeld N, et al: Ceftriaxone pharmacokinetics in newborn infants. Antimicrob Agents Chemother 23:341, 1983.

271. McDougall PN, Fleming PJ, Speller DCE, et al: Neonatal systemic candidiasis: A failure to respond to intravenous miconazole in two neonates. Arch Dis Child 57:884, 1982.

272. Morgan DJ, Ching MS, Raymond K, et al: Elimination of amphotericin B in impaired renal function. Clin Pharmacol Ther 34:248, 1983.

273. Munz D, Powell KR, Pai CH: Treatment of candidal diaper dermatitis: A double-blind placebo-controlled comparison of topical nystatin with topical plus oral nystatin. J Pediatr 101:1022, 1982.

274. Nahata MC, Powell DA: Comparative bioavailability and pharmacokinetics of chloramphenicol after intravenous chloramphenicol succinate in premature infants and older patients. Dev Pharmacol Ther 6:23, 1983.

275. Nahata MC, Powell DA, Gregoire RP, et al: Tobramycin kinetics in newborn infants. J Pediatr 103:136, 1983.

276. Neu HC: Adverse effects of new cephalosporins. Ann Internal Med 98:415, 1983.

277. Phillips AMR, Milner RDG: Clinical pharmacology of netilmicin in the newborn. Arch Dis Child 58:451, 1983.

278. Pickering LK, Cleary TG, Kohl S: Chloramphenicol toxicity—oral versus intravenous administration. J Pediatr 97:869, 1980.

279. Pyati SP, Pildes RS, Jacobs NM, et al: Penicillin in infants weighing two kilograms or less with early-onset group B streptococcal disease. New Engl J Med 308:1383, 1983.

280. Rajchgot P, Prober C, Soldin S, et al: Chloramphenicol pharmacokinetics in the newborn. Dev Pharmacol Ther 6:305, 1983.

281. Ralph ED: Clinical pharmacokinetics of metronidazole. Clin Pharmacokin 8:43, 1983.

282. Reed MD, Aronoff SC, Myers CM, et al: Developmental pharmacokinetics of moxalactam. Antimicrob Agents Chemother 24:383, 1983.

283. Ring JC, Cates KL, Belani KK, et al: Rifampin for CSF shunt infections caused by coagulase-negative staphylococci. J Pediatr 95:317, 1979.

284. Roe DA: Nutritional effects of antituberculous drugs. In Roe, DA: Drug-Induced Nutritional Deficiencies. Westport, Conn, Avi Publishing Co, Chapter 12, 1976.

285. Rosenfeld WN, Evans HE, Batheja R, et al: Pharmacokinetics of cefoperazone in full-term and premature neonates. Antimicrob Agents Chemother 23:866, 1983.

286. Russo J Jr, Russo ME: Comparative review of two new wide-spectrum penicillins: Mezlocillin and piperacillin. Clin Pharmacy 1:207, 1982.

287. Scholer JH: Flucytosin. In Speller (Ed), Antifungal Chemotherapy. Chichester, Wiley, 1980, p. 35.

288. Smith BR, LeFrock JL: Bronchial tree penetration of antibiotics. Chest 83:904, 1983.

289. Sohn CA: Evaluation of ketoconazole. Clin Pharmacy 1:217, 1982.

290. Steele RW, Eyre LB, Bradsher RW, et al: Pharmacokinetics of ceftriaxone in pediatric patients with meningitis. Antimicrob Agents Chemother 23:191, 1983.

291. Steele RW, Bradsher RW: Comparison of ceftriaxone with standard therapy for bacterial meningitis. J Pediatr 103:138, 1983.

292. Stein MT, Liang D: Clinical hepatotoxicity of isoniazid in children. Pediatrics 64:499, 1979.

293. Tessin I, Bergmark J, Hiesche K, et al: Renal function of neonates during gentamicin treatment. Arch Dis Child 57:758, 1982.

294. Thirumoorthi MC, Asmar BI, Buckley JA, et al: Pharmacokinetics of intravenously administered piperacillin in preadolescent children. J Pediatr 102:941, 1983.

295. Ward RM, Sattler FR, Dalton As Jr: Assessment of antifungal therapy in an 800-gram infant with candidal arthritis and osteomyelitis. Pediatrics 72:234, 1983.

296. Weitekamp MR: Prolonged bleeding times and bleeding diathesis associated with moxalactam administration. JAMA 249:69, 1983.

297. Whitley RJ, Alford CA Jr: Towards therapy and prevention of herpetic infections. Semin Perinatol 7:64, 1983.

298. Wise RI: The vancomycin symposium: Summary and comments. Rev Infect Dis 3:S293, 1981.

299. Wilson CB, Koup JR, Opheim KE, et al: Piperacillin pharmacokinetics in pediatric patients. Antimicrob Agents Chemother 22:442, 1982.

300. Wright AJ, Wilkowske CJ: The penicillins. Mayo Clin Proc 58:21, 1983.

301. Yee GC, Evans WE: Reappraisal of guidelines for pharmacokinetic monitoring of aminoglycosides. Pharmacotherapy 1:55, 1981.

302. Yeung CY: Intrathecal antiobiotic therapy for neonatal meningitis. Arch Dis Child 51:686, 1976.

FIVE

Anticonvulsants

SEIZURES IN THE INFANT

Seizures in the infant not only represent a significant therapeutic management problem but also have important prognostic implications. The reported incidence of neonatal seizures ranges from approximately 1 to 14 per 1000 live births. In one series, approximately 20% of infants weighing less than 2500 grams at birth were so affected.[93] Although a variety of disorders have been identified as causative factors in seizures in infants (Table 5–1), the most common is hypoxic–ischemic encephalopathy. Marshall and coworkers[65] determined in a prospective study that hypoxic–ischemic encephalopathy with or without intracranial hemorrhage accounted for 75% of seizures in infants admitted to a neonatal intensive care unit. Control of seizures in infants is important because the seizures themselves may result in further brain injury and may interfere with ongoing medical management, particularly when they involve major motor movements for considerable periods of time.

The etiology of the seizures must be established whenever possible to permit more specific and definitive therapy. Treatment of hypoglycemia-induced seizures with an anticonvulsant drug rather than IV glucose is hardly in the patient's best interest. The clinical manifestations of neonatal seizures can vary considerably, perhaps reflecting the status of neuroanatomic and neurophysiologic development in the perinatal period. Unlike older infants, newborns typically do not have well-organized, generalized tonic–clonic seizures. Premature infants have even less well-organized seizure activity than that seen in full-term infants. Apnea, for example, is known to be one of the more common manifestations of atypical neonatal seizures.[138] Volpe[107] has carefully reviewed the pathophysiologic aspects and clinical features of neonatal seizures and has emphasized the common subtle nature of this disorder in the neonate.

Although the exact mechanisms responsible for seizures in infants remain to be clarified, present knowledge suggests that the pathophysiologic disturbances result in excessive depolarization of CNS tissue. The underlying mechanism for the excessive depolarization can be a consequence of disturbance in energy production resulting in failure of the membrane potential, which is based on the sodium–potassium pump. Hypoxemia, ischemia, and hypoglycemia are examples of abnormalities that can produce such membrane disturbances from decreases in energy production. Alterations in the membrane potential can also result from changes in ion permeability, such as to calcium or sodium. Thus, hypocalcemia can result in changes in membrane potential. Finally, considerable evidence indicates that seizures may represent an imbalance between major inhibitory and excitatory influences in the CNS neurotransmitter systems.[46] It is this latter mechanism that is believed to be most vulnerable to anticonvulsant medications.

Decisions regarding the drug of choice and the duration of therapy have evolved largely on an empirical basis. Obviously, where etiologies can be identified, specific therapy is indicated (e.g., hypoglycemia: glucose; hypocalcemia: calcium; infection: antimicrobial drugs). In the remaining situations phenobarbital is generally regarded as the agent of choice for initiating anticonvulsant therapy. Careful examination of the older literature strongly suggests that a significant portion of the reported "failures" with phenobarbital therapy represent an inadequate dosing program rather than an inappropriate choice of drug. In legitimate cases of phenobarbital failure, phenytoin, diazepam, paraldehyde, and a variety of other agents have been utilized with varying degrees of success.

In choosing the appropriate therapeutic regi-

Table 5-1. CAUSES OF SEIZURES IN INFANTS

Disorder	Age at Onset	
	0-3 days	>3 days
perinatal asphyxia:ischemia	x	
metabolic disorders (e.g., deficiency of amino acid, glucose, calcium, magnesium)	x	x
intracranial hemorrhage	x	
intracranial infections	x	x
developmental CNS anomalies	x	x
toxicity (exogenous: drug or chemical; endogenous: bilirubin)	x	x
pyridoxine dependency	x	x
familial epilepsy (rare)		x

men for seizures in infants, the potential of all the anticonvulsant drugs to produce significant side-effects, some more easily recognized than others, must be recognized. For this reason alone, it is imperative to consider carefully the advantages and disadvantages of drug treatment in each case. Aggressive drug treatment of infrequently occurring seizures, particularly those associated with mild manifestations such as "jitteriness" or isolated focal twitching, may result in more adverse consequences than those anticipated from the seizures themselves. Obviously, seizures associated with respiratory compromise (hypoventilation, apnea, or both) as the sole sign of seizure disorder mandate immediate institution of rigorous anticonvulsant therapy. However, the worthy goal of total seizure control is often unobtainable without the use of anticonvulsants in sufficient dosage to produce side-effects or of a multidrug therapy program with its attendant problems. An appropriate balance must be maintained between the extent of seizure control deemed necessary and the side-effects associated with large-dose single-drug or multidrug therapy.

PHARMACOLOGIC PRINCIPLES OF THE ANTICONVULSANTS

An understanding of the pharmacologic properties of anticonvulsant drugs and of their application in seizures will enhance considerably the likelihood of optimal therapeutic benefit to the patient. For example, as can be seen from Table 5-3, the serum half-life values for phenobarbital can be expected to differ significantly among infants as well as in the same infant over time (age). As discussed in detail in

the first three chapters, the drug serum half-life reflects the time required for the drug concentration to decline by one half. This in turn is related to the time required for the drug to equilibrate in body tissues. Drugs with longer half-lives tend to require a longer period of time before steady state is reached. Steady-state concentration is of importance because it equates with the eventual therapeutic response. The longer the time required before steady state is reached, the longer the time anticipated before the therapeutic advantage is realized. In general, 4 to 6 half-lives represent the time required for steady-state tissue concentration to be achieved. From Table 5-3 and by simple calculations it can be determined that in infants in whom phenobarbital half-life is 100 hours, 2 to 3 weeks may be required to attain optimal steady-state serum levels if maintenance doses only are employed. This time required for steady state to be achieved can be significantly shortened by the employment of loading doses of the anticonvulsant. The **loading dose** is that amount of drug needed to achieve pharmacokinetic saturation of tissues into which the drug ordinarily slowly distributes and equilibrates, and therefore it is not dependent upon half-life. Although loading doses allow more rapid achievement of steady-state concentrations, the administration of large doses over a short period of time obviously can result in accentuation of certain pharmacologic effects, such as sedation.

The drug half-life also determines the frequency with which the drug should be administered to avoid large fluctuations in serum concentration. Peak and trough serum concentrations reflect toxicity and efficacy, respectively. By maintaining the drug serum concentration within a therapeutic "window," efficacy can be maximized and the toxicity minimized (see Fig. 2-7). In general, for those drugs (or neonates) demonstrating shorter drug half-lives, drug administration must be more frequent than for those drugs (or infants) where longer half-lives prevail. From a practical standpoint, in those situations in which seizures appear to "break through" the therapy during the period just preceding the next dose, consideration should be given to either an increase in dose or a shorter dosing interval. These dosage changes must be monitored carefully when steady state is again reached (4-6 times the $T\frac{1}{2}$) to avoid accumulation of toxic levels of drug.

The period of time required for steady-state drug concentrations to be reached is of great practical importance. Measurement of serum drug levels prior to the attainment of steady state will yield a false value; a change in dosage based on this value will result in adverse consequences. For example, if a blood level is measured 1 week into therapy with an agent that requires 2 weeks to attain steady-state levels, the concentration of drug in the serum will be significantly less than that normally achieved at steady state (see Fig. 2–6). An increase in dose in response to this pre–steady state determination could eventually lead to toxic levels of drug. It must also be appreciated that the lowering of toxic levels to optimal steady-state levels following dosage reduction will require the same length of time as that required for steady-state to be achieved following increase in dosage. Thus, adverse effects associated with toxic levels of drug cannot be expected to resolve immediately following dosage adjustment; the longer the half-life, the longer the toxicity will persist.

Anticonvulsant therapeutic monitoring has become a standard of care largely because of the evolution of sensitive analytical methods requiring very small samples of serum or plasma. There are two specific indications for therapeutic monitoring of anticonvulsant serum levels: One is the persistence of seizures in the face of drug therapy; in such cases, monitoring will reveal whether drug levels are inadequate despite appropriate choice of initial dosage. The second indication is the clinical suspicion of serious or significant drug toxicity; documentation of toxic serum levels of drug will confirm such findings to be side-effects of the drug and will help to rule out underlying disease as the cause. Routine serum level measurements without a specific purpose are to be discouraged. Inappropriate serum monitoring as discussed earlier (Chaps. 1 through 3) is also to be condemned. The usual time at which steady-state levels of drug are achieved is 2 to 4 weeks after institution of therapy; when loading doses of drug have been employed, however, steady-

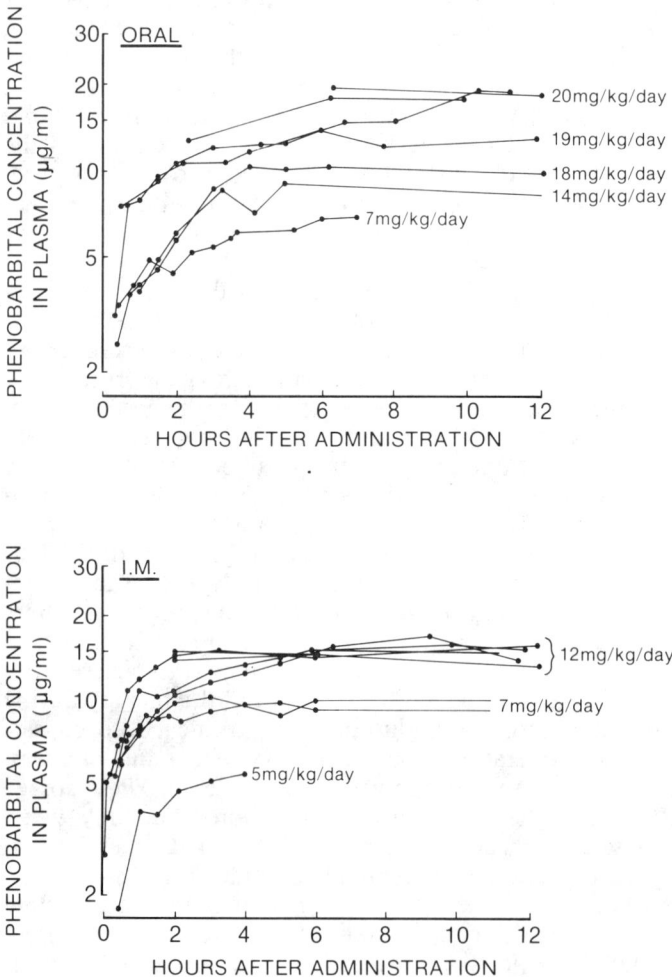

Figure 5–1. Plasma drug concentrations in neonates (aged 0–3 days at time of initial treatment) given a single dose of phenobarbital orally (*A*) or IM (*B*). The approximate doses used are shown by the respective curve of concentration vs. time. (Adapted from Jalling B: Acta Paediatr Scand 64:514, 1975.)

state levels can be anticipated to occur by 1 week. Exceptions to this generalization are discussed under the specific agents. Nevertheless, because of the variability among neonates in aspects of drug disposition (absorption, metabolism, excretion), monitoring of drug serum levels is appropriate at some point in time in all patients, particularly when long-term anticonvulsant therapy is necessary.

SPECIFIC ANTICONVULSANT AGENTS

Phenobarbital

Pharmacology. Phenobarbital is one of the oldest and most effective anticonvulsant agents in use. The absorption of phenobarbital is virtually complete after PO, IM, or rectal administration. Absorption is somewhat slower with oral than with parenteral administration. Maximum serum levels occur at 2 hours following IM administration and at 2 to 4 hours following PO administration. Studies by Lockman and colleagues[57] clearly show more variation in serum levels in infants receiving phenobarbital by IM administration. Thus, absorption from IM injection sites is less predictable and may cause more variation in serum levels than that with IV administration. The plasma phenobarbital concentrations resulting from differing doses given IM or PO are illustrated in Figure 5–1; the slower attainment of peak serum levels following PO administration can be appreciated by inspection of these results, but there is approximately equal scatter in the resulting plasma concentrations of phenobarbital among the different patients receiving equivalent doses. For initial dosing, therefore, it seems most reasonable to employ a parenteral route in infants with active seizure problems for the most rapid control of seizure activity; the greatest efficacy is realized with IV administration. Studies comparing the sodium salt of phenobarbital with the acid form have shown that, following a single IM injection, the absorption rates were significantly shorter with phenobarbital sodium than with phenobarbital acid.[69] Bioavailability studies in children and adults by Matsukura and coworkers[66] showed no significant differences among IV, IM, PO, and rectal routes of administration. Although similar studies have not been accomplished in neonates, there appears to be no therapeutic advantage to parenteral versus oral dosing for maintenance therapy.

Following absorption the volume of distribu-

tion of phenobarbital appears to be greater in newborns and infants than in adults; reported V_d values in neonates range from 0.6 to 1.0 l/kg.[10,44,57,76,124] On the other hand, plasma protein binding of phenobarbital is apparently significantly less in newborns than in adults; the bound fraction is equal to 10% to 30% of total plasma phenobarbital in neonates between 0 and 7 days of age.[99] By comparison, in adults the volume of distribution of phenobarbital is 0.60 to 0.75 l/kg, and the drug is about 46% to 48% bound to plasma proteins.[59,109] The fact that a higher percentage of plasma phenobarbital is non–protein bound (free) in neonates compared with that in adults suggests that diffusion of phenobarbital into the CNS might be greater. However, the brain/plasma phenobarbital ratio measured in children and adults is in the range of 0.6 to 0.9;[94,104] this correlates with a ratio of approximately 0.7 reported for neonates.[76] Two separate studies[44,99] have demonstrated that the CSF/plasma phenobarbital ratio achieved in the neonate is also approximately 0.7, confirming that there is reasonable correlation among plasma, CSF, and brain phenobarbital levels. The consistency of the correlations between plasma phenobarbital levels and brain and CSF phenobarbital levels gives further support to the use of plasma level monitoring in phenobarbital therapy to achieve optimal control of seizures. Studies by Painter and colleagues[76] indicate no accumulation of phenobarbital in the brain with increasing durations of treatment. These authors, however, have demonstrated that the phenobarbital brain/plasma ratios decrease with decreasing gestational age (28 vs. 40 wk); this finding suggests that higher plasma phenobarbital levels may be required for equal seizure control in small premature infants. Phenobarbital concentrations are actually higher in other tissues than in the brain. The tissue/plasma ratios of phenobarbital for liver, heart, and muscle are approximately 4, 6, and 3, respectively. Owing to its pK$_a$ value of 7.2, phenobarbital distribution in tissues is sensitive to pH variations in the plasma (Table 5-2): There is increased transfer of phenobarbital from plasma to tissues with decreases in blood pH (acidosis) and a redistribution from tissues to plasma with increases in blood pH (alkalosis). The magnitude of pH effect on phenobarbital distribution appears to be substantial, with the potential to alter clinical response to the drug.[109]

In the adult about 50% to 70% of the dose of phenobarbital is metabolized slowly by the liver and excreted in the urine, with another 20% to

Table 5–2. TISSUE/PLASMA RATIOS FOR PHENOBARBITAL AS AFFECTED BY CHANGES IN pH[a]

Treatment	Blood pH	Tissue/Plasma Ratio			
		Brain	Fat	Liver	Muscle
CO_2	6.76	1.2	1.0	2.4	1.0
CO_2	6.78	1.5		2.4	1.4
CO_2	6.80	1.4	1.0		1.1
CO_2	6.80	1.4	0.9	1.8	1.1
none	7.27	0.9	0.6		0.8
none	7.29	1.0	0.7		
none	7.42	0.9	0.6		0.8
respiratory pump	7.60	0.8	0.5	1.1	0.5
respiratory pump	7.70	0.7	0.6	1.1	0.6
$NaHCO_3$	7.70	0.6	0.4	1.0	0.5

[a]Data from studies in dogs by Waddell WJ, Butler TC: J Clin Invest 36:1217, 1957.

30% excreted in the urine unchanged. There is a similar pattern of renal excretion of unmetabolized phenobarbital and metabolites in the neonate.[10] The main metabolic pathway for phenobarbital metabolism in humans is via p-hydroxylation of the phenyl ring (Fig. 5–2). The p-hydroxy derivative of phenobarbital is believed to be devoid of anticonvulsant activity. Atypically high plasma levels of phenobarbital can be expected in patients with significant impairment of hepatic metabolism or renal disease. Because phenobarbital is reabsorbed at the tubular level, its renal clearance can be enhanced by increases in urinary pH (alkaline urine); thus, in patients with low urinary pH (acid urine), renal clearance may be diminished

and accumulation to toxic levels may occur. Of the two major metabolites of phenobarbital, conjugated p-hydroxy phenobarbital and unconjugated p-hydroxy phenobarbital, the conjugated form predominates in renal elimination in adults but not in neonates (Fig. 5–2). Studies by Garrettson[35] suggest that this difference is attributable to saturation of phenobarbital metabolism in neonates, as reflected by a constant rate of elimination of the p-hydroxy phenobarbital metabolite. Boreus and coworkers[10] have demonstrated that in neonates, only about 5% of a single dose of phenobarbital is excreted in conjugated form over an 8-day collection period, compared with about 15% in the adult. This relative deficit in conjugation is not clinically significant as long as the alternative mechanisms for elimination of phenobarbital remain intact; the low production of metabolites by neonates appears to be well compensated for by urinary output of nonmetabolized phenobarbital and unconjugated metabolite. Thus, for the newborn and the adult, the total renal elimination of administered phenobarbital is fairly equivalent regardless of the ability of the neonate to metabolize the drug. The prolonged plasma clearance of phenobarbital in neonates has been specifically ascribed to limited renal elimination.[40] The slow rate of renal elimination suggests that the use of 8- to 12-hour dosing intervals is unnecessary in the neonate.[21,35,111]

Peritoneal dialysis in neonates has been shown to remove significant amounts of phenobarbital.[16] The effect of dialysis may be sufficient to cause lessening of seizure control unless supplemental doses of phenobarbital are administered. During dialysis the dose may have to be doubled to maintain therapeutic serum levels.

Phenobarbital limits the spread of seizure activity and also appears to elevate the seizure

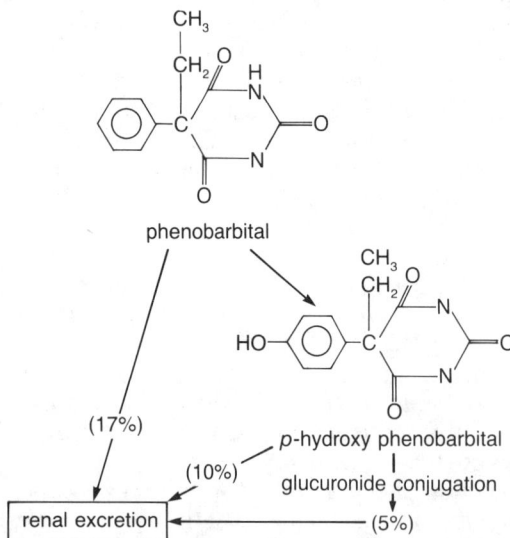

Figure 5–2. Phenobarbital: Structural formula and metabolism in neonates. The percentage of administered dose excreted in neonates is given in parentheses. (From Boreus LO et al: Acta Paediatr Scand 67:193, 1978.)

Table 5–3. SUMMARY OF CLINICAL PHARMACOLOGY STUDIES OF PHENOBARBITAL IN INFANTS

Author(s) of Published Study[a]	Study Group	Dose	Serum Concentration	Serum Half-life (T½)
Heinze and Kampffmeyer[41]	5 infants (1–3 mo old)	9–12 mg/kg IM × 1		47.1 ± 8 hr
Wallin et al[110]	11 neonates (33–37 wk)	5 mg/kg IM or PO (PO q 24 hr)	21–28 μg/ml (range over >6 days)	69–165 hr
Jalling[44]	18 neonates (36–43 wk)	5–21 mg/kg IM or PO q 24 hr	5–20 μg/ml (peak range) (CSF: 0–12.6 μg/ml with CSF/ plasma ratio of 0.5 to 0.8)	41–182 hr (range)
Pippenger and Rosen[79]	13 neonates (2.1–3.8 kg)	loading: 7.5–18 mg/kg IV maintenance: 5 mg/kg IM or PO q 24 hr	5–62 μg/ml (range)	
Gabriel and Albani[32]	7 neonates	5 mg/kg/24 hr × 3	19–35 μg/ml (range)	3–4 days (estimate)
Heiman and Gladtke[40]	30 infants (0–3 mo old)	5–10 mg/kg IV × 1	9.5 ± 1 μg/ml 0.4 wk 14 ± 1 μg/ml 2–3 mo Cl = 5.7 ml/kg · hr	119 ± 16 hr (0–4 wk old) 63 ± 5 hr (2–3 mo old)
Boreus et al[10]	4 neonates	11–20 mg/kg IM or PO	18–21 μg/ml (peak range)	61–173 hr
Painter et al[75]	32 neonates (27–>37 wk)	loading: 15–20 mg/kg IV maintenance: 2.5–5 mg/kg IV	21 ± 4 μg/ml (loading dose only, mean ± SD) 15–40 μg/ml (maintenance dose only, range of mean values)	Approx.: 100 hr, 2-wk treatment 70 hr, 3-wk treatment 50 hr, 4-wk treatment
Pitlick et al[80]	8 neonates (30–40 wk)	loading: 20 mg/kg IV maintenance: 2.5 mg/kg IV q 12 hr	2 wk: 20–37 μg/ml 3 wk: 15–20 μg/ml	115 hr, 1-wk treatment 67 hrs, 4-wk treatment
Gold et al[37]	18 neonates (37–41 wk)	loading: 20 mg/kg IV maintenance: 2.5 mg/kg IV q 12 hr	28–37 μg/ml (range of mean values)	
Lockman et al[57]	39 neonates	loading: 12–16 mg/kg IV or IM	14–20 μg/ml	
Donn et al[24]	30 neonates (26–34 wk)	loading: 10 mg/kg IV × 2 in 12 hr maintenance: 2.5 mg/kg IV q 12 hr	26.6 ± 6.5 μg/ml (mean ± SE) 15.9 – 39.6 μg/ml (range)	
Fischer et al[29]	40 neonates (31–40 wk)	loading: 13–21 mg/kg IM maintenance: 3–4 mg/kg IM q 24 hr	total body clearance: 6.4 ± 2.3 ml/kg · hr	103 ± 49 hr (mean) 43–217 hr (range)
Painter et al[76]	77 neonates (26–>37 wk)	loading: 5–30 mg/kg IV maintenance: 3–5 mg/kg q 24 hr	5–35 μg/ml (range-loading dose) 15–35 μg/ml (range-maintenance dose)	
Gal et al[33]	18 neonates (27–40 wk)	loading: 15 mg/kg IV maintenance: 2.5–5 mg/kg q 24 hr	total body clearance: 5.6 ml/kg · hr	
Morgan et al[70]	24 neonates (mean 30 wk)	20 mg/kg IM × 1	17 μg/ml (range 10–27 μg/ml)	144 hr (estimate)
Ouvrier and Goldsmith[74]	40 neonates (1.5–4 kg)	loading: 5–15mg/ kg IV or IM maintenance: 3 mg/kg IM or PO q 12 hr	21–27 μg/ml (range)	
Gilman et al[124]	16 infants (20–40 wk gestation; 0–94 days old)	loading: 7–15 mg/kg IV maintenance: 1.3–7.5 mg/kg IV once daily	26.3 ± 10.0 μg/ml (range: 13–45 μg/ml	244 ± 181 hr (range: 42–624 hr)

[a]Listed in order of publication; see References at end of chapter.

threshold. The exact mechanism responsible for this pharmacologic activity is not known, but Johnston and Singer[46] have speculated that it evolves by an increase in inhibitory neurotransmission via enhancement of the GABAergic (gamma-aminobutyric acid) systems. However, Macdonald and Barker[62] have proposed, on the basis of observations in cell cultures of mammalian spinal cord neurons, that the reduction by phenobarbital in seizure spread may depend on the potentiation of inhibitory pathways that are recruited during discharge of seizure foci, by means other than a GABA-type effect of phenobarbital. Staudt and colleagues[97] have examined the question of whether or not phenobarbital causes significant suppression of background EEG activity in neonates with seizure disorders. They concluded on the basis of their studies that suppression of EEG background activity in neonates with phenobarbital plasma levels as high as 60 μg/ml is secondary to brain pathology rather than produced by the medication. Similar conclusions were reached by Couto-Sales and coworkers[18] in studies during the first 24 hours of anticonvulsant therapy in neonates.

Clinical Pharmacology. Pharmacokinetic studies in infants reveal phenobarbital serum half-life to range from 40 to more than 200 hours (Table 5–3). This variation in phenobarbital kinetics among neonates can be explained on the basis of rate of hepatic metabolism, rate of renal elimination, and presence of endogenous or exogenous substances that may be competitive for phenobarbital metabolism or renal elimination. Studies by Heiman and Gladtke,[40] Painter and coworkers,[75] and Pitlick and colleagues[80] leave little doubt that the rate of elimination of phenobarbital increases with age. These observations reinforce the importance of careful definition and description of the study population when pharmacokinetic data are collected in neonates and infants.

Therapeutic Indications

Control of Seizures. Phenobarbital, with few exceptions, is the drug of choice for the control of seizures in infants. The amount of phenobarbital necessary to achieve seizure control will vary depending upon the pathophysiology of the seizure disorder and its impact on the wellbeing of the infant. Studies by Jalling[44] revealed the cessation of convulsions in neonates in whom serum levels of 12 to 30 μg/ml were attained; however, within the study population were neonates whose seizures could not be controlled despite the achievement of serum levels in this "therapeutic" range or higher. Lockman and coworkers[57] reported that serum levels

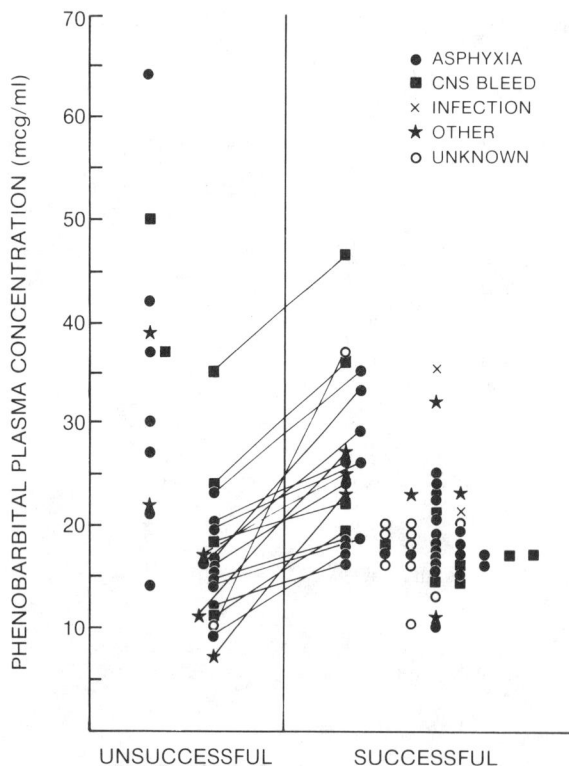

Figure 5–3. Relationship between phenobarbital plasma levels and anticonvulsant response in neonates with a variety of seizure etiologies. Points connected by a line represent the response of the same patient to increased phenobarbital plasma level. (Adapted from Gal P et al: Neurology 32:1401, 1982.)

Legend:
● ASPHYXIA
■ CNS BLEED
× INFECTION
★ OTHER
○ UNKNOWN

Y-axis: PHENOBARBITAL PLASMA CONCENTRATION (mcg/ml)

X-axis: UNSUCCESSFUL   SUCCESSFUL

above 16.9 $\mu g/ml$ were necessary for seizure control; their study population also included neonates who continued to demonstrate seizures although serum phenobarbital levels were above 16.9 $\mu g/ml$. Painter and colleagues[76] only occasionally observed anticonvulsant responses to phenobarbital therapy in newborns with levels below 15 $\mu g/ml$; in their series, only 28 of 77 patients with levels of approximately 20 $\mu g/ml$ responded. Studies by Ouvrier and Goldsmith[74] revealed seizure control in some neonates with plasma levels between 7 and 15 $\mu g/ml$. Bergman and coworkers[8] have estimated that in approximately 60% of high-risk newborns with seizures, control with phenobarbital alone can be expected. In studies by Gal and colleagues,[34] the success rate for controlling seizures with phenobarbital alone was 85%; failures occurred primarily in neonates with prolonged birth asphyxia. Of the 71 neonates in their series, 51% responded at plasma concentrations of 20 $\mu g/ml$ or less, 28% responded at levels between 20 and 30 $\mu g/ml$, and an additional 12% were controlled with levels higher than 30 $\mu g/ml$ (Fig. 5–3); 11 neonates (16%) required additional anticonvulsants.

There are no absolute minimal therapeutic concentrations of phenobarbital. Seizure control is dictated as much by the underlying extent of the abnormality producing the seizure as by the level of phenobarbital achieved. Since significant toxicities have not been reported with levels of phenobarbital below 25 to 30 $\mu g/ml$, the often-recommended therapeutic range of 15

to 30 $\mu g/ml$ appears appropriate for the neonate. Gal and coworkers[34] found continued benefit in some neonates in whom plasma phenobarbital levels reached 40 to 50 $\mu g/ml$ without encountering significant side-effects.

The dosing program for phenobarbital necessary to achieve the recommended serum levels for control of seizures has been the focus of numerous pharmacokinetic studies (Table 5–3). Rapid achievement of adequate therapeutic levels of phenobarbital can be accomplished with IV loading doses of phenobarbital. Studies by Lockman[57] and Fischer[29] and their colleagues indicate a peak serum concentration in $\mu g/ml$ equal to approximately 1.3 to 1.6 times the dose in mg/kg of phenobarbital. Therefore, the loading dose of approximately 15 mg/kg IM or IV will achieve a peak serum phenobarbital concentration of approximately 20 $\mu g/ml$. However, as can be seen in Table 5–4, both the route of administration (IV vs. IM) and the loading dose (9.5 mg/kg vs. 15 mg/kg) significantly affect the time required to achieve seizure control in neonates. The ideal initial loading dose is 15 to 20 mg/kg given IV (Table 5–5). Maintenance doses for phenobarbital of between 3 and 5.0 mg/kg per day usually result in phenobarbital concentrations in the therapeutic range of 15 to 30 $\mu g/ml$. Neither the loading dose nor the maintenance dose of phenobarbital required for seizure control in the newborn appears to be influenced by gestational age or birth weight.[8] Maintenance dosing should be begun no earlier than 12 hours after

Table 5–4. RELATIONSHIP BETWEEN PHENOBARBITAL DOSAGE AND TIME REQUIRED TO ATTAIN THERAPEUTIC SERUM LEVELS AND SEIZURE CONTROL IN NEONATES[a]

Phenobarbital Treatment	Time to Reach Therapeutic Levels (hr)[b]	Mean Serum Level ($\mu g/ml$)	Time to Achieve Seizure Control (hr)
Group I 9.5 mg/kg/day IM × 3 days, then 5.8 mg/kg/day IM or PO	38	21	60
Group II 9.5 mg/kg IV loading dose, then 6.8 mg/kg IM × 6 days, then PO	30	20.6	27
Group III 14.9 mg/kg IV loading dose, then 5.9 mg/kg/day IM or PO	<2	21.9	8
Group IV 15.2 mg/kg IM loading dose, then 5.9 mg/kg/day IM or PO	<2	26.5	32

[a]Neonates ($N = 40$ total) ranged in weight from 1.5 to 4 kg, and in age at time of study from 1 to 22 days. Etiologies for seizures included asphyxia, intracranial hemorrhage, congenital anomalies, and idiopathic.
[b]Therapeutic concentrations defined as 10–25 $\mu g/ml$.
Adapted from data of Ouvrier RA, Goldsmith R: Arch Dis Child 57:653, 1982.

Table 5-5. DOSAGE RECOMMENDATIONS FOR ANTICONVULSANTS EMPLOYED IN INFANTS

Drug	Recommended Dosage	Therapeutic Serum Level (μg/ml)	Toxicity
phenobarbital	[a] loading: 15–20 mg/kg IV [b] maintenance: 3–5 mg/kg IV, IM or PO q 24 hr (first dose given 12–24 hr after loading)	15–30	sedation, induce drug metabolism (interactions), sensitivity reactions
phenytoin	[c] loading: 20 mg/kg IV slowly over ½ to 1 hour (maximum rate of infusion 0.5 mg/kg/min) [d] maintenance: 4–8 mg/kg IV or PO q 24 hr (first dose given 24 hr after loading); if > 1 wk old may require increases in dosage up to or greater than 8 mg/kg IV q 12 or 8 hr	10–20[e]	see Table 5–7
diazepam	[f] 0.1 to 1.0 mg/kg given IV slowly; give in maximum increments of 0.2 mg/kg q 2 min; if seizures stop before completion of dosing, discontinue infusion rectal dose: 0.5–1.0 mg/kg	0.15–0.3	CNS depression, respiratory depression including apnea, phlebitis

[a]If seizures continue after the initial loading dose, additional 5 mg/kg bolus doses can be given (total loading dose employed should not exceed 35 mg/kg). Respiratory depression may develop with larger loading doses.

[b]Maintenance doses of 5 mg/kg/day may occasionally result in accumulation of serum levels to > 30 μg/ml in neonates less than 1 week of age. Unless undue sedation occurs (monitoring of phenobarbital serum levels will be of assistance in identifying and managing such patients), little adverse consequences should be anticipated from these higher serum levels.

[c]The complications of too rapid IV administration and phenytoin therapy include hypotension and bradycardia.[122]

[d]Maintenance doses of phenytoin are impossible to establish accurately because of marked individual variation (see Table 5–6). Frequent plasma phenytoin concentration measurements are essential particularly in the rapidly changing period of the first 3 weeks of age. The IM route should be avoided because of unpredictable absorption.

[e]If the therapeutic range is based on the premise that in the neonate there is a greater concentration of unbound phenytoin in plasma at any given total plasma concentration, then a total phenytoin plasma concentration of 6–14 μg/ml will provide the same concentration of unbound phenytoin as a 10–20 μg/ml total concentration in an adult. However, the actual relationship between serum levels and anticonvulsant activity of phenytoin (alone) has not been demonstrated in neonates. The plasma level 8 hr after dosing should be the most representative of the average phenytoin concentration.

[f]The total acute IV dose of diazepam necessary to control seizures in infants has ranged from less than 0.1 to 2.7 mg/kg. Based on the proposed therapeutic serum level of diazepam, a dose of 0.5 mg/kg should produce levels in excess of that ordinarily necessary. Only in very unusual circumstances should alternate routes of administration be considered. Evidence does exist to support the efficacy of rectal administration (see text). The parenteral injection form is used in conjunction with a syringe and catheter inserted 5 cm into the rectum.

the loading dose. If seizures continue after the initial IV loading dose or within 2 hours thereof, additional doses of 5 mg/kg of phenobarbital are appropriate, up to a total loading dose of 35 mg/kg. However, it is clear that absolute seizure control is often difficult, particularly in neonates with asphyxia-induced seizures, even when phenobarbital levels are in excess of 30 μg/ml.[33] In situations of continued seizures, the need for absolute seizure control must be weighed carefully against the consequences of adding drug toxicity or more complicated multidrug anticonvulsant therapy to existing clinical problems.

The need for dosing infants on an every-12-hour basis has been challenged by several clinical studies. Walson[111] and Davis[21] and their colleagues found no change in seizure activity or in incidence or severity of side-effects in infants and children when phenobarbital was given once daily compared with a dosing interval of 2 or 3 times per day. Although doses of 2.5 mg/kg given every 12 hours have been recommended, the pharmacokinetic justification for this frequent interval of administration is clearly nonexistent.

There is controversy regarding the duration of anticonvulsant therapy in neonates presenting with seizures. Hypoxic–ischemic encephalopathy–related seizures, for example, tend to remit spontaneously after 1 to 2 weeks,[8] suggesting that the course of therapy need not continue indefinitely. Fenichel[28] recommends discontinuing anticonvulsant therapy one week after achieving seizure control and points out the lack of evidence supporting more prolonged therapy. Another approach is to allow the neonate to outgrow the dosage, thus creating a gradual challenge to develop over time; subsequent documentation of plasma drug levels below those anticipated to be therapeutic, along with a seizure-free history, would be sufficient reasons to discontinue drug therapy. In a small series of 10 neonates, anticonvulsant therapy was stopped before they were discharged from the hospital; this constituted less than two weeks of therapy in 8 patients.[123] No recurrent seizure episodes developed.

Management of Apnea of Prematurity. Pharmacologic management of apnea of prematurity has included the use of phenobarbital.[32] The proposed mechanism for phenobarbital is a reduction in the ratio of the duration of active (REM) sleep to that of quiet sleep. Episodes of apnea or cardiac slowing occur predominantly, although certainly not entirely, during active sleep in neonates who otherwise appear healthy.[28,31] Alteration of the sleep cycle appears to coincide with reduction or prevention of apnea or bradycardia. In one study, phenobarbital (5 mg/kg q 24 hr × 3) decreased the percentage of active sleep by 75% and the incidence of apneic spells to about 50%.[32] The proposed importance of REM sleep for normal brain development and the more direct and specific pharmacologic effect of caffeine (see Chap. 6) in the management of apnea of prematurity has appropriately eliminated the use of phenobarbital as a first-line drug for this problem. It seems more reasonable to restrict the use of phenobarbital to management of apnea associated with seizures.[28]

Hyperbilirubinemia Prophylaxis. Another proposed therapeutic use of phenobarbital is prophylaxis against neonatal hyperbilirubinemia.[110] The mode of action of phenobarbital in reducing serum bilirubin levels may include facilitated uptake of bilirubin by hepatic cells, increased bilirubin conjugation, and increased biliary secretion of bilirubin. Significant reduction in serum bilirubin levels generally occurs after day 3 or 4 of age in term infants and later in premature infants. The clinical utility of this therapy is seriously questioned since more acceptable alternatives, such as phototherapy, are available.

Prevention of Intraventricular Hemorrhage. More recently, phenobarbital has been purported to prevent intraventricular hemorrhage in pre-term infants. Donn and colleagues[24] studied 60 infants weighing less than 1500 grams at birth and less than 6 hours of age who were randomly assigned to phenobarbital or placebo therapy; intraventricular hemorrhage occurred in 4 of 30 in the phenobarbital group

and 14 of 30 in the control group. Results of subsequent reports examining small numbers of infants were equivocal.[16,92] In a controlled study by Morgan and coworkers[70] 60 very-low-birth-weight infants were assigned alternately to placebo and to phenobarbital therapy; real-time ultrasonography of the head revealed no difference in phenobarbital-treated and untreated infants in incidence or severity of periventricular hemorrhage. Hope and colleagues[43] found an identical incidence of periventricular hemorrhage in 20 at-risk infants treated with phenobarbital compared with a "historical control" group.

The premise for these clinical investigations appears to be based on experimental animal studies that concluded that barbiturates reduce brain damage from a variety of insults. Close examination of the methodology employed in these experimental animal studies reveals the majority utilized short-acting barbiturates given in massive doses. Barbiturate protection of the CNS has been investigated in predominantly four types of experimentally induced acute cerebral lesions: focal ischemia, global ischemia, head injury, and acute metabolic and infective processes. Atlhough there is evidence that barbiturates can protect the ischemic brain in animals, particularly with focal lesions, the precise mechanism for this protective effect remains unclear. Pentobarbital without question can produce significant decreases in intracranial pressure, probably by reduction in both cerebral blood flow and intracranial blood volume.[64,90] These changes are believed to be associated with a reduction in oxygen demand by depression of the metabolic rate of CNS tissue and therefore could be of clinical value in head trauma. The importance of free-radical scavenging as a mechanism for barbiturate protection has been largely ruled out.[2] Godin and coworkers,[36] however, have recently reported that barbiturates may interact at the level of iron-catalyzed free-radical reactions. The clinical application of this experimental evidence remains to be accomplished. Steer[98] has recently reviewed the clinical experience with barbiturate therapy and the management of cerebral ischemia.

The exact etiology for periventricular hemorrhage in the small pre-term infant is unclear, although there is a strong association with prematurity, hypoxic events, and developmental aspects of the vascular bed found in the subependymal germinal matrix.[100,108] Thus, the appropriate rationale for employment of phenobarbital, if any, is difficult to determine. Wimberley and colleagues[113] have reported that phenobarbital sedation in infants reduced hypertensive peaks; such peaks have been proposed as a causative factor in the development of intraventricular hemorrhage. In 5 infants weighing more than 1.5 kg, phenobarbital (20 mg/kg loading dose, then 5 mg/kg q 24 hr) reduced motor activity and the number of mean arterial blood pressure peaks and their amplitude, although only for a short period after each injection. It seems most reasonable to conclude that the employment of barbiturates in ischemic anoxic insults in neonates remains an unestablished experimental consideration.

Clinical Toxicology. Although phenobarbital is relatively nontoxic at therapeutic levels, this drug is known to induce the synthesis and activity of hepatic mixed-function oxidase enzymes.[85] There is therefore a potential for phenobarbital to interact with exogenous and endogenous substances whose actions, including toxicity, are influenced by this system. Clinical evidence of such hepatic-based toxicity is indeed rare.[1]

Long-term therapy with phenobarbital has been reported to produce rickets in children with seizure disorders.[19,38,102] Several mechanisms have been proposed as causative factors,[51] including alteration of vitamin D metabolism.[68,71] Keck and coworkers[129] have re-examined the question of anticonvulsant drug effects on vitamin D metabolism, employing carefully matched control subjects. They found no evidence that anticonvulsants affect vitamin D metabolism. Vitamin D supplementation has been recommended for children receiving chronic (6 months or longer) anticonvulsant therapy,[38,68] but the need for such supplement has not been studied in infants or neonates.

Lethargy and sedation can be expected with plasma levels higher than 40 μg/ml, although these effects are sometimes difficult to distinguish from clinical signs of the underlying disorder. Severe lethargy has been noted with levels of 70 μg/ml.[75] Progression of lethargy to the point where artificial respiratory support is required, however, is unusual and should prompt measurement of serum phenobarbital levels to confirm the etiology of the CNS depression.

Scarlatiniform or morbilliliform rashes have been reported to occur in less than 2% of adults or children receiving the drug, but similar data for infants cannot be found in the literature. The effects of prolonged administration of phe-

nobarbital on the developing nervous system and learning ability remain unclear.[22]

The use of phenobarbital in conjunction with chloramphenicol has resulted in the development of subtherapeutic levels of chloramphenicol in some neonates and infants.[9,50a] The use of this drug combination is not uncommon in the neonate with meningitis who develops convulsions. Because phenobarbital has been shown experimentally to induce chloramphenicol metabolism, such an adverse drug interaction should not be unexpected.[50,77] Awareness of the potential adverse effect of phenobarbital on chloramphenicol metabolism and frequent determinations of chloramphenicol serum levels will preclude clinical difficulty. Other drug-drug interactions of phenobarbital, including phenytoin and valproate, increase phenobarbital plasma concentrations.[132]

Phenytoin

Pharmacology. Phenytoin, a weak acid (pK_a 8.3) with a very limited aqueous solubility, is probably the second most widely used anticonvulsant employed for the symptomatic treatment of seizures in infants. The absorption of phenytoin from the gastrointestinal tract is thought to be slow and variable, influenced by a variety of factors including the formulation of the pharmaceutical preparation. Although neonates and infants have been reported to absorb phenytoin poorly from the gastrointestinal tract,[75] plasma levels of phenytoin vary considerably regardless of the route of administration. In neonates, the oral route has been found to be adequate for phenytoin therapy;[58] less than 3% of an oral dose is recovered in the stool.[55] Studies in which the use of large bolus doses and the effects of overdosing were examined demonstrate that peak serum levels of phenytoin may not be reached until several days after oral administration, suggesting very slow rates of absorption from the gastrointestinal tract.[47] There is some evidence for enterohepatic recycling of phenytoin in adults.[4] Interruption of such recycling could explain the observations of poor or variable oral absorption of phenytoin and the striking intrapatient changes with age and interpatient variability in phenytoin kinetics. The IM route of administration should not be employed because the drug crystallizes in the muscle, resulting in unpredictable absorption.

Phenytoin is highly protein bound (> 70%), although less so in neonates than in infants and

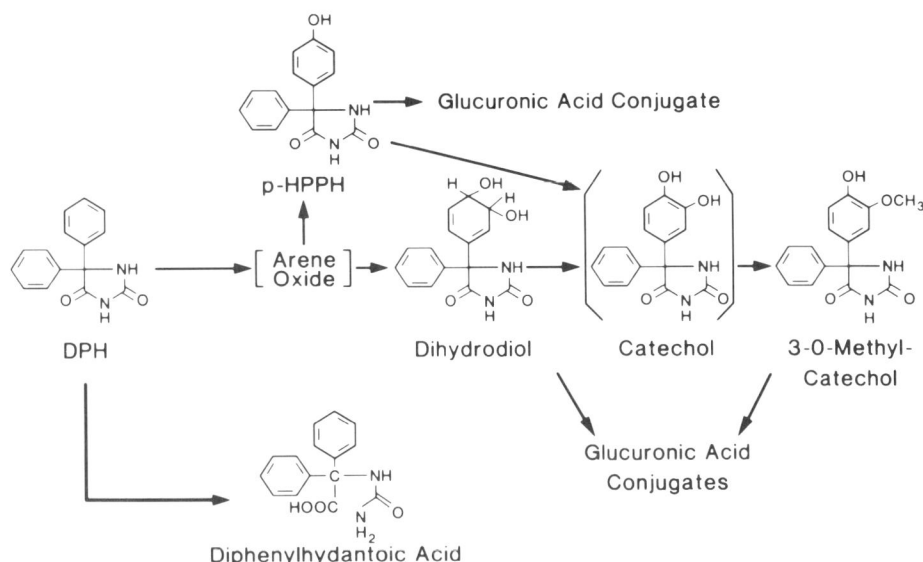

Figure 5 – 4. Summary of the proposed metabolism of phenytoin. Data in neonates are limited (see text). (From Chow SA and Fischer LJ: Drug Metab Dispos 10:156, 1982.)

adults.[25,83] Bilirubin effectively displaces phenytoin from albumin binding sites, resulting in an increased percentage of unbound drug in plasma. Thus, phenytoin therapy in a neonate with hyperbilirubinemia is unlikely to predispose to the development of kernicterus, but interpretation of phenytoin serum levels may be complicated (increased unbound phenytoin level relative to total serum phenytoin concentration). The drug distributes rapidly and widely throughout the body, with the volume of distribution in the neonate ranging from 0.7 to 2.0 l/kg; these values decline to those seen in the adult (0.6 l/kg) by 5 to 6 months of age.[72] The mean volume of distribution observed by Painter and coworkers[75] was 1.2 l/kg and did not differ among neonates of 27 to less than 37 weeks' gestation. Phenytoin levels in the brain rapidly reach 1.3 times plasma concentrations in the neonate,[76] significantly higher than the 0.8 mean value observed in adults.[104]

The metabolism of phenytoin has been incompletely studied in infants. The most important and major biotransformation step in humans is the *p*-hydroxylation of one of the phenol rings (Fig. 5 – 4), which leads to the formation of *p*-hydroxy diphenylhydantoin (*p*-HPPH). The *p*-HPPH is conjugated with glucuronic acid and excreted in the urine; this metabolite is essentially devoid of toxic and anticonvulsant effects. Several other minor metabolites of phenytoin have been identified, including dihydrodiol, catechol, methylated ca-

techol, *m*-HPPH, and diphenylhydantoic acid (DPHA), which is formed by opening of the hydantoin ring.[87] The precursor – product relationships for the various metabolites have not been completely elucidated, but the formation of an arene oxide (epoxide) is strongly suspected.[15] Folic acid given concurrently has been shown to affect serum phenytoin levels;[30] the mechanism involved is unclear, although enhanced metabolism and renal elimination of unchanged phenytoin and metabolite have been reported.

The metabolism of phenytoin occurs predominantly in the liver and is capacity-limited, with saturation occurring within the therapeutic range of plasma concentrations.[14,87] The large interpatient variability observed in phenytoin kinetics is believed to be associated with maturational changes in hepatic hydroxylation and conjugation activity.[72] In two separate studies, infants exposed to phenytoin transplacentally had negligible amounts of unmetabolized phenytoin in the urine; the major urinary metabolite was *p*-HPPH, with over 90% in the conjugate form.[84,86] Studies of phenytoin metabolism by examination of urinary metabolities of phenytoin have been accomplished in neonates treated directly;[55] no remarkable differences were found between neonates and adults in the pattern of urinary metabolites or in total recovery of drug-related substances in urine. Children excrete an average of 72% (range 59 – 86%) of the total daily phenytoin dose as *p*-HPPH, which is similar to reported adult values of 60% to 70%.[12]

Phenytoin limits the development of maximal seizure activity and reduces the spread of the seizure process from an active seizure focus.[45] It is superior to phenobarbital in blocking the spread of local seizure activity but inferior in suppressing focal activity. There is considerable evidence that the stabilizing effect of phenytoin results directly or indirectly from effects on the movement of ions (sodium, calcium) across cell membranes.[5]

Clinical Pharmacology. Numerous studies have demonstrated the dose-dependency of phenytoin pharmacokinetics. The kinetics of plasma disappearance of phenytoin change from first-order at levels less than 10 μg/ml to zero-order at higher plasma levels. Thus, there can be changes in pharmacokinetics (first-order to zero-order) over the normal therapeutic range (6–14 μg/ml). (See under Dose-Dependent or Zero-Order Kinetics, Chap. 2.) The saturable pharmacokinetics of phenytoin unfortunately undergo further change with the maturation of the infant (e.g., increased activity of hepatic hydroxylating enzymes, increased renal elimination) and with recovery from illness, making it extremely difficult for dosage prediction or adjustment. As can be seen from Table 5–6, striking differences in serum levels and half-lives have been reported within the infant population. Loughnan and colleagues [58] found values for half-life ranging from 7 to 42 hours in term infants and 20 to 160 hours in

Table 5–6. SUMMARY OF CLINICAL PHARMACOLOGY STUDIES OF PHENYTOIN IN INFANTS

Author(s) of Published Study[a]	Study Group	Dose	Serum Concentration	Serum Half-life[b] ($T\frac{1}{2}$; mean $\pm$ SD)
Albani[3]	2 neonates (<14 days old) 3 infants (4–5 mo old)	day 1: 9–13 mg/kg IV q 8 hr day 2: 5–9 mg/kg IV q 8 hr day 3: 3–5 mg/kg IV q 8 hr steady state: 7 mg/kg q 8 hr	neonates 20 μg/ml (mean) infants 12 μg/ml (mean steady state)	
Loughnan et al[58]	30 infants (2 days–96 wk old)	loading: 12 mg/kg IV maintenance: 4 mg/kg q 12 hr PO	steady state (mean $\pm$ SD) Age: <8 days: 11 $\pm$ 9.6 μg/ml 14–25 days: 2.2 $\pm$ 1.2 μg/ml 5–96 wk: 2.0 $\pm$ 1.5 μg/ml	75 $\pm$ 65 hr (premature) 20.7 $\pm$ 11.6 hr (<1 wk old) 7.6 $\pm$ 3.5 hr (>2 wk old)
Painter et al[75]	21 neonates (27 wk–term)	loading: 15–20 mg/kg IV maintenance: 5 mg/kg IV daily	14.5 $\pm$ 3.0 μg/ml (loading) 26 μg/ml (mean steady state) *average: peak–trough:*	104 $\pm$ 17 hr (>1 wk old)
Dodson[23]	4 infants (2–3 mo)	9 mg/kg q 12 hr PO 5 mg/kg q 12 hr PO 2 mg/kg q 12 hr PO	12 μg/ml 16–10 μg/ml 7 μg/ml 10–6 μg/ml 3 μg/ml 5–2 μg/ml	
Painter et al[76]	26 neonates (26–>37 wk)	loading: 15–20 mg/kg IV maintenance: <5 mg/kg IV daily	14.9 $\pm$ 2.8 μg/ml (loading dose only, mean $\pm$ SD)	194 $\pm$ 17 hr (9 infants at steady state)
Bourgeois and Dodson[120]	16 neonates (30–43 wk gestation, 2–36 days old)	loading: 20 mg/kg IV maintenance: 5–15 mg/kg/day IV or PO		ranges: 6–140 hr: <8 days old 5–80 hr: 9–21 days old 2–20 hr: 21–36 days old

[a]Listed in order of publication; see References at end of chapter.
[b]$T\frac{1}{2}$ values are known to be dependent upon the serum concentration (see text).

pre-term infants within the first week of life. Painter and coworkers[75] observed a mean steady-state serum phenytoin level of 26 μg/ml and a $T\frac{1}{2}$ of 104 hours in neonates; in a later study,[76] the mean half-life for 9 infants at steady state was 194 hours. The plasma clearance of phenytoin appears to be much more rapid between 2 weeks and 1 year of life than during the first week and after one year of life.[120] Genetic factors may also affect phenytoin metabolism: Kutt[52] and Vasko[106] and their colleagues have found evidence for an autosomal dominant defect resulting in hypometabolism of phenytoin.

Therapeutic Indications. Phenytoin is typically utilized along with phenobarbital when the seizures remain *refractory to phenobarbital therapy alone.* Although phenytoin plasma levels have been correlated with dose, toxicity, and seizure control in adults,[4] the utility of plasma level determinations is compromised by lack of similar correlative data in infants and by phenytoin's dose-dependent kinetics. In adults and children the serum level of phenytoin that has been demonstrated to correlate best with optimal seizure control and minimal toxicity is between 6 and 15 μg/ml.[12,60] The plasma level of phenytoin that gives complete seizure control varies among patients: Painter and coworkers[76] state that the therapeutic level for phenytoin is about 15 μg/ml. Patients not responding when phenytoin plasma levels are higher than 25 μg/ml (steady state) will generally not respond even with further increases in dosage.

The appropriate maintenance dose for phenytoin in infants is difficult to identify because of the paucity of information regarding the optimal therapeutic serum levels for seizure control in the infants and because of the rapidly changing and variable rate of elimination of phenytoin during the neonatal period. However, the loading dose of phenytoin required to achieve a known plasma level has been determined: An IV loading dose of 15 to 20 mg/kg rapidly produces a mean plasma drug concentration of approximately 15 μg/ml regardless of age (Fig. 5–5). The administration of this dose over a 15- to 30-minute infusion period has not been associated with toxicity. Earnest and colleagues[122] have examined the complications associated with acute IV administration of phenytoin in adults with seizures. The most serious complications included hypotension and bradycardia and other arrhythmias. The toxicities quickly resolved when the rate of infusion was slowed. The recommended maximum rate of infusion of phenytoin suggested by these authors for adults (40 mg/minute) equals approximately 0.5 mg/kg/minute. As with phenobarbital, loading and initial maintenance doses of phenytoin in the newborn infant are not influenced by birth weight or gestational age.[8]

Loughnan and colleagues[58] have determined from mean kinetic data for term infants less than 1 week of age that a maintenance dose of phenytoin of 5.9 mg/kg per day will achieve a mean steady-state plasma concentration of approximately 10 μg/ml. However, they remark that individual variation makes it impossible to recommend a fixed dosage regimen in this age group. Painter and coworkers[76] state that doses of phenytoin greater than 5 mg/kg per day given IV to the neonate will result in accumulation of toxic levels within a few days. In all infants there will be an increase in the rate of elimination of phenytoin over the first weeks of life, necessitating at least an increase in frequence of phenytoin administration. As can be seen from Table 5–5, a maintenance dose of 4 to 8 mg/kg IV per day may be necessary in neonates less than 1 week of age to maintain therapeutic phenytoin serum levels; infants older than 1 week of age may require doses of 8 mg/kg IV given every 12 hours or as often as every 8 hours. Rapid changes in the rate of elimination of phenytoin in individual neonates may occur; Loughnan and colleagues[58] determined the half-life values for one infant to be 42, 15, and 5.6 hours on days 2, 14, and 25 of life, respectively. These authors summarized the mean phenytoin plasma half-lives from the literature as follows: age 0 to 2 days, 80 hours; age 3 to 14 days, 15 hours; age 15 to 150 days, 6 hours. Whelan and coworkers[112] found that doses approaching 25 mg/kg per day were necessary to achieve therapeutic blood levels in one full term newborn

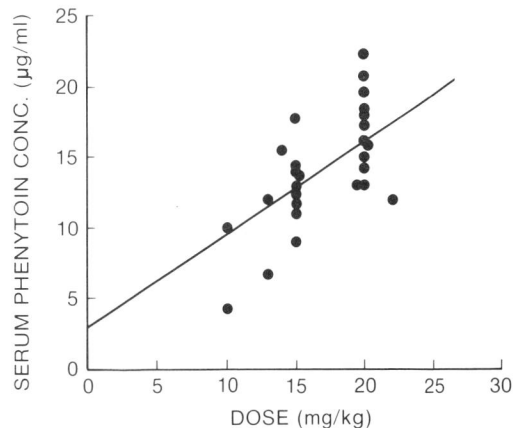

Figure 5–5. Phenytoin serum levels resulting from IV loading doses of 10 to 20 mg/kg. (Adapted from Bergman I et al: Semin Perinatol 6:54, 1982.)

over the first 4 weeks of life. Frequent monitoring of plasma phenytoin levels will greatly assist in identifying the need for dosage adjustments. Dodson[23] has determined by studies in infants and children that plasma levels obtained 8 hours after dosing, when the dose interval is every 12 hours, have the greatest accuracy and precision in determining the average phenytoin plasma level. It must be kept in mind, however, that marked fluctuations in phenytoin blood levels can occur in patients with rapid clearance rates. Evidence of seizures or signs of toxicity coincident with the periods of trough or peak drug levels, respectively, should prompt sampling of blood during these periods to document their etiology and to determine an appropriate remedy.

The ideal route of administration of phenytoin is unclear. However, in situations of difficult seizure control such as status epilepticus the IV route appears most reasonable. If the oral route is chosen, care must be taken to appreciate the possibilities of prolonged delay (in some cases, many hours) in absorption and of incomplete absorption.[76] The lack of uniform bioavailability in the various phenytoin preparations available commercially adds to the problem. It is also quite clear that the IV route does not eliminate the variability in kinetics seen among neonates or in any given neonate over the first few weeks and months of life.[112]

Liver dysfunction may significantly complicate phenytoin therapy since the elimination of phenytoin is predicated on its first being metabolized. Phenytoin intoxication has been reported in adult patients with liver disease. Uremic patients may have lower serum phenytoin concentrations than those in nonuremic patients receiving an equivalent dose; reduced binding to serum proteins appears to be the explanation.[87] Asconape and Penry[116] have reviewed the use of phenytoin in patients with liver and renal disease.

Comment

It appears that the complexities of establishing and maintaining adequate therapeutic levels of phenytoin sharply diminish the value of this drug in the long-term management of seizures in infants. A reasonable conclusion based on observed variability in pharmacokinetics is that optimal therapeutic benefits with the use of phenytoin alone are difficult to achieve, and that this drug is therefore less useful than phenobarbital in management of seizures in infants. Future studies to define more rigorously the pharmacokinetics of phenytoin in infants and the attendant dosage requirements will likely enhance the usefulness of this agent in treatment of seizures in infants.

Clinical Toxicology. The dose-dependent nature of phenytoin elimination from the body and the narrow "window" between therapeutic and toxic serum levels predispose to the development of toxic side-effects. The unpredictability and changing nature of phenytoin pharmacokinetics in the infant further complicate attempts at maximizing efficacy and minimizing toxicity. Although numerous reports have documented the toxic effects of phenytoin in adults and children, there have been few reports of phenytoin toxicity in infants. The likely explanation for this discrepancy resides not in the greater tolerance of the infant to phenytoin toxicity but in the greater difficulty of identifying on a clinical basis the presence of excess phenytoin levels. The availability of quantitative chemical monitoring of phenytoin has allowed correlations to be drawn between the progression of clinical manifestations of phenytoin intoxication and serum drug levels in children and adults: nystagmus, over 20 μg/ml; ataxia, over 30 μg/ml; and lethargy, over 40 μg/ml. In the case of neonates, infants, and young children, and for a few identified toxic manifestations, the relationship between toxicity and excessive serum levels of phenytoin appears to be less dependable. Thus, in young neonates, infants, and children, in whom the manifestations of toxicity may be subtle or not apparent clinically, careful monitoring to maintain phenytoin blood levels near or below the accepted peak therapeutic value of 15 to 20 μg/ml appears prudent. It must be appreciated, however, that there is a wide range of serum phenytoin levels associated with clinical toxicity. Borofsky and coworkers[11] studied patients ranging in age from newborns to 20 years and observed toxic manifestations with serum phenytoin levels between 14 and 40 μg/ml.

The clinical manifestations of phenytoin toxicity in children and adults have varied from the obvious to the occult (Table 5–7). The most obvious signs of toxicity are those that are extremely difficult to identify in the infant: ataxia, nystagmus, drowsiness, behavioral changes, slurred speech, diplopia, dizziness, headache, blurred vision, vomiting, gingivitis, and hirsutism. Another manifestation of phenytoin toxicity reported in children and adults is hypersensitivity reactions, characterized by rashes (including that seen with the Stevens-Johnson syndrome), fever, abnormal liver

Table 5-7. TOXICITIES ASSOCIATED WITH PHENYTOIN ANTICONVULSANT THERAPY

Signs or Symptoms	Hypersensitivity Reactions	Other Toxicities
nystagmus	rashes (morbilliform, erythema multiforme, Stevens-Johnson syndrome)	osteomalacia (rickets)
diplopia	fever	cardiac disturbances (arrhythmias)
incoordination	abnormal liver function	endocrine abnormalities (hyperglycemia, hypoinsulinemia)
ataxia	lymphoid hyperplasia	elevation of chloramphenicol levels to toxic levels
drowsiness	eosinophilia	
slurred speech	blood dyscrasias (leukopenia, thrombocytopenia, anemia)	
behavioral changes	serum sickness	
nausea: vomiting	albuminuria	
gum hypertrophy (gingivitis)		
hirsutism		
increased seizure activity		
encephalopathy, degenerative		
Peripheral neuropathy		

The fact that these observations have been largely confined to children and adults should not be interpreted to indicate that phenytoin is less toxic in the infant. See text for references.

function, lymphoid hyperplasia, eosinophilia, blood dyscrasias, serum sickness, albuminuria, or renal failure.[39,89] The hypersensitivity reactions including skin rashes and depression of the hematopoietic system appear to occur with the same incidence (approximately 5%) in children as in adults; no reports exist for infants. Osseous changes represented by calvarial thickening, osteomalacia, and rickets may also be associated with prolonged phenytoin therapy.[20,71,102] Hypocalcemia with radiologic and laboratory evidence of rickets may be of great relevance in the developing infant but has yet to be reported in neonates receiving phenytoin for seizure control, although many reports exist for children. The mechanism for the phenytoin effect on calcium metabolism is believed to be complex, involving several mechanisms, including altered vitamin D metabolism,[51] although possibly by a different alteration in metabolism from that discussed for phenobarbital.[68] However, alteration of vitamin D metabolism by anticonvulsants has been challenged by Keck and coworkers,[124] who observed no differences between children taking anticonvulsants and carefully matched control subjects. Phenytoin toxicity may also include endocrine disturbances such as hyperglycemia and hypoinsulinemia.[27]

It is well documented in children and adults that high phenytoin serum levels (> 20 μg/ml) may be associated with an increase in seizure activity.[103] This effect may occur in the absence

of other manifestations of phenytoin toxicity. This syndrome differs, therefore, from the phenytoin-induced encephalopathy that presents as a spectrum of CNS toxicity, including seizures. Vallarta and colleagues[105] reported that 10 patients who had received long-term phenytoin therapy later developed evidence of progressive encephalopathy indistinguishable from degenerative CNS disease. The toxicity was described as potentially irreversible with an onset ranging from months to years after the institution of phenytoin therapy. Since both clinical and laboratory studies strongly implicate chronic phenytoin toxicity in permanent cerebellar damage, routine monitoring of serum levels of phenytoin seems justified.

Wiriyathian and coworkers[114] reported the occurrence of cardiovascular toxicity resulting from the use of phenytoin (IV) in a premature infant of 32 weeks' gestation. These authors also noted the presence of profound neurologic abnormalities that were difficult to differentiate from underlying clinical problems. The reported signs of phenytoin-induced cardiac toxicity in children and adults have included atrial fibrillation, sinus bradycardia, sinus arrhythmia, incomplete right bundle branch block, and hypotension.

A variety of reports of interactions of phenytoin with other drugs exist in the literature.[53,132] The basis for these interactions includes drug metabolism, altered absorption, and competition for plasma proteins. Concurrent use with diazepam or phenobarbital has been reported to lower or raise the serum levels of phenytoin.[45] Phenobarbital may increase the biotransformation of phenytoin by an induction of the hepatic enzyme system, decrease the inactivation of phenytoin through competitive inhibition of phenytoin metabolism, or reduce the oral absorption of phenytoin.[82] In one series, potentially toxic chloramphenicol levels were reported in all 11 infants and children receiving phenytoin for control of seizures associated with CNS infection.[50a] Peak chloramphenicol levels averaged 41.7 μg/ml in patients receiving phenytoin, compared with 25.3 μg/ml in those receiving chloramphenicol alone. In contrast, patients receiving phenobarbital had peak chloramphenicol levels averaging 16.6 μg/ml. The increase in serum chloramphenicol levels associated with coadministration of phenytoin has been suggested to be due to competition for binding sites,[50a] although competition for hepatic metabolism may also be a factor. Of interest is the report in adults of elevation of phenytoin levels with concurrent administration of chloramphenicol.[50] (See under Chloramphenicol, Chap. 4.)

The development of folic acid deficiency and megaloblastic anemia with long-term phenytoin therapy has prompted the recommendation for supplemental folate therapy. The use of such supplements, however, has been reported to accentuate the seizure disorder in some patients.[30] The effect of folic acid on phenytoin metabolism (see under Pharmacology) has been incriminated as a causative factor in the exacerbation of seizures; moreover, folic acid itself may be epileptogenic. The etiology and clinical relevance of this interaction in the infant is unknown.

Diazepam

Pharmacology. Diazepam, a benzodiazepine, is well absorbed by all routes of administration including PO, IM, and rectal. The rate of absorption, however, differs, being most rapid with rectal administration and least rapid with PO administration.[54] Peak plasma concentrations generally are observed between 10 and 60 minutes after administration by the PO or rectal route. With IM administration, peak plasma concentrations are attained between 1 and 4 hours and are more variable.[72] Diazepam is highly bound to plasma protein (86%), with little difference observed between cord and adult serum.

Diazepam is metabolized primarily to the n-desmethyl derivative, which is pharmacologically active. Other metabolites include a ring-hydroxylated derivative (methyloxazepam) and oxazepam, which is a hydroxylated and demethylated pharmacologically active metabolite of diazepam. Conjugation of the metabolites with glucuronide can also occur (Fig. 5–6). The rate of metabolism of diazepam is lower in premature than in full-term infants, with hydroxylation and conjugation being more limited than demethylation.[63] Diazepam and metabolites are excreted slowly by the kidney.

Clinical Pharmacology. The plasma clearance rate of diazepam in the newborn is less than that in the infant or adult. This reduced rate of plasma disappearance appears to be associated with the slower rate of metabolism of diazepam. The apparent plasma half-life of diazepam is 40 to 400 hours in the premature and 20 to 50 hours in the full-term neonates.[72] IV administration of 0.5 mg/kg produces plasma levels of 2700 to 6500 ng/ml; a dose of 1 mg/kg results in levels between 5000 to 11,000 ng/ml. Estimates of anticonvulsive serum concentrations have ranged from 150 to 300 ng/ml.[54]

For tetanus therapy the minimum concentration of diazepam required in serum is approximately 3000 ng/ml in neonates; corresponding average levels of metabolites are 4000 ng/ml of n-desmethyl diazepam and 2850 ng/ml of oxazepam.[101] Accumulation of the primary metabolite, n-desmethyl diazepam, observed in infants receiving diazepam suggests slow elimination and potential accumulation of this active metabolite with repeated administration. Rectal administration of 0.5 or 1 mg/kg has produced anticonvulsant serum concentrations of diazepam within 5 minutes.[54]

Therapeutic Indications

Status Epilepticus. Diazepam given IV or rectally has been proposed by some authors to be an appropriate agent for effective short-term management of status epilepticus or prolonged resistant seizure activity in neonates.[7,54,67,96] Others discourage the use of diazepam for treatment of seizures in infants.[107] Conflicting reports exist regarding the efficiency of IM administration in infants.[49,54,67] The long-term use of diazepam is severely limited by the potential for accumulation and toxicity as well as the development of tolerance.[78] The doses employed in various studies range from 0.25 to 2.7 mg/kg given PO, IV, IM, or rectally. In one study,[96] the average dose employed was 0.7 mg/kg IV, which produced a clinical anticon-

diazepam
(active)

desmethyldiazepam
(active)

demethylation

hydroxylation

demethylation

methyloxazepam
(active)

oxazepam
(active)

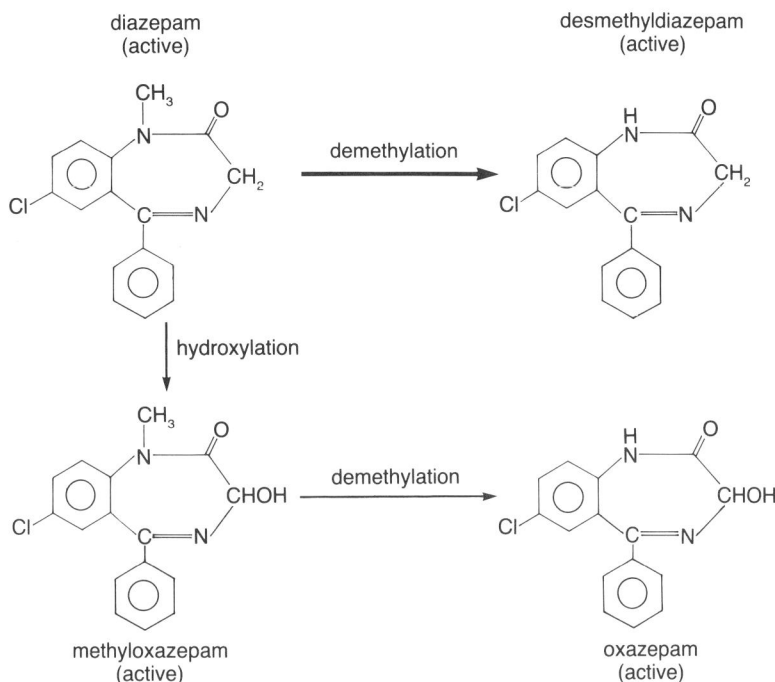

Figure 5-6. Diazepam and major metabolites: Structural formulas and biotransformation pathways. Conjugation of metabolites with glucuronide can also occur.

vulsant response in 70% of patients; the wide range of individual doses found to be effective (0.08 – 2.7 mg/kg) emphasizes the importance of titrating the dose administered (slow IV administration) to achieve the desired result. In another study,[67] equal efficacy was observed with IM and IV administration; the IV dose was delivered over a 2-minute period or until seizure manifestations ceased. The majority of patients who did respond did so in less than 3 minutes from the time of onset of administration. The recommended initial dose of diazepam in infants is 0.2 mg/kg, given as an IV infusion over 2 minutes. This dose can be repeated as needed, with the usual maximum required dose being 1.0 mg/kg (see Table 5–5).

Tetanus. Diazepam has assumed an increasingly important role in the clinical management of tetanus. Hendrickse and Sherman[42] employed oral diazepam (average dose, 1.1 mg/kg PO given every 6 hr) along with phenobarbital (4.4 – 6.6 mg/kg q 6 hr) and chlorpromazine (1.1 – 2.2 mg/kg q 6 hr) for treatment of 104 cases of neonatal tetanus; they concluded that although mortality rate was unaffected by diazepam, the drug was valuable in relieving trismus and opisthotonos. More recently, Khoo and colleagues[48] chose the IV route for diazepam administration in 43 cases of neonatal tetanus. Diazepam, 20 to 40 mg/kg per day, was given along with phenobarbital via a continuous IV infusion. This therapeutic regimen allowed avoidance of neuromuscular paralysis and the need for mechanical ventilation in 60% of the patients; by comparison, in the previous experience with more conventional doses of diazepam (0.5 – 2.5 mg/kg IV q 6 hr), only 20 percent improved. Tekur and coworkers[101] employed IV doses of diazepam of up to 50 mg/kg per day, given in divided doses every 2 hours. Others have found sedation alone inadequate for management of the tetanic spasms associated with tetanus neonatorum and therefore utilize neuromusclar blockade as the main therapy.[115]

General Sedative/Hypnotic. Diazepam has also been employed as a general sedative/hypnotic in neonates and infants. The validity of this use for diazepam should be questioned. The dosage required varies among patients, as does the duration of action. Although the therapeutic index (dose necessary to produce sedation/hypnosis vs. toxicity) is fairly wide, danger still exists for the development of respiratory depression in any given patient.[96]

Clinical Toxicology. Diazepam when administered IV has a propensity for producing phlebitis. This effect can be reduced but not eliminated by slow administration of the drug. The product information supplied by the manufacturer warns against mixing, diluting, or coadministration of the IV preparation with other IV solutions in order to avoid precipitation of the drug from solution. Very large bolus doses of diazepam have produced respiratory depression in the neonate, especially if other anticonvulsants have been given previously or if the infant is severely debilitated.[96] Repeated doses over time may result in severe hypotonia and CNS depression because of accumulation of toxic amounts of diazepam and the n-desmethyl metabolite.[54]

Other Anticonvulsants

Several other drugs have been employed infrequently in infants for management of more rare or difficult to control seizure disorders. The following drugs are agents for which there is some information in the literature regarding use in the infant.

ACTH

Adrenocorticotropic hormone (ACTH) has been the mainstay for treatment of *primary infantile spasms,* a disorder rarely seen in infants less than 3 months of age[134]. Although ACTH therapy may be less satisfactory in controlling symptomatic infantile spasms that are secondary to congenital cerebral malformations, metabolic diseases, or perinatal brain damage, over 50% of infants with primary or cryptogenic causes treated with ACTH appear to recover fully.[56] Other studies report less favorable results, and ACTH may not improve long-term prognosis regarding intellectual development.[130,133,134] Daily doses of ACTH from 5 to 180 units have been recommended, with the duration of treatment ranging from 2 weeks to 10 months.[88] According to the experience of Lerman and Kivity,[56] doses of ACTH of 80 units or more, continued for 6 to 9 months in tapering doses, produce the best seizure control and recovery. On the basis of their experience, Hrachovy and colleagues[126] recommend a 2 week course of therapy with ACTH gel (20 units/day), followed by a 1 week tapering-off period if the patient responds. Those who fail to respond are continued for an additional 4 weeks on ACTH gel (30 units/day), after which the dosage is reduced and discontinued over a 2 week period. Prednisone (1 to 2 mg/kg/day for 4 to 6 weeks) has also been used to treat infantile spasms. Although debate continues regarding the relative efficacies of ACTH and prednisone, a double-blind crossover study with placebo controls failed to demonstrate a major difference between the effectiveness of ACTH vs. that of prednisone.[126]

Side-effects associated with the large doses and long duration of therapy have been reported to be minimal to severe. In studies of 162 children by Riikonen and Donner,[88] 37% of the treated children had significant side-effects; the most common complications included hypertension, hypokalemic alkalosis, osteoporosis, and infections. The incidence of infections was significantly greater with doses of 120 units of ACTH than with doses of 40 units.

Clonazepam

Clonazepam is a benzodiazepine structurally related to diazepam. This agent has been useful in the treatment of myoclonic epilepsy and atonic seizures in children, although it is not the drug of choice. It has been also used as an adjunct to ACTH treatment of infantile spasms.[45] Its usefulness in neonates, however, remains unestablished.

Carbamazepine

Carbamazepine has been shown to be useful primarily against partial seizures and primary generalized seizures. Pharmacokinetic studies of carbamazepine in neonates have demonstrated half-lives ranging from 8 to 28 hours.[72] Doses in the range of 10 to 40 mg/kg given PO as a single daily dose or every 12 hours depending upon clearance rates have been associated with therapeutic levels of 6 to 12 μg/ml. Schain and coworkers[91] recommend a dose of 5 mg/kg every 12 hours, gradually increasing to a maximum of 15 mg/kg every 12 hours.

A wide variety of side-effects have been reported with carbamazepine, including hematologic (leukopenia) and neurotoxic abnormalities, particularly dystonia.[20] Water intoxication has been observed with the use of large doses, associated with the increase in the production of plasma antidiuretic hormone caused by this drug.[45] The indications for the use of this agent in neonates remain unclear.

Paraldehyde

In the past paraldehyde has been utilized in the newborn as an anticonvulsant, particularly in the treatment of status epilepticus. The plasma half-life of paraldehyde has been found to range from 3 to 10 hours in infants and children.[135] At steady state, the apparent volume of distribution ranges from 0.8 to 1.2 l/kg, and the serum levels are approximately 200 μg/ml. The majority of the dose is metabolized in the liver (70 to 80%), probably to acetaldehyde, which is subsequently oxidized to acetic acid and that in turn is metabolized to carbon dioxide and water. The remainder of paraldehyde is excreted in the expired air and a smaller amount in the urine. In patients with hepatic dysfunction, a larger proportion of paraldehyde is excreted in the expired air. It has been administered successfully rectally, intramuscularly, or as an intravenous drip of a 10% solution. The intramuscular dose for seizure control ranges from 0.07 to 0.35 ml/kg (1 gm/ml concentration). The recommended dose for seizure control is 0.15 ml/kg per dose, given IM every 4 to 6 hours. The recommended rectal dose is 0.3 ml/kg, given every 4 to 6 hours. For IV administration, a loading dose of 200 mg/kg followed by an IV infusion of 20 mg/kg/hr (10% solution) is recommended.[119] Side-effects of disagreeable taste and odor, local irritation, pulmonary edema, hemorrhage, and hypertension severely limit its value. Routine use in infants is discouraged except for in treatment of status epilepticus that is resistant to initial therapy with phenobarbital, phenytoin, or diazepam.

Primidone

Primidone has been utilized as an adjunct to other anticonvulsant drugs in the treatment of resistent seizure states.[8] Doses employed include a loading dose of 20 mg/kg PO followed by a maintenance dose of 15 mg/kg per day PO. Plasma levels of 8 to 15 μg/ml are considered to be maximum therapeutic concentrations.

Pyridoxine

Pharmacology. Pyridoxine-dependent seizures were first described by Hunt and colleagues in 1954,[127] and over 50 cases have been reported subsequently.[117] The seizure disorder (autosomal recessive trait in inheritance) results from a defective binding of pyridoxine to its apoenzyme, glutamate dicarboxylase, which catalyzes the conversion of glutamic acid to gamma-aminobutyric acid (GABA). GABA acts as an inhibitory neurotransmitter in the central nervous system. Seizure threshold is, therefore, lower in infants with reduced concentrations of GABA. Administration of pharmacologic doses of pyridoxine will correct the GABA deficiency.[131]

Clinical Pharmacology. Pyridoxine (B_6) in doses of 50 to 100 mg given intravenously or intramuscularly has successfully interrupted seizures in pyridoxine-dependent infants. The onset of seizures occurs on the average at approximately 4 hours of age, although a number of cases have been reported with onset of seizures as late as 3 months of age.[117] Seizures typically cease within 10 minutes after IV pyridoxine administration, with an occasional infant manifesting a delay in seizure control for up to an hour.[136] Normalization of EEG readings has varied from minutes to several weeks after the initiation of pyridoxine.[121,136] Discontinuation of pyridoxine results in the recurrence of seizures within 1 to 7 days in the neonate and 2 to 14 days in the older infant and child. The effective minimum daily requirement for pyridoxine has ranged from 2 to 200 mg.[121,125]

Therapeutic Indications. *Pyridoxine-dependent seizures* should be considered in the differential diagnosis in any infant who has intractable seizures regardless of the clinical history (e.g., sepsis, asphyxia), type of clinical presentation (e.g., infantile spasms), or response to conventional therapy. The routine use of pyridoxine as a diagnostic approach prior to the use of anticonvulsants in infants with seizures has been advocated by many (see Table 5-9).

The therapeutic dose of pyridoxine is 100 mg/kg IV, followed by a 30 minute observation period.[117] If severe seizures persist during this observation period, conventional anticonvulsant therapy should be instituted. When possible, the initial dosing with pyridoxine should be accompanied by EEG monitoring. Once a definite response to pyridoxine has been established, therapy should be continued for an indefinite period. The maintenance dose of pyridoxine is 50 to 100 mg PO given once daily. Increased doses may be required during periods of intercurrent illnesses. If questions remain regarding pyridoxine dependency, a period of withdrawal and EEG monitoring should produce evidence of recurrent seizures within one week in neonates.

Pyridoxine is also employed for the prevention or treatment of *isoniazid-induced deficiency states* (see Chapter 4). The recommended daily dosage (mg) should equal the mg amount of INH given daily (e.g., one to one ratio).[137]

Clinical Toxicology. Therapeutic doses of pyridoxine are virtually without toxicity.

Valproate

Pharmacology. Valproate represents a new category of anticonvulsant medication because of its unique chemical structure (*n*-dipropylacetic acid). It has been approved for the treatment

Table 5–8. PHARMACEUTICAL PREPARATIONS OF ANTICONVULSANTS COMMERCIALLY AVAILABLE FOR USE IN INFANTS

Drug	Available Preparation Form	Available Preparation Concentration	Comments
phenobarbital	drops	16 mg/ml	volume of dose for 1-kg
	elixir	4 mg/ml	infant: PO = 1.25 ml
	injection	$\geq$ 30 mg/ml	IV = 0.17 ml
			elixir is very bitter and may be rejected by some infants; have pharmacy prepare a more dilute stock solution for IV use in infants
phenytoin	suspension	6 mg/ml	volume of dose for 1-kg
		25 mg/ml	infant: PO = 0.67 ml
	injection	50 mg/ml	IV = 0.08 ml
			(manufacturer does not recommend dilution because of solubility of phenytoin)
diazepam	injection	5 mg/ml	volume of dose for 1-kg infant: IV = 0.04 ml
			(manufacturer does not recommend dilution because of solubility of diazepam; see under Clinical Toxicology)
carbamazepine	tablets	$\geq$ 100 mg	not commercially available as liquid preparation; stability of prepared suspension probably short
paraldehyde	solution	1 gm/ml	volume of dose for 1-kg infant: IM = 0.15 ml
	injection	1 gm/ml	
primidone	suspension	50 mg/ml	volume of dose for 1-kg infant: PO = 0.3 ml
valproate	syrup	50 mg/ml	volume of dose for 1-kg infant: PO = 0.4 ml

of absence seizures and as adjunctive therapy in multiple seizure types. It has also been employed in infants for treatment of refractory seizures and infantile spasms.[6,26,128] Absorption of valproate from the gastrointestinal tract is relatively slow but complete (86 to 100%), with peak plasma concentrations developing at 3 to 8 hours following administration in premature and full-term newborns. Valproate is highly bound to plasma protein (90 to 95%) and is largely metabolized before being excreted.

Clinical Pharmacology. Drug clearance rate is much slower in the newborn than in older infants; half-life values range between 10 and 67 hours in the first 2 weeks of life, compared with 9 to 22 hours in infants 2 weeks to 2 months of age and 7 to 13 hours in infants older than 2 months.[72,128] The drug is heavily dependent upon metabolism for elimination, which probably explains the delayed clearance seen in neonates. The reported values for volume of distribution in infants have ranged from 0.28 to 0.43 l/kg.[128]

Therapeutic Indications. Valproate should be used only in infants with seizures that are refractory to more traditional therapy. Dosage recommendations in neonates, based on preliminary data, are 15 and 40 mg/kg per day PO for premature and full-term newborns, respectively. The therapeutic serum values have been estimated to be between 50 and 100 μg/ml.[45]

Clinical Toxicology. A serious problem observed with the use of valproate is severe hepatotoxicity, which may be fatal. The onset of hepatotoxicity is associated with an elevation of serum transaminases. The drug has also been reported to provoke episodes of hyperglycinemia or hyperammonemia; such transient abnormalities must be distinguished from similar findings associated with genetically determined

Table 5–9. SEQUENCE FOR ACUTE THERAPY OF SEIZURES IN INFANTS

1. Correct and exclude metabolic abnormalities:
   a. hypoglycemia: 1–2 ml/kg of $D_{10}W$ given over 1 minute IV.
   b. hypocalcemia: 10–20 mg elemental calcium/kg over 30 minutes IV (see Table 10-4).
   c. hypomagnesemia: 25–50 mg/kg of $MgSO_4$ (10 mg/ml solution) IV.
   d. hypoxemia: O_2 and ventilation as required.
2. Pyridoxine: 100 mg IV.
3. Phenobarbital: loading dose, 15 to 20 mg/kg IV. If seizures continue, may repeat 5 mg/kg up to a total dose of 35 mg/kg (see Table 5-5).
4. Phenytoin: 20 mg/kg IV by slow infusion (see Table 5-5).
5. Diazepam: 0.1 to 1.0 mg/kg IV (see Table 5-5).
6. Neuromuscular blockade (see Chapter 10).

inborn errors of metabolism.[73,95] The hyperglycinemia resolves following discontinuation of valproate. However, MacDermot and colleagues[61] noted no change in CSF levels of glycine in nonketotic hyperglycinemic patients being effectively treated with valproate. Other toxicities include gastrointestinal disturbances, sedation, behavioral changes, alteration of coagulation (thrombocytopenia, increased platelet aggregation, hypofibrinogenemia), pancreatitis, and transient elevations of serum amylase levels.[13,81,118]

Precautions in Pediatric Dosage Preparation of Anticonvulsants

The commercial pharmaceutical anticonvulsant preparations available are inadequate for accurate delivery of recommended doses to the very small premature infant (Table 5–8). Phenobarbital is the *only* drug that can be safely diluted to allow more accurate dose measurement and delivery.

Summary

A logical sequence to therapy of neonatal seizures is outlined in Table 5–9.

References

1. Aiges HW, Daum F, Olson M, et al: The effect of phenobarbital and diphenylhydantoin on liver function and morphology. J Pediatr 97:22, 1980.
2. Aitkenhead AR: Do barbiturates protect the brain? Br J Anaesth 53:1011, 1981.
3. Albani M: An effective dose schedule for phenytoin treatment of status epilepticus in infancy and childhood. Neuropaediatrie 8:286, 1977.
4. Albert KS, Sakmar E, Hallmark MR, et al: Bioavailability of diphenylhydantoin. Clin Pharmacol Ther 16:727, 1974.
5. Ayala GF, Johnston D: The influences of phenytoin on the fundamental electrical properties of simple neural systems. Epilepsia 18:299, 1977.
6. Bachman DS: Use of valproic acid in treatment of infantile spasms. Arch Neurol 39:49, 1982.
7. Bailey DW, Fenichel GM: The treatment of prolonged seizure activity with intravenous diazepam. J Pediatr 73:923, 1968.
8. Bergman I, Painter MJ, Crumrine PK: Neonatal seizures. Semin Perinatol 6:54, 1982.
9. Bloxham RA, Durbin GM, Johnson T, Winterborn MH: Chloramphenicol and phenobarbital—a drug interaction. Arch Dis Child 54:76, 1979.
10. Boreus LO, Jalling B, Kallberg N: Phenobarbital metabolism in adults and in newborn infants. Acta Paediatr Scand 67:193, 1978.
11. Borofsky LG, Louis S, Kutt H, Roginsky M: Diphenylhydantoin: Efficacy, toxicity, and dose–serum level relationships in children. J Pediatr 81:995, 1972.
12. Borofsky LG, Louis S, Kutt H: Diphenylhydantoin in children. Neurology 23:967, 1973.
13. Browne TR: Valproic acid. N Engl J Med 302:661, 1980.
14. Chiba K, Ishizaki T, Miura H, Minagawa K: Michaelis-Menten pharmacokinetics of diphenylhydantoin and application in the pediatric-age patient J Pediatr 96:479, 1980.
15. Chow SA, Fischer LJ: Phenytoin metabolism in mice. Drug Metab Dispos 10:156, 1982.
16. Chow-Tung E, Lau AH, Vidyasagar D, John EG: Clearance of phenobarbital by peritoneal dialysis in a neonate. Clin Pharmacy 1:268, 1982.
17. Cooke RWI, Morgan MEI, Massey RF: Phenobarbitone to prevent intraventricular haemorrhage. Lancet 2:414, 1981.
18. Couto-Sales S. Rey E, Radavanyi MF, Dreyfus-Brisac C: Essay d'evaluation des therapeutics (diazepam, phenobarbital) sur l'EEG neonatal pendant les premiéres 24 heures du traitement. Rev EEG Neurophysiol 9:26, 1979.
19. Crosley CJ, Chee C, Berman PH: Rickets associated with long-term anticonvulsant therapy in a pediatric outpatient population. Pediatrics 56:52, 1975.
20. Crosley CJ, Swender PT: Dystonia associated with carbamazepine administration: Experience in brain-damaged children. Pediatrics 63:612, 1979.
21. Davis AG, Mutchie, KD, Thompson JA, Myers GG: Once-daily dosing with phenobarbital in children with seizure disorders. Pediatrics 68:824, 1981.
22. Diaz J, Schain RJ: Phenobarbital: Effects of long-term administration on behavior and brain of artificially reared rats. Science 199:90, 1978.
23. Dodson WE: Phenytoin kinetics in children. Clin Pharmacol Ther 27:704, 1980.
24. Donn SM, Roloff DW, Goldstein GW: Prevention of intraventricular haemorrhage in preterm infants by phenobarbitone: A controlled trial. Lancet 2:215, 1981.
25. Ehrnebo M, Agurell S, Jalling B, Boreus LO: Age differences in drug binding by plasma proteins: Studies on human foetuses, neonates, and adults. Eur J Clin Pharmacol 3:189, 1971.
26. Erenberg G, Rothner AD, Henry CE, Cruse RP: Valproic acid in the treatment of intractable absence seizures in children. Am J Dis Child 136:526, 1982.
27. Fariss BL, Lutcher CL: Diphenylhydantoin-induced hyperglycemia and impaired insulin release: Effect of dosage. Diabetes 20:177, 1971.
28. Fenichel GM, Olson, BJ, Fitzpatrick JE: Heart rate changes in convulsive and nonconvulsive neonatal apnea. Ann Neurol 7:577, 1980.
29. Fischer JH, Lockman LA, Zaske D, Kriel R: Phenobarbital maintenance dose requirements in treating neonatal seizures. Neurology 31:1042, 1981.
30. Furlanut M, Benetello P, Avogaro A, Dainese R: Effects of folic acid on phenytoin kinetics in healthy subjects. Clin Pharmacol Ther 24:294, 1978.
31. Gabriel M, Albani M, Schulte FJ: Apneic spells and sleep states in preterm infants. Pediatrics 57:142, 1976.
32. Gabriel M, Albani M: Rapid eye movement sleep, apnea, and cardiac slowing influenced by phenobarbital administration in the neonate. Pediatrics 60:426, 1977.
33. Gal P, Boer HR, Toback J, Erkan NV: Phenobarbital

dosing in neonates and asphyxia. Neurology 32:788, 1982.

34. Gal P, Toback J, Boer HR, et al: Efficacy of phenobarbital monotherapy in treatment of neonatal seizures—relationship to blood levels. Neurology 32:1401, 1982.

35. Garrettson LK: Phenobarbital disposition in the neonate. Addict Dis 2:179, 1975.

36. Godin DV, Mitchell MJ, Saunders BA: Studies on the interaction of barbiturates with reactive oxygen radicals: Implications regarding barbiturate protection against cerebral ischaemia. Can Anaesth Soc J 29:203, 1982.

37. Gold F, Bourin M, Granry JC, et al: Interet de la voie intraveineuse pour l'utilisation du phenobarbital chez le nouvau-ne a terme asphyxie. Arch Franc Pediatr 36:610, 1979.

38. Hahn TJ, Hendin BA, Scharp CR, et al: Serum 25-hydroxycalciferol levels and bone mass in children on chronic anticonvulsant therapy. N Engl J Med 292:550, 1975.

39. Haruda F: Phenytoin hypersensitivity: 38 cases. Neurology 29:1480, 1979.

40. Heimann G, Gladtke E: Pharmacokientics of phenobarbital in childhood. Eur J Clin Pharmacol 12:305, 1977.

41. Heinze E, Kampffmeyer HG: Biological half-life of phenobarbital in human babies. Klin Wschr 49:1146, 1971.

42. Hendrickse RG, Sherman PM: Tetanus in childhood: Report of a therapeutic trial of diazepam. Br Med J 2:860, 1966.

43. Hope PL, Stewart AL, Thorburn RJ, et al: Failure of phenobarbitone to prevent intraventricular haemorrhage in small preterm infants. Lancet 1:444, 1982.

44. Jalling B: Plasma concentrations of phenobarbital in the treatment of seizures in newborns. Acta Paediatr Scand 64:514, 1975.

45. Johnston MV, Freeman JM: Pharmacologic advances in seizure control. Pediatr Clin North Am 28:179, 1981.

46. Johnston MV, Singer HS: Brain neurotransmitters and neuromodulators in pediatrics. Pediatrics 70:57, 1982.

47. Jung D, Powell JR, Walson P, Perrier D: Effect of dose on phenytoin absorption. Clin Pharmacol Ther 28:479, 1980.

48. Khoo BH, Lee EL, Lam KL: Neonatal tetanus treated with high-dosage diazepam. Arch Dis Child 53:737, 1978.

49. Knudsen FU: Plasma-diazepam in infants after rectal administration in solution and by suppository. Acta Pediatr Scand 66:563, 1977.

50. Koup JR, Gibaldi M, McNamara P, et al: Interaction of chloramphenicol with phenytoin and phenobarbital. J Clin Pharmacol Ther 24:571, 1978.

50a. Krasinski K, Kusmiesz H, Nelson JD: Pharmacologic interactions among chloramphenicol, phenytoin and phenobarbital. Pediatr Inf Dis 1:232, 1982.

51. Kruse K: On the pathogenesis of anticonvulsant-drug-induced alterations of calcium metabolism. Eur J Pediatr 138:202, 1982.

52. Kutt, H, Wolk M, Scherman R, McDowell F: Insufficient parahydroxylation as a cause of diphenylhydantoin toxicity. Neurology 14:542, 1964.

53. Kutt H: Interactions of antiepileptic drugs. Epilepsia 16:393, 1975.

54. Langslet A, Meberg A, Bredesen JE, Lunde PKM: Plasma concentrations of diazepam and n-des-

methyldiazepam in newborn infants after intravenous, intramuscular, rectal and oral administration. Acta Paediatr Scand 67:699, 1978.

55. Leff RD, Roberts RJ, Fischer LJ, Charkowski DM, Berg MJ: Phenytoin disposition following intravenous and oral administration in the neonate. Drug Intell Clin Pharm. 17:448, 1983.

56. Lerman P, Kivity S: The efficacy of corticotropin in primary infantile spasms. J Pediatr 101:294, 1982.

57. Lockman LA, Kriel R, Zaske D, et al: Phenobarbital dosage for control of neonatal seizures. Neurology 29:1445, 1979.

58. Loughnan PM, Greenwald A, Purton WW, et al: Pharmacokinetic observations of phenytoin disposition in the newborn and young infant. Arch Dis Child 52:302, 1977.

59. Lous P: Blood serum and cerebrospinal fluid levels and renal clearance by phenemal in treated epileptics. Acta Pharmacol et Toxicol 10:166, 1954.

60. Lund L: Anticonvulsant effect of diphenylhydantoin relative to plasma levels. Arch Neurol 31:289, 1974.

61. MacDermot K, Nelson W, Weinberg JA, Schulman JD: Valproate in nonketotic hyperglycinemia. Pediatrics 65:624, 1980.

62. Macdonald RL, Barker JL: Anticonvulsant and anesthetic barbiturates: Different postsynaptic actions in cultured mammalia neurons. Neurology 29:432, 1979.

63. Mandelli M, Tognoni G, Garattini S: Clinical pharmacokinetics of diazepam. Clin Pharmacokinet 3:72, 1978.

64. Marshall LF, Smith RW, Shapiro HM: The outcome with aggressive treatment in severe head injuries. Part II. Acute and chronic barbiturate administration in the management of head injury. J Neurosurg 50:26, 1979.

65. Marshall R, Sheehan M, Escobedo M, et al: Seizures in a neonatal intensive care unit: A prospective study. Pediatr Res 10:450, 1976.

66. Matsukura M, Higashi A, Ikeda T, Matsuda I: Bioavailability of phenobarbital by rectal administration. Pediatr Pharmacol 1:259, 1981.

67. McMorris S, McWilliam PKA: Status epilepticus in infants and young children treated with parenteral diazepam. Arch Dis Child 44:604, 1969.

68. Mimaki T, Walson PD, Haussler MR: Anticonvulsant therapy and vitamin D metabolism: Evidence for different mechanisms for phenytoin and phenobarbital. Pediatr Pharmacol 1:105, 1980.

69. Minagawa K, Miura H, Chiba K, Ishizaki T: Pharmacokinetics and relative bioavailability of intramuscular phenobarbital sodium or acid in infants. Pediatr Pharmacol 1:279, 1981.

70. Morgan MEI, Massey RF, Cooke RWI: Does phenobarbitone prevent periventricular hemorrhage in very low-birth-weight babies? A controlled trial. Pediatrics 70:186, 1982.

71. Morijiri Y, Sato T: Factors causing rickets in institutionalised handicapped children on anticonvulsant therapy. Arch Dis Child 56:446, 1981.

72. Morselli PL, Franco-Morselli R, Bossi L: Clinical pharmacokinetics in newborns and infants: Age-related differences and therapeutic implications. Clin Pharmacokinet 5:485, 1980.

73. Murphy JV, Marquardt K: Asymptomatic hyperammonemia in patients receiving valproic acid. Arch Neurol 39:591, 1982.

74. Ouvrier RA, Goldsmith R: Phenobarbitone dosage in neonatal convulsions. Arch Dis Child 57:653, 1982.

75. Painter MJ, Pippenger C, MacDonald H, Pitlick W:

Phenobarbital and diphenylhydantoin levels in neonates with seizures. J Pediatr 92:315, 1978.

76. Painter MJ, Pippenger C, Wasterlain C, et al: Phenobarbital and phenytoin in neonatal seizures: Metabolism and tissue distribution. Neurology 31:1107, 1981.

77. Palmer DL, Despopoulos A, Rael ED: Induction of chloramphenicol metabolism by phenobarbital. Antimicrob Agents Chemother 1:112, 1972.

78. Penry JK, Newmark ME: The use of antiepileptic drugs. Ann Intern Med 90:207, 1979.

79. Pippenger CE, Rosen TS: Phenobarbital plasma levels in neonates. Clin Perinatol 2:111, 1975.

80. Pitlick W, Painter M, Pippenger C: Phenobarbital pharmacokinetics in neonates. Clin Pharmacol Ther 23:346, 1978.

81. Pruitt AW, Anyan WR, Hill RM: Valproic acid: Benefits and risks. Pediatrics 70:316, 1982.

82. Rall TW, Schleifer LS: Drugs effective in the therapy of the epilepsies. In AG Gilman, LS Goodman, and A Gilman (eds): The Pharmacological Basis of Therapeutics. Pp 448–467. Macmillan, New York, 1980.

83. Rane A, Lunde PKM, Jalling B, et al: Plasma protein binding of diphenylhydantoin in normal and hyperbilirubinemic infants. J Pediatr 78:877, 1971.

84. Rane A: Urinary excretion of diphenylhydantoin metabolites in newborn infants. J Pediatr 85:543, 1974.

85. Remmer H: Induction of drug metabolizing enzyme system in the liver. Eur J Clin Pharmacol 5:116, 1972.

86. Reynolds JW, Mirkin BL: Urinary corticosteroid and diphenylhydantoin metabolite patterns in neonates exposed to anticonvulsant drugs in utero. Clin Pharmacol Ther 14:891, 1973.

87. Richens A: Clinical pharmacokinetics of phenytoin. Clin Pharmacokinet 4:153, 1979.

88. Riikonen R, Donner M: ACTH therapy in infantile spasms: Side effects. Arch Dis Child 55:664, 1980.

89. Robinson HM Jr, Stone JH: Exanthem due to diphenylhydantoin therapy. Arch Derm 101:462, 1970.

90. Schaible DH, Cupit GC, Swedlow DB, Rocci ML Jr: High-dose pentobarbital pharmacokinetics in hypothermic brain-injured children. J Pediatr 100:655, 1982.

91. Schain RJ, Ward JW, Guthrie D: Carbamazepine as an anticonvulsant in children. Neurology 27:476, 1977.

92. Schub HS, Lazzara A, Ahmann PA, Dykes F: Phenobarbitone in neonatal intraventricular haemorrhage. Lancet 2: 869, 1981.

93. Seay AR, Bray PF: Significance of seizures in infants weighing less than 2,500 grams. Arch Neurol 34:381, 1977.

94. Sherwin AL, Eisen AA, Sokolowski CD: Anticonvulsant drugs in human epileptogenic brain: Correlation of phenobarbital and diphenylhydantoin levels with plasma. Arch Neurol 29:73, 1973.

95. Simila S, von Wendt L, Linna SL, et al: Dipropylacetate and hyperglycinemia. Neuropaediatrie 10:158, 1979.

96. Smith BT, Masotti RE: Intravenous diazepam in the treatment of prolonged seizure activity in neonates and infants. Dev Med Child Neurol 13:630, 1971.

97. Staudt F, Scholl ML, Coen RW, Bickford RB: Phenobarbital therapy in neonatal seizures and the prognostic value of the EEG. Neuropediatrics 13:24, 1982.

98. Steer CR: Barbiturate therapy in the management of cerebral ischaemia. Dev Med Child Neurol 24:219, 1982.

99. Taburet AM, Chamouard C, Aymard P, et al: Phenobarbital protein binding in neonates. Dev Pharmacol Ther 4(suppl 1):129, 1982.

100. Takashima S, Tanaka K: Microangiography and vascular permeability of the subependymal matrix in the premature infant. Can J Neurol Sci 5:45, 1978.

101. Tekur U, Gupta A, Tayal G, Agrawal KK: Blood concentrations of diazepam and its metabolites in children and neonates with tetanus. J Pediatr 102:145, 1983.

102. Tolman KG, Jubiz W, Sannella JJ, et al: Osteomalacia associated with anticonvulsant drug therapy in mentally retarded children. Pediatrics 56:45, 1975.

103. Troupin AS, Ojemann LM: Paradoxical intoxication —a complication of anticonvulsant administration. Epilepsia 16:753, 1975.

104. Vajda F, Williams FM, Davidson S, et al: Human brain, cerebrospinal fluid, and plasma concentrations of dephenylhydantoin and phenobarbital. Clin Pharmacol Ther 15:597, 1974.

105. Vallarta JM, Bell DB, Reichart A: Progressive encephalopathy due to chronic hydantoin intoxication. Am J Dis Child 128:27, 1974.

106. Vasko MR, Bell RD, Daly DD, Pippenger CE: Inheritance of phenytoin hypometabolism: A kinetic study of one family. Clin Pharmacol Ther 27:96, 1980.

107. Volpe JJ: Neonatal seizures. Clin Perinatol 4:43, 1977.

108. Volpe JJ: Neonatal intracranial hemorrhage. Pathophysiology, neuropathology, and clinical features. Clin Perinatol 4:77, 1977.

109. Waddell WJ, Butler TC: The distribution and excretion of phenobarbital. J Clin Invest 36:1217, 1957.

110. Wallin A, Jalling B, Boreus LO: Plasma concentrations of phenobarbital in the neonate during prophylaxis for neonatal hyperbilirubinemia. J Pediatr 85:392, 1974.

111. Walson PD, Mimaki T, Curless R, et al: Once-daily doses of phenobarbital in children. J Pediatr 97:303, 1980.

112. Whelan HT, Hendeles L, Haberkern CM, Neims AH: High intravenous phenytoin dosage requirement in a newborn infant. Neurology 33:106, 1983.

113. Wimberley PD, Lou HC, Pedersen H, et al: Hypertensive peaks in the pathogenesis of intraventricular hemorrhage in the newborn. Abolition by phenobarbitone sedation. Acta Paediatr Scand 71:537, 1982.

114. Wiriyathian S, Kaojarern S, Rosenfeld CR: Dilantin toxicity in a preterm infant: Persistent bradycardia and lethargy. J Pediatr 100:146, 1982.

115. Adams JM, Kenny JD, Rudolph AJ: Modern management of tetanus neonatorum. Pediatrics 64:472, 1979.

116. Asconape JJ, Penry JK: Use of antiepileptic drugs in the presence of liver and kidney diseases: A review. Epilepsia 23 (suppl):S65, 1982.

117. Bankier A, Turner M, Hopkins IJ: Pyridoxine-dependent seizures—a wider clinical spectrum. Arch Dis Child 58:415, 1983.

118. Batalden PB, Van Dyne BJ, Cloyd J: Pancreatitis associated with valproic acid therapy. Pediatrics 64:520, 1979.

119. Bostrom B: Paraldehyde toxicity during treatment of status epilepticus. Am J Dis Child 136:414, 1982.

120. Bourgeois BFD, Dodson WE: Phenytoin elimination in newborns. Neurology 33:173, 1983.

121. Clarke TA, Saunders BS, Feldman B: Pyridoxine-dependent seizures requiring high doses of pyridoxine for control. Am J Dis Child 133:963, 1979.

122. Earnest MP, Marx JA, Drury LR: Complications of intravenous phenytoin for acute treatment of seizures. Recommendations for usage. JAMA 249:762, 1983.

123. Gal P, Boer HR: Early discontinuation of anticonvulsants after neonatal seizures: A preliminary report. Southern Med J 75:298, 1982.

124. Gilman ME, Toback JW, Gal P, et al: Individualizing phenobarbital dosing in neonates. Clin Pharmacy 2:258, 1983.

125. Heeley A, Pugh RJP, Clayton BE, et al: Pyridoxol metabolism in vitamin B_6-responsive convulsions of early infancy. Arch Dis Child 53:794, 1978.

126. Hrachovy RA, Frost JD Jr, Kellaway P, et al: Double-blind study of ACTH vs prednisone therapy in infantile spasms. J Pediatr 103:641, 1983.

127. Hunt AD Jr, Stokes J Jr, McCrory W, et al: Pyridoxine dependency: Report of a case of intractable convulsions in an infant controlled by pyridoxine. Pediatrics 13:140, 1954.

128. Irvine-Meek JM, Hall KW, Otten NH, et al: Pharmacokinetic study of valproic acid in a neonate. Pediatr Pharmacol 2:317, 1982.

129. Keck E, Gollnick B, Reinhardt D, et al: Calcium metabolism and vitamin D metabolite levels in children receiving anticonvulsant drugs. Eur J Pediatr 139:52, 1982.

130. Kurokawa T, Goya N, Fukuyama Y, et al: West syndrome and Lennox-Gastaut syndrome: A survey of natural history. Pediatrics 65:81, 1980.

131. Minns R: Vitamin B_6 deficiency and dependency. Dev Med Child Neurol 22:795, 1980.

132. Pippenger CE: An overview of antiepileptic drug interactions. Epilepsia 23 (suppl):S81, 1982.

133. Pollack MA, Zion TE, Kellaway P: Long-term prognosis of patients with infantile spasms following ACTH therapy. Epilepsia 20:255, 1979.

134. Riikonen R: Infantile spasms: Some new theoretical aspects. Epilepsia 24:159, 1983.

135. Thurston JH, Liang HS, Smith JS, et al: New enzymatic method for measurement of paraldehyde: Correlation of effects with serum and CSF levels. J Lab Clin Med 72:699, 1968.

136. Waldinger C, Berg RB: Signs of pyridoxine dependency manifest at birth in siblings. Pediatrics 32:161, 1963.

137. Wason S, Lacouture PG, Lovejoy FH Jr: Single high-dose pyridoxine treatment for isoniazid overdose. JAMA 246:1102, 1981.

138. Watanabe K, Hara K, Miyazaki S, et al: Apneic seizures in the newborn. Am J Dis Child 136:980, 1982.

SIX

Methyl Xanthine Therapy:
Caffeine and Theophylline

APNEA IN THE PREMATURE INFANT

One of the more frustrating clinical problems in the neonatal intensive care unit is apnea in the premature infant. Concern regarding the contribution of this disorder to morbidity and mortality in the low-birth-weight infant has led to aggressive pharmacologic approaches in attempts to reduce or prevent its occurrence. In 1973, Kuzemko and Paala[55] observed a decrease in the frequency of apneic attacks in neonates treated with theophylline. Since that report many investigators have confirmed the effect of theophylline in decreasing the frequency or abolishing the occurrence of apneic spells (see Table 6–7). More recently, caffeine has been shown to have similar efficacy and has assumed the position of drug of choice for the treatment of apnea despite the lack of controlled trials for critical comparison of caffeine and theophylline. The potential advantages of employing caffeine in the treatment of apnea are reviewed in Therapeutic Indications under Caffeine later in this chapter.

Although **apnea** by strict definition means absence of respiratory movements, a variety of clinical definitions have been applied in the premature infant. The following definition of apnea is the most useful because it is both clear and interpretable: absence of respiratory effort for greater than 20 seconds with or without bradycardia or cyanosis.[75] **Periodic breathing,** which is sometimes included or confused with apnea, is thought to be a benign disorder that involves a respiratory pause lasting for 5 to 10 seconds alternating with breathing. Although heart rate has been shown to substantially decrease with true apnea and only slightly or not at all with periodic breathing,[25] transcutaneous

PaO_2 (arterial partial pressure of oxygen) monitoring has demonstrated reduced PaO_2 values in the absence of diminished heart rate. Interestingly, Fenichel and colleagues[32] have found that nonconvulsive neonatal apnea is more frequently associated with diminished heart rate than is convulsive neonatal apnea. The overall incidence of apnea in premature infants has been estimated to be 30% to 50%, with the incidence increasing dramatically to 90% in those infants who are 28 to 29 weeks or less in gestational age.[75]

Neonatal apnea is known to be associated with several underlying disorders, including sepsis, hypoglycemia, electrolyte imbalance, pneumonia, congestive heart failure, anemia, respiratory distress syndrome, intracranial bleeding, patent ductus arteriosus, and seizures. The exact pathogenesis of apnea and periodic breathing occurring in the absence of these diseases has been the subject of great debate and numerous investigations. Rigatto in a recent review[75] concluded that periodic breathing and neonatal apnea probably have a common physiopathogenic route, with apnea representing a greater degree of basic disturbance. The focus of most research on the mechanism of apnea has been on respiratory drive and the complexity of interactions that participate in maintaining respirations; disturbances of the respiratory center, central chemoreceptors, peripheral chemoreceptors, and reflexes from the lung and the performance of the respiratory pump have been examined. The origin of apnea in the premature infant appears to be related to an immaturity of the central respiratory control mechanisms, as reflected by a lack of dendritic arborization and a decreased number of synaptic connections in the CNS.[104] Several excellent review articles describe in detail the theories regarding the origin of apnea.[50,75,115]

In the considerations regarding treatment, priority must be given to the identification of known causes of neonatal apnea in order to effect their remedy as well as to control the apnea (e.g., infection). Another consideration is whether or not the apnea is sufficiently severe to mandate therapy. Late neurologic sequelae have been observed in infants with a history of repeated episodes of apnea.[9,10,109] It seems most reasonable to consider pharmacotherapy as an appropriate alternative to mechanical respiratory support.

THE METHYL XANTHINES

The **methyl xanthines** are a group of chemically related alkaloids, including caffeine and theophylline, that have been shown to reduce effectively the frequency and severity of neonatal apnea. Their use has a long and colorful history largely because of their various and potent pharmacologic properties, especially their effects on the CNS.

Caffeine

Pharmacology. Caffeine is a naturally occurring methylated xanthine, 1,3,7-trimethyl xanthine (see Fig. 6–1). Although the methyl xanthines in general are more soluble in lipid than in aqueous solutions, caffeine is more lipid-soluble than theophylline. It is rapidly and completely absorbed from the gastrointestinal tract with peak serum concentrations reached within 30 minutes to 2 hours.[6] Soluble preparations such as caffeine citrate are very acidic (pH 3 to 4) and should not be given by the IM route. Caffeine is distributed widely throughout the body after IV or PO administration, with fairly uniform concentrations being reached in various tissues. Warszawski and Gorodischer[98] observed greater concentrations of caffeine in tissues of newborn animals than those in adults given equivalent doses. They also measured caffeine concentrations in post-mortem tissues from two premature infants: For one infant, whose plasma concentration had been 70 μg/ml during therapy, tissue values were 84 μg/g in heart and 40 μg/g in spleen; in the other, whose plasma concentration had been 44 μg/ml, these values were 74 μg/g in heart, 18 μg/g in ileum, 32 μg/ml in CSF, and 19 μg/g in cerebrum. Other investigators have found that plasma concentrations of caffeine correlate closely with concentrations achieved in the CSF, the ratio of CSF to plasma levels being close to unity.[84,92] In animals, Sattin[80] observed that maximal brain concentrations of caffeine were reached at 5 minutes after intraperitoneal administration compared with 20 minutes with theophylline; accordingly, he speculated that the relative behavioral potency of caffeine and theophylline may be determined by the difference in rate of penetration into the forebrain. These results are consistent with the observations of Chu,[23] who concluded that caffeine is more epileptogenic than theophylline following systemic administration.

In neonates, the calculated mean volume of distribution for caffeine is approximately 0.8 to 0.9 l/kg;[7] this mean value is larger than that reported for adults (0.4–0.6 l/kg).[13,74] Caffeine is less bound to plasma protein than is theophylline, with values for percentage bound reported to be approximately 25%.[94]

Several investigations have demonstrated that the liver microsomal mixed-function mono-oxygenase system is involved in the metabolism of caffeine. Figure 6–1 depicts the metabolism of caffeine and theophylline in neonates and adults. Different forms of cytochrome *P450* have been proposed to be involved in the metabolism of caffeine and theophylline, thereby explaining the several-fold difference in rate of clearance of these two methyl xanthines in neonates.[41] Caffeine is excreted largely unchanged in the urine of neonates, in contrast to adults, who excrete less than 2% of the caffeine dose unchanged.[8] Horning and coworkers[46] found primarily unchanged caffeine in the urine of 1- to 3-day-old neonates who had acquired caffeine transplacentally. Aldridge and colleagues[1] found that caffeine accounted for 85% of the methylated xanthines in the urine in infants less than 1 month of age given caffeine. Caffeine remains the predominant urinary component for at least the first 3 months of life.[5] Adult plasma clearance rates appear to be achieved coincident with the increased capacity to produce demethylated metabolites of caffeine; this occurs at about 3 to 4 1/2 months of age.[5] The poor ability of the neonate to form *N*-demethylated metabolites of caffeine is nevertheless greater than that observed for other drugs, such as diazepam; this finding supports the existence of different forms of cytochrome *P450* mixed-function oxidases.[17] The urinary excretion pattern in neonates and the slow rate of clearance of caffeine from the plasma also suggest a deficiency in the capacity for oxidation, but less limited than that for demethyla-

Table 6–1. MAJOR PHARMACOLOGIC EFFECTS OF CAFFEINE AND THEOPHYLLINE

Effect	Estimated Relative Potency[a]	
	Caffeine	Theophylline
CNS		
stimulation of medullary respiratory centers	++++	+++
generalized (cortical) enhancement of CNS cellular response to stimulation	+++	+++
Cardiovascular		
heart: increased rate	− or +	++
vascular: decreased peripheral vascular resistance	+	+
increased cerebrovascular resistance	+	+
Smooth Muscle		
relaxation (i.e., bronchial)	+	+++
Skeletal Muscle		
stimulation	++	+
Kidney		
diuretic action	?	++
Gastrointestinal		
secretion (acid)	++	+
Cellular		
phosphodiesterase inhibition	+	++
competitive inhibition of adenosine	++	+++

[a]Comparative potency estimates are based on use of doses in the therapeutic range. Opposite or no effect: −; minimal effect: +; maximal effect: ++++. Very few critically controlled experiments have been conducted comparing the pharmacologic potency of caffeine and theophylline, particularly their CNS effects. No comparative studies have been done in neonates.

tion. One major urinary metabolite is believed to be 1,3,7-trimethyl dihydrouric acid;[41] however, in a recent study, neonates given theophylline who developed measurable caffeine levels did not excrete this metabolite.[91] Factors known to influence the metabolism and excretion of xanthines in adults, such as liver disease, diet, congestive heart failure, fever, and interactions with other drugs, have been studied to only a limited extent in neonates.[31]

Although caffeine and theophylline have in common several pharmacologic activities, there are differences in the intensity of these actions (Table 6–1). Caffeine is a potent CNS stimulant and is considered traditionally to be the most potent of the methyl xanthines. However, theophylline at plasma levels only two to three times the therapeutic level can produce a potent, potentially lethal stimulation of the CNS; the doses of caffeine necessary to result in seizure activity are far larger relative to the therapeutic

dose than those of theophylline—that is, caffeine has a greater therapeutic index. Nausea and vomiting resulting from methyl xanthine therapy probably involve CNS actions, since emesis occurs even after parenteral administration.[74] The cortical effects of caffeine in the CNS are reflected clinically as changes in alertness and enhanced performance of previously acquired abilities. Some investigators have suggested that the behavioral effects of methyl xanthines are related to an increase in turnover of monamines in the CNS.[49] The reticular formation may be an area of the CNS particularly sensitive to caffeine. As opposed to the cortex, where caffeine appears only to increase the CNS cellular response to receptive field stimulation, the spontaneous activity of the reticular formation is increased with caffeine.[33] These effects occur despite the vasoconstrictive action of caffeine on cerebral vessels.[63] Studies of cerebral blood flow in neonates exposed to caffeine have not been reported.

The respirogenic action of the methyl xanthines responsible for the alteration of neonatal apnea represents an excitation of the CNS. The proposed pharmacologic mechanisms responsible for methyl xanthine alteration of neonatal apnea are presented in Table 6–2 and in the Pharmacology section under theophylline. Caffeine produces marked stimulation of the respiratory center located in the medulla. There is an increase in the sensitivity of the medullary centers to the stimulatory actions of carbon dioxide, and respiratory minute volume is increased at any given value of $PaCO_2$ (alveolar partial pressure of carbon dioxide).[89] Animals rendered incapable of responding to peripherally sensed stimuli (via denervated carotid sinuses and sectioned vagi) remain responsive to caffeine-induced respiratory stimulation; this finding reinforces a primary central action.[59] In addition, caffeine appears to exert an additive effect on chemoreceptor sensitivity to carbon dioxide.[8] It has also been suggested that methyl xanthines may produce stimulation of the in-

Table 6–2. PHARMACOLOGIC MECHANISMS PROPOSED FOR METHYL XANTHINE ALTERATION OF NEONATAL APNEA

increased sensitivity of medullary respiratory center to CO_2
increased afferent nerve traffic to brain stem
increased catecholamine response
stimulation of central (inspiratory) drive
improved skeletal muscle contraction
improved metabolic homeostasis
improved oxygenation via increased cardiac output and decreased hypoxic episodes

trinsic activity of the respiratory drive mechanism, thus increasing respiratory drive without altering chemoreceptor sensitivity.[65] A great deal more work has been done on central respiratory influences of theophylline in neonates than on those of caffeine (see under Theophylline).

The effects of methyl xanthines on the cardiovascular system are complex, and some conflicting results have been reported, probably because the conditions prevailing at the time of administration in the particular system being examined have significant effects on the response observed. In addition, the capability of the methyl xanthines to stimulate vagal and vasomotor centers in the brain stem can complicate interpretations of the direct actions of methyl xanthines on vascular and cardiac tissues. Caffeine in therapeutic concentrations may produce small decreases in heart rate, presumably as a consequence of stimulation of the medullary vagal nuclei; at higher concentrations definite tachycardia occurs. In certain persons, sensitivity to methyl xanthines results in the development of arrhythmias, such as premature ventricular contractions. In adults, administration of 250 mg of caffeine has been reported to increase plasma renin activity by 57%, plasma norepinephrine by 75%, and plasma epinephrine by 207%.[77] The greater increase in plasma epinephrine than in norepinephrine may indicate a predominant effect of caffeine at the adrenomedullary level rather than an undifferentiated sympathetic stimulation. Another dose response study with IV aminophylline in adults showed dose-dependent increases in plasma catecholamines.[117] Studies in premature infants with apnea treated with caffeine revealed no change in urinary catecholamine excretion.[78] Bhat and coworkers[103] found no changes in biogenic amine metabolites in the CSF of neonates treated with theophylline for apnea. This would indicate that theophylline does not relieve apnea by stimulation of the central adrenergic system.

The controversial effect of caffeine on heart rate—both elevation and depression have been reported—may very well be a reflection of its multisystem actions (baroreceptor-mediated via change in blood pressure, direct effect at the level of the brain stem, direct cardiac muscle stimulation, sympathetic stimulation). The specific change in heart rate observed probably is directly related to the prevailing heart rate and the factors controlling this rate at the time of exposure to caffeine. Methyl xanthines given IV have been shown to produce peripheral vasodilation; the proposed mechanism is a direct relaxant effect on smooth muscle that is susceptible to modification by catecholamine release and stimulated homeostatic responses.[47] Howell and colleagues[47] have reported the occurrence of hypotension in one infant who received an IV dose of caffeine citrate over a 3-minute period. Effects of methyl xanthine therapy on patency of the ductus arteriosus are unlikely, as the doses required to produce relaxation in vitro far exceed those necessary to attain therapeutic plasma levels.[53]

Caffeine has been shown to increase the capacity for skeletal muscle work in humans.[74] Theophylline is considerably less potent in this regard. The effect of caffeine on skeletal muscle contraction has been proposed to occur by an increase in release of calcium from intracellular stores, increased intracellular concentrations of cyclic $3',5'$ AMP, and by a potentiation of calcium-induced release of acetylcholine at motor nerve terminals.[115]

Extensive studies in animals and adult humans have described the gastrointestinal effects of methyl xanthines, but similar studies have not been accomplished in neonates. Gastric acid secretion and pepsin secretion both increase with oral or parenteral doses of caffeine.[27] Maximal acid response is obtained with plasma caffeine levels of 20 μg/ml. Neither vagotomy nor atropine blocks gastric acid stimulation produced by caffeine. The administration of cimetidine, an H_2-receptor antagonist, completely prevents the caffeine-induced stimulation of gastric acid secretion in human adults; in animals, however, no effect on theophylline actions was observed.[22] Although these effects on the gastrointestinal tract have not been examined in neonates, no major gastrointestinal problems have been reported with caffeine given in therapeutic doses. Howell and coworkers[47] note that although caffeine can produce more severe gastroenteritis than that due to theophylline (also more pronounced in neonates than adult animals), neither vomiting nor diarrhea has been related to caffeine therapy in infants with known therapeutic serum levels. Occasional occurrence of transient abdominal distension, however, has been noted.

Caffeine has been shown to display anti-inflammatory activity in various model systems. Histamine release from isolated mast cells, including that augmented with the use of histamine-releasing agents, is reduced by methyl xanthines. Small doses of caffeine have also been shown to reduce the dosage required for anti-inflammatory effects of aspirin, indomethacin, and phenylbutazone by more than three-fold.[74]

Rothberg and colleagues[78] examined a variety of metabolic effects of caffeine in premature infants undergoing therapy with caffeine citrate for apnea. In contrast to findings in adults, there were no changes in mean heart rate and in urinary excretion of catecholamines, or of electrolytes in the 12-hour period following initial dosing with caffeine given IV; variable responses were observed for plasma glucose. Lazaro-Lopez and coworkers[58] reported a decline of plasma glucose levels in infants treated with caffeine that were formula-fed every 3 to 4 hours relative to levels in infants on continuous IV or gastric feedings. Normoglycemia has been observed in some cases of neonatal caffeine intoxication.[13,54] Of interest is the study by Spindel's group[87] demonstrating an effect of caffeine on anterior pituitary and thyroid function in experimental animals. Doses of caffeine that resulted in serum levels of 15 to 18 μg/ml lowered serum thyroid-stimulating hormone (TSH) and growth hormone in a dose-dependent manner. The decrease in serum TSH was followed by decreases in circulating thyroid hormones. These investigators speculated that the effect of caffeine on pituitary secretion may occur because of changes in the periphery, changes in the brain, or both. Comparable studies of caffeine have not been reported in humans. A biphasic response to a toxic dose of caffeine (50 mg/kg) has been reported in newborn rats: The plasma T_4 was increased at 4 hours and decreased at 24 hours.[47] In addition, there was a significant increase in growth hormone concentrations.

The cellular basis for the action of methyl xanthines, including caffeine and theophylline, has been the primary focus of attention in efforts to delineate the mechanism for their diverse pharmacologic effects. Three major cellular actions of the methyl xanthines have been studied: (1) translocation of intracellular calcium; (2) increasing accumulation of cyclic nucleotides, particularly cyclic 3',5' AMP; and (3) blockade of receptors for adenosine. Cyclic nucleotides probably contribute little to the pharmacologic activities because the concentrations of the methyl xanthines necessary to produce these effects have been shown to be far greater than normal therapeutic concentrations. For example, it has been frequently proposed that a variety of actions of methyl xanthines, particularly those in which the apparent potency of theophylline exceeds that of caffeine, are mediated by cyclic 3',5' AMP, which

accumulates as a consequence of the inhibitory effects of the methyl xanthines on phosphodiesterase. However, only about 10% or less of phosphodiesterase activity is inhibited at maximal therapeutic concentrations of theophylline and caffeine.[74]

In contrast, adenosine receptor blockade is undoubtedly of great importance in the effects of the methyl xanthines. One study has shown that adenosine is competitively inhibited by xanthines, with caffeine being a less potent inhibitor in vitro than theophylline.[79] Adenosine has been shown to have a wide variety of effects, including dilation of coronary and cerebral vessels, slowing of the rate of discharge of cardiac pacemaker cells and a variety of neurons in the CNS, inhibition of hormone-induced lipolysis, reduction in the release of norepinephrine from autonomic nerve endings, and inhibition of release of excitatory neurotransmitters in the CNS.[74] Activation of the receptors for adenosine are believed to result in either stimulation or inhibition of cyclic AMP synthesis. Methyl xanthines thus far have proved to be universal antagonists of adenosine. Accordingly, the antiadenosine action of methyl xanthines must be considered as a major mechanism for the variety of pharmacologic effects, although other factors probably play a role.

Clinical Pharmacology. Several excellent studies of the pharmacokinetics of caffeine in infants have been published (Table 6–3). Loading doses of caffeine (10 mg/kg) given PO produce peak serum levels of 6 to 10 μg/ml within 2 hours of administration.[6] IV loading doses of 10 to 15 mg/kg of caffeine result in peak serum levels ranging between 9 and 36 μg/ml. Steady-state serum levels resulting from maintenance doses of 2.5 mg/kg per day PO range from 8 to 14 μg/ml. Mean values for volume of distribution reported in the literature are 0.8 to 0.9 l/kg (Table 6–3). Half-life values in neonates are consistently prolonged compared with those in older infants and adults; most reported mean $T\frac{1}{2}$ values are greater than 60 hours, with a wide range of individual values (31–132 hr).

Therapeutic Indications. Caffeine has been demonstrated to effectively *decrease the frequency of neonatal apnea* (Table 6–4). The rationale for the employment of caffeine rather than theophylline for the treatment of apnea in the premature infant is based on the following advantages observed in adults: greater specificity of caffeine as a respirogenic agent with fewer peripheral effects, greater therapeutic index, once-daily-only dosing requirements, and no active metabolite to confuse the interpretation

Table 6-3. SUMMARY OF CLINICAL PHARMACOLOGY STUDIES OF CAFFEINE IN INFANTS

Authors of Published Study[a]	Study Group	Dose[b]	Serum Concentration (μg/ml)	Serum Half-life[c] (T½-hr)	Other Data[d]
Aranda et al[4]	18 prematures (28 wk)	5–10 mg/kg PO or IV q 8–24 hr		97.5 (range 41–231)	
Gorodischer et al[40]	18 prematures	15 mg/kg IV × 1		68 ± 3 (6 days old)	V_d = 0.8 l/kg
Bada et al[11]	5 prematures (<33 wk)	loading: 10 mg/kg PO maintenance: 5 mg/kg PO q 12 hr	5.6 ± 4.8 (<30 wk) 3.6 ± 2.1 (30–33 wk)		
Aranda et al[5]	7 infants (1–6 mo)	loading: 10 mg/kg IV or PO		1–2½ mo: 26 3–4½ mo: 14 5–6 mo: 2.6	
Aranda et al[6]	32 prematures (24–34 wk)	loading: 10 mg/kg IV 10 mg/kg PO maintenance: 11 mg/kg q 24 hr 2.5 mg/kg q 24 hr	12 ± 2 6–10 45 14	103 ± 18	V_d = 0.92 l/kg Cl = 8.9 ml/kg/hr (range 2.5–16.8)
Turmen et al[92]	4 prematures (25–32 wk)	loading: 10 mg/kg IV maintenance: 2.5 mg/kg q 24 hr	8 ± 2 (CSF = 8 ± 2)		
Parsons and Neims[72]	15 full-term infants	transplacentally acquired	5.5–0.03 (range)	82 (range 31–132)	
Somani and Khanna[84]	5 prematures (1.1–1.6 kg BW)	loading: 15 mg/kg IV maintenance: 5 mg/kg q 12 hr	9.2 (CSF = 8.8)		
Murat et al[64]	9 prematures (30 wk)	loading: 10 mg/kg IM maintenance: 2.5 mg/kg PO q 24 hr	9 ± 1 9.2 ± 0.2	66 ± 11 (range 36–105)	randomized control trial
Turmen et al[93]	7 prematures (30 wk)	loading: 10 mg/kg IV (in 2.5-mg/kg increments)	2.5 mg/kg: 3.6 5.0 mg/kg: 8.8 7.5 mg/kg: 11.5 10 mg/kg: 17.3		
Rothberg et al[78]	5 prematures (31 wk)	10 mg/kg IV × 1	13–14 (approx.)		
Gorodischer and Karplus[41]	13 prematures (25–34 wk)	15 mg/kg IV	12–36	65 ± 4 (range 48–88)	V_d = 0.78 l/kg Cl = 8.5 mg/kg/hr

[a]Listed in order of publication; see References at end of chapter.
[b]Dose is for caffeine base. Equivalent dosage values for caffeine citrate would be twice the caffeine base values shown.
[c]Values represent mean ±SE unless otherwise noted.
[d]V_d = volume of distribution; Cl = plasma clearance.

of the serum concentration measurements. These arguments have not been examined in a controlled fashion in premature infants with apnea. Several recent studies,[11,19,21] however, have clearly shown that theophylline is metabolized in part to caffeine in premature infants, suggesting the possibility that at least some of the activity of theophylline against apnea may in fact arise via conversion to caffeine. The minimal plasma concentration of caffeine demonstrated to be effective in neonatal apnea is as low as 2.9 μg/ml,[93] which is well within the plasma levels for caffeine reported in infants receiving theophylline.[17,19,21,91]

Only a few studies have actually attempted to establish the minimal or ideal dose or plasma

Table 6-4. STUDIES OF EFFICACY OF CAFFEINE IN THE TREATMENT OF APNEA

Authors of Published Study	No. of apneic episodes		Success Rate (No. of patients)	Serum Caffeine Concentration (μg/ml)
	Pretreatment	*Posttreatment*		
Aranda et al[4]	13.6/day	2.1/day	17 out of 19	7-16
Murat et al[64]	1-2.5/100 min	<1/100 min	9 out of 9	9

concentration of caffeine necessary for control of neonatal apnea. It is quite clear that there is a wide range of serum concentrations over which caffeine appears to be effective in altering the course of neonatal apnea. Serum concentrations as low as 3 μg/ml have been reported to be effective in some neonates,[93] whereas values as high as 24 μg/ml are subtherapeutic in other neonates.[41] It seems reasonable to conclude on the basis of experience to date that the desired serum concentration range for caffeine is probably 5 to 25 μg/ml. Infants with these serum caffeine levels generally will demonstrate a decrease in frequency of apneic spells and will have improvement in the regularity of their respiratory patterns; in some cases, however, reduction in the number of apneic episodes will not be seen even at the higher concentrations. What is unclear is whether further increase in serum caffeine concentration will result in added therapeutic benefit, or whether there is any benefit to the use of theophylline with treatment failure of caffeine.

The dosage of caffeine necessary to achieve serum levels in the range of 5 to 25 μg/ml is shown in Table 6-5. A loading dose of 10 mg/kg IV or PO of caffeine base, as recommended by Aranda and colleagues,[8] will result in plasma concentrations of caffeine of 8 to 14 μg/ml. This finding coincides with a report from Turmen and coworkers[93] that, as plasma concentrations approach 8 μg/ml, breathing patterns improve remarkably. Twenty-four hours following the loading dose a single daily maintenance dose of 2.5 mg/kg IV or PO of caffeine will produce serum steady-state levels of 7 to 20 μg/ml. Caffeine toxicity is generally not a problem if serum levels are less than 40 to 50 μg/ml. Thus, in neonates who fail to respond adequately to these recommended dosages, increases in dosage with careful monitoring of serum levels may be beneficial. Care must be taken to appreciate the very slow elimination rate in premature neonates; the time required to reach a new steady-state level subsequent to changes in maintenance dosage may exceed 2 weeks. The clinical benefit of raising serum caffeine levels to above 25 μg/ml for persistent neonatal apnea has not been reported and probably should not be anticipated.

The particular chemical form of caffeine employed has been discussed in a number of articles in the literature. The most frequently recommended form is **caffeine citrate**. Caffeine

Table 6-5. DOSAGE RECOMMENDATIONS FOR CAFFEINE AND THEOPHYLLINE IN NEONATES

	Recommended Dosage[a]		Serum Concentration (μg/ml)	
	Loading	*Maintenance*	*Therapeutic*	*Toxic*
Caffeine[b]	10 mg/kg IV or PO	2.5 mg/kg IV or PO q 24 hr (first dose given 24 hr after loading dose)	5-25	>40-50
Theophylline[c]	5 mg/kg IV	2 mg/kg IV q 12 hr[d] (first dose given 12 hr after loading dose)	2-15	>15-20

[a] Dosage recommendations provided are for the parent compounds (caffeine base and theophylline base) and not for the various salts and derivatives available.

[b] The amount of active caffeine base can range from 40% to 50% of the actual weight depending upon the chemical material utilized (e.g., caffeine citrate, caffeine sodium benzoate).

[c] The variety of oral preparations available contain from 50% to 100% theophylline base along with a variety of additives. Changing from IV to PO therapy may require an increase in dose.

[d] Maintenance dose requirements for theophylline will vary among neonates, generally ranging between 1 and 4 mg/kg per dose to achieve therapeutic serum concentrations. In older infants, the dose requirements may increase up to 20 to 25 mg/kg/day. The dosing interval may also need to be changed to every 4 to 8 hours (see text). Serum theophylline concentration monitoring should be accomplished within 48 hours of initiating the loading dose and maintenance therapy to avoid toxicity.

citrate can be prepared as an aqueous solution (20 mg/ml, equivalent to 10 mg/ml of caffeine base solution), which can be administered IV or PO. Because of its very acidic pH (3 to 4), caffeine citrate should not be given IM. The use of caffeine sodium benzoate has been discouraged because of concern regarding competitive inhibition of bilirubin albumin binding as well as variability in its caffeine content: The amount of active caffeine may range from 38% to 50%, depending upon the preparation used.[8] Gorodischer and Karplus[41] have suggested the use of caffeine base rather than caffeine salts to avoid the concerns regarding errors in calculation of amount of caffeine to be delivered. The 1% aqueous solution of caffeine employed by these investigators proved satisfactory.

The duration of therapy necessary for treatment of neonatal apnea has not been well studied. In the controlled study of caffeine therapy for apnea conducted by Murat and colleagues,[64] there were no significant differences between the treated and control groups by day 15 of the study. In the treated group the mean total duration of treatment was 24 days (range 15–40); the end of the treatment corresponded roughly to a gestational age of 36 weeks. No infant required treatment beyond the gestational age of 37 weeks.

Clinical Toxicology. A wide variety of adverse reactions has been reported with the methyl xanthines; such reactions largely represent exaggerations of the known pharmacologic effects previously discussed. In neonates no obvious cardiovascular, neurologic, or gastrointestinal toxicity has been observed at caffeine plasma concentrations less than 50 μg/ml. Transient jitteriness has been observed with plasma concentrations between 50 and 100 μg/ml.[6,54] Plasma concentrations above 100 μg/ml have been associated with tachycardia (200–260 beats/min) and mild glycosuria but no other adverse effects.[41] A number of clinical investigations report no adverse effects with serum levels in the therapeutic range. Acute caffeine overdose in three full-term infants has been reported by Banner and Czajaka;[13] following doses ranging from 36 to 136 mg/kg, they developed manifestations of tachypnea, fine tremor of the extremities, opisthotonus, tonic–clonic movements, and nonpurposeful jaw and lip movements. The plasma concentrations in two of the neonates were below 40 μg/ml at the time of these manifestations. Hypertension, hyperglycemia, ketonuria, and hematemesis were not present. Therefore, it appears important to consider the individual dosage as well as the duration of therapy (acute versus chronic) and

serum level at the time of the manifestations in interpretation of the relationship between caffeine and its toxicities.

Studies with caffeine demonstrating a constriction of cerebral vessels and a reduction in cerebral blood flow[114] prompted studies on the effect of caffeine on retinal vessels and the risk of development of retrolental fibroplasia in infants undergoing therapy for apnea. Gunn and coworkers[43] found no increase in incidence of retrolental fibroplasia in neonates receiving caffeine compared with control infants. Caffeine had no apparent harmful effects on growth and development as determined by follow-up examinations at 18 months, 2 years, and 3 years later. Howell and colleagues[47] have carefully reviewed the adverse effects of caffeine in infants.

Theophylline

Pharmacology. The chemical structure of theophylline is shown in Figure 6–1. A variety of complexes and true salts of theophylline have been utilized in various pharmaceutical preparations, the most common of which is **aminophylline,** the ethylene diamine complex. The rationale for the use of complexes or salts has been to increase the solubility of theophylline, which itself is only sparingly soluble in water. Of importance with respect to the pharmacologic actions is appreciation of the fact that it is the theophylline *base* that is the active form, and that the various complexes and salts contain less than 100% by weight of theophylline.

The absorption of theophylline is somewhat variable, depending upon the route of administration. PO administration has been found to result in variable rates of absorption, although 80 to 100% bioavailability is to be anticipated.[24] There is little direct information regarding theophylline absorption in pre-term infants in contrast to a large number of studies in older children and adults. Theophylline is erratically absorbed when given rectally, depending upon the particular preparation employed.[15] Local irritation of the gastrointestinal tract is believed to delay the rate of absorption, as does the presence of food. Heinmann and colleagues[107] observed the maximum serum theophylline concentrations 4.7 hours after administration in fed premature infants instead of 1.6 hours under fasting conditions. The amount absorbed was not affected by food intake. IM injection of theophylline preparations should not be utilized.

Theophylline distributes widely in the body after absorption. Bonati and colleagues[16] exam-

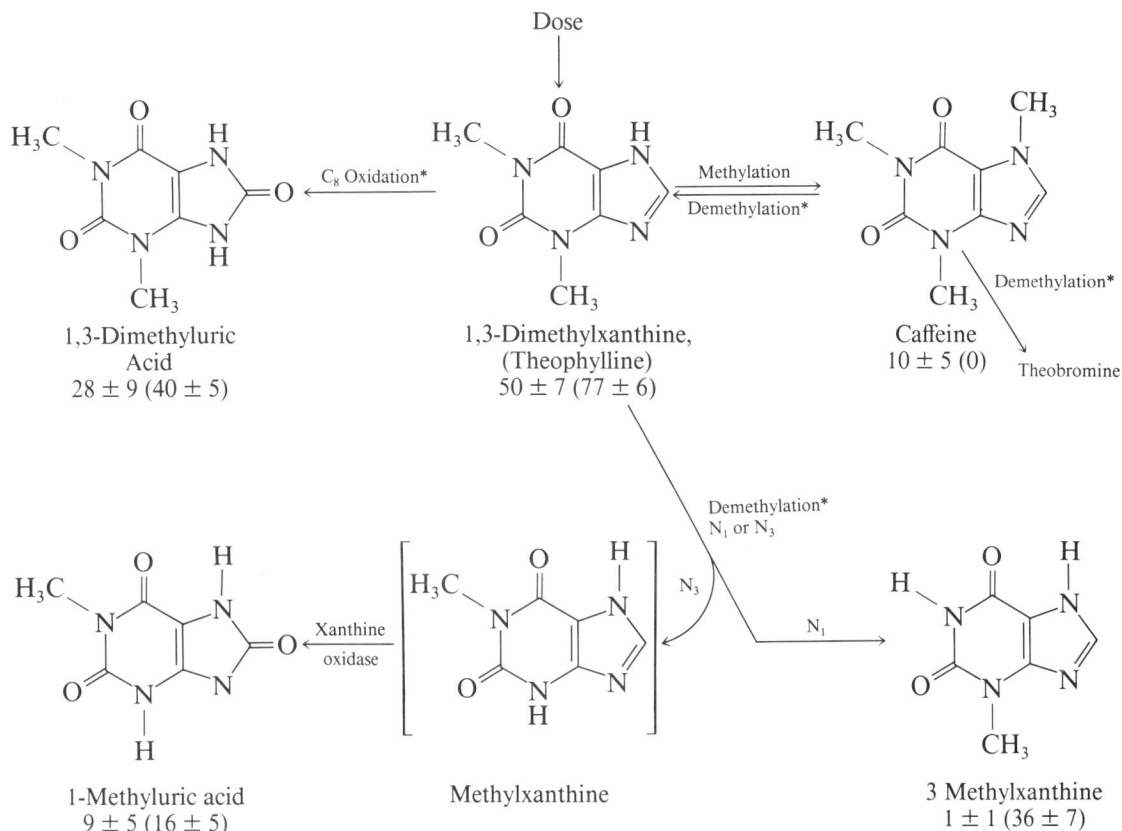

Figure 6 – 1. Proposed pathways for the metabolism of caffeine and theophylline in the neonate and adult (adapted from Takieddine et al, 1981).[90] The values shown under each compound indicate the percentage of administered theophylline excreted in the urine as theophylline and metabolites. The values in parentheses are those for adults. Asterisk denotes pathways assumed to be catalyzed by cytochrome P-450 mixed function oxidases.

ined theophylline concentrations in post-mortem tissues collected from premature neonates given theophylline; there was no apparent preferential accumulation in the tissues examined. Average tissue/blood ratios were lower for shorter-term courses of therapy (1 to 5 doses) than for therapy of longer duration, where the values approached unity. Plasma protein binding of theophylline in newborn infants (36%) is less than the 70% value reported in children and adults;[3,83] this reduced protein binding may in part explain the larger volume of distribution in pre-term infants compared with that in older infants and children. Reported V_d values range from 0.3 to 1.03 l/kg in neonates;[30] this wide variation probably reflects differences in the clinical situations and methodology of calculation.

Among the more fascinating discoveries of drug metabolism in neonates is that of theophylline (see Fig. 6 – 1). In neonates treated with theophylline, the mean ratio of caffeine to theophylline in plasma is about 0.3, although caffeine plasma levels may reach up to 50% of theophylline plasma levels. Soyka and Neese[85] first reported significant levels of caffeine in premature infants receiving aminophylline for apnea of prematurity. Similar findings have been reported by Bory,[18] Boutroy,[19] and Bada[11] and their coworkers. Brazier and colleagues[21] studied the metabolism of theophylline in premature neonates by the use of stable radioisotope-labeled material; they demonstrated unequivocally the biotransformation in vivo of theophylline to caffeine in premature infants. Using high-pressure liquid chromatography, Bory's group failed to identify any measurable caffeine levels following theophylline administration to four adult volunteers who were controlled for exogenous sources of caffeine.

Theophylline is metabolized by the cytochrome *P450* mono-oxygenase system. Based on a number of studies in human adults and neonates, the currently accepted pathway of theophylline metabolism includes oxidation to 1,3-dimethyluric acid and demethylation to 1-methyluric acid and 3-methyl xanthine, along with the unique metabolic pathway identified in the neonate: methylation of theophylline to caffeine (Fig. 6–1).

Examination of urine collected from premature infants treated with theophylline reveals excretion products remarkably different from those in adults. Grygiel and coworkers[42] found only unchanged theophylline and caffeine in urine from prematures treated with theophylline. Approximately 98% of the total theophylline administered was recovered unchanged in the urine; caffeine accounted for the remaining 2%. Oxidized and demethylated metabolites (1-methyluric acid 3-methyl xanthine, 1-methyl xanthine, and 1,3-dimethyluric acid) were not detected. In contrast, in adults and children approximately 20% of administered theophylline was excreted as 1-methyluric acid; 15%, as 3-methyl xanthine; a trace amount, as 1-methyl xanthine; and 55%, as 1,3-dimethyluric acid. Studies by Bonati and colleagues[17] confirmed the absence of demethylation of theophylline to 3-methyl xanthine; however, approximately 15% of the urine metabolite fraction was found to be excreted as 1-methyluric acid; 34%, as 1,3-dimethyluric acid; 45%, as theophylline, and 7% as caffeine. Studies by Tserng and coworkers[91] of theophylline metabolism in premature infants found that during steady state of a multidose regimen, the urinary metabolites of theophylline included caffeine, 9.6%; theophylline, 50%; 3-methyl xanthine, 1.3%; 1,3-dimethyluric acid, 27.7%; and 1-methyluric acid, 9.3%. More recent studies by these authors revealed urinary percentages of unchanged theophylline decreased from 61% in neonates at 28 to 32 weeks gestation to 43% at 38 to 42 weeks gestation.[116] These authors noted that previously popular methods for isolating theophylline from biological fluids did not extract most of the polar metabolites such as monosubstituted xanthines and uric acids. This may well be the explanation for the observed discrepancies in neonatal and adult urinary metabolite patterns for theophylline. In comparing the plasma and urine ratios of caffeine to theophylline (0.3 vs. 0.2, respectively), Tserng and coworkers[91] conclude that the difference represents greater reabsorption of caffeine from the renal tubules.

Apparently, at least two different cytochrome *P450* mono-oxygenases are responsible for the oxidation and oxidative demethylation of theophylline. In neonates, the enzyme system for *C8* oxidation of theophylline is relatively active (conversion to caffeine), while the cytochrome *P450* enzymes responsible for demethylation of theophylline are less active; the result is production and accumulation of caffeine following theophylline therapy, which is not seen in older infants and adults. The relatively small fraction of 3-methyl xanthine and 1-methyluric acid in the urine suggests underdeveloped demethylation pathways for N_1 and N_3. Theobromine, a product of demethylation of caffeine, has been identified in infants treated with theophylline.[21,116] The approximate age of transition of theophylline metabolism from the neonatal to the adult pattern is not clear, although infants of 16 months of age and older do not show any evidence of methylation to caffeine. The urinary fractions of theophylline and its oxidative metabolites are also similar to those for adults.[17,42] Rosen and coworkers[113] examined infants 4 to 18 months of age and found that childhood clearance rates for theophylline elimination were achieved by 6 months of age. Lönnerholm and colleagues[110] found a linear increase in theophylline plasma clearance between 2 and 10 weeks of age, with a plateau to childhood clearance rates at 6 to 7 months of age. Nassif's group[66] examined the clearance rates in infants 6 weeks to 48 weeks of age and found that the mean dose requirement among infants 6 weeks to 4 months of age was 12.4 mg/kg per day and increased to 22.4 mg/kg per day after 8 months of age. Takieddine and coworkers[90] examined the developmental aspects of theophylline metabolism in eight premature infants treated continuously to 42 weeks' postconceptional age. Methylation of theophylline to caffeine persisted during this period, although the fraction of 1,3-dimethyluric acid in the urine increased and correlated with a decrease in theophylline fraction.

It is clear that almost all organ systems can be influenced by the methyl xanthines, although the predominant sites of activity involve the CNS and the cardiovascular system (see Table 6–1). Since theophylline is converted to caffeine in the neonate, differentiation of the effects of theophylline alone from those of caffeine in the neonate is probably impossible. In general, the methyl xanthines, including theophylline, produce excitation throughout all levels of the CNS. The therapeutically desirable effect includes stimulation of the medullary respiratory centers. The CNS-stimulating effects of theophylline are well established in the adult, but only a few studies of these effects in the premature newborn have been accomplished. Gerhardt and colleagues[38] demonstrated that theophylline increased the respiratory center output as indicated by a 33% increase in esophageal pressure change per breath and by a 39% increase in expired volume per minute. In a later study, these investigators observed an increase in afferent impulses to the brainstem.[104] Their results were believed to be compatible with an increase in respiratory center drive in the premature infant, resulting in an increase of work of breathing and in capability of maintaining a normal alveolar ventilation. There is some controversy, however, with respect to carbon dioxide response.[115] The study by Gerhardt's group[38] provided evidence for a decrease in respiratory-center threshold to CO_2, leading to an increase in basal expired volume per minute and decreased $P_{A}CO_2$. The fact that the slope of the CO_2 curve remained unchanged indicates that the sensitivity of the respiratory center to CO_2 does not vary. However, Davi and coworkers[26] reported an increase in the slope of the CO_2 response curve in premature infants with apnea during treatment with aminophylline. Gerhardt and colleagues[38] suggested that the observed differences in the CO_2 response curve were related to the differences in theophylline serum levels in the two studies. Thus, the change in the slope of the CO_2 response curve may be dose-related, but a change in the slope is not necessary for an effective increase in expired volume per minute and a significant decrease in the incidence of apnea. Theophylline may render the respiratory center more sensitive to afferent impulses and, by shifting the CO_2 response curve to the left, may stabilize the output of the respiratory center. The failure of theophylline to affect directly lung function and oxygenation provides further evidence for a central mechanism responsible for its efficacy in apnea of prematurity.[26,38,115] Table 6–2 outlines the proposed mechanisms believed responsible for methyl xanthine alteration of apnea in premature infants.

Theophylline has been shown to alter the sleep state in premature infants.[28] A significant decrease in apneic episodes was associated with an increased wakefulness and an increased amount of active (REM) sleep. A similar hypothesis has been entertained for the effect of phenobarbital on apnea of prematurity (see under Phenobarbital, Chap. 5). Studies by Gabriel and colleagues.[34] found a decrease in number of apneic episodes in premature infants receiving theophylline that was closely related to the phases of active sleep. However, the amount of REM sleep remained unchanged during theophylline treatment. The relationship of the frequency of apneic episodes to the sleep state (REM versus non-REM) remains to be clarified .[62,104] The cellular mechanisms for the CNS effects of methyl xanthines are discussed under Caffeine.

The ability of theophylline to produce modest decreases in peripheral vascular resistance and marked cardiac stimulation was the basis for the traditional use of this agent in the emergency treatment of congestive heart failure. More specific and effective vasoactive and ionotropic agents are now preferred. The pharmacologic action of the methyl xanthines on the cardiovascular system is highly dependent upon the conditions prevailing at the time of their administration and the dose employed. In addition to producing direct effects on vascular and cardiac tissues, the methyl xanthines can affect the cardiovascular system indirectly by influencing vagal and vasomotor centers in the brain stem, and by peripheral actions mediated largely by catecholamine and renin–angiotensin systems. At plasma concentrations between 10 and 20 μg/ml, theophylline produces an increase in heart rate (via stimulation of medullary vagal nuclei) and a reduction in left ventricular ejection time index and in isovolumetric contraction time, both consistent with an increase in contractile force and a decrease in cardiac preload.[71] Some of these effects on the heart may be mediated through augmented release of catecholamines from the sympathetic–adrenal system.[74] In humans, following therapeutic doses of theophylline, vascular resistance declines. Thus, vasodilatation coupled with an increase in cardiac output results in an increase in blood perfusion.

In contrast to their dilating effect on systemic blood vessels, the methyl xanthines can cause a marked increase in cerebrovascular resistance with a decrease in cerebral blood flow and in oxygen tension in the brain.[63,99,114] The mechanism of the direct constrictor effect on cerebral blood vessels is unknown. Obviously, in premature infants with apnea who are at risk for ventricular hemorrhage, this effect on cerebrovasculature may be deleterious. The effects of the methyl xanthines on retinal vessels and retrolental fibroplasia and on the patency of the ductus arteriosus are discussed under Caffeine.

The pulmonary airway smooth muscle–relaxant effects of theophylline have been well appreciated and utilized in the treatment of asthma. In this regard, theophylline is more effective than caffeine and produces a definite increase in vital capacity and dilation of pulmonary arterioles.[115] The exact mechanism for

Table 6-6. SUMMARY OF CLINICAL PHARMACOLOGY STUDIES OF THEOPHYLLINE IN INFANTS

Authors of Published Study[a]	Study Group	Dose[b]	Serum Concentration[c] (μg/ml)	Serum Half-life[c] ($T\frac{1}{2}$ hr)	Other Data[d]
Shannon et al[81]	17 prematures (0.95–2.4 kg BW)	1.5–4 mg/kg PO q 6 hr	15 ± 7 (SD) (7–32)		
Aranda et al[3]	6 prematures (25–32 wk)	3.2–6 mg/kg IV q 8–12 hr	13–36 (range)	30 ± 7 (14–58)	V_d = 0.7 l/kg
Giacoia et al[39]	8 prematures (26–32 wk)	0.5–2 mg/kg PO q 6 hr	11–18	20 (13–29)	V_d = 0.9 l/kg (variable) Cl = 39 mg/hr/kg
Cottancin et al[24]	6 prematures (32 wk)	2.5–3 mg/kg PO or rectally q 12 hr	5–7 (approx. mean range)	28 (22–33)	V_d = 0.9 l/kg
Neese and Soyka[67]	12 prematures (28–36 wk)	loading: 6.4 mg/kg rectally at 0 and 12 hr maintenance: 3.2 mg/kg rectally q 12 hr	11.8 (6–20)	30 (12–54)	V_d = 0.3 l/kg
Peabody et al[73]	10 prematures (27–34 wk)	loading: 6.2 mg/kg rectally at 0 and 12 hr maintenance: 3.2 mg/kg rectally q 12 hr	10–16 2–3	(12–54)	
Dietrich et al[28]	9 prematures (26–32 wk)	loading: 5 mg/kg IV maintenance: 1.2 mg/kg IV q 8 hr	2.6 (0–12), trough levels		
Gabriel et al[34]	6 prematures (30–32 wk)	loading: 4.4 mg/kg IV maintenance: 0.9 mg/kg IV q 8 hr	11 ± 3.5 (5–15)	26 ± 7 (SD)	
Latini et al[57]	27 prematures (29–33 wk)	maintenance: 2.6–4.5 mg/kg IV	3–24 (approx.)	27 ± 7 (N = 7)	V_d = 0.4 l/kg (N = 7) Cl = 13 ± 3 mg/hr/kg (N = 7)
Boutroy et al[19]	27 prematures (31 ± 2 wk)	loading: 4 mg/kg + 3 mg/kg 6 hr later PO maintenance: 2 mg/kg PO q 6 hr	12 ± (4–43)	32 ± 13 (17–74)	K_{Cl} = 0.023
Gerhardt et al[37]	14 prematures (30 wk)	1.7 mg/kg IV q 6 hr	10.2 ± 0.7		
Brazier et al[20]	33 prematures	3 mg/kg PO q 6–8 hr	13–15 (mean)	30 ± 7	V_d = 1.0 l/kg Cl = 24 ± 5 mg/kg/hr
Bada et al[11]	8 prematures (<33 wk)	loading: 5 mg/kg IV maintenance: 1 mg/kg IV q 12 hr	<30 wk: 3.6 ± 2.5 30–33 wk: 2.5 ± 2.2		
Jones and Baillie[48]	14 prematures (25–30 wk)	loading: 5–8 mg/kg IV maintenance: constant IV infusion (4.4 mg/kg/q 24 hr)		34 ± 8 (N = 4)	V_d = 0.7 l/kg Cl = 18.6 ± 4.8 ml/hr/kg (N = 11)
King et al[52]	6 prematures (28–37 wk)	5 mg/kg PO × 1		35.5 (24–64)	
Bory et al[18]	7 prematures (26–33 wk)	0.5–2 mg/kg PO q 6 hr	11.0 ± 2.2 (4–19)		theophylline : caffeine ratio = 0.34
Hilligoss et al[45]	17 prematures (25–36 wk)	2 mg/kg PO q 6 hr		19 ± 4 hrs	V_d = 0.6 l/kg Cl = 23 ± 4 ml/hr/kg
Milsap et al[61]	11 prematures (27–32 wk)	loading: 2.5 mg/kg PO maintenance: 0.7 mg/kg PO q 8 hr	3.9 ± 0.2 (2.9–4.7)		
Myers et al[65]	7 prematures (28–34 wk)	loading: 2.5 mg/kg PO maintenance: 0.7 mg/kg PO q 8 hr	3.3 ± 0.2 (2.8 ± 3.9)		
Grygiel and Birkett[42]	6 prematures (28–32 wk)	4.1 mg/kg q 24 hr	11.4 ± 0.8		
Lagercrantz et al[56]	6 prematures (28–31 wk)	loading: 10–11 mg/kg IV maintenance: 2–3 mg/kg IV q 12 hr	7–15		
Kelly and Shannon[51]	22 full-term infants (4–47 days old)	7.5 mg/kg q 24 hr (6–12 mg/kg q 24 hr)	11 ± 4 (6–19)		
Bonati et al[17]	12 prematures (26–35 wk)	loading: 5.5 mg/kg IV maintenance: 1.1 mg/kg IV q 12 hr			Cl = 14.5 ml/hr/kg
Somani and Khanna[84]	7 prematures (26–35 wk)	loading: 5 mg/kg IV maintenance: 2 mg/kg IV q 12 hr	12.7 (CSF = 10.0) (saliva = 7.3)		
Gal et al[35]	30 prematures (25–34 wk)	loading: 6 mg/kg IV maintenance: asphyxiated: 2.1 mg/kg IV q 24 hr normal: 3.9 mg/kg IV q 24 hr			asphyxiated: Cl = 10.8 ± ml/hr/kg normal: Cl = 20.1 ± 2.6 ml/hr/kg V_d = 0.8 l/kg

Table 6-6. (Continued)

Authors of Published Study[a]	Study Group	Dose[b]	Serum Concentration[c] (μg/ml)	Serum Half-life[c] ($T^{1/2}$ hr)	Other Data[d]
Roberts et al[76]	10 prematures (26–34 wk)	loading: 6 mg/kg PO maintenance: 2 mg/kg PO q 8 hr	9.8 (6.6–13)		
Baley et al[12]	12 prematures (26–35 wk)	loading: 5 mg/kg IV maintenance: 1–2 mg/kg IV or PO q 24 hr	7.8 ± 0.4 (mean peak 11.8 ± 0.9)		
Lönnerholm et al[110]	17 prematures (28–34 wk)	loading: 4.74 mg/kg PO maintenance: 2.4 mg/kg PO q 12 hr	10–15 μg/ml		6–11 days old: Cl = 16.8 ± 0.4 ml/hr/kg 35–38 days old: Cl = 22.9 ± 1.3 ml/hr/kg 64–69 days old: Cl = 30.9 ± 2.5 ml/hr/kg

[a] Listed in order of publication; see References at end of Chapter.

[b] All doses are given as mg of theophylline base even though the original article may have used aminophylline (correction used was dose divided by 1.25 = theophylline dose).

[c] Values shown represent means ± SE (average concentration reached after dosing that may or may not be under steady-state conditions) or ranges of peak values attained. Values in parentheses are ranges unless otherwise noted.

[d] V_d = volume of distribution (determined by a variety of techniques); Cl = plasma theophylline clearance; K_{Cl} = elimination constant.

the effect on pulmonary airway smooth muscle is not clear but is believed to involve the release of or synergistic interactions with β-adrenergic agonists.[74] Theophylline is considerably less potent than caffeine in affecting skeletal muscle contraction; part of the explanation is the greater ability of caffeine to increase the calcium-mediated release of acetylcholine at the neuromuscular junction.

Theophylline in therapeutic doses has been shown to increase glomerular filtration rate in premature infants with apnea.[101] This effect on renal clearance occurs in conjunction with a significant increase in heart rate; no significant change is found in clearance of sodium and free water nor in urine volume. However, Nobel and Light[70] described a neonate who developed significant theophylline-induced diuresis associated with dehydration. Harkavy and colleagues[44] observed an increase in fractional excretion of sodium with a variable but nonsignificant change in creatinine and sodium clearance in neonates receiving theophylline. Shannon and Gotay[82] found no significant change in fractional excretion of sodium or free water clearance. Differences in study design, patient population, and clinical status of the patient, along with individual variation in response to theophylline, are reasonable explanations for the reported differences in the effect of theophylline on renal function in neonates. Observations to date suggest that the renal effects of methyl xanthines are usually not intense and do not compromise or complicate the routine care

of the neonate with apnea. The greatest danger occurs in the premature infant receiving excessive doses of theophylline.[47] In contrast, therapeutic or excessive caffeine levels have not been associated with enhanced excretion of water or electrolytes.

The metabolic effects of theophylline have been reviewed by Ward and Maisels.[97] The cellular effects of the methyl xanthines on cyclic AMP are reviewed under Caffeine. Theophylline can cause a significant increase in plasma glucose concentration in premature infants.[2,88] Its apparently variable effects on blood glucose levels in premature infants may be due to the type of nutritional intake of glucose (constant vs. intermittent) and variability in capacity for glucogenesis and glycogenolysis. The increase in blood glucose produced by theophylline has been attributed in part to the activation of hepatic glycogen phosphorylase by cyclic AMP. Cyclic AMP converts glycogen to glucose 1-phosphate and inactivates glycogen synthetase; these actions increase the output of glucose from the liver but only in the presence of adequate hepatic glycogen stores. Fasted prematures, therefore, would be unlikely to demonstrate an increase in blood glucose in response to theophylline therapy.[88] Insulin release has been found to increase following administration of theophylline; this increase has been attributed to a direct action of theophylline on the beta cells of the pancreas via cyclic AMP.[88] No change in glucagon levels has been reported. The effects of theophylline on plasma glucose, insulin, and glucagon levels have been studied only following a loading dose of this agent; similar studies with chronic theophylline therapy have not been done.

There is some concern regarding the potential for the methyl xanthines to impair lipid synthesis in the brain of neonates undergoing treatment for apnea.[96] This concern is based on observations of uncoupling of DNA and sterol synthesis in actively proliferating glial cells in vitro. The mechanism for this effect of methyl xanthines on lipid synthesis and its significance in the premature infant remain unknown. Only limited neurologic follow-up studies have been accomplished to date in infants given methyl xanthines for neonatal apnea.[68,69] Premature infants who had received theophylline were examined 9 months to 4 years later; no significant differences from normal were identified in Bayley scores, mental or physical developmental indices, and results of sensory and neurologic evaluations.

Clinical Pharmacology. A large number of pharmacokinetic studies has been accomplished with theophylline in infants (Table 6–6). The mean half-life values range from 19 to 32 hours, with overall ranges of 12 to 74 hours. Calculated clearance rates range from 10.8 to 39 ml/hr/kg, much lower than clearance rates in older infants and children. There appears to be a direct correlation between age and clearance in the first year of life. Rosen and coworkers[113] found plasma clearances from 46 to 156 ml/hr/kg in infants between the ages of 4 and 18 months. Lönnerholm and colleagues[110] observed a mean ($\pm$SE) plasma clearance of 16.8 ± 0.4 ml/hr/kg at a postnatal age of 6 to 11 days that increased to 30.9 ± 2.5 ml/hr/kg at 64 to 69 days. There are no reports of dose-dependent saturation kinetics for theophylline in preterm infants despite the fact that this is a known phenomenon in full-term infants by 1 month of age and in older children and adults.[83,100] Gardner and Jusko[36] examined a large number of data obtained from patients ranging in age from 1 to 30 years; plasma clearances generally were between 50 and 150 ml/hr/kg. The differences observed between and among neonatal and adult populations in half-life, clearance rate, and serum level determined for various dosage programs reflect several factors other than inherent differences in theophylline pharmacokinetics. For example, there are significant difficulties with the various analytical techniques that have been applied to theophylline measurements.[67,86] Very little work has been carried out to assess the influence of the clinical status of the neonate on theophylline pharmacokinetics. Gal and coworkers[35] have demonstrated that asphyxia of the neonate correlates with a clearance rate of approximately one half of that of nonasphyxiated newborns. These investigators calculate from the pharmacokinetic data that asphyxiated neonates should receive 2.1 mg/kg per day, and that nonasphyxiated neonates require 3.9 mg/kg per day, to maintain steady-state theophylline plasma concentrations of 8 μg/ml. Studies in adults have demonstrated that the rate of elimination of theophylline is reduced in congestive heart failure, acute pulmonary edema, liver disease, administration of a high-protein low-carbohydrate diet, fever, and macrolide antibiotic therapy.[83] Parenteral nutrition in the neonate has been shown not to affect theophylline elimination.[45] In adults, certain factors such as smoking have been shown to increase the rate of theophylline elimination. This increase has been attributed to stimulation of the cytochrome *P450* metabolism of theophylline.

The volume of distribution for theophylline has been reported to range from 0.3 to 1.0 l/kg (Table 6–6). A variety of techniques for calculating volume of distribution, use of different administration routes and extent of steady-state undoubtedly explain the range of values reported. The most consistent values range between 0.7 and 0.9 l/kg. Theophylline protein binding has been examined in neonates; the bound fraction is approximately 36%, somewhat below the range of 40% to 70% reported for adults.[3,83] In general, the binding of theophylline to serum protein in neonates is significantly less than that in adults; the significance of this finding may be reflected not only in the larger values for volume of distribution but also in the achievement of therapeutic effect with lower concentrations of theophylline than those established as optimal in the treatment of asthma in adults. When the lower plasma protein binding of theophylline in neonates is taken into consideration, the unbound effective concentrations appear to be in the same range as those for adults.

Loading doses of 5 mg/kg of theophylline given IV will generally produce peak serum concentrations of around 10 μg/ml (range 5–15 μg/ml). With clearance rates ranging between 15 and 30 ml/hr/kg, a maintenance dose of approximately 2 mg/kg of theophylline administered every 12 hours should maintain a steady-state serum concentration of approximately 10 μg/ml.[45] Table 6–6 shows the wide range of loading and maintenance doses that have been employed with theophylline in infants. Dosage recommendations for theophyl-

Table 6-7. STUDIES OF THE EFFICACY OF THEOPHYLLINE IN THE TREATMENT OF NEONATAL APNEA

Authors of Published Study[a]	No. of Apneic Episodes per Infant Pretreatment	Posttreatment	Success Rate (No. of Patients)	Serum Theophylline Concentration[b] (μg/ml)
Kuzemko and Paala[55]	5 "attacks"	"occasional to none"	24 out of 24	
Uauy et al[95]	11/day	<5/day	15 out of 15	
Shannon et al[81]	11.9/13 hr	0/13 hr	17 out of 17	6.6-32
Bednarek and Roloff[14]	1.7/hr	<0.5/hr	11 out of 13	
Gabriel et al[34]	21/24 hr	13/24 hr	5 out of 6	1.7-7.1
Peabody et al[73]	4-13/period	0-10/period	6 out of 6	5-16
Latini et al[57]			17 out of 27	3-24
Dietrich et al[28]	0.3/min	<0.1/min	9 out of 9	2-10
Davi et al[26]	55/hr	11/hr	8 out of 10	15-41
Brazier et al[20]			1 out of 33	13-15
Gerhardt et al[38]	29.7/day	4.4/day		10.2 ± 0.7 (average)
Milsap et al[61]	8.6/hr	1.6/hr	11 out of 11	2.9-4.7
Myers et al[65]	16/hr	5/hr	6 out of 7	2.8-3.9
Lagercrantz et al[56]	26/12 hr	3/12 hr		7.2-14.5
Roberts et al[76]	8.8/2 hr	3.2/2	10 out of 12	6.6-13

[a]Listed in order of publication; see References at end of chapter.
[b]Values are ranges unless otherwise noted.

line are given in Table 6-5; as noted, careful attention must be paid to the actual amount of active drug (theophylline) in the particular preparation being used.

Therapeutic Indications. Although no double-blind placebo-controlled study of theophylline in neonatal apnea has been performed, the large number of reports of clinical success, as listed in Table 6-7, provides overwhelming support for its efficacy in *decreasing the incidence and severity of neonatal apnea*. The dose-response characteristics of the effect on neonatal apnea remain unclear. Thus, an appropriate dosage recommendation and an optimal therapeutic range for serum theophylline concentration remain unestablished. Studies reported in neonates to date indicate that the upper limit of therapeutic levels of theophylline should be less than 15 μg/ml. In the early studies by Shannon and coworkers,[81] apneic spells were controlled with plasma theophylline concentrations in excess of 6.6 μg/ml, although tachycardia (heart rate >180/min) was noted with plasma concentrations of theophylline between 13 and 32 μg/ml. The association of recurrence of apnea with plasma concentrations of theophylline below 5 μg/ml prompted Jones and Baillie[48] to suggest that theophylline concentrations be maintained between 5 and 12 μg/ml. Dietrich and colleagues[28] noted a marked decrease in apnea attack rate with theophylline levels of 4 to 5 μg/ml. Boutroy and coworkers[19] commented on the difficulty of interpretation of the effect of minimal theophylline concentration because of the presence of the active

metabolite caffeine. In their series, the effective plasma level ranged from 1.3 to 17.7 μg/ml; there were no significant differences in the plasma levels of theophylline among infants with and without toxic signs (14.5 vs. 11 μg/ml), nor in the total amount of methyl xanthines (theophylline plus caffeine). In a recent study by Milsap and colleagues,[61] the employment of low-dose theophylline therapy (2 mg/kg q 24 hr) demonstrated therapeutic effect with plasma theophylline concentrations of 3.9 ± 0.2 μg/ml; with these low maintenance doses the caffeine plasma concentrations were less than 1 μg/ml in all neonates. Myers and coauthors[65] recommended a 2 mg/kg daily dose of maintenance theophylline as an effective treatment for apnea of prematurity. In their series, the plasma levels of theophylline associated with this theophylline dosage ranged from 2.8 to 3.7 μg/ml. In a study designed to explore the relationship between plasma level of theophylline and the effect on apnea, Lagercrantz and colleagues[56] concluded from regression-line analysis of a selected cut-off level for apnea (two episodes per 12-hr period) that the ideal plasma concentration is at least 7 μg/ml. Milsap and coworkers[62] have reviewed the efficacy of low-dose theophylline therapy: None of the infants receiving low-dose theophylline demonstrated statistically significant changes in resting heart rates, minute ventilation, arterial blood gas tension, total pulmonary compliance, serum sodium, serum potassium, or blood urea nitrogen. Normal growth was also maintained.

A loading dose of theophylline of 5 mg/kg IV

produces a plasma concentration of approximately 10 μg/ml (range 5-15 μg/ml). Since theophylline given PO may not be completely absorbed (80-100% bioavailability[24]), dose recommendations derived from IV pharmacokinetic data may not be valid. Maintenance doses used in the various studies range from 1 to 2 mg/kg every 6 to 8 hours to 1 to 4 mg/kg every 12 hours, or 4.5 mg/kg per day (Table 6-6). The recommended maintenance dose (Table 6-5) is 2 mg/kg IV given every 12 hours; this maintenance dose should be initiated 12 hours after the loading dose. Within 72 hours of initiating therapy, a 2 hour and trough serum theophylline level should be obtained to establish the appropriateness of the maintenance dose. It is clear that serious toxicities are most common with peak serum theophylline levels in excess of 15 to 20 μg/ml (Table 6-8). Under these circumstances the administration of theophylline should be stopped for a minimum of 24 hours or until evidence of apnea is observed, at which time a maintenance dose reduced to one half of the original can be restarted.

Theophylline is generally administered by the IV or PO route. The most commonly employed IV formulation of theophylline contains 78.9% theophylline as the ethylene diamine salt (aminophylline). Administration of rectal doses of theophylline is not recommended because of variable absorption.[15] IM injections are also to be avoided because of extreme pain. For PO administration, there are many commercial preparations available. These oral formulations, whose theophylline content ranges from 50% to 100%, may include any of several additives such as glucose, sodium cyclamate, dyes, or alcohol.[83] For each preparation, the dose prescribed must be calculated according to the anhydrous theophylline base content. It is essential to appreciate that the oral formulations have not been rigorously studied with respect to bioavailability in the neonatal patient.

In the infant, the frequency of theophylline administration should be in keeping with the rate of clearance. Since the half-life of theophylline in newborns is generally greater than 20 hours, there is no need to administer the drug more often than every 12 hours. However, the clearance of theophylline increases with age, which means that the dosage requirements will increase.[66,110,113] An increase in dose (up to 20 to 25 mg/kg/day) and a reduced dosing interval (4 to 8 hr) will be required in infants over 2 to 4 months of age.

Theophylline has been employed in infants with chronic lung disease, such as bronchopul-

Table 6-8. SIGNS OF TOXICITY IN INFANTS RECEIVING THEOPHYLLINE

Manifestation	Estimated Serum Theophylline Level Associated with Toxicity (μg/ml)
failure to gain weight	10-20
sleeplessness	
irritability	
tachycardia	
hyperglycemia	
vomiting	20
diuresis/dehydration	
jitteriness	>20
hyperreflexia	
cardiac arrhythmias	>40
seizures	

Data compiled from numerous sources; see especially Aranda and Dupont,[2] Nobel and Light,[70] Loughnan and McNamara,[60] Estelle et al,[29] Srinivasan et al,[88] and Howell et al.[47]

monary dysplasia (BPD), in an attempt to *improve pulmonary function*. The rationale for theophylline therapy in BPD is the achievement of relaxation of airway smooth muscle in hypertrophied small bronchioles. Its efficacy in increasing the success of weaning infants from respiratory support and oxygen requirements has not been uniform. The substantial variation in structural and functional lung abnormalities seen among infants with manifestations of chronic lung disease and the differences in other aspects of respiratory care practiced among medical care facilities present problems in interpretation of the results of such therapy. Theophylline has been shown to improve lung compliance and to reduce expiratory resistance in infants with BPD who are less than 1 month old;[112] it also facilitates more rapid weaning from mechanical ventilatory support in these infants and in neonates with RDS who are less than 2 weeks old.[102,106] Serum theophylline levels ranged between 5 and 10 μg/ml in infants in whom measurements were accomplished. A well-controlled study of theophylline therapy in infants with RDS or more chronic forms of lung disease remains to be carried out.

Clinical Toxicology. The toxic effects of theophylline have not been fully explored in the neonate in any systematic fashion. The large experience with the drug, however, has identified certain aspects of theophylline toxicity that should be anticipated in its use in the neonate. Subtle toxic symptoms, such as failure to gain weight, sleeplessness, and irritability, along with tachycardia, should be considered serious warning signs of the more ominous toxicities well appreciated in older patients: tremor, seizures, hypertension, and cardiac arrhythmias (see Table 6–8). Tachycardia has occurred with serum theophylline concentrations ranging from 13 to 32 μg/ml.[81] Other side-effects associated with the use of theophylline in neonates include hyperglycemia,[2] diuresis and dehydration,[70] hyperreflexia, jitteriness, and seizures.[29] Employment of appropriate doses and maintenance of serum theophylline levels below 15 to 20 μg/ml will be associated with negligible overt CNS excitation and other major complications. Low serum protein levels will increase the risk of theophylline toxicity.[3] More recently, theophylline therapy has been implicated in the development of necrotizing enterocolitis.[108,111,118] These clinical reports do not clearly demonstrate a cause and effect relationship, although the known pharmacologic actions of theophylline provide a plausible mechanism for such a toxic role.[105] Howell and colleagues[47] have carefully reviewed the adverse effects of theophylline in the newborn infant.

References

1. Aldridge A, Aranda JV, Neims AH: Caffeine metabolism in the newborn. Clin Pharmacol Ther 25:447, 1979.
2. Aranda JV, Dupont C: Metabolic effect of theophylline in the premature neonate. J Pediatr 89:833, 1976.
3. Aranda JV, Sitar DS, Parsons WD, et al: Pharmacokinetic aspects of theophylline in premature newborns. N Engl J Med 295:413, 1976.
4. Aranda JV, Gorman W, Bergsteinsson H, Gunn T: Efficacy of caffeine in treatment of apnea in the low-birth-weight infant. J Pediatr 90:467, 1977.
5. Aranda JV, Collinge JM, Zinman R, Watters G: Maturation of caffeine elimination in infancy. Arch Dis Child 54:946, 1979.
6. Aranda JV, Cook CE, Gorman W, et al: Pharmacokinetic profile of caffeine in the premature newborn infant with apnea. J Pediatr 94:663, 1979.
7. Aranda JV, Turmen T: Methylxanthines in apnea of prematurity. Clin Perinatol 6:87, 1979.
8. Aranda JV, Grondin D, Sasyniuk BI: Pharmacologic considerations in the therapy of neonatal apnea. Pediatr Clin North Am 28:113, 1981.
9. Bacola E, Behrle FC, Schweinitz L, et al: Perinatal and environmental factors in late neurogenic sequelae. I. Infants having birth weights under 1,500 grams. Am J Dis Child 112:359, 1966.
10. Bacola E, Behrle FC, Schweinitz L, et al: Perinatal and environmental factors in late neurogenic sequelae. II. Infants having birth weights from 1,500 to 2,500 grams. Am J Dis Child 112:369, 1966.
11. Bada HS, Khanna NN, Somani SM, Tin AA: Interconversion of theophylline and caffeine in newborn infants. J Pediatr 94:993, 1979.
12. Baley JE, Ruuskanen O, Miller K, Pittard WB III: Effects of theophylline on the neonatal immune response. Pediatr Res 16:649, 1982.
13. Banner W Jr, Czajka PA: Acute caffeine overdose in the neonate. Am J Dis Child 134:495, 1980.
14. Bednarek FJ, Roloff DW: Treatment of apnea of prematurity with aminophylline. Pediatrics 58:335, 1976.
15. Bolme, P, Edlund PO, Eriksson M, et al: Pharmacokinetics of theophylline in young children with asthma: Comparison of rectal enema and suppositories. Eur J Clin Pharmacol 16:133, 1979.
16. Bonati M, Latini R, Marra G, et al: Theophylline distribution in the premature neonate. Dev Pharmacol Ther 3:65, 1981.
17. Bonati M, Latini R, Marra G, et al: Theophylline metabolism during the first month of life and development. Pediatr Res 15:304, 1981.
18. Bory C, Baltassat P, Porthault M, et al: Metabolism of theophylline to caffeine in premature newborn infants. J Pediatr 94:988, 1979.
19. Boutroy MJ, Vert P, Royer RJ, et al: Caffeine, a metabolite of theophylline during the treatment of apnea in the premature infant. J Pediatr 94:996, 1979.
20. Brazier JL, Renaud H, Ribon B, Salle BL: Plasma xanthine levels in low birth weight infants treated or not treated with theophylline. Arch Dis Child 54:194, 1979.
21. Brazier JL, Salle B, Ribon B, et al: In vivo N_7 methylation of theophylline to caffeine in premature infants. Dev Pharmacol Ther 2:137, 1981.
22. Cano R, Isenberg JI, Grossman MI: Cimetidine inhibits caffeine-stimulated gastric acid secretion in man. Gastroenterology 70:1055, 1976.
23. Chu NS: Caffeine- and aminophylline-induced seizures. Epilepsia 22:85, 1981.
24. Cottancin G, Baltassat P, Bory C, Challamel MJ, Frederich A: Pharmacocinetique de la theophylline chez le nouveau-né de petit poids de naissance. Paediatrie 32:677, 1977.
25. Daily WJR, Klaus M, Meyer HBP: Apnea in premature infants: Monitoring, incidence, heart rate changes, and an effect of environmental temperature. Pediatrics 43:510, 1969.
26. Davi MJ, Sankaran K, Simons KJ, et al: Physiologic changes induced by theophylline in the treatment of apnea in preterm infants. J Pediatr 92:91, 1978.
27. Debas HT, Cohen MM, Holubitsky IB, Harrison RC: Caffeine-stimulated acid and pepsin secretion: Dose-response studies. Scand J Gastroenterol 6:453, 1971.
28. Dietrich J, Krauss AN, Reidenberg M, et al: Alterations in state in apneic pre-term infants receiving theophylline. Clin Pharmacol Ther 24:474, 1978.
29. Estelle F, Simons R, Friesen FR, Simons KJ: Theophylline toxicity in term infants. Am J Dis Child 134:39, 1980.
30. Estelle F, Simons R, Rigatto H, Simons KJ: Pharmacokinetics of theophylline in neonates. Semin Perinatol 5:337, 1981.
31. Estelle F, Simons R, Simons KJ, et al: The pharmacokinetics of theophylline in an infant with hepatic failure. Dev Pharmacol Ther 4:132, 1982.
32. Fenichel GM, Olson BJ, Fitzpatrick JE: Heart rate changes in convulsive and nonconvulsive neonatal apnea. Ann Neurol 7:577, 1980.
33. Foote WE, Holmes P, Pritchard A, et al: Neurophysiological and pharmacodynamic studies on caffeine and on interactions between caffeine and nicotinic acid in the rat. Neuropharmacoly 17:7, 1978.
34. Gabriel M, Witolla C, Albani M: Sleep and

aminophylline treatment of apnea in preterm infants. Eur J Pediatr 128:145, 1978.

35. Gal P, Boer HR, Toback J, et al: Effect of asphyxia on theophylline clearance in newborns. South Med J 75:836, 1982.

36. Gardner MJ, Jusko WJ: Effect of age and sex on theophylline clearance in young subjects. Pediatr Pharmacol 2:157, 1982.

37. Gerhardt T, McCarthy J, Bancalari E: Aminophylline therapy in idiopathic apnea in premature infants: Effects on lung function. Pediatrics 62:801, 1978.

38. Gerhardt T, McCarthy J, Bancalari E: Effect of aminophylline on respiratory center activity and metabolic rate in premature infants with idiopathic apnea. Pediatrics 63:537, 1979.

39. Giacoia G, Juskoi WJ, Menke J, Koup JR: Theophylline pharmacokinetics in premature infants with apnea. J Pediatr 89:829, 1976.

40. Gorodischer R, Karplus M, Worszawski D, et al: Caffeine pharmacokinetics in the neonate: Human and animal studies. Pediatr Res 11:1013, 1977.

41. Gorodischer R, Karplus M: Pharmacokinetic aspects of caffeine in premature infants with apnoea. Eur J Clin Pharmacol 22:47, 1982.

42. Grygiel JJ, Birkett DJ: Effect of age on patterns of theophylline metabolism. Clin Pharmacol Ther 28:456, 1980.

43. Gunn TR, Metrakos K, Riley P, et al: Sequelae of caffeine treatment in preterm infants with apnea. J Pediatr 94:106, 1979.

44. Harkavy KL, Scanlon JW, Jose P: The effects of theophylline on renal function in the premature newborn. Biol Neonate 35:126, 1979.

45. Hilligoss DM, Jusko WJ, Koup JR, Giacoia G: Factors affecting theophylline pharmacokinetics in premature infants with apnea. Dev Pharmacol Ther 1:6, 1980.

46. Horning MG, Butler CM, Nowlin J, Hill RM: Minireview: Drug metabolism in the human neonate. Life Sci 16:651, 1975.

47. Howell J, Clozel M, Aranda JV: Adverse effects of caffeine and theophylline in the newborn infant. Semin Perinatol 5:359, 1981.

48. Jones RAK, Baillie E: Dosage schedule for intravenous aminophylline in apnoea of prematurity, based on pharmacokinetic studies. Arch Dis Child 54:190, 1979.

49. Karasawa T, Kurukawa K, Yoshida K, Shimizu M: Effect of theophylline on monoamine metabolism in the rat brain. Eur J Pharmacol 37:97, 1976.

50. Kattwinkel J: Neonatal apnea: Pathogenesis and therapy. J Pediatr 90:342, 1977.

51. Kelly DH, Shannon DC: Treatment of apnea and excessive periodic breathing in the full-term infant: Pediatrics 68:183, 1981.

52. King DM, Heeley AF, Kuzemko JA: Half-life of theophylline in the preterm baby with apnoeic attacks. Arch Dis Child 54:238, 1979.

53. Kreil E, Zapol W, Sharp G, et al: Effect of cyclic AMP on isolated ductus arteriosus. Pediatr Res 7:300, 1973.

54. Kulkarni PB, Dorand RD: Caffeine toxicity in a neonate. Pediatrics 64:254, 1979.

55. Kuzemko JA, Paala J: Apnoeic attacks in the newborn treated with aminophylline. Arch Dis Child 48:404, 1973.

56. Lagercrantz H, Rane A, Tunell R: Plasma concentration–effect relationship of theophylline in treat-

ment of apnea in preterm infants. Eur J Clin Pharmacol 18:65, 1980.

57. Latini R, Assael BM, Bonati M, et al: Kinetics and efficacy of theophylline in the treatment of apnea in the premature newborn. Eur J Clin Pharmacol 13:203, 1978.

58. Lazaro-Lopez F, Colle E, Dupont C, Aranda JV: Metabolic effects of caffeine in the preterm neonate. Pediatr Res 14:468, 1980.

59. LeMessurier DH: The site of action of caffeine as a respiratory stimulant. J Pharmacol Exp Ther 57:458, 1936.

60. Loughnan PM, McNamara JM: Paroxysmal supraventricular tachycardia during theophylline therapy in a premature infant. J Pediatr 92:1016, 1978.

61. Milsap RL, Krauss AN, Auld PAM: Oxygen consumption in apneic premature infants after low-dose theophylline. Clin Pharmacol Ther 28:539, 1980.

62. Milsap RL, Krauss AN, Auld PAM: Efficacy of low-dose theophylline. Semin Perinatol 5:321, 1981.

63. Moyer JH, Tashnek AB, Miller SI, et al: The effect of theophylline with ethylenediamine (aminophylline) and caffeine on cerebral hemodynamics and cerebrospinal fluid pressure in patients with hypertensive headaches. Am J Med Sci 224:377, 1952.

64. Murat I, Moriette G, Blin MC, et al: The efficacy of caffeine in the treatment of recurrent idiopathic apnea in premature infants. J Pediatr 99:984, 1981.

65. Myers TF, Milsap RL, Krauss AN, et al: Low-dose theophylline therapy in idiopathic apnea of prematurity. J Pediatr 96:99, 1980.

66. Nassif EG, Weinberger MM, Shannon D, et al: Theophylline disposition in infancy. J Pediatr 98:158, 1981.

67. Neese AL, Soyka LF: Development of a radioimmunoassay for theophylline. Application to studies in premature infants. Clin Pharmacol Ther 21:633, 1977.

68. Nelson RM, Resnick MB, Holstrum WJ, Eitzman DV: Developmental outcome of premature infants treated with theophylline. Dev Pharmacol Ther 1:274, 1980.

69. Nelson RM Jr, Resnick MB: Long-term outcome of premature infants treated with theophylline. Semin Perinatol 5:370, 1981.

70. Nobel PA, Light GS: Theophylline-induced diuresis in the neonate. J Pediatr 90:825, 1977.

71. Ogilvie RI, Fernandez PG, Winsberg F: Cardiovascular response to increasing theophylline concentrations. Eur J Clin Pharmacol 12:409, 1977.

72. Parsons WD, Neims AH: Prolonged half-life of caffeine in healthy term newborn infants. J Pediatr 98:640, 1981.

73. Peabody JL, Neese AL, Philip AGS, et al: Transcutaneous oxygen monitoring in aminophylline-treated apneic infants. Pediatrics 62:698, 1978.

74. Rall TW: Central nervous system stimulants: The xanthines. In Gilman AG, Goodman LS, Gilman A (eds): The Pharmacological Basis of Therapeutics, 6th ed. New York, Macmillan, 1980, p 592.

75. Rigatto, H: Apnea. Pediatr Clin North Am 29:1105, 1982.

76. Roberts JL, Mathew OP, Thach BT: The efficacy of theophylline in premature infants with mixed and obstructive apnea and apnea associated with pulmonary and neurologic disease. J Pediatr 100:968, 1982.

77. Robertson D, Frolich JC, Carr RK, et al: Effects of caffeine on plasma renin activity, catecholamines and blood pressure. N Engl J Med 298:181, 1978.

78. Rothberg AD, Marks KH, Ward RM, Maisels MJ: The metabolic effects of caffeine in the newborn infant. Pediatr Pharmacol 1:181, 1981.

79. Sattin A, Rall TW: The effect of adenosine and adenine nucleotides on the cyclic adenosine 3′,5′-phosphate content of guinea pig cerebral cortex slices. Molec Pharmacol 6:13, 1970.

80. Sattin A: Increase in the content of adenosine 3′,5′-monophosphate in mouse forebrain during seizures and prevention of the increase in methylxanthines. J Neurochem 18:1087, 1971.

81. Shannon DC, Gotay F, Stein IM, et al: Prevention of apnea and bradycardia in low-birth-weight infants. Pediatrics 55:589, 1975.

82. Shannon DC, Gotay F: Effects of theophylline on serum and urine electrolytes in preterm infants with apnea. J Pediatr 94:963, 1979.

83. Simons KJ, Simons FER, Briggs CJ, Lo L: Theophylline protein binding in humans. J Pharmaceut Sci 68:252, 1979.

84. Somani SM, Khanna NN: Methylxanthines in serum, saliva, and spinal fluid of premature infants. Semin Perinatol 5:346, 1981.

85. Soyka LF, Neese AL: Perinatal exposure to methylxanthines: Possible effects on pregnancy outcome. Clin Pharmacol Ther 23:130, 1978.

86. Soyka LF: Monitoring of serum theophylline concentrations. Semin Perinatol 5:406, 1981.

87. Spindel E, Arnold M, Cusack B, Wurtman RJ: Effects of caffeine on anterior pituitary and thyroid function in the rat. J Pharmacol Exp Ther 214:58, 1980.

88. Srinivasan G, Pildes RS, Jaspan JB, et al: Metabolic effects of theophylline in preterm infants. J Pediatr 98:815, 1981.

89. Stroud MW, Lambertsen CJ, Ewing JH, et al: The effects of aminophylline and meperidine alone and in combination on the respiratory response to carbon dioxide inhalation. J Pharmacol Exp Ther 114:461, 1955.

90. Takieddine FN, Tserng KY, King KC, Kalhan SC: Postnatal development of theophylline metabolism in preterm infants. Semin Perinatol 5:351, 1981.

91. Tserng KY, King KC, Takieddine FN: Theophylline metabolism in premature infants. Clin Pharmacol Ther 29:594, 1981.

92. Turmen T, Louridas TA, Aranda JV: Relationship of plasma and CSF concentrations of caffeine in neonates with apnea. J Pediatr 95:644, 1979.

93. Turmen T, Davis J, Aranda JV: Relationship of dose and plasma concentrations of caffeine and ventilation in neonatal apnea. Semin Perinatol 5:326, 1981.

94. Tyrala EE, Dodson WE: Caffeine secretion into breast milk. Arch Dis Child 54:787, 1979.

95. Uauy R, Shapiro DL, Smith B, Warshaw JB: Treatment of severe apnea in prematures with orally administered theophylline. Pediatrics 55:595, 1975.

96. Volpe JJ: Effects of methylxanthines on lipid synthesis in developing neural systems. Semin Perinatol 5:395, 1981.

97. Ward RM, Maisels MJ: Metabolic effects of methylxanthines. Semin Perinatol 5:383, 1981.

98. Warszawski D, Gorodischer R: Tissue distribution of caffeine in premature infants and in newborn and adult dogs. Pediatr Pharmacol 1:341, 1981.

99. Wechsler RL, Kleiss LM, Kety SS: The effect of intravenously administered aminophylline on cerebral circulation and metabolism in man. J Clin Invest 29:28, 1950.

100. Weinberger M, Ginchansky E: Dose-dependent kinetics of theophylline disposition in asthmatic children. J Pediatr 91:820, 1977.

101. Zakauddin S, Leake RD, Trygstad CW: Theophylline increases glomerular filtration rate in preterm infants. Dev Pharmacol Ther 1:333, 1980.

102. Barr PA: Weaning very low birthweight infants from mechanical ventilation using intermittent mandatory ventilation and theophylline. Arch Dis Child 53:598, 1978.

103. Bhat AM, Scanlon JW, Lavenstein L, et al: Cerebrospinal fluid concentration of biogenic amine metabolites in idiopathic apnea of prematurity. Biol Neonate 43:16, 1983.

104. Gerhardt T, McCarthy J, Bancalari E: Effects of aminophylline on respiratory center and reflex activity in premature infants with apnea. Pediatr Res 17:188, 1983.

105. Grosfeld JL, Dalsing MC, Hull M, et al: Neonatal apnea, xanthines, and necrotizing enterocolitis. J Pediatr Surg 18:80, 1983.

106. Harris MC, Baumgart S, Rooklin AR, et al: Successful extubation of infants with respiratory distress syndrome using aminophylline. J Pediatr 103:303, 1983.

107. Heimann G, Murgescu J, Bergt U: Influence of food intake on bioavailability of theophylline in premature infants. Eur J Clin Pharmacol 22:171, 1982.

108. Jones RAK: Xanthines and necrotising enterocolitis. Arch Dis Child 56:3, 1981.

109. Jones RAK, Lukeman D: Apnoea of immaturity. 2. Mortality and handicap. Arch Dis Child 57:766, 1982.

110. Lönnerholm G, Lindström B, Paalzow L, et al: Plasma theophylline and caffeine and plasma clearance of theophylline during theophylline treatment in the first year of life. Eur J Clin Pharmacol 24:371, 1983.

111. Robinson MJ, Clayden GS, Smith MF: Xanthines and necrotising enterocolitis. Arch Dis Child 55:494, 1980.

112. Rooklin AR, Moomjian AS, Shutack JG, et al: Theophylline therapy in bronchopulmonary dysplasia. J Pediatr 95:882, 1979.

113. Rosen JP, Danish M, Ragni MC, et al: Theophylline pharmacokinetics in the young infant. Pediatrics 64:248, 1979.

114. Rosenkrantz TS, Oh W: Reduction of cerebral blood flow (CBF) in low birth weight (LBW) infants after aminophylline administration. Pediatr Res 16:306, 1982.

115. Trippenbach T: Effects of drugs on the respiratory control system in the perinatal period and during postnatal development. Pharmacol Ther 20:307, 1983.

116. Tserng KY, Takieddine FN, King KC: Developmental aspects of theophylline metabolism in premature infants. Clin Pharmacol Ther 33:522, 1983.

117. Vestal RE, Eiriksson CE Jr, Musser B, et al: Effect of intravenous aminophylline on plasma levels of catecholamines and related cardiovascular and metabolic responses in man. Circulation 67:162, 1983.

118. Williams AJ: Xanthines and necrotising enterocolitis. Arch Dis Child 55:973, 1980.

SEVEN

Cardiovascular Drugs

A number of drugs are capable of regulating, inhibiting, or stimulating the cardiovascular system of the infant. To employ these drugs effectively, physicians must understand how cardiovascular pathophysiology contributes to infant disease.[103,104,136] The development of invasive and noninvasive diagnostic techniques has aided greatly in furthering the understanding of cardiovascular dysfunction in infant disease. This chapter reviews the pharmacology of and the clinical experience with cardiovascular drugs used in the care of infants.

INOTROPIC AGENTS

Inotropic drugs improve cardiac output by augmenting myocardial contractility. Drugs considered to be inotropic agents include the **digitalis glycosides** and the **sympathomimetic amines.** The latter group includes naturally occurring catecholamines—epinephrine, norepinephrine, and dopamine—and synthetic drugs that mimic their actions. Inotropic drugs are one of the most extensively studied groups of pharmacologic agents. Besides their inotropic effects, these drugs may possess other prominent pharmacologic actions including peripheral excitatory and inhibitory action on smooth muscle, metabolic actions (glycogenolysis), endocrine actions (modulation of insulin, renin, and pituitary hormones), and CNS actions.[179] The pharmacologic properties of the various agents differ primarily in a quantitative respect, but some important qualitative differences exist as well.

Inotropic agents are used primarily in acute cardiovascular resuscitation and in chronic support of the damaged myocardium. The appropriate use of these agents along with volume expansion can restore and maintain sufficient cardiac output and vascular perfusion to preserve life under even the most adverse circumstances. However, the proper selection of drug or drugs requires an understanding of the hemodynamic abnormality. Perkin and Levin recently reviewed normal hemodynamics and shock in the pediatric patient.[154,155] Detailed discussions of the pharmacologic properties and clinical use of inotropic agents are presented in the following sections. Though valuable, pharmacologic information alone cannot be effectively employed for selection and use of appropriate inotropic drugs without an understanding of the relationships between pathophysiology and drug actions.

Digitalis Glycosides: Digoxin

Pharmacology. Digoxin is one of several cardiac glycosides in clinical use. Digoxin consists of an aglycone and three molecules of digitoxose (Fig. 7–1). The enteral absorption of digoxin is influenced by a variety of factors including gastrointestinal function or dysfunction, presence and composition of food, and bioavailability of the pharmaceutical preparations employed. All currently available formulations of digoxin used for PO administration are variably and completely absorbed from the gastrointestinal tract.[57] In infants, the extent of absorption of digoxin given PO has been found to average 72% (range 52–79%) of an equivalent dose given IV.[91] These results agree with oral bioavailability studies conducted in adults showing 76% absorption.[57] The rate of oral absorption of digoxin is rapid; detectable levels are observed as early as 5 minutes after administration, and peak levels occur by 1 to 3 hours.[30,50,91] Other than the potential loss of drug dose through vomiting or regurgitation, digoxin elixir given either shortly before or after feeding the infant is absorbed to the same ex-

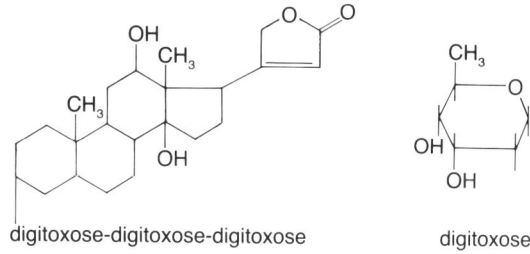

Figure 7–1. Digoxin: Structural formula (*upper left*) and various metabolites. Along the major route of metabolism (*heavy arrow*), digoxin reduction products (DRPs) are formed. DRPs (i.e., dihydrodigoxin) contain a saturated lactone ring and are inactive. Other metabolic products are formed by hydrolysis of one or more of the sugar (digitoxose) groups, which may remain active. (Adapted from Peters U et al: Arch Intern Med 138:1074, 1978.)

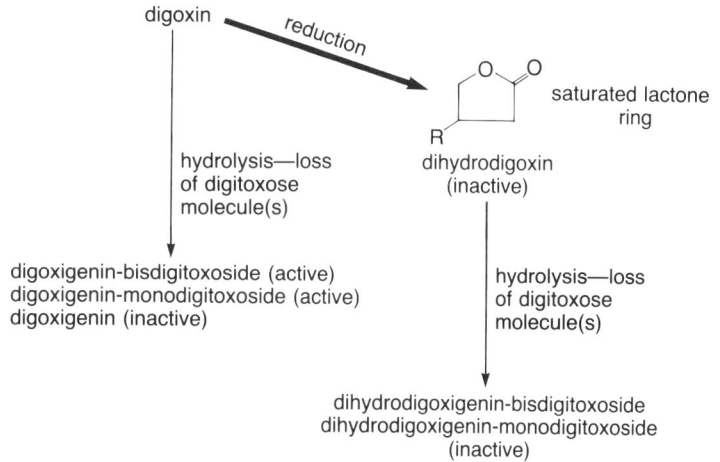

tent. Diminished absorption of digoxin given PO has been reported in infants with severe cardiac failure,[14] although other reports indicate that gastrointestinal absorption is adequate for therapeutic purposes.[30,50]

IM administration of digoxin clearly does not eliminate variability in absorption. The PO and IM routes of administration result in similar pharmacokinetics, but because IM injection causes pain and local tissue injury,[86] most authorities recommend avoiding this administration route.[24,30,50] It is unlikely that differences in rate or extent of absorption of digoxin explain the higher doses (dose per unit body weight) required in infants to maintain serum levels equivalent to those in adults.

The distribution half-life of digoxin into peripheral tissue compartments following absorption is 0.4 to 0.7 hour, but the time to reach steady state is much slower, reflecting the large volume of distribution of digoxin.[92] Digoxin levels measured in tissue obtained post mortem show the same relative distribution of digoxin for both infants and children (Table 7–1):

choroid plexus > ventricular myocardium
> kidney > liver > skeletal muscle

While kidney, liver, skeletal muscle, and brain digoxin concentrations are similar, myocardial

digoxin levels appear to be significantly higher in infants than in adults. There is considerable variation in absolute values for digoxin concentrations among patients[1] and among clinical studies (Table 7–1). Park and colleagues recently demonstrated that the myocardium from infants accumulates digoxin more avidly than does myocardium from adults; the mean myocardial-to-serum ratio was 149:1 in infants and 28:1 in adults, a more than fivefold difference. Similar findings were reported in earlier studies, although the magnitude of difference between infants and adults was not as great (Table 7–1). Studies in patients between 9 months and 18 years of age revealed a mean ratio (atrial appendage/serum) of 78, which is intermediate to those reported in infants and adults.[384]

The reason for the apparent increased affinity of neonatal myocardium for digoxin compared with that in the adult is unknown. No age-related differences in the cellular localization of digoxin within the heart have been identified in animal studies.[5] The higher concentration of myocardial $Na^+–K^+$ ATPase found in neonates and infants has been proposed as the explanation, since it binds the cardiac glycosides and may in fact constitute the "digitalis receptor."[94] However, only a small fraction of digoxin present in the myocardium is believed to be actually bound to active receptor sites.[92]

Table 7–1. SERUM AND TISSUE DIGOXIN CONCENTRATIONS IN NEONATES, INFANTS, AND ADULTS[a]

Authors of Published Study[b]	Study Group[c]	Serum Concentration (ng/ml)	Tissue Concentration (ng/g wet weight)				
			Heart (V = ventricle; A = atrium)	Skeletal Muscle	Kidney	Liver	Brain
Hernandez et al[30]	20 infants (1 wk–5.5 mo)		150 ± 20		170 ± 10	110 ± 20	
Coltart et al[11]	18 adults[d]	1.2 ± 0.8 (SD)	78 ± 43 V	11 ± 5			
Krasula et al[44]	18 children (1–16 yr)	1.2 ± 0.1	*digitalized:* 109 ± 9 *chronic:* 62 ± 6	*digitalized:* 8 ± 1 *chronic:* 24 ± 7			
Jusko and Weintraub[37]	15 adults	2.9 ± 0.4	97 ± 16 V				
Karjalainen et al[38]	13 adults	4.6 ± 2.3 (SD) (whole blood[e])	112 ± 66 (SD) V 43 ± 26 (SD) A	20 ± 13 (SD)	123 ± 65 (SD)	68 ± 51 (SD)	
Andersson et al[1]	12 infants (5 days–8 mo)	1.7 ± 0.1	245 ± 33 V 165 ± 25 A	31 ± 4	167 ± 24	82 ± 12	30 ± 5 (choroid plexus: 287 ± 51)
	17 adults	1.6 ± 0.2	133 ± 16 V 65 ± 9 A	30 ± 4	128 ± 20	72 ± 13	32 ± 6 (choroid plexus: 211 ± 23)
Kim et al[40]	7 prematures (2–24 days)	1.9 ± 0.4	190 ± 70	37 ± 33	73 ± 43	56 ± 34	7 ± 8
	4 full-term infants (2–11 days)		185 ± 60	32 ± 17	198 ± 69	50 ± 34	14 ± 15
	4 children (1.5–7 yr)	0.6 ± 0.3	67 ± 25	8 ± 6	232 ± 27	41 ± 25	21 ± 12

Reference							
Gorodischer et al[22]	8 infants (1 day–26 mo)	3.5 ± 3.3	386 ± 321 V	42 ± 42			
Hartel et al[27]	12 adults	1.3 ± 0.6	89 ± 43 (SD) V				
Lang et al[48f]	13 prematures (1–30 days)	2.4	165 V	38	90	94	
	6 full-term infants (2–26 days)	2.8	171	66	211	73	
	5 infants (2–14 mo)	2.2	104	24	108	26	
Park et al[72]	12 infants (1.5–36 mo)	1.3 ± 0.3	212 ± 72 A				
	17 adults	1.3 ± 0.1	35 ± 8				
Wagner et al[384]	25 infants and children (9 mo–18 yr)	0.5–0.8 (mean range, two different assays)	48 (range 1–178)				
Hastreiter and Van Der Horst[379]	36 infants and children						
	(premature)	2.3 ± 1.0 (SD)	235 ± 97	28 ± 13	155 ± 128	86 ± 39	
	(full term)	2.6 ± 0.7	296 ± 135	46 ± 14	171 ± 69	103 ± 55	<20
	(<2 yr)	1.2 ± 0.3	127 ± 94	48 ± 55	291 ± 397	77 ± 76	
	(>2 <18 yr)	0.9 ± 0.3	86 ± 54 (left vent)	31 ± 37	131 ± 118	39 ± 28	

[a] Values shown are mean ± SE unless otherwise noted. There are considerable differences in these studies with respect to the amount of digoxin administered, duration of therapy, and the analytic technique employed.

[b] Listed in order of publication; see References at end of chapter.

[c] Age at time of study is given in parentheses.

[d] At steady state.

[e] Note that whole blood values are about 30% higher than serum values.

[f] Mean values have been recalculated from data presented by the authors.

Binding studies in erythrocytes have demonstrated two and one-half times as many digoxin binding sites on erythrocytes obtained from neonates as those on adult erythrocytes.[39] In addition, binding of digoxin to tissue can be altered by changes in concentrations of potassium and magnesium. Differences in digoxin serum-to-myocardium ratios, however, have not been associated with differences in concentrations of potassium or magnesium.

Myocardial tissue concentrations of digoxin have been demonstrated to be higher in neonates and infants shortly after administration of loading doses of digoxin (i.e., digitalized) than in those on chronic maintenance digoxin therapy.[1,44] Thus, the safety and therapeutic advantage of loading doses of digoxin (digitalization) versus initiating maintenance therapy without digitalization must be seriously questioned. Moreover, a nonsaturation linear relationship between myocardium and serum digoxin concentration has been demonstrated in neonates; this finding suggests that after initial distribution, the higher the serum digoxin level, the greater will be the myocardial concentration.[22] Why ventricular digoxin levels are greater than atrial levels (Table 7–1) in both infants and adults is not known, although differences in blood flow per gram of tissue may be responsible. Greater blood flow would result in delivery of significantly greater quantities of drug to the ventricular tissue over a period of time.

Figure 7–2 illustrates the serum concentration–time curve for digoxin following PO and IV administration to four neonates. The rapid decline in serum levels after IV administration coincides with the movement of digoxin into tissue (Fig. 7–3). The time required to complete the distribution phase (α phase) of digoxin is approximately 4 to 6 hours in neonates,[9] when peak digoxin tissue levels are reached. The 4- to 6-hour distribution time is consistent with other published observations on elapsed time before maximum hemodynamic response to digoxin following its administration.[53,70]

The volume of distribution of digoxin appears to be age-dependent. In low-birth-weight neonates, mean values range from 4.3 to 5.7 l/kg (Table 7–2). In full-term neonates, the average V_d is 12 to 16 l/kg, about twice that in low-birth-weight infants;[94] the explanation for this difference is not clear. The larger volume of distribution in neonates and infants compared with that in adults (5 l/kg) has been attributed to the greater tissue binding of digoxin in infants. The data of Lang[48] and Kim[40] and their colleagues demonstrate greater concentrations

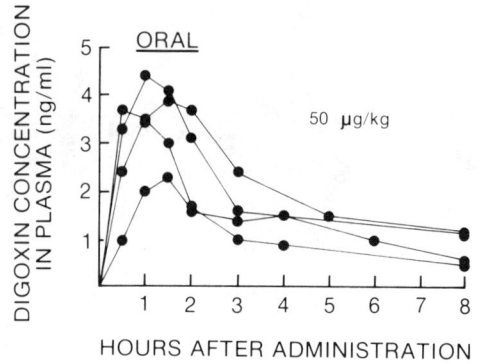

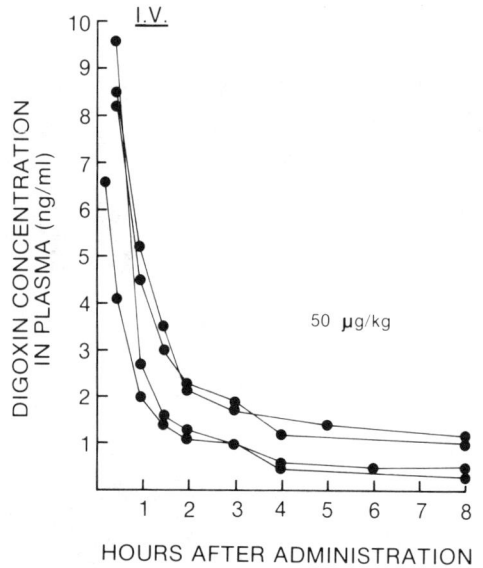

Figure 7–2. Serum concentration–time curves in four infants after a single oral dose (*A*) or rapid IV injection (*B*) of 50 μg/kg of digoxin. (Adapted from Wettrell G, Andersson KE: Eur J Clin Pharmacol 9:49, 1975.)

of digoxin in skeletal muscle of premature and full-term neonates than those in older infants and children (Table 7–1). Since skeletal muscle accounts for 20% to 25% of body mass in neonates and infants, this tissue contains the largest store of digoxin in the body. The difference in skeletal muscle digoxin levels could in part explain the age-related differences in volume of distribution of digoxin. Changes in body composition (ratio of extracellular fluid volume and tissue weight to body weight) may be an additional contributing factor.[64]

Digoxin in serum is about 20% protein bound in neonates, a value similar to that reported for adults.[21] No significant interaction occurs between digoxin and other protein-bound substances such as bilirubin or other drugs.

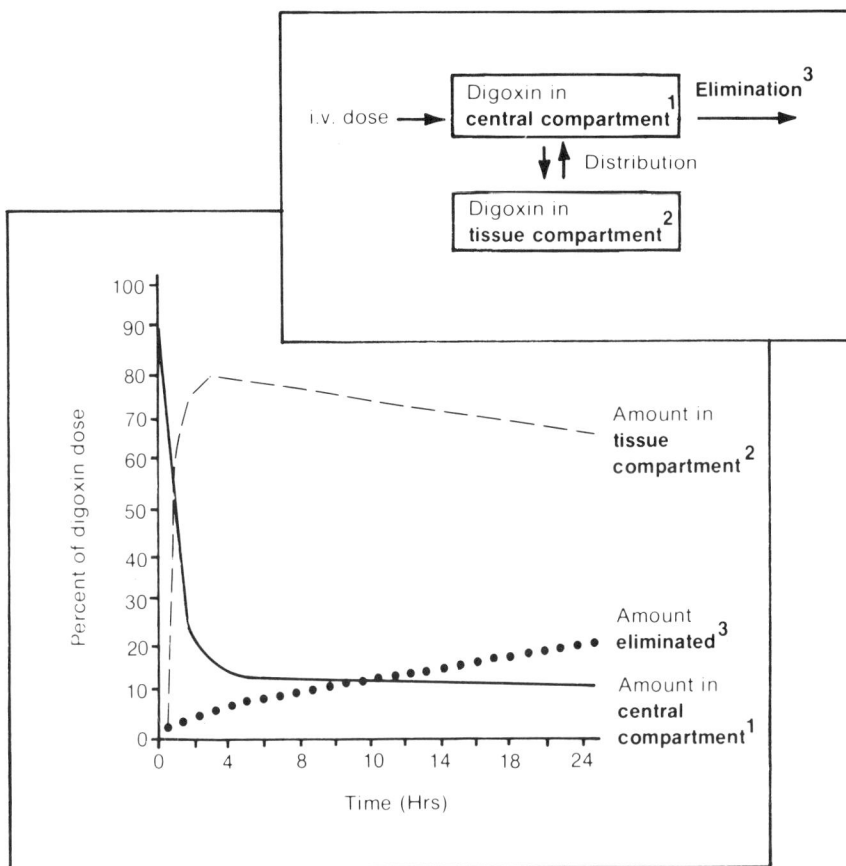

Figure 7 – 3. Computer-simulated curves for distribution and elimination of digoxin in the neonate over a 24-hour period following a single IV injection. *Inset,* The open two-compartment model describing distribution and elimination of digoxin. (Adapted from Collins-Nakai RL et al: Dev Pharmacol Ther 5:86, 1982.)

Digoxin is known to be metabolized to a limited extent in adults, although it has been recognized that some adults will metabolize digoxin extensively.[55,56,374] When the lactone ring on the digoxin molecule is reduced, dihydrodigoxin (or its aglycone) and dihydrodigoxigenin are formed; these metabolites have very little cardiac activity (see Fig. 7 – 1). Active metabolites include digoxigenin bisdigitoxoside and digoxigenin monodigitoxoside. It has been estimated that one out of ten adult patients receiving digoxin will excrete 30% to 40% or more of the total dose as metabolites in the urine. The origin of these metabolites has been suggested to be the enteric flora;[55,374] findings indicating that approximately 30% of each dose of digoxin may undergo enterohepatic recirculation provide strong evidence for metabolism by gut flora.[8] Changes in the state of the gut flora by administration of certain antibiotics can markedly affect the production of digoxin reduction products and as a consequence alter the serum level of digoxin.[55] Studies of this phenomenon have not been accomplished in neonates. Conventional radioimmunoassay (RIA) methods for analyzing digoxin cannot differentiate digoxin from some of these metabolites.[42] This is a particularly significant finding, since the cardiac activity of these metabolites is different from that of digoxin.

Gibson and Nelson[20] demonstrated that in adults on digoxin therapy from 6% to 42% of the measured serum digoxin concentration represented compounds other than digoxin that cross-reacted with RIA materials commonly employed for determination of digoxin serum levels. An endogenous digitalis-like substance, termed endotoxin, which inhibits $Na^+ - K^+$ ATPase, as does digitalis, and reacts with antibodies to digoxin, has been identified in adults with congestive heart failure or renal failure and in the plasma of volume-expanded dogs.[377,378] Godfraind and coworkers[376] identified an endogenous digitalis-like material, termed cardiodigin, isolated from mammalian heart. In studies in premature and full-term infants *not*

Table 7-2. SUMMARY OF DIGOXIN PHARMACOKINETIC STUDIES IN NEONATES AND INFANTS

Author(s) of Published Study[a]	Patients Study Group[b]	Digoxin Dosage	Serum Digoxin Concentration[c] (ng/ml)	Other Data[c]
Rogers et al[76]	7 neonates (3–30 days)	loading: 40–60 µg/kg IV; maintenance: 7.5–10 µg/kg q 12 hr PO	neonates: 1.8 ± 1.2; infants: 2.1 ± 0.7	
Krasula et al[43]	9 infants (6–24 mo)	11 µg/kg q 12 hr PO	peak: 3.2 ± 0.3; plateau: 1.0 ± 0.2	
Hayes et al[29]	31 infants (1 wk–11 mo)	14–20 µg/kg q 24 hr PO or IM	IM: 3.5 ± 1.3; PO: 2.8 ± 1.4; PO: 2.2 ± 1.1	
O'Malley et al[71]	13 infants (12–225 days)	infants: 24 µg/kg q 24 hr; adults: 5 µg/kg q 24 hr	<1 mo: 3.8 ± 1.2 (SD); >1 mo: 1.4 ± 0.5 (SD); 1.4 ± 1.1 (SD)	
Iisalo and Dahl[34]	26 infants and children (12 days–7 yr)	10 µg/kg q 24 hr PO	<1 mo: 2.1 ± 0.3; 1–3 mo: 12.6 ± 0.2; 4–6 mo: 1.1 ± 0.1; 7–12 mo: 0.8; 1–7 yr: 1.4 ± 0.3	Cl (ml/min/1.73 m²): 53, 69, 87, 106; 36–55% of dose excreted in urine
Larese and Mirkin[50]	15 infants and children (7 days–12 yr)	5 µg/kg q 12 hr PO; 11 µg/kg q 12 hr PO; 10 µg/kg q 12 hr IM; 9 µg/kg q 12 hr IV	1.0 ± 0.4; 2.5 ± 0.4; 2.2 ± 0.6; 2.4 ± 0.3	
Wettrell et al[90]	12 neonates (3–30 days)	loading: 50 µg/kg PO maintenance: 6 µg/kg q 12 hr PO	2.1 ± 0.5 (range 1.2–3.1)	$Cl = 47.5$ ml/min/m² (range 18–94)
	24 infants (1–12 mo)	loading: 70 µg/kg PO maintenance: 6–10 µg/kg q 12 hr PO	low dose: 1.2 ± 0.5 (range 0.4–1.9); high dose: 2.1 ± 0.6 (range 1.1–2.9)	
	17 children (1–10 yr)	loading: 50 µg/kg PO maintenance: 6 µg/kg q 12 hr PO	1.4 ± 0.4 (range 0.6–2.4)	
	25 adults	maintenance: 5–10 µg/kg/day	1.2 ± 0.3 (range 0.7–1.9)	

Morselli et al[64]	5 neonates	11 µg/kg IV × 1	1.5 ± 0.3	$T\frac{1}{2}$ = 69 ± 25 hr Cl = 1.8 ± 0.6 ml/min/kg V_d = 7.5 ± 0.9 l/kg
	7 infants (1–11 mo)	high dose: 23 µg/kg IV × 1	1.5 ± 0.2	$T\frac{1}{2}$ = 18 ± 3 hr Cl = 10.7 ± 0.7 ml/min/kg V_d = 16.3 ± 2.1 l/kg
		low dose: 10 µg/kg IV × 1	0.8 ± 0.1	$T\frac{1}{2}$ = 33 ± 4 hr Cl = 4.5 ± 0.5 ml/min/kg V_d = 13.2 ± 1.5 l/kg
	3 children (18–60 mo)	17 µg/kg IV × 1	0.9 ± 0.2	$T\frac{1}{2}$ = 37 ± 9 hr Cl = 5.6 ± 1.7 ml/kg/min V_d = 16.1 ± 0.8 l/kg
Lang and von Bernuth[47]	9 prematures 10 full-term infants	loading: 26 µg/kg IV or 35 µg/kg PO maintenance: 3.6 µg/kg q 12 hr IV or PO	2.4 (range 1.5–4.5) 2.3 (range 1.2–3.5)	$T\frac{1}{2}$ = 57 hr (range 38–88) $T\frac{1}{2}$ = 35 hr (range 17–52)
Gorodischer et al[23]	11 infants (0.6–5 mo)	loading: 30–60 µg/kg IM maintenance: 12–21 µg/kg q 24 hr PO	2.2 ± 0.4	Cl = 88 ± 11 ml/min/1.73 m² (range 37–143)
Neutze et al[66]	53 neonates and infants (<1–18 mo)	high dose: 9–11 µg/kg q 12 hr PO low dose: 7–8 µg/kg q 12 hr PO	0–1 mo: high dose: 2.9 ± 0.4 low dose: 2.9 ± 0.5 1–4 mo: high dose: 2.5 ± 0.2 low dose: 1.8 ± 0.2 4–18 mo: high dose: 1.4 ± 0.2 low dose: 1.1 ± 0.2	
Wettrell[93]	7 neonates and infants (full-term; 2–81 days)	14–22 µg/kg IV × 1	predicted: 0.9–1.7 observed: 0.8–1.6	$T\frac{1}{2}$: <1 mo: 44 hr (mean) infants: 19 hr (mean) Cl: (ml/min/1.73 m²) <1 mo: 65 infants: 236 V_d = 12.1 l/kg

Table continued on following page

145

Table 7-2. SUMMARY OF DIGOXIN PHARMACOKINETIC STUDIES IN NEONATES AND INFANTS (Continued)

Author(s) of Published Study[a]	Patients Study Group[b]	Digoxin Dosage	Serum Digoxin Concentration[c] (ng/ml)	Other Data[c]
Halkin et al[25]	34 infants (1 wk – 2 yr)	maintenance: 0.22–0.29 mg/m² body surface q 24 hr PO	<1 mo: 3.4 ± 0.9 (SD); 1–3 mo: 1.9 ± 0.9 (SD); 3–12 mo: 1.1 ± 0.5 (SD); 1–2 yr: 0.9 ± 0.4 (SD)	Cl: (ml/min/1.73 m²) 1–2 wk: 33; 7–12 wk: 60; 33–51 wk: 88; 128 wk: 144
Berman et al[3]	46 neonates (24–35 wk at 1–20 days)	loading: 30–58 µg/kg IV maintenance: 5–23 µg/kg q 24 hr IV	5.9 ± 1.7; 3.8 ± 1.4	$T\frac{1}{2}$ = 1.4–4.75 days (range)
Nyberg and Wettrell[68]	5 full-term infants (2–21 days)	loading: 25 µg/kg PO maintenance: 9 µg/kg q 24 hr PO	2.4 (range 1.7–3.4)	
Pinsky et al[74]	37 neonates (26–35 wk at 2–14 days)	loading: 20 or 30 µg/kg IV maintenance: 2.5 or 3.75 µg/kg q 12 hr IV	high dose: 3.5 ± 0.4; low dose: 1.7 ± 0.2	$T\frac{1}{2}$ = 72 ± 5.2 hr (range 56–88)
Sandor et al[79]	18 neonates (1–25 days)	loading: 18–60 µg/kg maintenance: 2–10 µg/kg q 12 hr	2.0–3.6 (mean range)	
Warburton et al[89]	9 neonates (27–33 wk at 2–39 days)	loading: 20 or 40 µg/kg IV over 24 hr	1.8–7.0 (24-hr level, range)	$T\frac{1}{2}$ = 15.3 ± 3.6 hr; V_d = 3.3 ± 1.1 l/kg
Ng et al[67]	7 prematures (1–9 days)	loading: 40 µg/kg IV maintenance: 5 µg/kg q 12 hr IV		Cl = 10.4 ml/min/1.73 m²
Krivoy et al[46]	12 infants (1–12 mo)	17 µg/kg q 24 hr PO	1.5 ± 0.8 (saliva: 1.0 ± 0.6)	
Hastreiter et al[28]	6 neonates (29–40 wk at 4–7 days)	20 µg/kg IV × 1		$T\frac{1}{2}$ = 45.5 ± 7.3 hr; Cl = 1.34 ± 0.24 ml/kg/min; V_d = 5.37 ± 1.01 l/kg
Collins-Nakai et al[9]	15 neonates (26–40 wk)	loading: 40 µg/kg IV over 24 hr maintenance: 5 µg/kg q 12 hr IV	3.7 ± 0.9	Cl: (ml/min/1.73 m²) 0.8–1.0 kg: 22.5 ± 5.5; 1.0–1.5 kg: 29.5 ± 5.6; 1.5–2.3 kg: 59.0 ± 16.2

146

Reference	Subjects (age)[b]	Dosage	Serum digoxin[c]	Pharmacokinetic data[c]
Collins-Nakai et al[10]	5 neonates (29–32 wk)	loading: 15 µg/kg IV over 24 hr maintenance: 5–6 µg/kg q 12 hr IV	1.7 ± 0.4 (range 1.4–2.3)	
	13 neonates (26–38 wk)	loading: 40 µg/kg over 36 hr maintenance: 5 µg/kg q 12 hr IV	4.7 ± 1.4	$T\frac{1}{2}$ = 47 ± 21 hr Cl = 29.8 ± 14.7 ml/min/173 m² V_d = 5.7 ± 1 l/kg
Patterson et al[382]	29 neonates (0.78–1.5 kg)	loading: 20–60 µg/kg IV maintenance: 1–5 µg/kg q 12 hr	1.5–4.0 ng/ml (estimated from data)	
Berman et al[6]	21 infants (1–7 mo)	loading: 40 µg/kg IV over 24 hr maintenance: 13 ± 5 µg/kg q 24 hr (range 5–23 µg/kg)	1.6 ± 0.3 (range 0.9–2.2)	$T\frac{1}{2}$ = 20.9 ± 6.1 hr (range 13–34) V_d = 9.8 ± 2.6 (SD) l/kg (range 6.8–16.2 l/kg)
Lundell and Boreus[380]	16 neonates (26–33 wk)	loading: 20 µg/kg IV maintenance: 2.5 µg/kg IV q 12 hr	1.9 + 0.6 nmol/L 2.6 ± 1.1 nmol/L	$T\frac{1}{2}$ = 87 ± 17 hr

[a] Listed in order of publication; see References at end of chapter.

[b] Approximate age at time of study is given in parentheses. For neonates, gestational age is given if available.

[c] Serum digoxin and other pharmacokinetic values shown represent mean ± SE unless otherwise noted. $T\frac{1}{2}$ = half-life of elimination (β phase); V_d = volume of distribution (β phase); Cl = rate of clearance from the body, with m² indicating body surface.

receiving cardiac glycosides, Pudek and co-workers[75] and Valdes and coworkers[383] found an endogenous substance in serum that also cross-reacts with conventional RIA materials. Concentrations of this digoxin-like substance in neonates ranged from 0.3 to 4.1 ng/ml (mean $\pm$ SD $= 1.4 \pm 0.8$). Conflicting observations have been made on the presence of the digoxin-like immunoequivalent substance in plasma in infants over 2 months of age.[75,383] The endogenous digitalis-like substance has been proposed to play an active role in the regulation of $Na^+ - K^+$ ATPase and in certain pathologic conditions (e.g., hypertension, congestive heart failure, and renal failure).[75,376,378,383]

In adults digoxin is eliminated mainly by glomerular filtration, although tubular secretion and reabsorption from the tubular lumen can affect digoxin clearance.[19,85] Passive reabsorption in the proximal tubule may alter the apparent rate of active renal clearance of digoxin. In neonates, digoxin clearance increases in parallel to the maturation of renal function; thus, premature infants have a lower digoxin clearance than that in full-term neonates.[67] In premature neonates glomerular filtration of digoxin is predominant, with some degree of tubular secretion occurring; in full-term and older infants renal tubular secretion is predominant. The literature in general supports the concept that digoxin clearance is equal to creatinine clearance, but in older infants up to 2 years of age, tubular secretion further enhances renal digoxin clearance.[25,54] Renal clearance of digoxin is a major determinant of the steady-state serum level, especially in full-term and older infants.

In neonates and infants on digoxin maintenance therapy, the urinary excretion of digoxin averages 31% of the daily oral dose, the range being 18% to 43%.[92] Although no obvious differences in percentage of dose excreted have been noted among the various pediatric age groups studied, marked individual variations have been found.

Nonrenal elimination of digoxin is believed to occur in very premature infants.[67] Szefler and coworkers[97] observed a serum digoxin half-life that was surprisingly short (1.5 days) in an infant with markedly impaired renal function, suggesting alternative routes of elimination. In comparing the amount of digoxin excreted in the urine to the total elimination calculated from the pharmacokinetic parameters, Wettrell[93] concluded that nonrenal elimination of considerable magnitude may occur in certain infants. In healthy adults about 25% of the total

elimination of digoxin has been estimated to be nonrenal.[41] Caldwell and Cline[8] concluded that enterohepatic recirculation of digoxin occurs: Although 30% of an administered dose of digoxin reaches the intestinal tract via biliary excretion within 24 hours of administration, only a very small fraction of digoxin is actually eliminated in the stool. Dungan and colleagues[15] found that about 50% of stool excretion of digoxin represented metabolites, while metabolites were virtually absent from the urine. No significant differences in metabolism or excretion have been observed among the PO, IM, and IV routes of administration of digoxin.[30]

The main pharmacodynamic property of digoxin is its ability to increase the force of contraction of the myocardium — the so-called **positive inotropic action.** The mechanism responsible for the inotropic effect of digoxin on the heart has been the focus of research efforts for many years. Currently, the majority of evidence supports two dose-dependent actions: (1) At low digoxin doses or levels, myocardial catecholamine levels increase (positive inotropy based on local myocardial catecholamine elevation); and (2) increasing digoxin levels inhibit sarcolemmal $Na^+ - K^+$ ATPase (the $Na^+ - K^+$ pump). Some of the confusion regarding the mechanism of the inotropic effects of digoxin relates to the fact that at low doses, the digoxin inhibition of the $Na^+ - K^+$ pump is offset by the increase in catecholamine release, which stimulates the $Na^+ - K^+$ pump.[49] An elevation of intracellular Na^+ activates the trans-sarcolemmal $Na^+ - Ca^{2+}$ exchange system, which increases the influx of Ca^{2+}, producing further positive inotrophy.[49,80] The amount of free intracellular calcium is proportional to myocardial contractility.[31] This scheme of biochemical cellular events affected by digoxin is illustrated in Figure 7-4. The intracellular concentrations of sodium and potassium are normally maintained by the activity of the $Na^+ - K^+$ pump. The intracellular concentration of calcium is primarily determined by the exchange mechanism with sodium (*exchange site* in the figure).

This hypothesis for digoxin action assumes that the $Na^+ - K^+$ ATPase is a pharmacologic receptor for the drug, and that when digoxin binds to this transport enzyme, active transport of sodium decreases. Studies show that digoxin binds to the ATPase in a specific and saturable manner. In addition, the rate of digoxin binding to the enzyme is increased by sodium and decreased by potassium. Thus, potassium and digoxin appear to compete for myocardial binding sites, although potassium binding affinity is

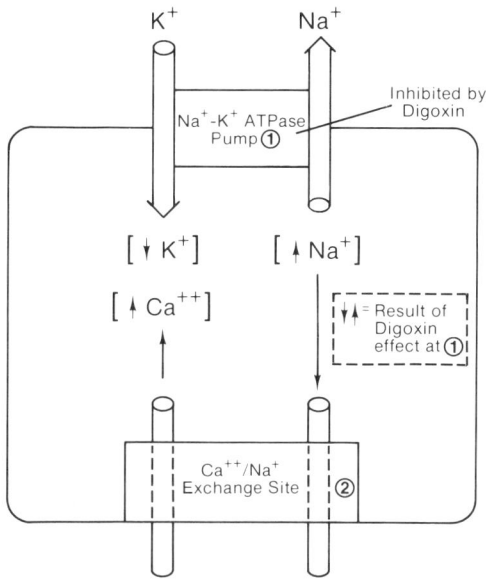

Figure 7-4. Schematic representation of the influence of digoxin on the normal flux of Na^+, K^+, and Ca^{2+} across cardiac cell membrane. Normally the intracellular concentration of Na^+ and K^+ is maintained by the activity of the Na^+–K^+ ATPase pump. Digoxin inhibits Na^+–K^+ ATPase at ①, resulting in decreased active extrusion of Na^+. Consequently, intracellular $[Na^+]$ increases, producing a rise in intracellular $[Ca^{2+}]$ because of increased rate of exchange with Na^+ at the exchange site, ②.

less than that of digoxin. As a consequence, potassium has little effect on digoxin already bound to myocardial tissue and therefore will not alter the toxic and contractile effects of this bound fraction of dose.[61] In this situation, additional inhibition of the Na^+–K^+ pump by digoxin can lead to a large net loss of cellular K^+, with resulting toxic effects.

The quantitative effect of digoxin on myocardial contractility depends in part on the levels of digoxin present and the condition of the cardiac muscle. Normal as well as abnormal myocardium is capable of an inotropic response (Fig. 7–5).[60] The concentrations of a number of cations, including potassium, sodium, calcium, and magnesium, can affect the magnitude and rate of onset of the inotropic effect of digoxin.[81] In addition, the effect of digoxin may be age-related.[4] The difference between newborn and adult myocardial contractility is in part related to the proportion of myocardial tissue consisting of contractile myofilaments.[117] However, it remains to be established whether the immature myocardium has a diminished quantitative response to digoxin compared with the mature myocardium. An alternative consideration is that the newborn myocardium operates at peak contractile function and cannot further increase contractility.[4] Investigators no longer believe that neonates and infants are "resistant" to digoxin.[97]

Digoxin can exert a **negative chronotropic effect** on the heart. This effect — slowing of the heart rate — is mediated indirectly through the vagus nerve[31] and produces prominent changes in the activity of the sinoatrial (S-A) node, the atria, and the atrioventricular (A-V) node. The increase in vagal activity arises from digoxin-induced sensitization of peripheral baroreceptors that influence efferent vagal activity arising centrally, and via a direct effect of digoxin on central vagal nuclei. Digoxin-induced increases in efferent vagal impulses decrease the atrial sinus rate and reflexly induce decreases in sympathetic tone. Atropine can abolish the vagal-induced slowing of the atrial sinus rate. Digoxin can also directly affect the S-A node and the specialized atrial fiber system. The sensitivity of the S-A node to the negative chronotropic effects of acetylcholine is increased by digoxin. A normal heart at rest will generally not slow in response to digoxin, but with exercise the maxi-

Figure 7-5. Effects of digoxin on ventricular function as determined by cardiac output and left ventricular end-diastolic pressure (LVEDP). The highest curve represents normal function for comparison; the lowest curve, congestive heart failure (CHF). The middle curve shows improved function following treatment of CHF with digoxin. Starting at point N, the following sequence of events is depicted: A, depression of contractility; B, Frank-Starling compensation; C, increased contractility with digoxin therapy; D, digoxin-induced reduction in Frank-Starling compensation. Points N, D, and B represent the same cardiac output but at different LVEDPs. High LVEDP causes congestive symptoms; low cardiac output results in fatigue (*hatched areas on ordinate and abscissa*). (Adapted from Mason DT: Am J Cardio 32:437, 1973.)

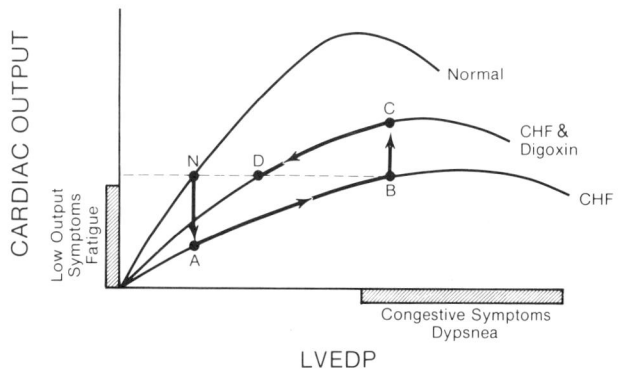

mal heart rate will be less.[33] With congestive heart failure, the sinus rate is usually increased so that the negative chronotropic effect of digoxin is apparent.

The A-V node is strongly influenced by both indirect and direct actions of digoxin. The enhanced vagal activity caused by digoxin slows conduction through the A-V node and prolongs the repolarization phase of the cardiac cycle. At high concentrations, digoxin can also decrease A-V as well as S-A node sensitivity to catecholamines and efferent sympathetic impulses. This direct effect of digoxin augments or intensifies the indirect vagal effects on the A-V node. A-V node conduction is impaired and can progress to complete heart block. Even though the effect of digoxin on the atria increases the rate at which impulses enter the atrial margin of the A-V node, its direct and indirect inhibitory effects on the A-V node decrease the ventricular response rate. Neurally mediated indirect effects of digoxin on the ventricular tissue are minor compared with the effects on S-A node, atria, and A-V node. Table 7–3 summarizes the mechanisms for the pharmacologic actions of digoxin on the heart.

The ability of the entire cardiovascular system to respond to digoxin ultimately determines its overall effect. Changes in systemic arterial pressure, cardiac output, heart size, and end-diastolic and venous pressure are variable from patient to patient. When congestive heart failure is due to poor myocardial contractility,

Table 7–3. MECHANISMS RESPONSIBLE FOR INOTROPIC AND CHRONOTROPIC ACTIONS OF DIGOXIN ON THE HEART[a]

Inotropic Action (Increased Myocardial Contractility)

increase in local myocardial catecholamine levels: enhances myocardial contractile activity
inhibition of sarcolemmal Na^+-K^+ ATPase: results in net increase in intracellular Ca^{2+}, which enhances contractile activity

Chronotropic Action (Antiarrhythmic Action/Decrease in Heart Rate)

Indirect Effect

vagal stimulation
parasympathetic and sympathetic slowing of S-A node firing
slowing of conduction through A-V node
delay in recovery of excitability of A-V node

Direct Effect

decreased sensitivity of S-A and A-V nodes to catecholamines and efferent sympathetic impulses

[a] See text for further details.

digoxin can increase cardiac output and decrease cardiac filling pressure, heart size, and venous and capillary pressures (Fig. 7–6). As circulation improves, sympathetic activity as well as arterial resistance and venous tone decreases. A change in peripheral resistance may lead to a decrease in afterload, which will further improve cardiac function. On the other hand, the inotropic effect of digoxin can be opposed by both direct and reflex vasoconstrictor effects, particularly in patients with normal left ventricular function.[83] Thus, the inotropic effect of digoxin can be offset by an increase in peripheral resistance (afterload).

The central and peripheral effects of digoxin are determined by the degree of left ventricular dysfunction. Since myocardial work (oxygen consumption) depends on afterload, preload, systolic ejection time, and contractility, the dominant vasoconstrictor effect of digoxin in persons with normal hearts results in an increase in myocardial work. In patients with congestive heart failure and poor contractility, digoxin decreases the afterload (reduction in the heart failure-induced sympathetic overactivity), the preload (shift of the Frank-Starling curve; see under Antihypertensives and Vasodilators), and the systolic ejection time. These effects of digoxin in the failing heart result in a net decrease in myocardial work (oxygen consumption).[61]

Digitalis glycosides, including digoxin, have characteristic *effects on the electrocardiogram* (ECG), specifically on the ST segment and the T wave. The T wave typically becomes diminished in amplitude, isoelectric, or inverted. The ST segment may also demonstrate depression. These ECG changes are a result of transmembrane potential effects of digoxin. The exact mechanisms are not known.[77] The slowed conduction through the A-V node produces the prolongation of the P–R interval. This effect of digoxin is related primarily to an increase in vagal activity. Atropine can reverse primary, secondary, or tertiary A-V block produced by digoxin but will not affect its direct actions (decreased sensitivity to catecholamines and efferent sympathetic impulses). The Q–T interval is shortened by digoxin because ventricular repolarization is accelerated.

It is important to appreciate that essentially every type of ECG abnormality associated with cardiac disorders has been reported to be caused by digoxin. In neonates, depression of S-A and A-V nodal function are more common than the disturbances in cardiac automaticity seen in adults.[35,36] In low-birth-weight neonates, brady-

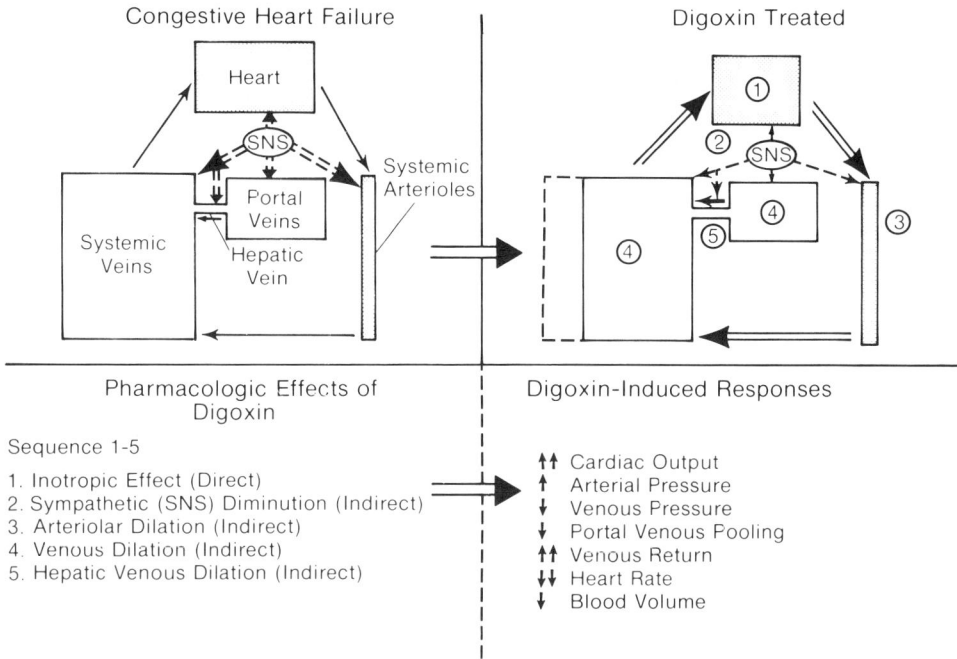

Figure 7-6. Hemodynamic actions of digoxin in patients with congestive heart failure. *Left,* The typical congestive heart failure state (myocardial failure). *Right,* The hemodynamic alterations resulting from digoxin therapy. The circled numbers refer to the pharmacologic effects of digoxin listed in the lower portion, with the corresponding hemodynamic responses. The width of the solid arrow lines reflects the relative amount of blood flow. The interrupted arrows represent the sympathetic nervous system (SNS) activity, with the double line (congestive heart failure) denoting a more active state than the single interrupted line following digoxin therapy. (Adapted from Mason DT et al: Prog Cardiovas Dis 11:443, 1969.)

cardia and prolongation of the P–R interval by more than 50% of control are good indices of digoxin toxicity.[3]

Digoxin has pharmacologic effects in tissues other than the myocardium: The drug induces *peripheral vasoconstriction* by a local direct action on vascular smooth muscle, and indirectly through effects on the CNS.[82] It increases intracellular calcium concentration in peripheral arterial and venous smooth muscle. The CNS (neural) effect is mediated through α receptor stimulation and appears to be the major mechanism responsible for digoxin-induced increase in skeletal muscle vascular resistance. As previously noted, in the normal patient the peripheral vasoconstrictor action of digoxin can cause sufficient increased afterload to oppose any potential increase in cardiac output. Figure 7–6 illustrates the reflex-mediated effects of digoxin on the peripheral vascular bed in the patient with congestive heart failure due to inadequate cardiac output.[59] In this situation, digoxin improves cardiac output, which reflexly reduces sympathetic activity, resulting in decreased vascular tone; this decrease is the opposite of the result of digoxin therapy in the normal myocar-

dial-output state. Comparable studies have not been done in neonates.

Digoxin also causes *splanchnic vasoconstriction* and has been implicated in the pathogenesis of mesenteric vascular disease.[63] Milstein and coworkers[62] demonstrated in newborn lambs that digoxin *increased pulmonary vascular resistance;* this effect would be beneficial in patients with left-to-right ductal shunts but detrimental in patients with pulmonary hypertension. Noteworthy in this regard is the study by Warburton and colleagues[89] in low-birthweight neonates with left-to-right ductal shunts. They concluded that digoxin reduced circulatory volume overload by extracardiac effects of the drug rather than by a primary myocardial effect.

A marked *stimulation of respiration* has been demonstrated following administration of digoxin in animal studies;[88] minute volume increased largely as a result of an increase in respiratory rate. The mechanisms proposed for this effect include alteration of peripheral chemoreceptor activation and CNS stimulation.

Digoxin in normal doses produced as much as a 78% *reduction in CSF production* in three adult patients requiring ventricular drainage in a study by Neblett and colleagues.[65] These investigators proposed that digoxin inhibits the sodium–potassium ATPase pump in the choroid plexus. Interestingly, the choroid plexus has the highest tissue concentration of digoxin in the body (see Table 7–1).[1]

Diuresis is characteristic of a successful response to digoxin in a patient with congestive heart failure. Although digoxin can impair renal tubular function by inhibiting renal tubular $Na^+–K^+$ ATPase, such impairment is seen only with very large doses. Therefore, it is unlikely that digoxin produces diuresis by a direct effect on the kidney. Diuresis is more likely a result of improved cardiac output and renal perfusion.

Clinical Pharmacology. The fundamental aspects of digoxin disposition are presented in the preceding section. The relative rate of absorption and resulting serum concentration after PO and IV administration are illustrated in Figure 7–2. Analysis of reported clinical experience with digoxin in neonates (Table 7–3) reveals important variations in digoxin pharmacokinetics for premature and full-term neonates and during the first years of life. In premature infants, the total body clearance of digoxin (20–30 ml/min/1.73 m^2 of body surface) is significantly less than in other age groups;[9,28,67] their renal blood flow and number of glomeruli are also less, which may account for the reduced renal excretion.[28,67] Although digoxin clearance rate is higher in full-term infants than in older children and adults,[34,64] renal excretion rates are the same in these three age groups.[94] Therefore, nonrenal elimination of digoxin may be the major determinant of its clearance rate.[67,87,94]

Variation in digoxin metabolism could play a significant role in the observed age-related differences in its pharmacokinetics. Lindenbaum and colleagues[55] demonstrated a twofold increase in serum digoxin subsequent to inactivation of digoxin by gut flora in adults. Pinsky and coworkers[74] showed that when infants were digitalized with a total dose of 30 μg/kg, smaller, more immature infants had higher serum concentrations than those in larger more mature prematures. However, no differences were seen in serum concentration among these same groups of infants when doses of 20 μg/kg were employed. These data suggest saturation of a clearance mechanism for digoxin (tissue uptake, renal or intestinal elimination). Some of the reported differences in digoxin pharmacokinetics are undoubtedly due to the fact that the

blood or urine samples were taken prior to achievement of steady state. For digoxin, steady state can be calculated to occur after a period of 4 to 6 half-lives ($\approx 1–2$ wk); the time to equilibration will be less when digitalization procedures are employed ($\approx 4–7$ days).

Therapeutic Indications. Digoxin is used in two major clinical situations, decreased myocardial contractility and arrhythmias. *Diminished myocardial contractility* with attendant clinical signs and symptoms of congestive heart failure is a major indication for the inotropic action of digoxin. Whether digoxin is effective in treating myocardial failure depends on the cause of the failure and on the severity of the myocardial damage. The direct positive inotropic effect of digoxin increases cardiac output, decreases cardiac filling pressures, and decreases heart size and venous and capillary pressure. With the improvement in circulation, sympathetic activity is reduced, which in turn decreases systemic arterial resistance and venous tone. The decrease in systemic arterial resistance decreases the afterload on the left ventricle and permits further improvement in cardiac function. As shown in Figure 7–5, the result is a shift from one ventricular function curve to another. Myocardial dysfunction occurs in neonates following ischemic insults associated with perinatal asphyxia;[17] these neonates present with ECG evidence of myocardial ischemia, decreased ventricular function by echocardiography or cardiac catheterization, elevated myocardial specific fractions of creatinine phosphokinase (CPK-MB), and abnormal thallium uptake by the myocardium.

The therapeutic value of cardiac glycosides, including digoxin, in any type of circulatory shock (cardiogenic, hypovolemic, septic) is questionable.[155] Digoxin does not improve cardiac output in patients in cardiogenic shock.[137] In addition, digoxin may aggravate myocardial ischemia and increase peripheral vascular resistance, particularly in the splanchnic bed, leading to mesenteric ischemia and necrosis.[18]

The dosage requirements for optimal inotropic action of digoxin in infants are unclear. Some reports in the literature suggest that high-dose digoxin therapy is often necessary to achieve adequate control of myocardial failure; others suggest clinical effectiveness with much lower dosages. Levy and coworkers[53] demonstrated that maximal inotropic effects were achieved with doses of 30 μg/kg using pre-ejection period shortening and ejection time as the evaluation criteria. Doses of 80 μg/kg of digoxin produced no greater effect. These results were corroborated by adult echocardiographic studies, by Hoffstetter and colleagues,[32] using low-dose digoxin, which produced a mean plasma digoxin level of 2.2 ng/ml (range 0.7–4.4 ng/ml). Sahn and coauthors[78] described echocardiographic evidence of improvement in congestive heart failure in infants and children treated with a loading dose of 35 to 45 μg/kg of digoxin; the inotropic effect was present 6 to 12 hours after digitalization had been completed. Levy and coworkers[53] showed changes in ratio of preejection period to left ventricular ejection time (PEP/LVET) 4 hours after administration of digoxin, 30 μg/kg; systolic time intervals did not change further after the administration of additional amounts of digoxin. Pinsky and colleagues[74] also failed to observe improvement of PEP/LVET in premature infants with patent ductus arteriosus who received loading doses of digoxin (20 or 30 μg/kg). Lundell and Boreus[380] studied digoxin therapy in 16 premature infants with symptomatic PDA. Digoxin treatment was not associated with significant changes in heart rate, pre-ejection intervals, or LVET in spite of adequate serum digoxin levels. Sandor and coworkers[79] studied 18 neonates in heart failure with high and low serum digoxin levels; digoxin produced measurable changes in the indices of left ventricular function, but the magnitude of these changes was no different in the high-level (3.6 ± 1.0 ng/ml) and low-level (2.0 ± 0.4 ng/ml) serum digoxin groups. In studies in low-birth-weight neonates Warburton and coworkers[89] observed no echocardiographic differences in patients given either 20 or 40 μg/kg of digoxin over a 24-hour period; there was an inotropic effect within 30 minutes of the initial dose. Unfortunately, a wide variety of diseases and clinical conditions are represented in these studies, making comparisons and extrapolation to other patients difficult and sometimes hazardous (see following section).

Digoxin is also used for the *treatment of arrhythmias,* primarily reentry *supraventricular tachycardia (SVT).* Digoxin suppresses SVT by both autonomic (indirect) and direct actions: It slows the sinus node rate via vagal mechanisms and can change the critical refractory period, thus decreasing the chance of reentry supraventricular tachycardia. This agent can also modify refractoriness and enhance intra-atrial conduction, which may alter propagation through reentrant pathways in the atrium. Prolongation of A-V nodal refractoriness and slowing of A-V node impulse conduction are largely responsi-

ble for the slowed ventricular response that occurs when digoxin is used in the treatment of *atrial flutter or fibrillation:* Rapidly occurring atrial impulses are prevented from initiating ventricular responses at the same frequency.[77]

Other aspects of digoxin therapy of arrhythmias are discussed under Antiarrhythmic Agents at the end of this chapter.

The *recommended dose of digoxin* for prematures, full-term neonates, or older infants depends upon age-related differences in its pharmacokinetics. Although a variety of dosages have been proposed over the years,[371] those based on pharmacokinetic data obtained during steady-state maintenance digoxin therapy are probably most valid. Nyberg and Wettrell[69] published dosage recommendations that are supported by studies by Berman,[3] Halkin,[25,26] Pinsky,[74] and Warburton[89] and their coworkers (Table 7–4). Because the volume of distribution and clearance rate are low in premature infants, both the loading and maintenance doses of digoxin are less in this group.

However, these schedules are based on average pharmacokinetic values determined for each age group. Differences in drug disposition or drug response in the individual patient can alter the relationship between digoxin dose, serum concentration, and effect. Each patient's clinical response must be considered along with the digoxin serum concentration measurements to establish an optimal maintenance dose. Since renal function increases in the first few weeks of life (glomerular filtration rate increases more dramatically in full-term infants than in premature infants), dosage requirements for digoxin will increase with postnatal age. Information available in this regard is shown in Table 7–2.

Table 7–5 outlines clinical problems known to influence digoxin dosage requirements. Determination of renal function is imperative because of its importance in digoxin elimination. Generally, patients with one-half normal renal clearance should receive one-half the maintenance dose of digoxin along with frequent monitoring of serum digoxin levels.[41] Because of the large volume of distribution, only small amounts of digoxin are removed by exchange transfusions (<6% of dose) even if the procedure is performed shortly after digoxin administration.[92] Creatinine clearance rate is 21 to 60 ml/1.73 m²/min in full-term infants (neonates up to those 3 to 5 weeks of age), compared with 16 to 37 ml/1.73 m²/min in premature infants.[2] Thus, by 1 month of age premature infants

Table 7–4. RECOMMENDED DIGOXIN DOSES IN PREMATURE AND FULL-TERM NEONATES AND INFANTS

	Loading Dose (total)[a]	Maintenance Dose
prematures		
<1.5 kg	10–20 μg/kg IV or PO[b]	4 μg/kg q 24 hr IV[c]
1.5–2.5 kg		8 μg/kg q 24 hr IV[d]
full-term neonates	30 μg/kg IV or PO	5 μg/kg q 12 hr PO[e]
infants (1–12 mo)	35 μg/kg IV or PO	7–12 μg/kg q 12 hr PO

[a] The total loading (digitalizing) dose is administered in three equally divided doses or in three unequally divided doses (½, ¼, ¼) given every 8 hours. The first maintenance dose should not be given any earlier than 24 hours after the last loading dose in premature infants and 12 hours in full-term neonates and infants (1–12 mo old).

[b] Conversion to oral doses traditionally involves increasing the IV dose employed by 20% to 30% because of the assumed bioavailability differences (see under Pharmacology for details). Whether this dose modification from IV to PO administration translates to meaningful pharmacologic equivalency in patients is unknown.

[c] The 24-hr dosing interval in premature infants is based on their prolonged plasma clearance of digoxin. It can be anticipated that renal function will increase sufficiently by approximately 1 month of age to necessitate the same recommended dose every 12 hours (see under Clinical Pharmacology for details). Measurement of serum digoxin levels will confirm the need for such dosing changes.

[d] Dose should be increased at 1 month of age to that of full-term newborn (5 μg/kg q 12 hr). Measurement of serum digoxin levels will confirm the need for such dosing changes.

[e] Dose should be increased at 1 month of age to that of infant (7–12 μg/kg q 12 hr). Measurement of serum digoxin levels will confirm the need for such dosing changes.

Dosages for prematures were derived from studies by Berman,[3] Pinsky,[74] and Warburton[89] and their coworkers and by Nyberg and Wettrell[69] and Collins-Nakai;[10] for full-term neonates, by Wettrell and Andersson[94] and Nyberg and Wettrell;[69] and for infants, by Nyberg and Wettrell.[69]

Table 7–5. DIGOXIN DOSAGE CONSIDERATIONS IN SPECIAL CLINICAL PROBLEMS

Clinical Problem	Anticipated Dosage Adjustment
renal disease	decrease (maintenance dose proportional to creatinine clearance; e.g., ½ dose if creatinine clearance ½ of normal)
electrolyte abnormalities (all increase digoxin toxicity)	
hypokalemia	decrease
hypercalcemia	decrease
hyper- or hypomagnesemia	decrease
thyroid disease (alters digoxin clearance)	
hyperthyroidism	increase
hypothyroidism	decrease
liver disease	usually no change necessary; monitor serum levels
gastrointestinal disease	monitor serum levels
drug interactions	
antacids (decrease absorption)	increase
quinidine (decreases excretion and volume of distribution)	decrease
β blockers	
negative inotropic action	increase
increase sensitivity to chronotropic action of digoxin	decrease
diuretics, amphotericin B (predispose to hypokalemia)	decrease
spironolactone (decreases digoxin clearance)	decrease
amiodarone (increases digoxin serum levels)	decrease
hypoxemia (may predispose to toxicity because of decreased renal digoxin clearance)	decrease
myocarditis (may predispose to digoxin toxicity)	decrease

Data from studies by Smith and Haber,[81,82] Mintz and Bharadwaja,[63] Hesslein,[454] and Brown[7], Cogan,[372] and Ochs[381] and their colleagues.[7]

should receive a dose equivalent to that recommended in the full-term newborn (12-hr rather than 24-hr dosing interval). Serum digoxin determinations to confirm this dosing requirement are recommended.

Loading Doses. Review of the literature suggests that many cases of digoxin intoxication occur in infants during or immediately after digitalization. Therefore, it is recommended that digoxin loading doses (digitalization) be eliminated, except for the management of arrhythmias or in emergency situations of impending death. Krasula and coworkers[45] found by ECG that 25% of children rapidly digitalized before open-heart surgery had arrhythmias, whereas all those on maintenance therapy were in normal sinus rhythm. Other studies have shown that myocardial digoxin levels are higher after loading doses than during maintenance therapy.[1,44] Higher myocardial digoxin levels correlate with greater likelihood of toxicity. The observations regarding equivalent inotropic response with high and low digoxin doses (see above—Therapeutic Indications) further diminish the theoretical value of digitalization. One report associated digitalization with acute hemorrhage and necrosis of the intestines.[18] Unfortunately, no well-designed controlled study in infants has been done to evaluate the results of maintenance-only versus digitalization-plus-maintenance therapy.

Frequency of Dosing. Since digoxin half-life is prolonged in neonates (Table 7–2), a 24-hour dosing interval would be adequate for therapeutic benefit. However, most authors suggest an every-12-hour regimen (except in the low-birth-weight infant) to minimize the possibility of toxic peak levels and subtherapeutic trough levels.[10] Cree and colleagues[12] found that serum digoxin concentrations frequently fell below 1 ng/ml in children placed on once-a-day maintenance digoxin therapy. Similar studies have not been done in neonates on maintenance therapy. Dosing frequency should be increased in premature infants, from every 24 hours to every 12 hours, as renal function increases, probably by 1 month of age (see Table 7–4).

Controversial Aspects of Digoxin Therapy. The importance of distinguishing between myocardial failure and circulatory congestion secondary to a large left-to-right shunt has been stressed by White and Lietman.[96] The inotropic stimulation of the myocardium by digoxin may be of little value in circulatory congestion resulting from acute volume or pressure overload. Several studies have in fact failed to demonstrate a substantial improvement in echocardio-

graphic parameters of myocardial contractility in neonates with congested circulatory state after digoxin therapy;[6,58,95] these studies included neonates with left ventricular overload, patent ductus arteriosus, and ventricular septal defect. The use of digoxin in these clinical circumstances is questionable because (1) resting level of myocardial function normally is higher in the neonate than the adult, and (2) left ventricular function is usually normal or above normal in neonates with left ventricular overload, thus minimizing the potential inotropic benefit from digoxin. In fact, digoxin can increase peripheral vascular resistance and afterload in such patients, which would aggravate circulatory congestion. On the other hand, some neonates clinically improve without measurable improvement in echocardiographic function, suggesting that a noninotropic action of digoxin ameliorates the symptoms of congestive heart failure.[6,58,89] The direct and indirect effects of digoxin on several peripheral vascular resistance beds are discussed in this regard under Pharmacology. The potential for management of myocardial failure and circulatory congestion with alternative types of therapy including peripheral vasodilation (preload, afterload reduction) is discussed later in this chapter.

There also is substantial controversy about the chronic use of digitalis glycosides.[84] Digoxin can be discontinued without adverse effects in over 85% of adult patients who have "recovered" from nonarrhythmia-associated congestive heart failure.[375] Thus, whether the benefits of long-term maintenance digoxin therapy outweigh the risk of toxicity is unclear.

Clinical Toxicology. Toxicity is the most serious limitation to the use of digoxin. Reported incidence of digoxin toxicity (listed in Table 7–6) ranges from 0% to 43%. Three mechanisms are believed to be involved in digoxin-induced cardiotoxicity: (1) an indirect effect of digoxin via the adrenergic nervous system affecting cardiac rhythm and conduction; (2) release of catecholamines from the adrenal medulla; and (3) a direct action on the cardiac tissues. These mechanisms have been reviewed by Lathers and Roberts.[51] The arrhythmias associated with use of digoxin in neonates are similar to those reported for older infants and children and include S-A node depression with ectopic escape beats and A-V block (Table 7–6). Premature infants in particular develop bradycardia even with "therapeutic" digoxin serum levels.[35] ECG abnormalities appear to be the most reliable clue to digitalis intoxication in young infants.

Table 7-6. TOXIC EFFECTS REPORTED WITH DIGOXIN USE IN INFANTS

Cardiac Effects
arrhythmias
  premature ventricular contractions
  ventricular bigeminy, trigeminy, or tachycardia
  nonparoxysmal atrioventricular tachycardia
  A-V dissociation
  atrial fibrillation
  A-V block
  paroxysmal atrial tachycardia with A-V block
bradycardia (sinus node): major manifestation in low-birth-weight infants
congestive heart failure: secondary to arrhythmia

Gastrointestinal Effects
feeding intolerance/diminished appetite
vomiting (questionable in infants)

Other Adverse Effects
lethargy
drug interactions (undesirable): see Table 7-5

Data from studies by Joos and Johnson[36] and by Krasula,[45] Halkin,[26] and Johnson[35] and their coworkers.

Although infants are reportedly more tolerant to digoxin than older patients, there can be no question that infants of any age or size can develop digoxin toxicity (Table 7-7).[26] In full-term neonates and infants, *serum concentrations of digoxin exceeding 3.5 ng/ml during maintenance therapy are considered to be in a toxic range and may be extremely hazardous.* In such cases, ECG monitoring is essential, and the dose of digoxin should be reduced unless very critical clinical states dictate a continuation of the regimen.

Serum digoxin concentrations obviously do not determine the diagnosis of digoxin toxicity nor negate it. The elements of individual sensitivity to the drug, the pharmacokinetic variability among patients, and the overlap between the nontoxic and toxic ranges of digoxin discourage the selection of a single maximal-threshold serum digoxin concentration for toxicity. The presence of an endogenous digoxin-like substance, which reacts with the clinical immunoassays used to measure digoxin, further discourages the use of rigid toxic threshold values. It is generally agreed, however, that when therapeutic effect is not optimal and serum digoxin is less than 2 ng/ml, an increase in dose can be instituted if the patient is carefully observed for evidence of digoxin toxicity. Depletion of body potassium and magnesium, which can occur in conjunction with long-term diuretic therapy[373] and elevated serum calcium levels, should be avoided because of the known aggravation of digoxin cardiotoxicity. A number of other serious interactions have been identified and are summarized in Table 7-5.[7]

Treatment of Digoxin Toxicity. Early recognition of digoxin toxicity is of utmost importance, not only for immediate discontinuation of the drug but also for appropriate treatment of any serious arrhythmias induced by digoxin. Sinus bradycardia, S-A arrest, and A-V block of second or third degree may be treated effectively with **atropine,** 10 μg/kg per dose. Repeated single doses of up to 40 μg/kg may be given within 2 minutes with ECG monitoring. **Phenytoin** is effective in reversing digoxin-induced ventricular arrhythmias, including bigeminy, unifocal and multifocal ventricular premature contractions, and ventricular tachycardia; however, it does not depress and may actually increase A-V node or intraventricular conduction. The recommended dose of phenytoin is 2 to 5 mg/kg IV slowly over a 5-minute period, repeated every 5 to 10 minutes up to a total dose of 20 mg/kg.

Although therapy of digoxin toxicity predominantly involves close monitoring of the ECG and serum electrolytes and specific antiarrhythmic therapy with atropine and phenytoin, other agents have been employed: **Lidocaine** has also been used successfully in treating ventricular tachyarrhythmias, premature contractions, and ventricular bigeminy. Its effects are similar to those of phenytoin, but lidocaine does not alter atrial activity or improve conduction through the A-V node, which may limit its value in the treatment of acute digoxin intoxication. **Propranolol** has been used successfully to treat some digoxin toxicities including premature ventricular contractions and ventricular tachycardia; however, it is contraindicated in atrial tachycardia with block, since it depresses conduction velocity and therefore may intensify the block and induce bradycardia. The use of these agents in digitalis toxicity has been reviewed by Smith and Haber[82] and Ekins and Watanabe.[16]

Sympathomimetic Agents

Epinephrine, norepinephrine, dopamine, dobutamine, and isoproterenol are catecholamines with potent sympathomimetic activity. The pharmacologic actions of the sympathomimetic agents are categorized according to their effects on "receptors" in the body.[138,148,151] Sympathetic-system agonists (stimulators) and

Table 7-7. SUMMARY OF CLINICAL STUDIES OF DIGOXIN DOSAGE, SERUM LEVELS, AND TOXICITY

Authors of Published Study[a]	Study Group	Digoxin Dosage	Serum Digoxin Concentration (ng/ml)	
			Nontoxic	Toxic (% or No. of Patients with Manifestations)
Levine and Blumenthal[52]	prematures	loading: 30–75 µg/kg	no serum levels reported	(30-µg/kg dose: 2.5%) (50-µg/kg dose: 9.4%) (75-µg/kg dose: 33%)
Hayes et al[29]	31 infants 33 children 24 adults	maintenance PO or IM: 14–28 µg/kg q 24 hr 6–17 µg/kg q 24 hr 1–11 µg/kg q 24 hr	2.8 ± 1.9 1.3 ± 0.4 1.3 ± 0.6	4.4 (5/31) 3.4 (10/33) 2.9 (4/24)
Krasula et al[45]	34 infants (2 days–5 mo) 57 children (5–12 yr)	loading: 80 µg/kg PO 45 µg/kg IM maintenance, PO: < 9 kg: 20 µg/kg q 12 hr 9–18 kg: 15 µg/kg q 12 hr	(levels at maintenance dosages) 1.7 ± 0.9 (infants) 1.1 ± 0.6 (children)	3.6 ± 0.9 (12/34) 2.9 ± 0.9 (4/57)
Halkin et al[26]	34 infants (1 wk–2 yr)	maintenance: 0.22–0.29 mg/m² body surface q 24 hr		> 2.0 (4/30)
Berman et al[3]	46 prematures	loading: 30–40 µg/kg maintenance: 10 µg/kg q 24 hr		10.0 ± 1.7 (9/30) 5.4 ± 0.8 (5/16)
Johnson et al[35]	18 prematures	loading: 20–30 µg/kg maintenance: 3–5 µg/kg q 12 hr	not done	> 2.5 (9/18)

[a] Listed in order of publication; see References at end of chapter.

antagonists (inhibitors) have provided evidence for classification of receptors as either α (alpha) or β (beta) receptors. The development of drugs with even more selective agonist and antagonist activity has resulted in further subclassifications (α_1, α_2, β_1, and β_2 receptors) and in the identification of dopaminergic receptors, which have also been subclassified (see Table 7–8).[102] Activation of α receptors in vascular and other smooth muscle results in constriction, while activation of β_2 receptors in these same tissues results in dilation.

Sympathomimetic agents are important modulators of several renal functions. The receptors mediating these effects are not fully defined.[130] Stimulation of α_1 receptors causes vasoconstriction and increased renal vascular resistance in most portions of the intrarenal vasculature. The α-adrenergic vasoconstriction predominates over the weak β-adrenergic vasodilation. Catecholamine release of renin from juxtaglomerular cells is believed to be a result of β_1 receptor stimulation, although indirect effects (vascular resistance, reabsorption of ions) also contribute. Releases of kallikrein and erythropoietin and control of gluconeogenesis in the kidney is thought to be regulated by adrenergic receptors. A role for dopaminergic receptors in the renal vascular remains speculative.

In the pancreas, α receptor stimulation decreases insulin secretion; β_2 receptor stimulation increases insulin secretion. Both the α_2 and β_2 receptors diminish gastrointestinal tract motility and tone. Activation of cardiac β_1 receptors increases heart rate and contractility. The effects of α, β, and dopaminergic receptors are summarized in Table 7–8.

The response resulting from the administration of any particular sympathomimetic amine requires consideration of several factors in addition to the intrinsic receptor-stimulating activity and the dose of the drug: First, the response is dependent upon the proportion and density of the α and β receptors present in the tissue, particularly in the neonate since the sympathetic and parasympathetic systems are still maturing.[146,180] Second, sympathomimetic drugs can affect reflex homeostatic mechanisms; an example is the compensatory reflexes associated with a rise in arterial pressure (i.e., bradycardia). Finally, chronic exposure to sympathomimetic agents diminishes the responsiveness of α and β receptors; this phenomenon is referred to as refractoriness, desensitization, down-regulation, or tachyphylaxis. The

Table 7–8. CLASSIFICATION, LOCUS, AND PREDOMINANT ACTION OF ADRENERGIC RECEPTORS

Receptor	Location	Predominant Action
α-adrenergic		
α_1	smooth muscle (postsynaptic effector sites)	
	vascular (arterioles and veins)	constriction
	sphincters (stomach and intestine)	contraction
α_1	liver	gluconeogenesis
α_1	pancreas	decreased insulin secretion
α_2	nerve terminals	
	intestine and stomach (presynaptic feedback inhibition)	decreased motility and tone
β-adrenergic		
β_1	heart	
	myocardium	increased contractility
	S-A node	increased heart rate
	A-V node, conduction tissue	increased automaticity and conduction velocity
β_1	kidney	renin secretion
β_2	smooth muscle	
	vasculature (arterioles and veins)	dilation
	lung (bronchial)	relaxation
	intestine	decreased motility and tone
β_2	liver	glycogenolysis
β_2	pancreas	increased insulin secretion
dopaminergic	vascular smooth muscle	dilation
	renal	
	mesenteric	
	cerebral	
	coronary	

mechanisms responsible for the diminished response are multiple and complex.[127]

Since the sympathomimetic amines have similar chemical structures, it is not surprising that a spectrum of activities ranging from almost pure α activity (norepinephrine) to an almost pure β activity (isoproterenol) can be found among the various agents. In addition, these agents demonstrate a range of activities relative to a direct action on adrenergic receptors as well as indirect effects through the release of norepinephrine. Table 7–9 summarizes the various pharmacologic activities of the major sympathomimetics used in the care of infants.

The sympathomimetic drugs are frequently used in cardiovascular resuscitation. Unfortunately, their use sometimes represents automatic recourse to a pressor or inotropic agent for treatment of hypotension rather than a thoughtful effort to improve tissue perfusion. Adequate tissue perfusion depends on sufficient cardiac output and appropriate vascular resistance. Impaired tissue blood flow can be the result of reduced cardiac output, severe vasoconstriction or vasodilation (inadequate perfusion pressure), hypovolemia, or a combination of these factors; this wide variety of possible derangements mandates selecting the proper sympathomimetic agent for the patient's particular pathophysiologic disorder. The following sections present pharmacologic details for each sympathomimetic drug along with a summary of clinical experience.

Epinephrine

Pharmacology. Epinephrine is the terminal product in biosynthesis of the endogenous catecholamines (Fig. 7–7). Epinephrine must be given parenterally to reach pharmacologically effective concentrations because it is rapidly metabolized in the gastrointestinal tract and liver. Its vasoconstrictor properties account for the slow rate of absorption from subcutaneous (SQ) or IM administration sites. Following direct administration into the respiratory tract (via an endotracheal tube), its effect is rapid in onset and has a comparatively long duration[162,163] (Fig. 7–8); this route is often utilized for emergency resuscitation, particularly when the IV route is not immediately available.[123,391]

The major portion of administered epinephrine is rapidly metabolized by the same enzyme systems that metabolize endogenous catecholamines (see Fig. 7–9). Catechol-O-methyltransferase (COMT) and monoamine oxidase (MAO) metabolize epinephrine to metabolites that are widely distributed throughout the body, with the highest concentration occurring in the liver and kidney. COMT is found largely in the cytoplasm and, in contrast to MAO, is not selectively associated with the adrenergic nerves. MAO is located primarily in mitochondria, including those associated with adrenergic nerve terminals. Thus, circulating and exogenously administered catecholamines are metabolized primarily by COMT, whereas endogenously released norepinephrine at nerve terminals is metabolized by MAO.

Epinephrine activates α and β receptors, but its most prominent action is on β receptors in the heart and in vascular and other smooth muscle.[99,121] Low doses of epinephrine cause a fall in blood pressure; larger doses cause a biphasic response: disproportionate increase in systolic versus diastolic pressure followed by a below-normal mean pressure. Increases in blood pressure following administration of epinephrine occur as a result of cardiac stimulation (positive inotropic and chronotropic action), vasoconstriction of many precapillary resistance vessels, and constriction of veins. However, if epinephrine is administered slowly in lower doses, α and β receptor stimulation may be proportional, and little if any change occurs in mean blood pressure. Under these conditions the increase in cardiac output is offset by a decrease in peripheral resistance resulting from a dominant β_2 receptor stimulation.[118] Very large doses of epinephrine will cause primarily an increase in total peripheral resistance (Table 7–9).

Epinephrine increases blood flow to skeletal muscle, brain, liver, and myocardium (coronary). In contrast, renal blood flow is reduced by as much as 40%. Pulmonary resistance may increase, although the major effect of epinephrine is to redistribute blood from the systemic to the pulmonary circulation and thereby increase pulmonary pressure.

Epinephrine is a very potent stimulant of the heart by the activation of β_1 receptors. The drug also affects the cells of the S-A node and the conducting tissues. The inotropic and chronotropic stimulatory actions increase cardiac work and oxygen consumption, and cardiac efficiency (work done relative to oxygen consumption) is reduced.

Epinephrine also decreases gastrointestinal smooth muscle tone and frequency and amplitude of spontaneous contractions. In the lung, it produces a potent bronchodilation, which is particularly pronounced if bronchoconstriction is present prior to administration.

Table 7–9. PHARMACOLOGIC ACTIONS OF THE SYMPATHOMIMETIC DRUGS[a]

Drug	Agonist Activity[b,c]				Vascular Effects[c]					Cardiac Effects[c]			Intensity of Cardiovascular Effects
	α (↑ SVR)	β₁ (cardiac)	β₂ (↓ SVR)	dopaminergic (↓ SVR)	BP	TPR	PVR	BBF	RBF	HR	CO	CBF	
epinephrine	+	+++	++	0	↑	↓,↑	↑	↑	↓	↑↑	↑↑↑	↑	cardiac = VC > VD
norepinephrine	+++	++	0	0	↑	↑	0,↓	0,↓	↓	↓	0,↑,↓	↑	VC > cardiac
dopamine	++	+++[d]	+	+++	0,↑	↓	0,↑	↑	↑	0,↑	↑	↑	cardiac = VD = VC (dose-dependent)
dobutamine	+	++	++	0	0	↓	0,↓		0,↑	0,↑	↑↑↑	↑	cardiac > VD > VC
isoproterenol	0	+++	+++	0	0,↓	↓	0,↓	0,↓	↓,0	↑↑↑	↑↑↑	0,↓	VD > cardiac

[a] Data have been summarized from a large number of literature sources, most of which represent information derived from human adults; extrapolation of this information to the sick infant requires caution.
↑ = increase; ↓ = decrease; + = stimulates (the more + signs, the greater the intensity of effect); 0 = no effect. SVR = systemic vascular resistance; BP = blood pressure; TPR = total peripheral resistance; PVR = pulmonary vascular resistance; BBF = brain blood flow; RBF = renal blood flow; HR = heart rate; CO = cardiac output; CBF = coronary blood flow; VC = vasoconstriction; VD = vasodilation.
[b] The α- and β₂-agonist activities represent only peripheral vascular receptors and not organ receptors. See under the specific agents for further details.
[c] The vascular and cardiac responses to sympathomimetic drugs are dependent upon the dose of the drug and the relative state of activity or inactivity at the time of drug administration. For example, if maximum vasoconstriction or heart rate exists, further increases will not occur.
[d] Part of the inotropic action of dopamine is produced by the release of catecholamines from neural tissue (myocardium and possibly elsewhere). Dobutamine does not cause a release of catecholamines.

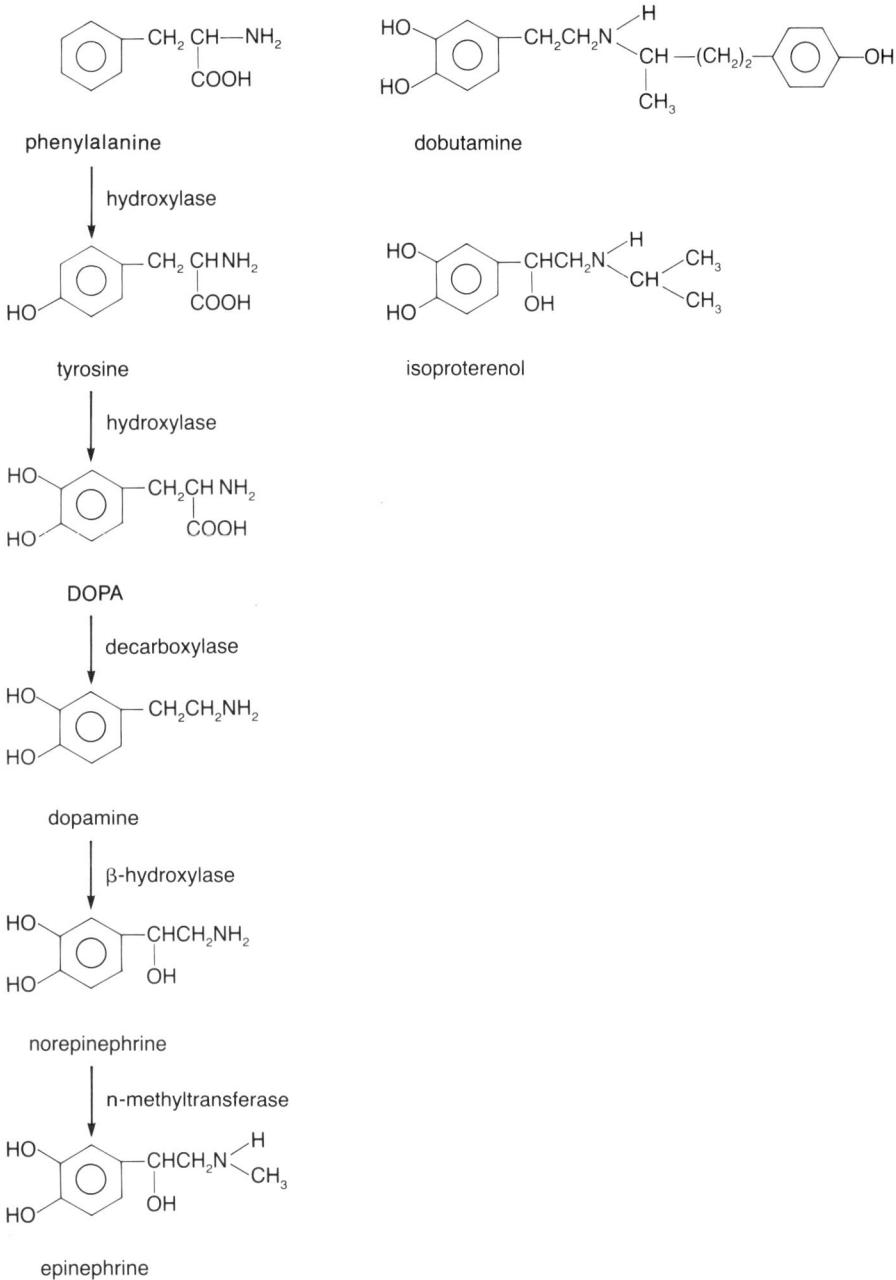

Figure 7-7. Structural formulas of endogenous catecholamines, in order of biochemical synthesis, and of related inotropic agents. The enzymes involved in biosynthesis are shown at the arrows.

Among the important metabolic effects of epinephrine is the inhibition of insulin secretion. Insulin release is inhibited by α receptors and stimulated by β receptors. The predominant action of epinephrine is on α receptor activity in the pancreatic beta cell. The concentration of free fatty acids is increased following epinephrine administration as a result of activation of triglyceride lipase, which accelerates the breakdown of triglycerides to form free fatty acids.

Clinical Pharmacology. There is a surprising paucity of published reports critically evaluating the clinical use of epinephrine in neonates, even though it is widely recommended and used in acute cardiovascular collapse.[105,125] Rudolph and coworkers[166] gave epinephrine by infusion to three infants with severe left ventricular fail-

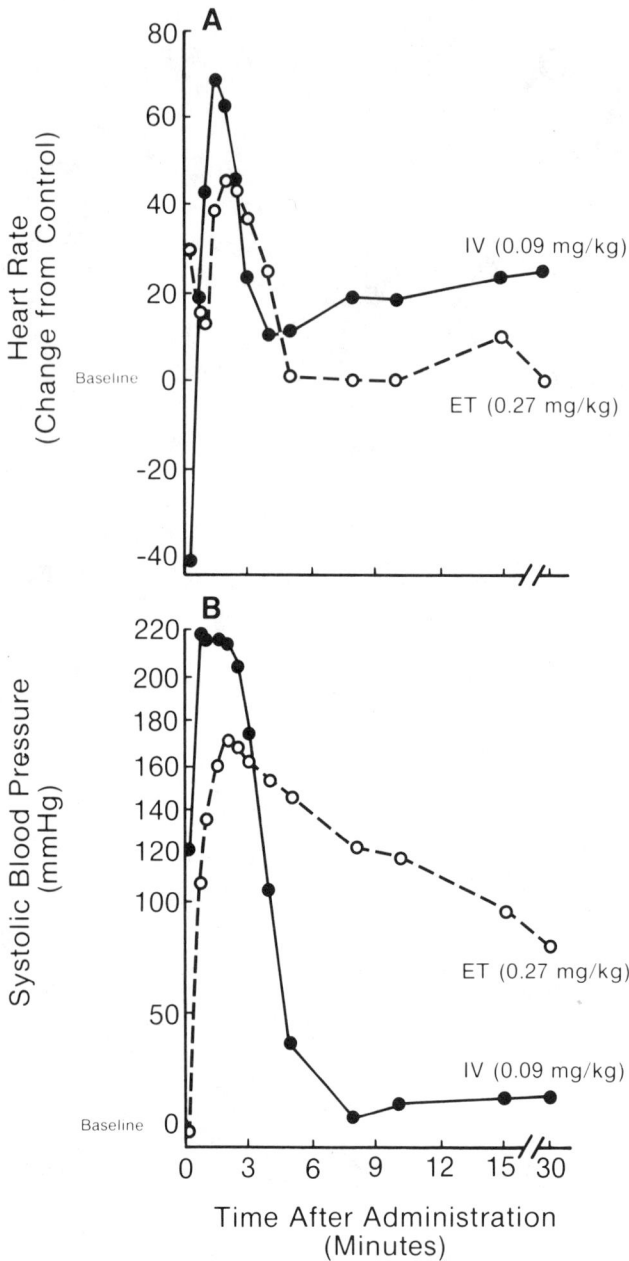

Figure 7-8. The effects of epinephrine administered by intravenous (IV) vs. endotracheal (ET) routes on heart rate (*A*) and blood pressure (*B*). (Adapted from Roberts JR et al: JACEP 7:260, 1978; and from Roberts JR et al: JACEP 8:53, 1979.)

ure, large left-to-right shunts, and pulmonary edema who had failed to improve on the standard regimen of digoxin and diuretics. Epinephrine infusion, 0.5 to 0.9 µg/kg/min, resulted in clinical improvement as evidenced by an increased heart rate, improved peripheral circulation and peripheral pulses, and decreased pulmonary rales. The infusions were continued for 4 to 6 hours. No adverse effects were observed, and renal output appeared unimpaired. However, the authors cautioned against routine use of epinephrine in the man-

agement of cardiac failure. Reimenschneider and colleagues[160] infused epinephrine (0.5 to 1.0 µg/kg/min) in seven infants with myocardial dysfunction associated with right-to-left shunting (via foramen ovale, ductus arteriosus, or both); In six of the infants, systemic pressures increased by 7 to 18 mm Hg, and descending aortic oxygen saturations improved, indicating a decrease in the right-to-left shunt. Lindemann[391] reported on the successful use of epinephrine by endotracheal administration in resuscitation of newborn infants.

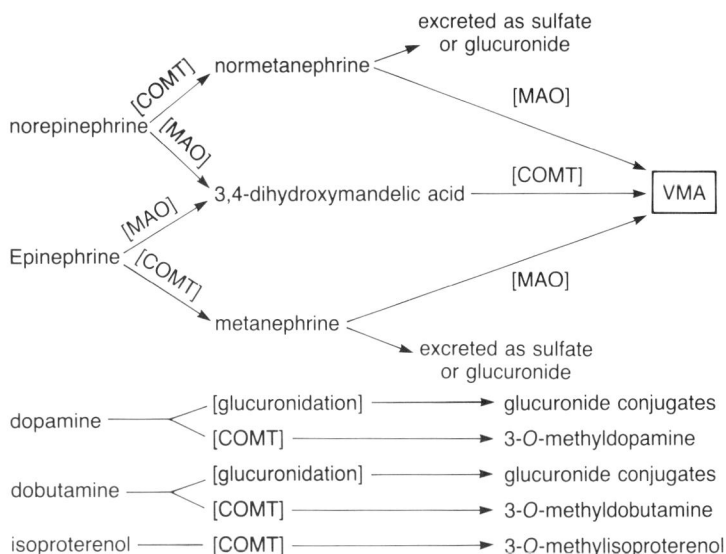

Figure 7-9. Metabolism of endogenous catecholamines and related inotropic agents. The two major enzymes involved in catecholamine metabolism are monoamine oxidase (MAO) and catechol-*O*-methyltransferase (COMT). COMT is primarily responsible for metabolism of circulating and exogenously administered catecholamines. VMA is vanillylmandelic acid. The metabolites are primarily excreted in the urine.

The IV infusion of 0.25 to 0.30 μg/kg/min of epinephrine in adults increases cardiac contractile force and heart rate and decreases total peripheral resistance.[118,142] The major limitation of epinephrine infusion is the likelihood of severe vasoconstriction in the renal vascular bed.

Therapeutic Indications. The effects of epinephrine on the heart, vascular bed, and bronchial smooth muscle are used in a variety of clinical conditions. In neonates, the use of epinephrine has largely been confined to *cardiac resuscitation.* The single bolus dose of epinephrine is 0.1 to 0.2 ml/kg of a 1:10,000 solution given IV, intratracheally, or by direct intracardiac administration (Table 7-10). Accidental injection into the myocardial tissue will result in necrosis. Atropine may also be administered intratracheally, but this route is contraindicated for other drugs used in resuscitation, such as bicarbonate, because of toxicity to lung tissues and poor bioavailability.[123]

The short-term use of epinephrine infusion for *severe cardiac failure resistant to other drug management* requires careful monitoring of the cardiovascular response, since peripheral vascular resistance effects are dose-dependent (Table 7-10). Doses greater than 2.0 μg/kg/min will cause renal vascular ischemia. In older infants and children, epinephrine is used for the relief of *bronchospasm* and *hypersensitivity reactions.*

Clinical Toxicology. Serious reactions to epinephrine include cardiac arrhythmias, renal vascular ischemia, and severe hypertension with cerebral hemorrhage. The most common complication is premature ventricular beats and ventricular tachycardia; these are most likely to develop in patients with heart disease or hypoxemia, or during halogenated hydrocarbon anesthesia. Local infiltration of epinephrine, including infusion of distal extremities, may cause tissue ischemia and necrosis. Therapeutic doses of epinephrine can cause hypokalemia through a specific β_2 receptor effect.[386]

Norepinephrine

Pharmacology. Norepinephrine is the endogenous neurotransmitter released from postganglionic adrenergic nerves. Like epinephrine, the drug is ineffective when given PO and is poorly absorbed from SQ injections. It is rapidly metabolized by MAO and COMT (Fig. 7-8), with less than 20% of an administered dose excreted unchanged in the urine.

The β_1 cardiac-stimulating properties of epinephrine and norepinephrine are approximately equal. However, norepinephrine is a potent α receptor agonist in vascular tissue (epinephrine is weak) but has little β_2 receptor agonist activity. As a consequence, the major effect of norepinephrine is to increase total peripheral resistance, which initiates an elevation in blood pressure that induces a reflex bradycardia. Despite an increase in cardiac contractility (inotropy), the simultaneous increase in peripheral vascular resistance and reflex bradycardia may diminish cardiac output. The net result is a decrease in blood flow through organs such as the kidney, liver, and usually skeletal muscle.[99,121] Coronary blood flow, however, is

Table 7–10. DOSAGE RECOMMENDATIONS FOR SYMPATHOMIMETICS[a] AND ASSOCIATED INOTROPIC AND VASCULAR RESPONSES

Drug	Dose[b]	Cardiac Output	Predominant Vascular Effect[c] — Constriction	Predominant Vascular Effect[c] — Dilation	Comment	Available Commercial Preparations[d]
epinephrine (Adrenalin)	*cardiac resuscitation:* 0.1 ml/kg of 1:10,000 solution given IV, IC, or ET (10 µg/kg), as needed[e]	+++				injection: 1:1,000 (never give IV, IC, or ET) 1:10,000
	infusion: initial 0.05 µg/kg/min	++		++	vasoconstriction predominates over vasodilation at higher doses; may cause renal ischemia	
	1.0 µg/kg/min	+	++			
norepinephrine (Levophed)	*infusion:* initial 0.05 µg/kg/min	±	++		vasoconstriction predominates over inotropic effect at all doses, so cardiac output may be unchanged or decreased; may cause renal ischemia	injection: 0.2% solution (equivalent to 0.1% nor-epinephrine base)
	0.5 µg/kg/min (dose of drug base)	±	+++			
dopamine (Inotropin)	*infusion:* initial 0.5–4 µg/kg/min			+ (renal)	dose-dependent effects on renal and peripheral resistance (see text)	injection: 40 mg/ml
	5–10 µg/kg/min	+		++		
	>10 µg/kg/min (max. 20–50 µg/kg/min)	++	++			
dobutamine (Dobutrex)	*infusion:* initial 1–2 µg/kg/min	+			larger doses result in decreased peripheral resistance	injection: 250-mg vials (powder for reconstitution)
	3–10 µg/kg/min (max. 15–40 µg/kg/min)	++		+		
isoproterenol (Isuprel)	*infusion:* initial 0.05–0.1 µg/kg/min	++		++	dose-dependent inotropic and vasodilator effect; may decrease coronary and renal blood flow	injection: 0.2 mg/ml (1:5,000 vials)
	0.2–0.5 µg/kg/min (max. 2 µg/kg/min)	+++		+++		

[a] Cardiac and vascular effects are expectations based on a wide variety of clinical situations that may not pertain to individual infants. Significant departures from the suggested doses may be necessary in selected patients The maximum doses will largely be determined by adverse effects.

[b] Suggested method for calculation of drug solutions:

Method: select desired drug dose
select desired IV fluid rate

Calculation: mg drug/100 ml IV solution = weight [kg] $\times$ 6 $\times$ $\dfrac{\text{desired dose } [\mu g/kg/min]}{\text{desired IV fluid rate } [ml/hr]}$

[c] Although constriction and dilation may occur simultaneously (see Table 7–9), only the predominant effect is given.

[d] Not intended to be an exhaustive list of available preparations.

[e] IC = intracardiac; ET = endotracheal.

substantially increased, owing to increases in driving pressure (elevation of blood pressure) and coronary vasodilation. Although norepinephrine increases cardiac work, this effect is balanced by improved coronary perfusion.[176] The metabolic and endocrine effects of norepinephrine are not as great as those of epinephrine in the liver and pancreas (Table 7–9).

Therapeutic Indications. Since norepinephrine stimulates both α- and β-adrenergic receptors, the hemodynamic effects can vary depending upon the clinical status of the patient and the dose administered. Norepinephrine has only limited therapeutic value in the treatment of hypotension. It has been used in adults with low cardiac output states following cardiac surgery or myocardial infarction.[124] Its use in combination with phentolamine (an α blocker that minimizes the adverse α-stimulating effects of norepinephrine) has been demonstrated to improve cardiovascular dynamics in adults.[131a] Norepinephrine would be most likely to improve hemodynamics in patients with primary problems of low arterial mean or diastolic pressures where volume expansion has been ineffective or is unacceptable. The decrease in renal blood flow to already hypoperfused tissues seriously compromises the value of norepinephrine as an inotropic agent.

Clinical Toxicology. Signs of norepinephrine toxicity are similar to those produced by epinephrine. When norepinephrine is infused over prolonged periods, monitoring of the ECG for arrhythmias and of blood pressure for hypertension is critical. Care must be taken to avoid prolonged reduction of blood flow to organs (liver, kidney) and other vital tissues. Elevation of blood pressure can result in excessive cardiac work without improvement in tissue perfusion. Norepinephrine has been shown to aggravate rather than to improve hypoperfusion associated with hemorrhagic shock.[137] In addition, care must be exercised to prevent local infiltration or infusion of distal extremities or digits with high concentrations of norepinephrine since the potent vasoconstrictor activity will lead to vasospasm and eventually tissue necrosis; in the event of such mishaps, however, an α blocker such as **phentolamine** can be administered locally into the region of the infiltration or infusion.

Dopamine

Pharmacology. Dopamine is the immediate precursor in the synthesis of norepinephrine and epinephrine by the body (Fig. 7–7). It is found in high concentrations in sympathetic nerves, adrenal glands, and the basal ganglia of the CNS, where it probably serves as a neurotransmitter. Because dopamine is metabolized by both MAO and COMT, it is effective only when administered intravenously by constant infusion. The half-life of dopamine effect is about 2 minutes, which is the same as the other catecholamines.[159]

Because dopamine has several different dose-dependent pharmacologic actions, there is a divergent clinical experience and opinion on its use. Studies in developing pigs demonstrate that dopaminergic responses change with maturation, and that the rate of change follows a different time course in renal, mesenteric, and peripheral vascular beds.[122] Dopamine has a positive inotropic effect on the myocardium through the release of norepinephrine from myocardial nerve terminals and secondarily by direct stimulation of β_1 receptors. Inotropic response to equivalent doses of dopamine is diminished in isolated myocardium obtained from neonatal animals and in the intact neonatal animal compared with the adult.[110] This observation suggests that maturational differences in endogenous norepinephrine stores and β receptor maturation diminish the cardiac response to dopamine in the neonatal animal. Coronary artery vasodilation has been reported experimentally, although the mechanism responsible is unclear. Large doses of dopamine cause vasoconstriction of arteries and veins in all vascular beds; this action is attributed to α-adrenergic and serotonin-type activities. In addition to these effects on α, β, and serotonin receptors, dopamine is believed capable of neurogenic stimulation. Because it crosses the blood–brain barrier poorly, no central effects of dopamine are usually observed. However, its neurogenic-stimulating properties are believed to participate actively in the production of its peripheral vascular effects, such as the vasodilation observed in the skeletal muscle vascular bed.

The effects of dopamine on the adult kidney and various parameters of renal function have been fully described in the literature.[119,392] Dopamine dilates the renal arteries by a direct effect on dopaminergic receptors, resulting in an increase in renal blood flow, in urinary volume, and in excretion of sodium and potassium. The glomerular filtration rate is only moderately increased, if at all. The effects on the kidney are dose-dependent. At doses over 6 μg/kg/min, the renal vasodilating (dopaminergic) effects are less pronounced or even reversed by the α-adrenergic actions. In the kidney of the neonate, the density of α and β receptors has not yet been demonstrated. It is conceivable that in the neonate, dopamine may produce less renal vasodilation and perhaps vasoconstriction, particularly with doses greater than 6 μg/kg/min.[98]

Dopamine can increase sodium excretion without changing the total renal blood flow.[167] The mechanism may be a redistribution of intrarenal blood flow from the outer two thirds to the inner one third of the cortex,[126] as well as a direct action on the renal tubule.

Studies of the effect of dopamine on the pulmonary circulation have demonstrated variable effects. The effect on the pulmonary circulation may be partially mediated by α receptors.[114] In isolated pulmonary vascular strips, α blockade with phentolamine attenuates the dopamine-induced constriction.[150]

Dopamine evokes a variety of hormonal and metabolic responses. Prolactin release is inhibited, but the growth hormone secretory system responds to dopaminergic stimulation.[135] Release of both glucagon and insulin, along with renin and parathyroid hormone, is stimulated by dopamine.[134] The effects of dopamine on glucagon, insulin, and prolactin secretion are not mediated through adrenergic mechanisms but are under dopaminergic control.[141]

A comparison of the pharmacologic properties of dopamine and other inotropic agents is presented in Table 7 – 9. These properties represent estimates of pharmacologic potency on selected parameters. The α-adrenergic receptor agonist activity of dopamine is less than that of epinephrine and norepinephrine. The effect of dopamine on heart rate is less than that of isoproterenol at doses producing equivalent increases in cardiac output. Also, isoproterenol, although a potent peripheral dilator, does not produce an increase in renal blood flow because of redistribution of blood flow to skeletal muscle (see under Isoproterenol). Myocardial efficiency is improved by dopamine because coronary arterial blood flow increases more than does myocardial oxygen consumption. Thus, for dopamine, the pharmacologic property of greatest value is the selective dilation of renal, mesenteric, cerebral, and coronary vessels (at low doses) coupled with an increase in cardiac output (at moderate doses).

Clinical Pharmacology. Because of the multiple actions of dopamine, different doses of dopamine can be expected to produce both quantitative and qualitative differences in the resulting cardiovascular response (Table 7 – 11). At infusion rates less than 2 μg/kg/min, dopamine receptors that decrease vascular resistance in mesenteric, renal, coronary, and cerebral

Table 7 – 11. CARDIOVASCULAR RESPONSE TO DOPAMINE AT DIFFERENT DOSES

Low Dose (<2 μg/kg/min)
dopaminergic stimulation: decrease in vascular resistance in mesentary, renal, and cerebral vessels

Intermediate Dose ($2-10$ μg/kg/min)
β_1-receptor stimulation: inotropic response in myocardium resulting from the release of norepinephrine from nerve terminals

High Dose (>10 μg/kg/min)
α-adrenergic stimulation: increase in peripheral and renal vascular resistance

vessels are activated. At low doses, dopamine increases glomerular filtration, renal blood flow, and sodium excretion. Dopamine is especially useful in the management of cardiogenic, traumatic, or hypovolemic shock, where increases in sympathetic activity may compromise renal function. Moderate doses of dopamine (<10 μg/kg/min) have a positive inotropic effect on the myocardium, resulting from a direct effect on β_1 receptors in the myocardium and from the release of norepinephrine from nerve terminals located in the myocardium. Little change occurs in heart rate, and there is either reduction or no change in total peripheral resistance. At doses greater than 10 μg/kg/min, α-adrenergic receptors are stimulated.[120] Blood pressure and peripheral resistance increase, and heart rate may increase or decrease, but renal blood flow decreases because of α receptor – mediated renal vasoconstriction.

The clinical studies of dopamine in neonates and children are summarized in Table 7 – 12. Hoshino[388] administered dopamine to six neonates in shock, in doses of 10 or 20 μg/kg/min. A more favorable hemodynamic response was obtained with the higher dose of dopamine. Driscoll and colleagues[108] evaluated the effect of dopamine in 24 patients (aged 2 days – 18 yr; mean 39 mo) with manifestations of circulatory hypotension; 13 responded favorably with an increase in blood pressure and urine output. In acute studies conducted over a 10-minute experimental period, Lang and coworkers[133] observed an increase in heart rate, systemic arterial pressure, and cardiac index in five infants with low cardiac output following repair of congenital cardiac defects (doses >15 μg/kg/min). They observed no change in right or left atrial pressure, pulmonary pressure or resistance, or systemic vascular resistance. Fiddler and colleagues[116] described clinical improvement in

Table 7–12. SUMMARY OF CLINICAL STUDIES OF DOPAMINE USE IN INFANTS AND CHILDREN

Author(s) of Published Study[a]	Study Group	Diagnosis	Dopamine Dose	Clinical Response[b]	Side-effects	Other Data
Hoshino[388]	6 neonates	shock	10–20 μg/kg/min	hemodynamic improvement, more favorable with 20 μg/kg/min		
Driscoll et al[108]	24 infants and children (2 days–18 yr)	shock: 20 congestive heart failure 4 infection	0.3–25 μg/kg/min (mean 9 μg/kg/min)	↑ SAP and urine output, no change in CVP or HR; favorable response in 13/24 survival: 9/24	none	
Lang et al[133]	5 infants (2–24 mo)	congenital heart disease (post-operative)	5–25 μg/kg/min	↑ SAP, HR, and cardiac index at >15-μg/kg doses; no change in peripheral or pulm. vasc. resistance or pulm. pressure		study periods: 10 min each
Fiddler[116]	4 newborns	myocardial dysfunction, pulmonary hypertension	2–5 μg/kg/min	all patients improved		multiple drugs used
DiSessa et al[107]	14 neonates	asphyxia (not hypotensive)	2.5 μg/kg/min	5/5: ↑ SAP; 4/6: ↑ cardiac function; no change in HR survival: 7/7 dopamine, 5/7 placebo	none	prospective, placebo, double-blind study

[a] Listed in order of publication; see References at end of chapter.
[b] SAP = systemic arterial pressure; CVP = central venous pressure; HR = heart rate.

167

four newborns with myocardial dysfunction associated with persistent fetal circulation. In a prospective double-blind study conducted in neonates with asphyxia (ECG changes of myocardial ischemia), DiSessa and coworkers[107] observed increases in systolic blood pressure without evidence of changes in systemic or pulmonary vascular resistance. Inulin clearance doubled in the dopamine-treated neonates, indicating a significant increase in glomerular filtration rate with doses of 2.5 μg/kg/min. A number of clinical studies have been published involving the use of dopamine in conjunction with vasodilating agents; see under Totazoline.

The effect of dopamine on the pulmonary vascular bed is controversial. In adults, dopamine has produced both vasoconstriction and vasodilation.[100,128,129,157] Few studies of pulmonary circulation have been done in children and neonates. Lang and coworkers[133] found no significant change in pulmonary pressure or resistance, although one patient with preexisting pulmonary hypertension had a significant increase in pulmonary resistance following dopamine administration. DiSessa and colleagues[107] found no evidence of changes in systemic or pulmonary vascular resistance in neonates who responded to dopamine with an increase in systemic blood pressure. Drummond and coworkers[114] observed a variable response in pulmonary resistance in neonatal lambs following infusion of dopamine; the pulmonary resistance tended to increase in parallel with the systemic resistance, although variability among animals was extremely high.

Therapeutic Indications. Dopamine is used to treat *refractory congestive heart failure* and *shock* resulting from a variety of causes.[119,120,159] Most clinical experience is in adults. However, in a survey the majority of neonatologists reported using dopamine for treatment of "shock" in neonates,[181] in spite of inadequate documentation of its efficacy in various etiologies of shock.

The usual starting dose for dopamine is 2 to 5 μg/kg/min given as a constant infusion IV (Table 7–10). Goldberg and coworkers[120] recommend starting doses of 0.5 to 1 μg/kg/min in adults, with gradual increases in infusion rate until urine flow is augmented or until increases in diastolic pressure and heart rate are observed. This recommendation is based on variability of individual response to the vasoconstrictor effect of dopamine. Increases up to 25 μg/kg/min and greater have been employed, but such large doses will result in adrenergic stimulation, which will increase vascular smooth muscle

tension, along with further dopaminergic effects (see under Clinical Pharmacology). Drummond and colleagues[115] found dopamine to be ineffective in neonates at doses below 6 μg/kg/min; these investigators frequently used doses in excess of 20 μg/kg/min ($\geq$ 125 μg/kg/min) to achieve the desired increases in systemic arterial pressure or urine output. The neonates in their series were also receiving tolazoline for pulmonary hypertension, which may account for these dose requirements (see under Tolazoline). There are striking differences between newborns and adults in responsiveness to vasoconstrictors and vasodilators;[146] these differences may be relevant to the apparent dose–response differences observed in clinical experiences with dopamine in adults and neonates.

In summary, in critically ill infants suffering from cardiovascular dysfunction, careful attention to identifying the ideal rate of infusion of dopamine for each patient is more likely to result in appropriate increases in cardiac output, urine output, peripheral perfusion, and blood pressure. The demonstrated pharmacologic properties of dopamine indicate that it is less likely than isoproterenol to cause either excessive vasodilation and hypotension, and that it is less likely than norepinephrine to cause excessive vasoconstriction and increased cardiac work.

Controversial Aspects of Dopamine Therapy. The major areas of controversy surrounding the use of dopamine have been presented by Kliegman and Fanaroff.[132] One major concern is the fact that much of the pharmacology of dopamine has been examined in mature animals, which may not represent the circumstances in the newborn. As an example, the sympathetic innervation of the heart and other tissues is incomplete at birth.[117,180] Therefore, the inotropic effect of dopamine mediated by release of norepinephrine from nerve terminals in the myocardium may be reduced in the maturing heart.

Loeb and colleagues[140] emphasize the value of the increase in peripheral resistance induced by dopamine in hypotensive patients with clinical shock and in normotensive patients with chronic low-output cardiac failure. High-dose dopamine is indicated in patients with septic shock who have low systemic vascular resistance; the effect of increased afterload can be anticipated to enhance rather than to antagonize the inotropic response to the drug. In addition, restoration of arterial pressure will favor improved coronary and systemic perfusion.

Because isoproterenol was found to be more

potent than dopamine in isolated neonatal dog myocardium, isoproterenol was originally recommended as the drug of choice to increase cardiac output.[108] Subsequent studies in intact neonatal animals, however, showed that dopamine is more potent than isoproterenol;[110] moreover, the fact that isoproterenol can cause blood to be shunted away from critical organs cannot be ignored (see under Isoproterenol).[178] Other studies indicate that dopamine may also be more potent than dobutamine in improving cardiac function.[174]

Experiments in neonatal models or randomized controlled trials comparing dopamine, dobutamine, and isoproterenol are required to resolve these concerns and to identify the role of each drug in the treatment of low cardiac output.

Clinical Toxicology. Dopamine is a safe drug when used in conjunction with meticulous monitoring of blood pressure and the ECG. The most common side-effect is cardiac arrhythmia. Few other adverse effects have been reported in infants. Maggi and colleagues[145] described gangrene lesions in the extremity of a neonate who was given 5 to 7 μg/kg/min IV for about 24 hours. Supraventricular tachycardia was reported in another infant receiving 17 μg/kg/min.[169] An accidental bolus dose of dopamine (675 μg/kg) produced an increase in systemic pressure with no other consequence.[115]

A potential interaction between digoxin and dopamine has been proposed because of the ability of each drug to increase peripheral vasomotor tone.[172] Aggravation of peripheral ischemia and pregangrenous changes could theoretically result. No evidence for such toxic interactions has been reported in infants.

Dobutamine

Pharmacology. Dobutamine is a synthetic catecholamine similar in structure to dopamine except for a bulky aromatic substitution on the amino group (Fig. 7–7). It was synthesized by systematic modification of the isoproterenol structure in an attempt to reduce the chronotropic, arrhythmogenic, and vascular side-effects of this drug while preserving the inotropic activity.[177] As with other catecholamines, dobutamine is not effective when given PO because of rapid metabolism in the liver to inactive conjugates with glucuronic acid and to 3-O-methyldobutamine (Fig. 7–9).[179] As a consequence, dobutamine must be administered by continuous IV infusion. Dobutamine is a β_1 agonist, but unlike dopamine it does not appear

to stimulate the heart indirectly by releasing norepinephrine from nerve endings in the myocardium.[173] Thus, dobutamine would be expected to be more effective in increasing the contractile force of the heart than in increasing the heart rate. However, clinical studies have failed to substantiate consistently this difference.[101] Clinical observations do suggest a more favorable effect of dobutamine than that of dopamine during prolonged infusions in patients in heart failure, although some tolerance does develop.[396] One explanation offered is that the indirect component of dopamine action (release of norepinephrine) is attenuated over time, whereas the pure direct action of dobutamine does not change.[144]

Dobutamine activates both α-adrenergic and β_2-adrenergic receptors in arterial vessels in the peripheral circulation.[173] In small doses very little effect occurs on these receptors, but with larger doses both α and β_2 receptors are activated, with the β_2 effect predominating. The result is a decrease in total peripheral resistance. At equally potent doses in terms of effect on myocardial contractility, dobutamine exerts a much weaker β_2-adrenergic action than that of isoproterenol and a much weaker α-adrenergic action than that of norepinephrine.[164] Dobutamine is about four times as potent as dopamine when contractile potency is compared at low doses.[197] At higher doses, however, dobutamine decreases peripheral resistance, in contrast to the α-adrenergic pressor actions of dopamine, which increase peripheral resistance.[139,174] This difference with larger doses resides in the predominant β_2 effect of dobutamine as opposed to the α effect of dopamine (Table 7–9).

Clinical Pharmacology. The mean plasma half-life of dobutamine in patients with congestive heart failure is about 2 minutes.[390] The volume of distribution is about 0.2 ± 0.08 l/kg and the mean body clearance is 0.06 ± 0.03 l/min/kg. Dobutamine causes a dose-related increase in cardiac output in patients with heart failure. Although the majority of clinical studies have been done in adults, some data for infants and children are available (Table 7–13). Driscoll and coworkers[109] studied the cardiovascular responses to dobutamine (2–7.75 μg/kg/min) during diagnostic cardiac catheterization in 12 children (2–16 yr old) with various cardiac problems; although heart rate and pulmonary and systemic vascular resistance were unchanged during dobutamine infusion, the cardiac output, cardiac index, stroke volume, stroke index, and systemic mean pressure increased significantly. Studies by Bohn and col-

Table 7-13. SUMMARY OF CLINICAL STUDIES OF DOBUTAMINE USE IN INFANTS AND CHILDREN

Authors of Published Study[a]	Study Group	Diagnosis	Dobutamine Dose	Clinical Response[b]	Side-effects
Driscoll et al[109]	12 children (2.3–16.7 yr)	congenital heart disease	2–7.75 μg/kg/min	↑ cardiac index, CO, SAP; no change in HR, PAP, SVR, PVR	none
Bohn et al[101]	11 infants and children (2.5 mo–11 yr)	congenital heart disease (postoperative: cardiopulmonary bypass)	1–10 μg/kg/min	↑ HR, SAP, cardiac index; no change in SV index, SVR, LAP	tachycardia
Schranz et al[168]	12 infants and children (1 day–14 yr)	low cardiac output: trauma, sepsis, shock	7.5–10 μg/kg/min	↑ cardiac index, CO, HR, SAP; ↓ SVR; no change or ↓ in PVR	none
Perkin et al[155]	33 infants and children (4 wk–17 yr)	septic or cardiogenic shock	2.5–10 μg/kg/min	no change in HR, SAP, PAP; ↑ cardiac index, PWP; ↓ SVR; mortality 67%	dysrhythmias hypotension hypertension ↑PWP symptomatic chest pain

[a] Listed in order of publication; see References at end of chapter.
[b] CO = cardiac output; SAP = systemic arterial pressure; HR = heart rate; PAP = pulmonary artery pressure; SVR = systemic vascular resistance; PVR = pulmonary vascular resistance; SV = stroke volume; LAP = left atrial pressure, PWP = pulmonary wedge pressure.

leagues[101] of the hemodynamic effects of dobutamine in 11 children (aged 2.5–11 yr) after cardiopulmonary bypass demonstrated the drug to be an effective inotropic agent. Significant increases in cardiac index by 19% to 23% were seen at doses of 4 and 7 μg/kg/min in association with an increase in heart rate. The tachycardia prompted discontinuation of dobutamine in four patients. In the series of Perkin and coauthors,[156] dobutamine at doses of 2.5 to 10 μg/kg/min significantly increased cardiac index, left ventricular stroke work index, and pulmonary wedge pressure in 33 infants and children with cardiogenic or septic shock. No significant changes occurred in heart rate, mean systemic arterial pressure, mean pulmonary arterial pressure, right atrial pressure, or pulmonary arteriolar resistance index. These investigators postulated an attenuated response to the action of dobutamine in patients 12 months of age or younger. They also observed a wide variance in action, as has been noted for other inotropic agents. Schranz and coworkers[168] administered dobutamine (7.5–10 μg/kg/min) to 12 patients (aged 1 day–14 yr) with low cardiac output syndromes. They observed an increase in cardiac index, stroke volume index, and cardiac output. The mean heart

rate changed only slightly, suggesting that the increase in cardiac output was mainly due to the alteration of stroke volume. The mean systemic arterial pressure increased significantly, but the mean pulmonary artery pressure and pulmonary resistance were unchanged.

In adults, an inotropic response to dobutamine has been uniformly demonstrated. The hemodynamic effects of dobutamine and other sympathomimetics have been compared in patients with heart failure and during emergence from cardiopulmonary bypass procedures: In general, dobutamine is preferable to dopamine for patients with ventricular failure because high doses of dopamine increase afterload (vasoconstriction).[139,140] In studies in adults emerging from cardiopulmonary bypass procedures,[174] dopamine was judged to be about twice as potent as dobutamine in improving cardiac function; dobutamine, dopamine, and epinephrine were found to be superior to isoproterenol. Dobutamine increased the cardiac index by 15% to 25% at doses of 5 to 10 μg/kg/min. No change was observed in peripheral vascular resistance with either dobutamine or epinephrine; however, dopamine caused an increase in peripheral vascular resistance, but this occurred in less than half of the patients. Dobutamine has been used effectively in adults with septic shock associated with fluid overload or cardiac failure.[131]

Therapeutic Indications. The clinical experience with dobutamine in neonates is limited. In older infants and children, dobutamine is effective for the treatment of *low output cardiac failure.*[101,156,168] Significant increases in cardiac output may or may not be associated with increases in heart rate. Dobutamine is less likely to increase peripheral vascular resistance than are isoproterenol and norepinephrine. Whether dobutamine has any consistent advantages over dopamine in the treatment of the neonate with myocardial dysfunction remains to be established. Dobutamine does not appear to be of value in initial therapy of cardiac arrest.[152]

The dose of dobutamine used in the majority of the clinical studies was between 1.0 and 10 μg/kg/min (Table 7–13). The onset of action occurs within 2 min of the beginning of infusion, with the maximal effect being reached by 10 min.[390] Perkin and coworkers[156] observed optimal cardiac effects at doses up to 7.5 μg/kg/min; complications more commonly occurred with higher doses. Therefore, the initial recommended dose is 1 to 2 μg/kg/min, and the expected maximum effective dose without significant toxicity is 7.5 to 10 μg/kg/min (Table 7–10).

Clinical Toxicology. The side-effects of dobutamine are similar to those of other sympathomimetic amines. However, the incidence of arrhythmias is lower than that reported for isoproterenol or dopamine.[173] Dobutamine may cause a marked increase in heart rate or change (increase or decrease) in systolic blood pressure, which will generally rapidly resolve with reduction in the infusion rate.[174] Patients with atrial fibrillation may be at risk of development of a rapid ventricular rate, because dobutamine facilitates A-V conduction. Perkin and coworkers[156] observed an increase in pulmonary wedge pressure with dobutamine use that was associated with pulmonary congestion and edema in one patient. Shranz and colleagues[168] reported no adverse side-effects in infants and children receiving dobutamine.

Isoproterenol

Pharmacology. Isoproterenol is a β_1- and β_2-adrenergic agonist with almost no action on α receptors. It is readily absorbed when administered parenterally, but absorption following PO administration is unpredictable.[179] Sublingual doses have been found sufficiently bioavailable

to be useful in the treatment of pulmonary hypertension.[143] Isoproterenol is primarily metabolized in the liver and other tissues by COMT (see Fig. 7–9).

An IV infusion of isoproterenol increases cardiac output through a positive inotropic and chronotropic action and an increase in venous return to the heart. Peripheral resistance is generally reduced, primarily as a result of vasodilation in skeletal muscle and mesenteric vascular beds. Renal blood flow usually does not increase following IV administration, although administration of isoproterenol directly into the renal artery causes renal vasodilation.[149,165] Blood pressure will remain unchanged or diminish, depending on the relative change in cardiac output and peripheral resistance. The skeletal muscle vasodilation may be sufficient to actually decrease mean blood pressure, thereby diverting blood flow away from critical tissues such as myocardium, kidneys, and brain.[174] Since myocardial oxygen consumption is directly dependent on heart rate, peripheral resistance, and contractile state, drugs such as isoproterenol that increase heart rate may have a deleterious effect on the ischemic ventricle.[161]

In studies on immature dogs, Driscoll and colleagues[113] found that isoproterenol does not increase cardiac output. These investigators speculate that the high resting cardiac output may have limited the capacity for further inotropic response to occur despite β-adrenergic stimulation. Manders and coworkers[146] found that vasoconstrictors and vasodilators, including isoproterenol, induced smaller responses in conscious newborn lambs than in adult sheep. Driscoll and colleagues[112,113] also observed reduced systemic vascular resistance following isoproterenol in adult dogs but not in puppies, although heart rate increased similarly. In vitro studies have also suggested that the developing cardiovascular system may be less responsive to adrenergic stimulation. Park and coworkers[155] showed that newborn rabbit papillary muscle was less sensitive than that of the adult to the inotropic effect of isoproterenol and calcium. The potentially favorable actions of isoproterenol on myocardial function may, therefore, be less in neonates than in adults.

Isoproterenol decreases pulmonary artery pressure and resistance in experimental animals and in clinical studies in adults.[170] Isoproterenol also relaxes bronchial and gastrointestinal smooth muscle. Insulin secretion is stimulated both by the hyperglycemic effect of isoproterenol and by the direct β-adrenergic action on pancreatic islet cells. The pharmacologic properties of isoproterenol are summarized in Table 7–9.

Clinical Pharmacology. Isoproterenol has been used in neonates to augment cardiovascular function.[104] However, there are few reports evaluating critical cardiovascular parameters before and after isoproterenol therapy in neonates. Cabel and coworkers[104] found that isoproterenol increased heart rate and decreased arterial and central venous pressure in four newborns diagnosed as having heart failure due to severe perinatal asphyxia (the authors did not specify dose used). Three patients also received digoxin or diuretics, oxygen, calcium gluconate, and other supportive care. Holloway and coworkers[128] used isoproterenol to improve cardiac output in postoperative low cardiac-output syndrome in adults. Following a dose of 0.0125 to 0.025 μg/kg/min, cardiac output increased by as much as 37%, and heart rate increased up to 28% of control; systemic vascular resistance decreased by as much as 29%. Rigaud and colleagues[161] observed in adult patients with or without congestive heart failure (with a variety of underlying diseases) that isoproterenol caused a significant fall in mean aortic pressure, peripheral vascular resistance, and mean pulmonary arterial pressure. Cardiac stroke work remained unchanged, while minute work was significantly increased. In other studies, short- and long-term reductions in pulmonary artery hypertension in adults have also been observed in association with isoproterenol therapy.[106,143] Significant reductions in pulmonary artery pressure and resistance, along with increases in cardiac index, occurred following administration of this agent.

Therapeutic Indications. Isoproterenol is used in a variety of *cardiovascular shock* states,[175] including those seen following cardiopulmonary bypass procedures[128] and cardiogenic shock associated with perinatal asphyxia.[104] This agent has also been used to treat *primary pulmonary hypertension.*[106,143,170] Isoproterenol may be useful in conditions of poor cardiac output associated with aortic regurgitation because it produces a decrease in afterload.[142] It also is useful for treatment of bradycardia associated with myocardial dysfunction, particularly when pulmonary vascular resistance is elevated.[111]

In general, isoproterenol is considered a second-choice agent because of its marked chronotropic and arrhythmogenic effects. Extension of myocardial ischemic injury, as well as preferential decrease in perfusion of critical tissues (kidney, heart, brain), is an additional disadvantage of the drug. Isoproterenol is of no value in cardiac resuscitation[158] and is ineffective in shock associated with myocardial infarction.[124]

The recommended dose of isoproterenol is 0.05 to 0.5 μg/kg/min (Table 7–10). Because of the systemic vasodilation produced by isoproterenol, venous return to the heart is reduced. Therefore, central venous pressure should be carefully monitored, and fluid volume given as needed to maintain this pressure.

Clinical Toxicology. Cardiac arrhythmias and myocardial necrosis are the most serious adverse effects associated with isoproterenol therapy. Steen and colleagues[174] found that isoproterenol-induced arrythmia and tachycardia limit the value of its inotropic effect. Maroko and coworkers[147] have shown experimentally that isoproterenol-induced increase in oxygen demand (due to tachycardia) exacerbates preexisting myocardial infarctions. Rapidly fatal cardiovascular deterioration has been reported with the use of isoproterenol.[124,171]

Bipyridines — Amrinone and Milrinone

Pharmacology. Efforts to discover more potent, orally active inotropic agents have led to the development of the bipyridine compounds. These nonsympathomimetic, nonglycoside inotropes produce major dose-dependent increases in tension and the rate of tension development in myocardial muscle.[385] The pharmacologic inotropic effects are not inhibited by blockade of β-adrenergic and histamine receptors and do not involve alterations of Na^+–K^+ ATPase. The mechanism responsible for the inotropic action of amrinone and milrinone has been postulated to involve cyclic AMP or direct effects on membrane handling of calcium. Both drugs also produce a decrease in systemic and pulmonary vascular resistance.[385,389] Milrinone has been estimated to be 10 to 30 times more potent as an inotropic agent than amrinone.

Clinical Pharmacology. A number of clinical trials have been conducted that demonstrate the beneficial inotropic effects of the bipyridines in adult patients with congestive heart failure.[385,387,393,395,397,398] Oral bioavailability of amrinone is greater than 90%, and the reported half-life in normal subjects is approximately 2 to 4 hr compared with 8 hr in adults with chronic congestive heart failure.[394] The half-life for milrinone in adults is about 2 hr.[385] A 50% increase in cardiac index has been observed in adults with serum concentrations of amrinone averaging 3700 ng/ml.[387] A similar response was observed with milrinone in patients who had an average blood concentration of 166 ± 23 ng/ml.[385] There have not been any studies reported in infants.

Therapeutic Indications. The bipyridine derivatives appear to have great potential in the treatment of myocardial failure. They are orally effective and have a much wider therapeutic index than the digitalis glycosides. There is no reported experience with the bipyridine derivatives in infants.

Clinical Toxicology. Observations in over 200 adult patients have revealed up to a 15% incidence of thrombocytopenia or fever. A 5 to 10% incidence of gastrointestinal side-effects has been reported, including vomiting, dyspepsia, cramps, and diarrhea. These side-effects can be sufficiently severe to require dose reduction or drug withdrawal. Limited experience with milrinone suggests a lower incidence of side-effects compared with amrinone.[385,393]

Selection of the Appropriate Agent

Selection of the appropriate inotropic or sympathomimetic agent requires an understanding of the patient's cardiovascular abnormality. Cardiovascular and septic shock are complex pathophysiologic states of circulatory dysfunction that trigger a variety of compensatory mechanisms.[154] Confusion regarding rational drug therapy of the various shock states is the result of the complex hemodynamics and anecdotal reports of clinical experience with drugs often selected at random. Although helpful, the pharmacologic information outlined in Tables 7–9 and 7–10 will not necessarily apply to every sick infant with circulatory shock. It must also be remembered that much of the data on the pharmacology of the inotropic drugs, especially the sympathomimetics, have been collected from experimental animals and adults. Despite the seriousness of these considerations, guidelines for the employment of the inotropic agents have been cautiously summarized in Table 7–14.

ANTIHYPERTENSIVES AND VASODILATORS

Antihypertensive–vasodilator therapy has been employed with success in infants and children with a variety of underlying cardiovascular

Table 7–14. DRUGS OF CHOICE FOR MYOCARDIAL DYSFUNCTION AND SHOCK IN INFANTS

Manifestations of Myocardial Dysfunction	Drug(s) of Choice[a]
inadequate cardiac output (myocardial dysfunction)	
with hypoperfusion only	digoxin[b] dobutamine
with vasoconstriction	dopamine (low to moderate doses) vasodilators (see following section) dobutamine (high dose) isoproterenol
with hypotension	dopamine (high doses) epinephrine[c] norepinephrine + phentolamine
with bradycardia only	atropine isoproterenol[c] epinephrine[c]
adequate or increased cardiac output	
with systemic hypotension[a]	dopamine (high doses) epinephrine[c]
cardiac arrest	epinephrine

[a] Correction of hypovolemia, acidosis, and hypoxemia must precede or accompany all drug therapy.
[b] Digoxin is not a drug of choice in acute circulatory shock (see Therapeutic Indications under Digoxin).
[c] May seriously aggravate existing tissue hypoperfusion.

abnormalities. These clinical experiences are reviewed under the specific agents. In this section, the drugs are grouped according to their principal mechanisms of action (see Tables 7–15 and 7–17) rather than their clinical use; the therapeutic indications are summarized in Table 7–16.

Selection of the appropriate agent requires an understanding of the disease process and of the therapeutic rationale. Accordingly, some general considerations in the use of antihypertensive–vasodilator drugs are presented here, prior to discussion of specific agents.

Principles of Antihypertensive–Vasodilator Therapy

Antihypertensive and vasodilator drugs are used to normalize blood pressure in hypertensive patients, to alter vascular resistance or capacities (preload, afterload) in refractory congestive heart failure, and to reduce pulmonary

Table 7 – 15. CLASSIFICATION AND MECHANISM OF ACTION OF ANTIHYPERTENSIVE AND VASODILATOR DRUGS

Classification	Drugs	Mechanism of Action[a]
diuretics	chlorothiazide furosemide	reduces extracellular fluid volume by promoting renal excretion of sodium and water (see Chap. 8)
direct vasodilators	diazoxide hydralazine minoxidil nitroglycerine nitroprusside	direct action on vascular smooth muscle, causing vasodilation; may affect mainly arteriolar, venous, or both vascular beds (see Table 7–17)
α-adrenergic blockers	prazosin	selective blocker of postsynaptic α-adrenergic receptors
	tolazoline	multiple actions including H_1 and H_2 receptor stimulation, histamine release, parasympathomimetic, direct vasodilation, α-adrenergic blocker
β-adrenergic blockers	propranolol	reduces heart rate and cardiac contractility; lowers plasma renin activity
CNS sympathetic agonist	clonidine methyldopa	central α-adrenergic stimulation of vasomotor centers, causing vasodilation
calcium-channel blockers	nifedipine verapamil	interfere with the movement (entry) of Ca^{2+}
renin–angiotensin system inhibitors	captopril	inhibition of conversion of angiotensin I to angiotensin II; increase levels of vasodilators (bradykinin, prostaglandins)

[a] There may be more minor mechanisms of action in addition to those presented.

vascular resistance in conditions associated with pulmonary hypertension. Although many drugs are capable of altering vascular tone, the mechanism varies considerably. Table 7–15 summarizes the major antihypertensive–vasodilator drugs and their mechanisms of action. For selection of the appropriate drug, the patho-

Table 7 – 16. THERAPEUTIC INDICATIONS FOR ANTIHYPERTENSIVE AND VASODILATOR DRUGS

Clinical Problem	Drug(s) of Choice
	Antihypertensives
acute hypertensive crises	diazoxide nitroprusside: requires continuous infusion and arterial blood pressure monitoring
hypertension nonacute but continuous or progressive	diuretics (see Chap. 8) hydralazine (add propranolol if β-adrenergic side-effects prominent; see Fig. 7–13)
	propranolol methyldopa prazosin nifedipine clonidine } all orally effective
resistant to standard therapy	minoxidil captopril } particularly effective for hypertension of renal origin
	Vasodilators[a]
refractory congestive heart failure	
with major afterload component	hydralazine nitroprusside prazosin
with major preload (pulmonary) component	nitroglycerin prazosin
with combined preload and afterload components	nitroprusside prazosin hydralazine
pulmonary hypertension	tolazoline nitroglycerin prazosin hydralazine + nitroglycerin nifedipine

[a] These indications for vasodilator therapy are rational considerations based on pharmacologic activity of the drugs and results from use in adults. Experience in infants has been limited to investigational studies.

physiology for the hypertension or refractory congestive heart failure should be matched to the mechanism of drug action. Several excellent articles have been written regarding the pathophysiology of hypertension in pediatric patients[184,193,275] and the role of preload and afterload in congestive heart failure.[210,264,271,279,286,294,314,343]

Hypertension in the Neonate

Systemic hypertension in the neonate is largely associated with renovascular abnormalities: In Adelman's series,[184] the cause of the hypertension was renal artery thrombosis in

Table 7 – 17. **PRINCIPAL SITE OF ACTION, DURATION OF ACTION, AND HEMODYNAMIC EFFECTS OF VASODILATOR DRUGS**

Drug	Principal Site of Action	Duration of Action	Hemodynamic Effect			
			BP	*CO*	*HR*	*PAWP*
diazoxide	arteriolar	6 hr (2 – 36 hr)	↓↓[a]	↑	0, ↑	↓
hydralazine	arteriolar	3 – 6 hr	↑, ↓	↑↑↑	↑ (↓BP) 0 (CHF)	↑, ↓
minoxidil	arteriolar	1 hr to 3 – 4 days	↓↓	↑	↑	↓
nifedipine	arteriolar	2 – 12 hr	↓↓	↑	↑	↓↓
nitroglycerine	venous	min to hr[b]	↓	↑	0	↓↓
nitrates	venous	min to hr[b]	↓	↑	0	↓↓
nitroprusside	arteriolar/venous	min	↓↓	↑↑	0	↓
prazosin	arteriolar/venous	~6 hr	↓	↑↑	0	↓
tolazoline	arteriolar/venous	1 – 7 hr	↓	↑	↑	↓↓

[a] ↓ = decrease; ↑ = increase; 0 = no change or effect. The number of arrows indicates relative potency of effect. BP = blood pressure; CO = cardiac output, HR = heart rate; PAWP = pulmonary artery wedge pressure; CHF = congestive heart failure.

[b] Duration of action is dependent upon the particular dosage form employed.

75% of infants and renal artery stenosis in 18%; no clear etiology was found in 7%. In the same study, the presence of hypertension was documented in 2.5% of infants admitted to intensive care. Unfortunately, very little literature exists with respect to the natural history of hypertension in neonates, or regarding the effectiveness and benefits of antihypertensive therapy in this age group. Although these voids of information exist for older infants and children as well,[275] awareness of the problem is increasing, and there is a general consensus that effective therapy should be initiated to prevent associated organ damage. There is no reason to believe that neonates are immune to the potential ad-

verse consequences of hypertension. Therefore, an understanding of the pathophysiology of hypertension in the neonate is of importance, particularly since rational drug therapy is dependent upon treatment of the basic mechanism of the hypertension.[193] Diagnosis of hypertension requires definition of normal blood pressure distribution curves for the infant population (full-term and premature infants). Use of this information requires rigid adherence to details of blood pressure measurement.[224,275,337] The selected data on "normal" blood pressures for neonates and infants shown in Figure 7 – 10 are in general agreement with results reported in various studies.[229,257,258,269]

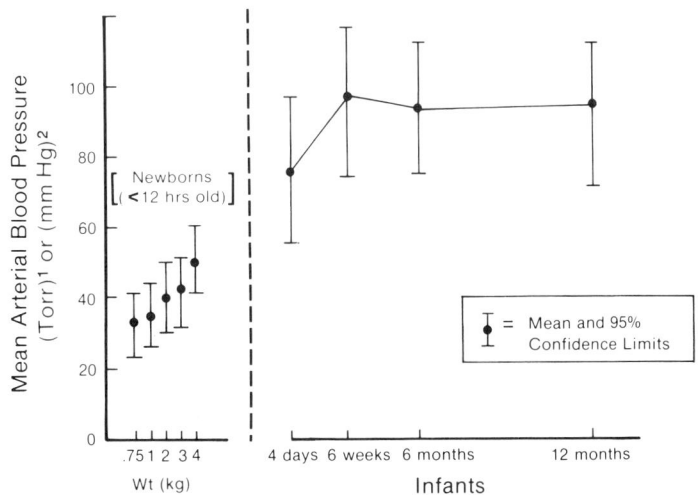

Figure 7 – 10. Average arterial blood pressures in newborns (premature to fullterm <12 hrs old) and infants. [1]Data for new borns represent mean aortic blood pressures obtained via an umbilical artery catheter during the first 12 hours of life (torr). [2]The values for infants 4 days to 1 year old were obtained by Doppler/pressure cuff technique (mm Hg). (Data compiled from deSweit M et al: Pediatrics 65:1028, 1980; and from Versmold HT et al: Pediatrics 67:607, 1981.)

Congestive Heart Failure

Pathophysiology. The use of vasodilating drugs for treatment of congestive heart failure requires a complete understanding of the pathophysiology of heart failure. The major factors that regulate cardiac performance are myocardial contractility, preload, afterload, and heart rate and cardiac rhythm (Fig. 7–11). In contrast to inotropic agents, which can increase cardiac output by influences on contractility and heart rate, vasodilator drugs alter preload and afterload. In isolated cardiac muscle, **preload** refers to the fiber length prior to contraction.[271] Increases in preload result in the development of a greater contractile force — the **Frank-Starling effect** (see Fig. 7–5). In the intact heart, preload is proportional to end-diastolic ventricular volume and is most often measured as mean left ventricular filling pressure or left ventricular end-diastolic pressure (LVEDP). Pulmonary wedge pressure also reflects left ventricular preload in the absence of mitral valve dysfunction.

Afterload is the tension developed in a cardiac fiber before shortening occurs. In the intact heart, afterload reflects the tension that must be developed by the ventricular wall to overcome the forces opposing ventricular ejection. These forces include arterial (aortic) impedance, which depends on stroke volume; peripheral vascular resistance; and arterial compliance (Fig. 7–11).[271] The term **impedance** refers to properties of blood vessels and blood that oppose flow. Because an enlarged heart must develop a greater muscular force than that of a small heart to produce the same systolic pressure (the Laplace relationship), afterload will be greater for a large heart than for a small heart.[314]

In general, increases in myocardial contractility, preload, or both result in an increase in ventricular output, whereas an increase in afterload reduces cardiac stroke volume. In patients with congestive heart failure, both preload and afterload are increased to compensate for depressed myocardial contractility. Retention of salt and water (subsequent to poor cardiac perfusion of the renal vasculature) is responsible for the increases in venous blood volume that elevate the preload. The development of peripheral edema and pulmonary congestion limits the increased cardiac output associated with the increase in preload. Insufficient cardiac output results in increased sympathetic reflex arteriolar constriction,[262] increase in blood viscosity and in vascular smooth muscle "stiffness" and reactivity,[283] and the accumulation of vasoactive substances such as renin in the circulation,[212] all of which contribute to the increase in afterload. Blood pressure may still be maintained despite the low cardiac output.

Principles of Correction by Vasodilators. The normal heart is considered to have a given level of preload and contractility, with substantial reserve to increase both. In acute and chronic heart failure, the peripheral vascular resistance is often elevated (reflex sympathetic response; see Fig. 7–6), thus maintaining blood pressure in the face of low cardiac output. The increase in peripheral vascular resistance along with cardiac dilation (increase in afterload) accounts for the potential benefits of afterload reduction. In patients with congestive heart failure and increased afterload, drug-induced vasodilation can result in increased stroke volume, decreased myocardial wall tension, and increased work and power of contraction. As a consequence, greater myocardial efficiency may result.[264] In contrast, the use of inotropic agents, which cause peripheral vasoconstriction, further compromises cardiac output by causing additional increases in afterload.

Preload can be reduced by lowering intravascular volume through restricting sodium and fluids, by administering diuretics, or by administering venous vasodilators. The latter group of drugs reduces ventricular diastolic pressure and end-diastolic fiber length.[264] Although such therapy may reduce symptoms of congestion and reduce afterload by reducing ventricular size, impaired left ventricular function may de-

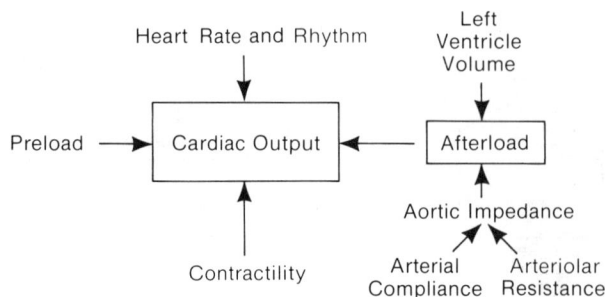

Figure 7–11. Major factors determining cardiac output.

pend on an increased preload to maintain adequate systolic output. These and other considerations with respect to the use of vasodilators in congestive heart failure are depicted in Figure 7–12.

Vasodilator drugs are classified on the basis of site of action. As shown in Table 7–17, the primary effect may be on arterioles (e.g., hydralazine) or on veins (e.g., nitroglycerin), or there may be a balanced effect on arteries and veins (e.g., nitroprusside). None of the currently available vasodilator drugs have purely arteriolar or venodilatory effects. Circulating blood volume can be effectively redistributed by vasodilators that predominantly dilate systemic veins. Vasodilators with a predominant effect on arteriolar resistance beds decrease systemic vascular resistance and increase cardiac output with little or no change in systemic or pulmonary venous pressures. Drugs with balanced effects on arteriolar and venous beds cause an increase in cardiac output and a decrease in systemic and pulmonary venous pressures. However, the response to vasodilator drugs may vary among patients. The potential for adverse consequences with vasodilator therapy requires careful monitoring to ensure accurate determi-

nation of the cardiovascular status and quantification of the response to vasodilator therapy.

In adult patients with diminished cardiac output, there is a downward and rightward shift of the ventricular function curve—that is, a decrease in stroke volume at a given level of LVEDP, as shown in Figure 7–12. A decrease in afterload shifts the curve up and to the left, meaning that there is an increase in stroke volume at the same filling pressure (curve ① or ② in the figure). As long as filling pressure remains adequate, a decrease in filling pressure with the use of a venodilator drug (e.g., nitrates) will cause only a small reduction in cardiac output, since this portion of the ventricular function curve is relatively flat (A to D or C). By careful correction of ventricular filling pressure using volume expansion (C to B on curve ①), maximum enhancement of cardiac output can be achieved. Knowledge of the initial left ventricular filling pressure is necessary for proper evaluation and management of vasodilator-induced changes in performance.[210,279] Any change in cardiac output will be directly related to the baseline ventricular filling pressure as well as the systemic resistance but inversely related to baseline cardiac output.[236]

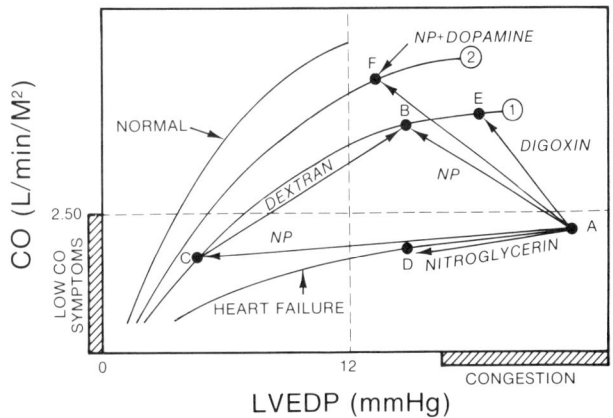

Figure 7–12. Effects of various therapeutic agents on ventricular function as determined by cardiac output (CO) and left ventricular end-diastolic pressure (LVEDP). The highest curve represents normal function for comparison. The lowest curve represents congestive heart failure (CHF); A is the point at which the dysfunctioning left ventricle begins to operate. Intermediate curve ① demonstrates the improved relation between CO and LVEDP after the administration of digoxin (E), as well as the effects of nitroprusside (NP) given alone when LVEDP = >12 mm Hg (B) and when LVEDP = <12 mm Hg (C); in the latter case, the addition of dextran at C produces the result seen at B, with NP alone. Prazosin or combined hydralazine–nitrate therapy gives the same result as that with NP therapy (A to B); hydralazine therapy alone produces the effects of digoxin therapy (A to E). The improvement from A on the lowest (CHF) curve to B on intermediate curve ① after NP administration is not the result of increased contractility; rather, it is due to the enhanced CO–LVEDP relationship that follows the reduction of impedance to left ventricular ejection seen with NP therapy. D on the lowest (CHF) curve is the LVEDP after diuretic or nitroglycerin therapy. Intermediate curve ② demonstrates the improvement in CO and decrease in LVEDP achieved with combined NP–dopamine therapy (A to F). The horizontal broken line indicates the lower limit of normal for CO; the vertical broken line, the upper limit of normal for LVEDP. CONGESTION = pulmonary congestion. (Adapted from Mason DT: Am J Med 65:106, 1978.)

Direct Vasodilators

The direct vasodilators are well-known useful agents in the treatment of hypertension. However, the more potent agents induce reflex sympathetic changes undesirable in hypertensive patients. The administration of sympatholytic drugs in combination may be necessary.

Diazoxide

Pharmacology. Diazoxide is related chemically to the thiazide diuretics (Chap. 8). For maximum antihypertensive effectiveness the drug must be administered by the IV route. The drug is highly bound to plasma protein (90%);[307] the extensive protein binding may explain the association between the degree of antihypertensive response and the rate at which the drug is administered,[321] although this concept has been challenged.[202,414] The drug is metabolized, the majority of the metabolites being excreted in the urine.[307] About one third of the administered dose is found unchanged in the urine, but considerable tubular reabsorption is believed to occur. Although diazoxide can affect small postcapillary resistance vessels and large veins, its primary effect is on arterioles (Table 7–17). Diazoxide not only directly relaxes vascular smooth muscle but also inhibits the spontaneous activity of other smooth muscle.[198]

Diazoxide has similar effects to those of the thiazides on the peripheral vascular bed but has opposite effects on fluid and electrolyte balance. Because it causes marked retention of sodium and water and expands the plasma volume, the drug produces fluid overload and edema in patients with myocardial dysfunction. Although these effects can occur as a consequence of the reduction in blood pressure, glomerular filtration rate, and renal plasma flow, sodium retention can occur without any change in hemodynamics.[253] In addition, diazoxide can increase plasma glucose by decreasing insulin secretion from the pancreas, by increasing epinephrine secretion, and by directly increasing glucose production as well as inhibiting its uptake.[185]

Clinical Pharmacology. Pharmacokinetic studies of diazoxide in children indicate a half-life of 9.5 to 24 hours. In a study by Pruitt and coworkers,[307] children receiving maintenance diazoxide therapy for control of hypoglycemia (5 to 19 mg/kg q 24 hr PO) had a blood diazoxide level of 15 to 50 μg/ml. These authors speculated that diazoxide blood concentrations of 300 to 400 μg/ml would be expected with rapid IV injection of these doses.

Diazoxide can significantly reduce elevated systemic pressure associated with a wide variety of disorders. McLaine and Drummond[285] treated hypertension with this drug in 17 infants and children without encountering side-effects. The mean arterial pressure in their patients fell below 115 mm Hg in 82% of the hypertensive episodes; the mean duration of action was 5 hours. Boerth and Long[202] administered diazoxide to 16 infants and children (2–7.5 mg/kg IV over 10–20 sec, or as two or three smaller doses injected at 15- to 20-min intervals); a significant dose–response relation was observed in reduction of diastolic blood pressure

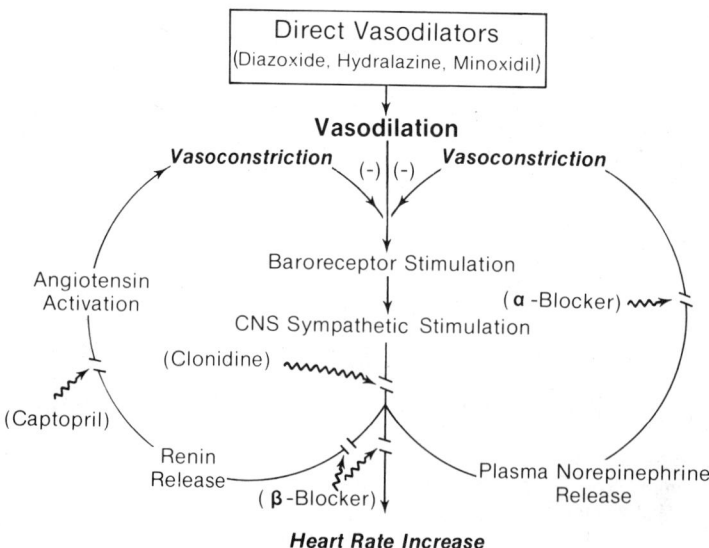

Figure 7–13. Reflex sympathetic changes induced by vasodilator drugs. Illustrated are the sympatholytic inhibition of reflex-initiated vasoconstriction and increased heart rate (broken lines). Not represented is the potential for β-blockade to influence several other undesirable side-effects associated with direct-vasodilator therapy. (Adapted from Pettinger WA: N Engl J Med 303:922, 1980.)

(average 30 mm Hg). McCrory and colleagues[282] studied the antihypertensive effect of diazoxide in 36 infants and children ranging in age from 2 months to 18 years who had severe symptomatic hypertension; a prompt and marked decrease in systolic and diastolic blood pressure occurred in all patients within 10 minutes after an initial injection (5 mg/kg IV given over 30 sec or less). The maximum antihypertensive effect was reached by 30 minutes and persisted for at least 6 hours. A slightly greater effect was observed in older children, perhaps related to the higher absolute pressures. No serious persistent hypotension developed. Individual variability in the antihypertensive responsive to diazoxide has been attributed to differences in plasma and extracellular fluid volumes and plasma protein binding.[202] Studies of the influence of rate of diazoxide administration on the antihypertensive effect indicate that slow infusion (over 20 to 30 min) is as effective as rapid IV bolus (<30 sec).[414,418]

Therapeutic Indications. Diazoxide is effective for *rapid reduction of acute elevations of blood pressure.* Its use should be restricted to acute emergency situations rather than prolonged maintenance programs. The recommended dose is 2 mg/kg given IV over at least 15 to 30 seconds or over 15 to 30 minutes; this dose can be repeated every 10 to 15 minutes to a maximum total dosage of 5 mg/kg (Table 7–18). Slow infusion will not influence the antihypertensive effect (see under Clinical Pharmacology) and will minimize the possible dangers of ischemic injury to the heart and brain resulting from sudden precipitous decreases in blood pressure.[414,430] The duration of the antihypertensive effect ranges from 2 to 36 hours.[308] Therefore, the dosing interval required to control blood pressure will vary, with the usual being every 2 to 6 hours. Neonates with hypoproteinemia or contracted intravascular volume may be unusually sensitive to the antihypertensive effect of the drug.

Diazoxide use in adult patients with *pulmonary hypertension* produced mixed clinical and hemodynamic effects in the study by Klinke and Gilbert.[259] Pulmonary vascular resistance decreased, and cardiac output increased in association with improvement in clinical manifestations of the disease. Use of diazoxide for treatment of elevated pulmonary resistance in neonates has not been reported.

Diazoxide has been found useful for the management of selected cases of *hypoglycemia* associated with hyperinsulinism.[319,399] The recommended dose is 3 to 8 mg/kg PO every 8 to 12 hours (Table 7–18). The appropriate dose and dosing interval can be determined by the magnitude and duration of the blood glucose increase.

Clinical Toxicology. A variety of side-effects occur with the administration of diazoxide.[202,282] A non-dose-related hyperglycemia has been noted in some patients. Other side-effects include tachycardia, nausea and vomiting, flushing, and burning or pain at the site of administration. Interactions with hydralazine or propranolol may cause development of extreme hypotension.[260] Chronic use of diazoxide can lead to sodium or water retention.

Hydralazine

Pharmacology. Hydralazine causes direct relaxation of the smooth muscle in the peripheral vascular bed. When given PO, hydralazine is subject to high first-pass clearance by the intestinal wall and liver, resulting in reduced systemic bioavailability. The metabolism of hydralazine in humans is complex because both enzymatic and nonenzymatic processes are involved.[287] The activity of the enzymatic acetylation pathway is determined by the phenotype of the patient with respect to acetylation rate.[312,426] During chronic therapy with identical doses of hydralazine, slow acetylators achieve higher plasma concentrations of hydralazine than those in rapid acetylators; this finding has implications with respect to toxicity. The acetylated metabolite probably undergoes further metabolism, since little is recovered in the urine. The reported values for volume of distribution of hydralazine range from 0.3 to 10.6 l/kg; the values from more specific analytic assays are between 4 and 8 l/kg.[426] About 85% of the circulating hydralazine is believed to be bound to serum albumin.[260] Less than 15% of the administered dose is excreted unchanged in the urine in adults. There is no evidence that dosage adjustment is necessary in the presence of renal failure, although this has been recommended by some.[426]

Hydralazine predominantly affects the precapillary arteriolar resistance bed; the relaxation of the venous capacitance vessels is far less pronounced (Table 7–17).[260] The vasodilation is not uniform, as the coronary, cerebral, splanchnic, and renal vasculature are more affected than vessels in the skin and muscle. The major hemodynamic effects following both PO and IV administration are a decrease in systemic vascular resistance (afterload) and an increase in cardiac output; the latter also appears

Table 7 – 18. RECOMMENDED DOSAGES OF ANTIHYPERTENSIVE – VASODILATOR DRUGS IN NEONATES

Drug	Recommended Dosage	Available Dosage Forms
Direct Vasodilators		
diazoxide (Hyperstat)	*hypertensive crisis:* 2 mg/kg IV given over at least 15 – 30 sec or over 15 to 30 min. Repeat dose until desired BP effect achieved; maximum total dose: 5 mg/kg; repeat effective dose q 2 – 6 hr as required for control	capsules: 50, 100 mg injection: 15 mg/ml suspension: 50 mg/ml
	hypoglycemia: 3 – 8 mg/kg PO or IV (over 1 hr) q 8 – 12 hr as required for control	
hydralazine (Apresoline)	*antihypertensive:* 0.1 – 0.5 mg/kg IV, IM, or PO q 3 – 6 hr as required for BP control; dose may be gradually increased to maximum of 2 mg/kg q 6 hr; PO dose generally twice the effective IV dose Note: combination with other antihypertensives is expected to reduce dose requirements to < 0.15 mg/kg	tablets: 10, 25, 50, 100 mg injection: 20 mg/ml
	vasodilation: 0.1 – 0.5 mg/kg IV q 6 hr; maximum dose: 2 mg/kg q 6 hr	
minoxidil (Loniten)	*antihypertensive:* 0.1 – 0.2 mg/kg PO q 12 – 24 hr as required for BP control, increasing to maximum daily dose of 5 mg/kg	tablets: 2.5, 10 mg
nitroglycerin	*vasodilation:* 0.5 – 20 μg/kg/min (experimental; see text)	paste, capsules, tablets, injection
nitroprusside (Nipride)	*hypertensive crisis:* 1 μg/kg/min IV, increasing as necessary to control BP (maximum 10 μg/kg/min for 10 min); maximum infusion rate for prolonged therapy: 2 μg/kg/min.	injection: 50 mg powder for reconstitution
	vasodilator therapy: 0.5 – 10 μg/kg/min (see above)	
α-Adrenergic Blockers		
prazosin (Minipress)	*antihypertensive:* initial dose 5 μg/kg PO; observe for severe hypotension; increase dose as needed to control BP up to 25 μg/kg q 6 hr (experimental; see text)	capsules: 1, 2, 5 mg
	vasodilator: as for antihypertensive	
tolazoline (Priscoline)	*pulmonary vasodilator:* 2 mg/kg IV bolus; then 1 – 2 mg/kg/hr (doses > 5 mg/kg/hr not likely to be of additional benefit)	injection: 25 mg/ml
β-Adrenergic Blockers		
propranolol (Inderal)	*antihypertensive and antiarrhythmic:* PO: 0.25 mg/kg q 6 – 8 hr; increase dose daily as needed to control BP (maximum: 1 – 4 mg/kg) IV: 0.01 – 0.15 mg/kg q 6 hr	tablets: 10, 20, 40, 80 mg injection: 1 mg/ml
	thyrotoxicosis: initial dose 0.25 mg/kg PO q 6 hr; increase daily to maximum of 1 mg/kg PO q 6 hr as needed to control symptoms	
CNS Sympathetic Antagonists		
clonidine (Catapres)	*antihypertensive:* 3 – 5 μg/kg PO q 6 – 12 hr; increase dose for BP control (experimental; see text)	tablets: 0.1, 0.2 mg
methyldopa (Aldomet)	*antihypertensive:* PO: 2 – 3 mg/kg q 6 – 8 hr; increase dose as needed for control of BP (maximum 12 – 15 mg/kg/dose) IV: 5 – 10 mg/kg q 6 – 8 hr as required for BP control	tablets: 125, 250, 500 mg injection: 50 mg/ml
Calcium-channel Blockers		
nifedipine (Procardia)	*antihypertensive:* 0.25 – 0.50 mg/kg sublingual (experimental; see text)	capsules: 10 mg
verapamil (Calan, Isoptin)	*antiarrhythmic:* 0.1 – 0.2 mg/kg IV over 2 min; repeat dose if necessary	tablets: 80, 120 mg injection: 2.5 mg/ml
Renin – Angiotensin System Inhibitors		
captopril (Capoten)	*antihypertensive:* initial dose 0.5 mg/kg PO; maintenance doses range from 0.1 to 1.0 mg/kg PO q 6 – 12 hr as required for BP control (experimental; see text)	tablets: 25, 50, 100 mg

to result from a direct, positive inotropic action on the myocardium.[256] With hydralazine therapy, pulmonary vascular resistance tends to decrease in patients with left ventricular failure. In experimental animal studies of hypoxemic-induced pulmonary vasoconstriction, hydralazine-induced pulmonary vasodilation was inhibited by indomethacin pretreatment, suggesting that the vasodilator effect of hydralazine is mediated by prostaglandins.[439] Arterial pressure, heart rate, and ventricular filling pressures do not change in any consistent fashion, although tachycardia subsequent to hydralazine therapy is generally more common in patients with hypertension than in those with heart failure (Table 7–17).

Clinical Pharmacology. Attempts to describe the pharmacokinetics of hydralazine have been hampered by analytical difficulties due largely to instability of the drug and its metabolites.[426] Acetylator phenotype has no detectable effect on hydralazine pharmacokinetics after intravenous administration, but it does after oral dosing. Therefore, acetylator phenotype determines bioavailability but not the rate of systemic clearance of hydralazine. Slow acetylators have higher serum concentrations of hydralazine than rapid acetylators for a given oral dose. In adults, the half-lives range from 0.6 to 6 hours in normal individuals and from 2 to 6 hours in slow acetylators.[312] Significant hemodynamic effects of hydralazine have been observed as early as 5 minutes following IV administration, with the peak effect reached by 35 minutes.[194] Hydralazine was used successfully to control hypertension in one group of neonates.[184] Blood pressure was well controlled in the majority of infants receiving hydralazine alone or in combination with other antihypertensive drugs. In contrast, in another series, six infants with hypertension as a complication of umbilical arterial catheterization responded poorly to antihypertensive therapy that included hydralazine (0.3–1 mg/kg/dose) in combination with other medication.[302]

Fried and coauthors[238] reported marked improvement in clinical status following the administration of hydralazine in a 12-year-old child with cardiac failure due to adriamycin therapy. Linday and colleagues[270] observed no beneficial effect of hydralazine or phentolamine in infants and children with left-to-right shunts. The patients ranged in age from 3 months to 13 years; five had ventricular septal defects, one had an atrial septal defect, and one had a patent ductus arteriosus. The dose of hydralazine ranged from 0.15 to 0.30 mg/kg administered as a single dose IV over 3 minutes. Hydralazine produced an increase in both systemic and pulmonary blood flow, with the predominant increase occurring in pulmonary flow. Heart rate increased by only about 5% to 7% and aortic pressure decreased. The findings in this report

differ from those of Beekman and coworkers.[194] These investigators studied 7 infants (aged 2.5–11 mo) with large ventricular septal defects who were in congestive heart failure. Hydralazine 0.2 mg/kg administered as a bolus IV over 1 minute decreased systemic resistance, but pulmonary resistance remained unaffected. Systemic blood flow increased, and the left-to-right shunt decreased by 24%. These results are in general agreement with experimental animal studies (artificially created left-to-right shunt) that demonstrated reduced left-to-right shunting with afterload reduction.[204,335] The benefits of afterload reduction in neonates with left-to-right shunts are most likely when myocardial failure coexists with elevation of systemic resistance. Long-term hydralazine therapy for chronic heart failure in adults has had mixed success.[411,412,429]

Because potent vasodilation triggers activation of the peripheral sympathetic nervous system by way of the carotid and aortic baroreceptor reflexes, combination therapy with sympatholytic agents (e.g., propranolol, clonidine, phenoxybenzamine) has been recommended. The therapeutic rationale for such combinations is illustrated in Figure 7–13. The fact that these reflex responses directly oppose the desired antihypertensive result sought emphasizes the potential value of combination therapy. When hydralazine is used in combination with sympatholytic agents, the usual parenteral dose of this drug may be remarkably reduced (Table 7–18).

Therapeutic Indications. Hydralazine is an effective antihypertensive agent that should be considered a drug of choice in the treatment of *hypertension in infants.* The usual starting dose is 0.1 to 0.5 mg/kg given IV every 3 to 6 hours. The oral dose required is generally larger since the liver effectively clears the drug, thus preventing significant amounts from reaching the systemic circulation. When a change from IV to oral dosing is instituted, an increase of up to twice the effective IV dose may be necessary. Doses may be gradually increased every 2 to 3 days to achieve the desired antihypertensive effect, to a maximum dose of 2 mg/kg given every 6 hours (Table 7–18). Hydralazine should be used in combination with other antihypertensive agents[260] (see under Pharmacology); the dose of this agent necessary when used with propranolol or other β blockers will probably be substantially less (0.15 mg/kg/dose).[308] Hydralazine is not a drug of choice for treatment of hypertensive emergencies.

The use of hydralazine for *afterload reduction*

in infants with left-to-right intracardiac shunts is experimental. Whether the adult experience with hydralazine in the treatment of ventricular failure (secondary to septal defects, primary pulmonary hypertension, or tricuspid, mitral, pulmonary, or aortic regurgitation) has any application in the infant awaits further clinical and experimental laboratory investigation.[277,279,315,317]

Clinical Toxicology. A wide variety of side-effects have been observed in patients treated with hydralazine, and the incidence is high.[260] Many of the side-effects may be reduced or prevented by the concurrent administration of a β-adrenergic antagonist (Fig. 7–13).[198] In adults, headache, palpitation, anorexia, nausea, dizziness, and sweating are common; nasal congestion, flushing, lacrimation, conjunctivitis, paresthesias, edema, tremors, and muscle cramps occur less frequently. Drug fever, urticaria, skin rash, polyneuritis, gastrointestinal hemorrhage, anemia, agranulocytosis, and pancytopenia are rare, but when they do occur, hydralazine therapy must be stopped. About 10% to 20% of adult patients develop a lupus-like syndrome; the most prone are slow acetylators. This adverse reaction is reversible and is less likely to occur with use of lower doses of hydralazine. In neonates, hydralazine therapy has been associated with diarrhea and emesis and, in one case, temporary agranulocytosis.[184]

Minoxidil

Pharmacology. Minoxidil is a potent vasodilator used for the treatment of severe hypertension. At least 95% of a dose given PO (tablet or solution) is absorbed, with peak concentrations reached within 1 hour.[276] Nearly 90% of an administered dose is metabolized by the liver, primarily to minoxidil-O-glucuronide, which is subsequently excreted in the urine along with the remaining 10% or so of the dose as unmetabolized drug. There is some evidence that the major metabolite has antihypertensive activity. Dosage adjustment is not required in patients with renal disease.

Like diazoxide and hydralazine, minoxidil is a direct vasodilator of systemic arterioles. Both diazoxide and minoxidil have been demonstrated to block calcium uptake into vascular smooth muscle membranes; this mechanism is believed responsible for the vasodilating action.[276] The potent vasodilator effect results in the triggering of reflex sympathetic activity, causing release of renin and norepinephrine (see Fig. 7–13). Most of the increase in cardiac

rate and output produced by minoxidil can be suppressed by **propranolol. Clonidine** can also minimize the compensatory reflex effects of minoxidil.

Clinical Pharmacology. In adults the antihypertensive effect may occur within 4 hours and persist for 3 or 4 days. The plasma half-life in contrast, is about 4 hours. This disparity between the pharmacokinetics and pharmacodynamics is believed to be due at least in part to the drug's high-affinity binding to vascular smooth muscle and at other sites.[300] Ideal control of blood pressure in hypertensive infants and children occurs gradually over 1 to 3 weeks.[299,324,325] The hemodynamic effect of minoxidil in adult patients with heart failure is very similar to that of hydralazine. In the majority of patients with heart failure, minoxidil causes a marked reduction in systemic vascular resistance with a reflex increase in cardiac output and stroke volume; there is typically no increase in pulmonary or systemic venous pressure. In adults, pulmonary artery pressure and pulmonary vascular resistance remain unchanged. Experimentally, minoxidil has been shown to inhibit hypoxic pulmonary vasoconstriction.[402]

Therapeutic Indications. Treatment with minoxidil should be limited to patients with *moderate to severe hypertension* who are refractory to more conventional therapy. It is more effective as an antihypertensive than hydralazine, particularly in hypertensive pediatric patients with advanced renal disease.[325] The drug should be used in combination with β-blocking drugs and a diuretic to minimize dosage requirements.[219]

The usual starting dose is 0.1 to 0.2 mg/kg given PO every 12 to 24 hours as determined by the blood pressure response. The dose can be increased by 0.3 to 0.5 mg/kg each day until satisfactory control of blood pressure is achieved (maximum dose 5 mg/kg over a 24-hr period; see Table 7–18). There is only limited reported experience with minoxidil in infants, and therefore, the use of minoxidil in this age group should be considered experimental. However, it has been effectively employed in short-term and long-term management of childhood hypertension.[222,325]

Clinical Toxicology. A variety of toxicities have been associated with the use of minoxidil. Increased hair growth (hypertrichosis) is an unpleasant side-effect that occurs in almost all patients and has predisposed to poor compliance, particularly in female patients. Fluid retention is another frequent complication. Pericardial effusion has been reported in some patients, particularly those with uremia, collagen vascular disease, cardiac failure, or infections.[276] Pulmonary hypertension has also been noted,[191] but this finding may be related more to case selection than to a predilection. Hepatic, renal, hematologic, or CNS toxicity has not been reported.[300] Rebound hypertension following minoxidil withdrawal manifesting as hypertensive encephalopathy has been reported in three children; the concomitant administration of β-adrenergic blockers (propranolol) may have predisposed the patients to this phenomenon.[278]

Nitroglycerin

Pharmacology. Nitroglycerin and organic nitrates have a direct vasodilatory effect on vascular smooth muscle, primarily in large veins (capacitance vessels), with a lesser effect on arteriolar resistance vessels (Table 7–17). Nitroglycerin, as well as organic nitrates, has little effect on precapillary arteriolar sphincters but causes dilation of postcapillary vessels.[210] These hemodynamic effects are seen with IV, sublingual, and topical nitroglycerin. Isosorbide dinitrate has been shown to be pharmacologically active following IV, sublingual (or chewable), and PO administration. These drugs are metabolized in the liver and probably in many other tissues to mono and dinitro metabolites, which are inactive.[189] Much larger doses are required with the oral route than with sublingual administration because of liver metabolism. Whether liver disease alters metabolism of nitroglycerin and nitrates is unknown. The nitrates released by partial denitration may form methemoglobin, but the clinical significance of this phenomenon in patients receiving nitroglycerin has not been studied.[248]

Clinical Pharmacology. The half-life of nitroglycerin is between 2 and 4 minutes in adults.[189] The reported therapeutic blood concentrations range between 1 and 11 ng/ml, with the average level during therapy of 1 to 3 ng/ml. Nitroglycerin produces qualitatively similar hemodynamic effects in patients with both acute and chronic heart failure. Systemic and pulmonary vascular pressure reduction is a consistent finding. Pulmonary artery pressure and pulmonary vascular resistance tend to decrease in the majority of adult patients.[210,435] In adults, nitroglycerin produces a greater decrease in pulmonary capillary wedge pressure than that caused by nitroprusside.[188] Arterial pressure changes are minor, and systemic vascular resistance,

cardiac output, and stroke volume responses are variable. The hemodynamic effects of isosorbide dinitrate are similar to those of nitroglycerin. A vasoconstrictive effect has been noted on the splanchnic circulation.[234] Nitroglycerin does not exert any direct inotropic effect on the myocardium. A degree of tolerance to the effects of nitrates given PO and sublingually has been described, apparently the result of alterations at the receptor site.[183]

The effects of nitroglycerin given IV were studied by Benson and colleagues[195] in 10 children who had undergone hypothermic cardiopulmonary bypass. Although myocardial preload was adequate, some of the children were treated with volume expansion to maintain the left atrial pressure within pretreatment levels. Cardiac index increased significantly, being further increased by reestablishment of control preload levels. Total peripheral resistance decreased significantly, but mean arterial pressure and heart rate did not change throughout the study. These investigators concluded that vasodilator therapy with nitroglycerin, in conjunction with maintenance of filling pressure, can improve myocardial function significantly in children following intracardiac surgery.

Therapeutic Indications. The role of nitroglycerin therapy in neonates is unclear and remains experimental. However, in adults nitroglycerin is a valuable therapy for *congestive heart failure* associated with myocardial infarction or severe chronic heart failure with acute exacerbation.[189,331,416] The drug reduces pulmonary capillary wedge pressure and raises cardiac index and stroke volume. A small fall in mean arterial pressure may occur without evidence of serious compromise to coronary perfusion.[331] There is a wide variation in patient response, and a degree of tolerance to the effects of nitrates given PO and sublingually occurs. Nitroglycerin can cause relaxation of pulmonary vascular smooth muscle; in adults with severe congestive heart failure, this effect may result in a decrease in arterial PaO_2, suggesting an alteration in ventilation/perfusion balance.[301] Problems with toxic metabolites and rebound hypertension as seen with other vasodilating agents evidently do not occur with nitroglycerin. Whether nitroglycerin will be a useful vasodilator agent in infants remains to be established.

Nitroglycerin doses in children have not been established. Benson and colleagues[195] employed doses ranging from 0.4 to 60 μ/kg/min, with an average infusion rate of 20 μg/kg/min (Table 7–18). In adults, doses of nitroglycerin given IV that have demonstrated therapeutic success are usually less than 5 to 7 μg/kg/min.

Clinical Toxicology. The potent rapid-acting hemodynamic effects of nitroglycerin demand that it be used only under conditions of continuous hemodynamic monitoring. Nausea, vomiting, hypotension, hypoxemia, decreased cardiac output, and tachycardia have been reported. IV filters, plastic containers, and the IV administration sets commonly employed are known to decrease nitroglycerin concentration by as much as 80% (function of infusion rate, length of tubing exposure, and tubing material).[192]

Nitroprusside

Pharmacology. Sodium nitroprusside is a potent, direct-acting vasodilator that relaxes arteriolar and venous smooth muscle equally (Table 7–17). The chemical structure of nitroprusside is unusual; the molecule is an iron core surrounded by five cyanide groups and a nitroso moiety. The drug must be given by continuous IV infusion to achieve pharmacological effects on vascular smooth muscle. Nitroprusside is rapidly broken down to cyanide by nonenzymatic reactions involving free and intracellular hemoglobin and other molecules with free SH groups.[444] Some of the cyanide is subsequently metabolized to thiocyanate by the enzyme rhodanase. Thiocyanate is cleared very slowly by the kidney (half-life $\approx$ 4 days), which can account for some of the toxicity problem associated with prolonged nitroprusside therapy (see under Clinical Toxicology).

Nitroprusside has little effect on gastrointestinal or uterine smooth muscle (Table 7–17) and even less effect on the autonomic nervous system or CNS. Thus, the drug appears to be uniquely specific for effects on vascular smooth muscle.[295]

Clinical Pharmacology. Twenty children (aged 7–17 yr) with severe arterial hypertension of renal origin responded to nitroprusside administered IV within 1 to 20 minutes (average dose 1.4 μg/kg/min);[243] no undesirable effects were noted. Applebaum and colleagues[187] studied 16 infants ranging in age from 2 weeks to 17 months who had undergone intracardiac surgery performed with cardiopulmonary bypass and profound hypothermia; only patients with elevated mean arterial blood pressures were selected. Nitroprusside was infused at a rate sufficient to return the mean arterial blood pressure to approximately normal for age (2.5–12

μg/kg/min). Cardiac index increased from 17% to 41% of the control value in all but two patients; the greatest increases occurred in those patients given boluses of fluid to return atrial filling pressures to initial levels. Systemic and pulmonary vascular resistance decreased with the infusion of nitroprusside. Benzing and coworkers[196] observed similar effects in 11 children (aged 1–12 yr) who received nitroprusside because of low cardiac index and high systemic resistance following open heart surgery. Abbott and coauthors[182] reported a marked improvement in arterial oxygenation in a 3-kg (38-wk gestation) neonate with right-to-left shunting. Nitroprusside was infused at a dose of 2 to 5 μg/kg/min over a period of 120 hours. Blood gas values showed improvement within 30 seconds of initiation of the infusion, along with improvement in peripheral perfusion blood pressure and urine flow. No apparent side-effects were noted.

Dillon and colleagues[225] employed nitroprusside in six children and adults (aged 1–28 yr) who had severe congestive heart failure due to left ventricular disease. The initial dose was 0.5 μg/kg/min and was increased until a fall in mean arterial pressure of 5 to 10 mm Hg or evidence of substantial clinical improvement occurred. The final dosage ranged from 1.1 to 3.5 μg/kg/min (mean 2.3 μg/kg/min), which was infused continuously for 20 to 216 hours (mean 76 hr). Four of the six patients showed significant improvement, including a twofold increase in urine output. Serum thiocyanate levels ranged from 0.6 to 1.9 mg/dl. No adverse side-effects were observed.

In another study, nitroprusside was administered to 14 patients (aged 3 mo–16 yr) following cardiac surgery for repair of atrial septal defect, ventricular septal defect, tetralogy of Fallot, or mitral, aortic or pulmonary stenosis.[316] The nitroprusside infusion was started at 1 μg/kg/min and adjusted until the mean arterial systemic pressure showed a 10% fall; infusion rates ranged from 0.6 to 8.7 μg/kg/min. The systemic and pulmonary vascular indices fell, and the cardiac index increased significantly in these patients. No differences in response were identified when the results were evaluated for age or by postoperative pulmonary artery pressures. Subramanyam and coworkers[333] studied the effect of nitroprusside in 10 patients between the ages of 1 1/2 and 5 years with ventricular septal defect and congestive heart failure. The rate of nitroprusside infusion was adjusted until a 20% to 25% reduction in systemic arterial pressure was obtained. The average rate of infusion was 8 μg/kg/min over a 20-minute period. In patients with elevated left ventricular filling pressures, sodium nitroprusside infusion decreased pulmonary artery pressure and left ventricular filling pressure and decreased the left-to-right shunt. Patients without pulmonary artery hypertension showed an increase in the magnitude of the left-to-right shunt, suggesting that those most likely to benefit were patients with pulmonary arterial hypertension and elevated left ventricular filling pressures. The data indicate a direct pulmonary vasodilator effect of nitroprusside.

Stephenson and colleagues[328] studied the hemodynamic effects of nitroprusside and dopamine, alone and in combination, in 28 children (aged 3 mo – 16 yr) subsequent to intracardiac repair of various congenital heart lesions. With nitroprusside alone a greater fall occurred in pulmonary vascular resistance than in systemic vascular resistance. The greatest percentage of decrease in pulmonary vascular resistance occurred in patients with elevated pulmonary vascular resistances. Dopamine caused a significant increase in cardiac output and heart rate but no notable change in peripheral or pulmonary vascular resistance. When used together, nitroprusside and dopamine demonstrated mutually beneficial effects on cardiac index (13% increase), peripheral vascular resistance (23% decrease), and pulmonary vascular resistance (21% decrease).

In the study by Pierpont and coworkers[301] in adults with evidence of left ventricular failure, nitroprusside reduced pulmonary capillary pressure and increased cardiac output. In addition, PaO_2 decreased, and A-a gradient increased without a change in pulmonary mechanical function. Because of the increased cardiac output, calculated oxygen delivery was enhanced. These investigators concluded that nitroprusside causes an increase in blood flow to the lung by dilating all pulmonary vessels, including those perfusing poorly ventilated alveoli.

Therapeutic Indications. The immediate and pronounced reduction in systemic pressure produced by sodium nitroprusside makes it a drug of choice for the treatment of *hypertensive crisis.* The starting dose is 1 μg/kg/min, with subsequent adjustment based on clinical response (Table 7 – 18). Although as much as 400 μg/kg/min for short periods may be utilized to achieve the desired hypotensive effect,[295] the manufacturers' recommendation is not to exceed 10 μg/kg/min for more than 10 minutes. To avoid toxicity with more prolonged therapy,

the dose should not exceed 2 μg/kg/min (Table 7 – 18).[433]

Sodium nitroprusside therapy for treatment of *severe congestive heart failure through afterload reduction* has been effective in selected cases in infants, children, and adults. In some patients, the balance between arteriolar and venous vasodilation may be more valuable than the more selective vasodilation produced by agents such as hydralazine (arteriolar) or nitroglycerin (venous). Nitroprusside vasodilation therapy in infants should be considered experimental therapy. Nitroprusside is sensitive to light, necessitating precautions to prevent photochemical degradation from occurring during the infusion process; as much as 50% of the initial nitroprusside material can be degraded by 6 hours.[237]

For safe employment, continuous blood pressure measurements, along with other measurements to detect evidence of toxicity (metabolic acidosis, increasing venous Po_2, serum lactate and serum thiocyanate levels on a daily basis) are indicated in all patients.[444]

Clinical Toxicology. The primary acute toxicity of nitroprusside is associated with its marked vasodilator activity. With continued nitroprusside infusion, major toxicities can develop due to the liberation of free cyanide from degradation of the nitroprusside molecule in the blood, which occurs through nonenzymatic reduction processes involving hemoglobin and molecules with free SH groups.[433] About 60 to 70% of the released cyanide binds to cytochrome oxidase in the tissue, and the remainder is bound to RBCs in the blood. The RBC-bound cyanide is subsequently metabolized by the enzyme rhodanase in the liver and kidneys.[444] The rate of this reaction is limited by the quantity of endogenous sulfur available. Concentrations of RBC cyanide of about 40 nmol/ml of RBCs are associated with increased base deficit and an elevated mixed venous blood oxygen content. At levels of 200 to 250 nmol/ml, severe clinical symptoms develop (increasing tolerance to antihypertensive effects even with increasing dose, tachycardia, dyspnea, vomiting, headache, dizziness, loss of consciousness); and concentrations greater than 400 – 500 nmol/ml are considered lethal. Other principal manifestations of nitroprusside toxicity are fatigue, nausea, and anorexia, progressing to disorientation and psychotic behavior and muscle spasms.[295] These effects are attributable to accumulation of thiocyanate. Thiocyanate is removed almost exclusively by the kidney, with a half-life of approximately 4 to 7 days in patients with normal renal function. Toxic symptoms with thiocyanate begin to appear at plasma levels of 5 to 10 mg/dl, and fatalities have been reported with levels of 20 mg/dl. Thus, nitroprusside poisoning can develop as a consequence of gross disturbances in the usual rapid conversion of cyanide to thiocyanate (hepatic or renal failure) or from accumulation of thiocyanate.[221] Because of the potential for accumulation of cyanide and thiocyanate, long-term therapy with doses > 2 μg/kg/min of nitroprusside should be avoided. Daily monitoring for clinical and laboratory evidence of cyanide poisoning, including measurements of RBC cyanide or serum thiocyanate levels, is indicated, particularly with protracted use. It is important to appreciate that thiocyanate levels do not accurately reflect cyanide intoxication.

Combined administration of thiosulfate with sodium nitroprusside has been proposed as a means of reducing the high levels of cyanide that otherwise develop with continued administration of nitroprusside.[433] The infusion consists of a mixture of nitroprusside and thiosulfate in a ratio of about 1 : 10 by weight. The use of hydroxocobalamin as prophylaxis against cyanide toxicity is based on the belief that it combines with cyanide to form cyanocobalamin (vitamin B_{12}).[408] The use of hydroxocobalamin cannot be recommended, however, because of the very large quantities required to decrease cyanide levels and because its therapeutic value has not been established.

α-Adrenergic Blockers

Prazosin

Pharmacology. Prazosin is a postsynaptic α_1-adrenergic blocker. The drug is well-absorbed from the gastrointestinal tract, producing peak plasma concentrations within 2 to 3 hours after administration. The drug is extensively metabolized in the liver mainly by O-dealkylation and glucuronide conjugation. The metabolites have little or no pharmacologic activity. Over 90% of the administered dose is eliminated via biliary secretion and subsequent fecal excretion.

Despite early reports of direct vasodilation, prazosin appears to possess only α_1-adrenergic blocking capability.[244] The drug selectively inhibits postsynaptic (vascular) α_1-adrenergic receptors. Since prazosin does not block presynaptic α_2 receptors, tachycardia and renin release do not occur when the drug is used in hypertension; this finding also reflects the drug's combined action on both arterial and venous beds. In this respect, prazosin resembles the direct-acting vasodilator compounds such as nitroprusside.

Prazosin appears to lack any CNS, ganglionic, vagal, β receptor, or reflex sympathetic effects.[244] Prazosin can inhibit the enzyme phosphodiesterase, being more potent in this effect than either theophylline or hydralazine; it is doubtful, however, that concentrations required for phosphodiesterase inhibition can be achieved with therapeutic doses.

Clinical Pharmacology. The half-life of prazosin in adults ranges between 2 1/2 and 4 hours, although it may be as long as 6 hours in patients in severe chronic congestive heart failure.[209] Following PO administration of prazosin to hypertensive patients, arterial blood pressure, arterial resistance, and venous tone (afterload and preload) decrease, with little change in right atrial pressure, cardiac output, or heart rate. In patients with congestive heart failure, prazosin reduces pulmonary artery and pulmonary capillary wedge pressures and arterial and right atrial pressures and increases cardiac output, stroke volume, and stroke work.[210] Five patients ranging in age from 1 to 28 years were given oral prazosin following improvement in congestive heart failure subsequent to nitroprusside therapy.[225] A dose of 25 μg/kg/min given PO every 6 hours sustained the improvement in congestive heart failure initiated by nitroprusside, but one patient developed orthostatic hypotension with the first dose. Plasma levels for prazosin of 12.6 ± 1.2 ng/ml are equated with therapeutic effects.[410] The development of tachyphylaxis due to the hemodynamic effects of prazosin in patients with chronic congestive heart failure has been reported, although considerable controversy exists in the literature.[410,428]

Therapeutic Indications. Oral prazosin is effective in the *treatment of hypertension* in adults as well as children, whether utilized alone or as an adjunct to other antihypertensive medications. There have been very few published reports on the use of prazosin in infants. The adverse effects associated with hydralazine (marked increase in heart rate, vascular headaches, flushing) are uncommon with prazosin therapy. However, in most reported clinical experiences, prazosin has been used as an adjunct to one of the more established antihypertensive drugs.

A more recent application of the preload- and afterload-reducing properties of prazosin has been in the treatment of *severe congestive heart failure*[231] (Table 7-16). The effectiveness of oral prazosin makes it attractive for long-term support of patients with severe congestive heart failure.

Initial therapy should begin with a low dose to avoid the marked reduction in arterial pressure that can occur with the onset of therapy. In adults the recommended initial oral dose is 20 to 30 μg/kg, with an increase in dose at 6-hour intervals until satisfactory clinical response is achieved. Dillon and coworkers[225] employed doses of up to 25 μg/kg given every 6 hours.

The use of prazosin in infants is experimental, and extreme caution should be exercised in the initial dosing. The dose recommended in Table 7-18 (5 μg/kg) is an estimate based on a conservative extrapolation of adult experience and on results with the limited use in pediatric patients. Since the drug is highly metabolized by the liver, including via glucuronidation, the required dosing interval may be longer than the 6-hour period used for adults; frequent blood pressure measurements will assist in this determination. Renal dysfunction does not appear to necessitate an alteration in dosage.

Clinical Toxicology. The side-effects associated with chronic use of prazosin are mild and rarely require discontinuation of the drug. The major side-effect is the first-dose phenomenon characterized by manifestations of hypotension.[207]

Tolazoline

Pharmacology. Although classified as an α blocker, tolazoline has a wide range of pharmacologic actions, including adrenergic blockade and sympathomimetic, antihypertensive, antihistaminic, histaminic, and cholinergic effects (Table 7-19). Tolazoline is completely absorbed following both parenteral and oral administration. However, rapid renal excretion, coupled with a slow rate of absorption from the gastrointestinal tract, precludes the development of therapeutic activity when the PO route is used. The drug is excreted unchanged in the urine, with about 30% of administered dose excreted per hour.[206] The short duration of action of tolazoline is related to its rapid renal clearance and the small amount of drug distributed outside the vascular compartment. The important role of renal tubular secretion in the elimination of the drug suggests that accumulation may occur with impaired renal function.

The IV administration of tolazoline produces cardiac stimulation and vasodilation. The

Table 7 – 19. PHARMACOLOGIC ACTIONS OF TOLAZOLINE

Cardiac, Vascular Smooth Muscle, GI
sympathomimetic effect: cardiac stimulation (increased cardiac output)
parasympathomimetic effect: gastrointestinal tract stimulation (hyperperistalsis)
"histamine-like" effect: gastrointestinal tract stimulation (secretion of acid and pepsin) and peripheral vasodilation
direct vasodilation: major effect
α-adrenergic blockade:[a] peripheral vasodilation (at high doses)
Pulmonary Vascular Resistance (PVR)
H_1, H_2, and direct (?) vasodilating action: decrease PVR
α-adrenergic agonist activity (?) (at high doses): increase PVR

[a] Although classified as in α-adrenergic blocking agent, tolazoline produces very little α-adrenergic blockade at usual therapeutic doses.

blood pressure response will therefore be determined by the relative contributions of these two effects. The cardiac effects of tolazoline can be blocked by H_2 (histamine) blockers[341] but not by β blockers. The peripheral vasodilation is predominantly due to a direct action of tolazoline on vascular smooth muscle. Only at very high doses does the drug have an α-adrenergic blockade effect. The stimulatory activity of tolazoline on gastric acid secretion is also mediated through H_2 receptors. It is not clear whether the H_2 receptor activation is intrinsic to the tolazoline molecule or is mediated by release of endogenous histamine.[342] In newborn lambs, Goetzman and Milstein[242] demonstrated that the pulmonary vasodilator action of tolazoline is mediated via histamine receptors, since blockade of both H_1 and H_2 receptors was required to inhibit the vasodilator response to tolazoline. They concluded that the α-adrenergic blocking action of tolazoline is not involved in its lowering of elevated pulmonary vascular resistance.

Clinical Pharmacology. There is considerable clinical experience with tolazoline in the management of pulmonary hypertension and persistent fetal circulation in neonates (Table 7-20). The first pharmacokinetic studies of tolazoline in neonates were reported by Monin and coauthors:[288] Following a bolus dose of 2 mg/kg and a continuous infusion of 2 mg/kg/hr, the plasma levels of tolazoline increased progressively during the first 12 hours of therapy and then remained relatively stable. Plasma concentrations ranged between 5 and 20 μg/ml. Plasma disappearance of the drug followed a

Table 7–20. SUMMARY OF CLINICAL STUDIES OF TOLAZOLINE USE IN NEONATES

Author(s) of Published Study[a]	Drug(s) Employed[b]	Dosage Employed	Study Group No. of Patients	Diagnosis[c]	Patients Improved with TZ Treatment (%)	Survival Rate (%)	Comments
Cotton[215]	TZ	2 mg/kg bolus	5	HMD	100	?	no criteria provided for improvement; no control groups
Korones and Eyal[261]	TZ	2 mg/kg bolus	5	PFC	100	100	no control groups
Goetzman et al[241]	TZ / P, M	1–2 mg/kg bolus, 1–2 mg/kg hr	46 / 10, 36	RV, RDS: HMD, MA, Pn, others	80, 60	70, 36	response to TZ noted in 16 infants of < 30-wk gestation; volume expansion used for ↓ BP; no control groups
Levin et al[268]	TZ, C	1 mg/kg bolus (infused in 1 patient)	11 (only 4 given TZ)	PPHN	50	91	not clear which patients received TZ vs. C; no control groups
Purohit et al[309]	TZ	2 mg/kg bolus, 2 mg/kg/hr	27 / 13, 8, 3, 1, 1	HMD, PFC, MA, CDH, Pn	89 (13/13)(8/8)(1/3)(1/1)(1/2)	63	volume expansion used for ↓ BP; no control groups
Moodie et al[289]	TZ	1–3 mg/kg bolus (infused in 3 patients)	12 / 6, 2, 2, 2	HMD, CDH, MA, ?	92	45	volume expansion used for ↓ BP; no control groups
Peckham and Fox[297]	TZ	2 mg/kg over 10 min, 1–2 mg/kg/hr	10 (only 6 given TZ)	PPHN	33 (↑ PaO$_2$), 50 (↓ PAP)	80	variable response to TZ; continuous pulmonary pressure measured; hyperventilation effective; no control groups
McIntosh and Walters[284]	TZ	1–2 mg/kg bolus	20	HMD	50	55	volume expansion used for ↓ BP; no control groups
Stevenson et al[330]	TZ / DA / P, M	2 mg/kg bolus, 1–10 mg/kg/hr, 5–20 μg/kg/min	39 / 15, 15, 89	HMD, MA, ?	66, 87, 44	46	volume expansion and DA used for ↓ BP; no control groups
Johnson et al[254]	TZ	2 mg/kg bolus, 2–5 mg/kg/hr	16 / 4, 4, 8	HMD, MA, Pn	50	44	no control groups; responders to TZ had increased LPEP/LVET and RPEP/RVET ratios
Stevens et al[329]	TZ	1–2 mg/kg bolus, 1–2 mg/kg/hr	57 / 47	HMD, MA, PFC, Sep, others	60	57	volume expansion or DA used for ↓ BP; patients given DA or T not specified; no control groups; 80% of survivors normal at 1 yr

Study[a]	Drugs[b]	Dose	n	Diagnosis[c]			Comments
Ein et al[230]	DA, T		10	CDH	57	20	variety of drugs used
	TZ IP, NP, DA, CPZ, ACh	1 mg/kg bolus (repeated as needed)	19 (8 enrolled for drug study)	CDH	38 (3/8)	63 (5/8)	retrospective control group utilized
Bloss et al[199]	TZ P	2 mg/kg bolus, 1–6 mg/kg/hr	12	CDH	33	33	no control groups; TZ effect variable and unpredictable; DA: effective
Drummond	TZ DA	2 mg/kg/hr 7–28 μg/kg/min	6/3, 1, 1, 1	PH, Pn, MA, HL	variable	67	
Sumner and Frank[334]	TZ	1–2 mg/kg bolus, 1–2 mg/kg/hr	10	CDH	100	100	included only patients with potential for adequate oxygenation
Jones et al[255]	TZ	1–2 mg/kg bolus, 1–2 mg/kg/hr	15/6, 4, 5	CD, VSD, TA, APVD	100	53	older infants and children (2 mo–10 yr) with episodes of severe pulmonary vasoconstriction after surgical correction
Monin et al[288]	TZ	2 mg/kg bolus, 2 mg/kg/hr	26/12, 4, 4, 1, 4, 1	HMD, MA, Sep, PFC, CD, ?	90	40	$T\frac{1}{2}$ for TZ: 7.2 ± 3.4 hr (range 3–33); plasma concentration: 5–20 μg/ml (range); nonresponders: pH < 7.2

a Listed in order of publication; see References at end of chapter.

b Drugs given in addition to tolazoline (TZ): P = pancuronium; M = morphine; C = curare; DA = dopamine; T = tubocurarine; IP = isoproterenol; NP = nitroprusside; CPZ = chlorpromazine; ACh = acetylcholine.

c HMD = hyaline membrane disease; PFC = persistent fetal circulation; PV = pulmonary vasospasm; RDS = respiratory distress syndrome; MA = meconium aspiration, Pn = pneumonia; PPHN = persistent pulmonary hypertension, newborn; CDH = congenital diaphragmatic hernia; Sep = sepsis; PH = pulmonary hypertension; HL = hypoplastic lung; CD = cardiac disease; VSD = ventricular septal defect; TA = truncus arteriosus; APVD = anomalous pulmonary venous drainage.

one-compartment model, with an elimination half-life of 7.7 ± 3.4 hours (range $3.3-33$ hr). All patients except one had a plasma half-life between 3 and 10 hours. This mean half-life is approximately four times greater than the 2-hour adult value. No correlation was found between tolazoline half-life and gestational age or postnatal age, or between changes in oxygenation and plasma level of the drug. Monin's group concluded that infants who respond do so rapidly and that the steady-state drug levels achieved with the doses employed (at 12 hr) exceeded those necessary for pharmacologic effect.

The first published report of the use of tolazoline in neonates appeared in 1965.[215] Since that time tolazoline has been used for a variety of neonatal diseases (Table 7-20). Goetzman and coworkers[241] examined 46 newborns with evidence of increased pulmonary artery pressure at catheterization and PaO_2 levels that remained unchanged despite mechanical ventilation and administration of 100% oxygen; there was an increase in PaO_2 following tolazoline administration in 63% of these neonates. Stevens and coauthors[329] reported their experience with tolazoline therapy in 10 patients with diaphragmatic hernia and 47 neonates with multiple causes of persistent fetal circulation, including hyaline membrane disease, meconium aspiration, idiopathic persistent fetal circulation, and sepsis. They observed an increase in PaO_2 (> 20 mm Hg by 1 hr) in 28 infants (59%). This response rate is similar to that previously reported (63%). Drummond and coworkers[228] measured pulmonary artery pressure in five infants with pulmonary hypertension utilizing an indwelling pulmonary artery catheter. Separate and combined effects of hyperventilation and administration of dopamine and tolazoline produced variable responses. Tolazoline failed to selectively lower pulmonary pressure in any infant; the decrease in systemic arterial pressure during drug therapy equaled or exceeded pulmonary pressure. They concluded that diverse biochemical or perhaps anatomic derangements contribute to abnormal pulmonary vasospasm, and that specific pharmacologic therapy must be individualized for each patient according to the underlying disease.

Most of the early investigations noted the importance of prevention and treatment of systemic hypotension subsequent to tolazoline therapy. A variety of approaches have been used in an attempt to prevent the systemic hypotension, including volume expansion and the administration of dopamine or epinephrine.

Other measures employed to improve the pulmonary vasodilating effects of tolazoline have included the induction of muscular paralysis[329] and blood pH manipulation (e.g., via hyperventilation).[228]

Variability in individual patient response to tolazoline has been ascribed to a variety of causes, including the multiple pharmacologic effects of the drug, the amount of endogenous histamine stores present in the lung and in the circulation of the infant with respiratory problems,[227,228] the status of the pulmonary vascular resistance in the neonate at the time of tolazoline administration,[272] and the presence of irreversible structural abnormalities of the pulmonary vascular bed.[230,334]

The difficulties associated with the employment of tolazoline therapy in newborns with diaphragmatic hernia are compounded by the presence of pulmonary hypoplasia. The most lethal combination of abnormalities would be elevated pulmonary vascular resistance, persistent fetal circulation, and pulmonary hypoplasia. Ein and coworkers[230] used tolazoline and a variety of other agents in an attempt to control and regulate the right-to-left shunt present postoperatively in neonates born with diaphragmatic hernia. They emphasize the frustration of attempting to regulate a vascular bed (pulmonary) with fixed high resistance while having to deal with the problem of existing anatomic shunts (intracardiac as well as patent ductus arteriosus) that allow dilution of oxygenated blood.

In one of the earliest studies on the employment of tolazoline as a pulmonary vasodilator in children, Grover and coworkers[247] infused 1 mg/kg of tolazoline into the pulmonary artery of normal persons (aged 6-45 yr) and of 8 children with isolated ventricular septal defects (aged 5 mo-12 yr). In normal persons, cardiac output remained unchanged, and pulmonary and systemic arterial pressures decreased by only 2 to 4 mm Hg. An obvious reduction in pulmonary and systemic vascular resistance occurred only in patients with increased cardiac output. In patients with increased pulmonary vascular resistance associated with ventricular septal defect, tolazoline produced an average reduction in mean pulmonary artery pressure of 28 mm Hg versus 9 mm Hg in systemic pressure. Pulmonary blood flow increased in six patients and modestly increased in two others as a result of shunting left to right across the ventricular septal defect. The calculated pulmonary vascular resistance decreased in all patients with isolated ventricular septal defect.

Jones and colleagues[255] employed tolazoline to treat severe episodes of pulmonary hypertension in 15 children (aged 2–10 yr) immediately following open-heart surgery for various congenital heart lesions (Table 7–20). All 15 patients responded to tolazoline treatment (1–2 mg/kg bolus dose into the pulmonary artery followed by continuous infusion of 1–2 mg/kg/hr). Continuous measurement of pulmonary artery pressure postoperatively demonstrated episodic elevations of pulmonary artery pressure, implicating pulmonary vasoconstriction as a cause of profound clinical deterioration. Tolazoline was highly effective in the management of these acute pulmonary vasoconstrictive episodes. Serious adverse outcomes following attempts to lower pulmonary vascular resistance postoperatively in 3 children with congenital cardiac defects have been reported.[420] Paradoxical pulmonary hypertension was theorized to have been responsible, possibly as a consequence of a drug-induced reflex response resulting in an increase in pulmonary vascular resistance.

The overall efficacy of tolazoline as a pulmonary vasodilator is impossible to judge, since in the reports of clinical experience, a variety of ailments were treated, and complete hemodynamic measurements are often lacking; moreover, additional measures, including the use of inotropic drugs, neuromuscular paralysis, and volume expansion, were frequently employed. It could be argued that patients who appear to respond maximally to therapeutic manipulations are those maintained at an optimal status of cardiac output with volume expansion and inotropic therapy combined with specific efforts to decrease pulmonary vascular resistance. The effect of tolazoline has been reported to be directly proportional to the extent of elevation of pulmonary vascular resistance. Using echocardiography, Johnson and colleagues[254] observed that infants who responded to tolazoline had echocardiographic evidence of elevated right ventricular afterload. Lock and co-workers[272] calculated that even in the absence of an ideal change in ratio of pulmonary to systemic resistance (decrease in pulmonary resistance relative to systemic), an increase in cardiac output occurring in conjunction with tolazoline therapy can improve arterial oxygenation (Fig. 7–14).

Therapeutic Indications. Tolazoline has been employed with mixed success in patients who are manifesting *elevations of pulmonary vascular resistance or pressure with or without a right-to-left shunt.* In these cases, tolazoline therapy must be accompanied by adequate ventilatory support. In addition, extreme care and vigorous monitoring is required for the prevention and treatment of systemic hypotension, which will aggravate a right-to-left shunt condition. Volume expansion and the co-infusion of dopamine or dobutamine are recommended to minimize this problem.[409]

The dosages employed in studies with tolazoline in neonates are presented in Table 7–20. The usual initial dose is 2 mg/kg given as a bolus IV, followed by an infusion of 1 to 2 mg/kg/hr. Although higher doses have been employed,

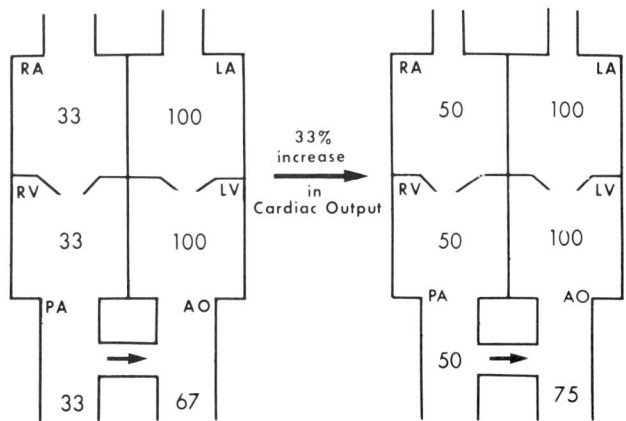

Figure 7–14. Changes in oxygenation induced by increasing cardiac output in a hypothetical case of neonatal right-to-left shunting: $\dot{V}O_2 = 200$ ml/min/m²; systemic index = 3.0 l/min/m²; pulmonary index = 1.5 l/min/m²; hemoglobin (Hgb) = 15 g/dl. With a 33% increase in cardiac output (both systemic and pulmonary), there is a rise in systemic arterial O_2 saturation from 67% to 75%. *RA* and *LA* = right and left atria; *RV* and *LV* = right and left ventricles; *PA* = pulmonary artery; *AD* = aorta. (From Lock JE et al: J Pediatr 95:600, 1979.)

they apparently do not produce significant further pulmonary vasodilation, and other modes of therapy should be considered. Optimal therapy can be achieved with constant monitoring of pulmonary artery pressures and by the delivery of the drug directly into the pulmonary artery distal to the ductus.[255] When administered by means of a peripheral IV system, the drug may preferentially cross into the systemic circulation by means of a right-to-left shunt. The consequence is peripheral vasodilation rather than pulmonary vasodilation, since tolazoline is not a specific vasodilator of the pulmonary vascular bed. Preferential reduction of systemic vascular resistance will aggravate right-to-left shunting and further exaggerate hypoxemia. The importance of selective administration of tolazoline into the pulmonary artery and for the maintenance of systemic pressures is obvious.

Clinical Toxicology. A variety of side-effects may be seen with tolazoline therapy (Table 7–21). Stevens and colleagues[329] noted that many, if not all, of the reported side-effects of the drug could be ascribed to the underlying disease state. As is evident in Table 7–21, the incidence of any reported complication associated with tolazoline use varies widely; this inconsistency may reflect the variety of diseases present in patients receiving tolazoline. Nonetheless, certain adverse reactions, such as gastrointestinal disturbances (histamine release) and hypotension (vasodilation of peripheral vascular smooth muscle), are specific for the drug. In general, the clinical significance of tolazoline side-effects is often less than that of the existing illness. The development of hypotension, however, is a definite exception, because it can jeopardize the drug's efficacy. Cohen and coworkers[211] concluded from long-term follow-up studies that the morbidity in survivors of respiratory failure treated with tolazoline is related not to the use of the drug but to the degree of perinatal asphyxia.

Tolazoline vs. Other Agents in Correction of Pulmonary Perfusion Abnormalities. Reducing pulmonary resistance is an important strategy for the treatment of a variety of respiratory and cardiac illnesses in the neonate. The dynamic changes that occur in the pulmonary vascular bed with the onset of breathing are remarkable and complex.[252] When this delicate and complex process is asynchronous or perturbed by disease,[311,313,316] pharmacologic restoration of perfusion (pulmonary vasodilation, ductal patency manipulation, increased cardiac output) can be life-saving. Therefore, it is important that progress be made in identifying and understanding disease processes that involve a significant component of abnormal pulmonary hemodynamics (e.g., increased pulmonary vascular resistance, ineffective pulmonary perfusion or hypoperfusion, pulmonary vascular abnormalities), and the appropriate drug(s) for correction of the problem. Unfortunately, the difficulty of extrapolating from animal-model experiments, as emphasized by many investigators, complicates acquisition of this critical information.

Tolazoline is without question effective in reversing pulmonary perfusion problems in neonates. The large number of factors that can alter pulmonary blood flow, including endogenous substances (Table 7–22), however, suggests that more than one drug will be useful in approaching these problems. Some currently available drugs that can alter pulmonary resistance (blood flow) are listed in Table 7–23; any one of these drugs, which differ in pharmacologic action and locus of effect (preload, afterload), could have a major impact on a variety of causes of abnormal pulmonary hemodynamics. Clearly, failure with tolazoline therapy should not terminate pharmacologic manipulation in any neonate with serious compromise of pulmonary perfusion.

β-Adrenergic Blockers

The β-adrenergic blocking agents are important drugs for management of certain cardiovascular disorders, including hypertension and cardiac arrhythmias.[214] Propranolol was the first clinically successful β-adrenergic antagonist; compared with some of the newer agents of

---

Table 7–21. TOLAZOLINE SIDE-EFFECTS

Side-effects	Estimated Occurrence in Various Studies[a] (% of Patients)
erythema	100, 60, 0
oliguria	42, 30, 15, 11, 0
hypotension	67, 50, 20, 19, 0
thrombocytopenia	45, 31, 6, 4, 0
gastric bleeding	55, 33, 12, 8, 4, 0
increased gastric secretion	100, 36, 0
gastrointestinal perforation	10, 0
pulmonary hemorrhage	12, 2, 0

[a] Reported by Goetzman et al,[241] Peckham and Fox,[297] Purohit et al,[309] Stevenson et al,[330] Bloss et al,[199] Johnson et al,[254] Stevens et al,[329] Matsuo et al.[280]

Table 7–22. PULMONARY VASCULAR EFFECTS OF VARIOUS ENDOGENOUS AGENTS AND FACTORS[a]

Effect	Agent/Factor
vasoconstriction	angiotensin
	histamine: H_1[b]
	hypoxemia
	leukotrienes
	$PGF_{2\alpha}$
	serotonin
	catecholamines: norepinephrine, epinephrine
vasodilation	acetylcholine
	β-agonists
	bradykinin
	histamine-H_2 (H_1 in newborn)[b]
	oxygen
	PGI_2, PGE_2
	surfactant

[a] Species variation may be an important consideration; much of this information was derived from experimental animal studies.

[b] Activation of either H_1 or H_2 receptors produces vasodilation in the newborn lung. Histamine itself is a direct constrictor but an indirect vasodilator of the pulmonary vascular bed in the neonate.[273]

this class, it is highly potent, but its activity is nonselective (Table 7–24).

Beta receptors are present in the heart, in selected vascular beds, including the coronary arteries, and in renal vessels, as well as in bronchial smooth muscle and the uterus; they also mediate liver and muscle glucose release and insulin secretion. The β receptors have been subclassified according to their responses to sympathomimetic amines: β_1 receptors are those responsible for lipolysis and cardiac stimulation; those controlling bronchodilation, catecholamine-induced insulin release, glucose mobilization, and vasodilation are classified as β_2 receptors.[422]

The mechanism by which β-adrenergic blocking agents lower blood pressure (i.e., antihypertensive action) is unclear.[320,427] The generally accepted hypothesis is a major reduction in sympathetic tone, but the site of action for this effect remains in debate. A central or peripheral effect or an indirect effect through afferent pathways are all possible sites for antihypertensive action. It is possible that more than one of these sites of action is involved, and that a multiplicity of mechanisms is responsible for the gradual development of an antihypertensive effect.[320] Results from studies involving β blockers with differing pharmacologic actions indicate the nonessentiality of cardiodepression, renin suppression, and blockade of central β receptors.[427] These observations implicate blockade of presynaptic β receptors as the cause of the vasodilatory and antihypertensive effects of these drugs, a theory supported by the observations on the changes in concentrations of norepinephrine in plasma.

Table 7–23. MECHANISM OF ACTION AND HEMODYNAMIC EFFECTS OF VARIOUS VASODILATOR AGENTS

Vasodilator	Mode of Action	Hemodynamic Effect[a]		
		Arterial (Afterload)	Venous (Preload)	Pulmonary Resistance
tolazoline	H_1, H_2 receptor activation (sympathomimetic, parasympathomimetic, direct)	↓	↓	↓
chlorpromazine[b]	α receptor blockade	↓	↓	↓
PGE_1, PGE_2[c]	direct	(↓)	(↓)	↓
hydralazine	direct	↓		↓
isoproterenol	β receptor activation	↓		↓
nifedipine	Ca^{2+} channel blocker	↓		↓
nitroglycerine	direct		↓	↓
nitroprusside	direct	↓	↓	↓
prazosin	α receptor blockade	↓	↓	↓

[a] Responses presented are summary estimations of the potential each drug has for producing reduction (↓) in hemodynamic parameters. Individual patients may or may not demonstrate these effects. Therefore, rigorous monitoring (ideally, invasive) of cardiovascular status before and subsequent to initiation of drug therapy is important.

[b] Data from studies by Borman[203] and Larsson[265] and their coworkers. For other drugs, see individual discussions in the text.

[c] The effects of PGE are dependent on access to the systemic vascular bed. Ordinarily, most of the dose would be destroyed by metabolism in the lung. (See Chap. 9.) For other drugs, see individual discussions in the text.

Table 7–24. PHARMACOLOGIC PROPERTIES OF β-ADRENERGIC BLOCKING AGENTS

Drug	Serum Half-life (T½:hr)	β₁ Receptor Activation (heart)	β₂ Receptor Activation (lung, kidney, peripheral vascular)	Intrinsic Sympatho-mimetic Activity	Membrane Activity (quinidine-type local anesthetic)
propranolol	3–6	+	+	0	++
nadolol	20	+	+	0	0
metoprolol	3–4	+	0	0	+
practolol	5–10	+	0	++	0

++ = extremely active; + = active; 0 = little or no effect. This information is largely from studies in adults and may or may not relate to infants.

Propranolol

Pharmacology. Propranolol is a highly potent, nonselective β-adrenergic blocking agent with no intrinsic sympathomimetic activity (Table 7–24). The drug is completely absorbed following PO administration but is susceptible to high first-pass clearance by the liver, so that only about one third of the dose reaches the systemic circulation. Clearance of propranolol by the liver diminishes with repeated administration, probably as a consequence of the reduced cardiac output caused by the drug itself.[292] Protein binding of propranolol in infants (70%) is significantly less than in adults (90%). The liver metabolizes virtually all of the propranolol dose prior to its excretion in the urine. At least four of the more than 18 metabolites appear to retain β-adrenergic blocking activity.[442] A relatively short half-life of one active metabolite, 4-hydroxypropranolol, ordinarily reduces its concentration below therapeutic levels. Other metabolites include glucuronide conjugates of propranolol and 4-hydroxypropranolol, and α-naphthoxylactic acid. The variability in plasma concentrations observed among adult patients following identical oral dosing may relate to differences in hepatic metabolism, hepatic blood flow, or plasma protein binding.[292] Silber and colleagues[442] have demonstrated in adults that the elimination of propranolol is saturable at doses from 40 to 320 mg/day.

At least three pharmacologic mechanisms have been proposed for the effect of propranolol in the management of hypertension.[306] Propranolol reduces cardiac output rapidly after administration. This effect on cardiac output, along with a reduction in heart rate, is more dramatic under conditions of increased demand and sympathetic tone. There is also an impairment of the release of norepinephrine from adrenergic nerve terminals following sympathetic nerve stimulation, which possibly contributes to the antihypertensive effects of the drug. Blockade of β receptors in the kidney can be expected to influence renal blood flow and glomerular filtration rate by intrarenal mechanisms, as well as by reduction in cardiac output and blood pressure.[340] These effects can significantly reduce elevated plasma renin activity by inhibition of secretion of renin by the kidney and may contribute to the drug's antihypertensive action.

Propranolol can inhibit the vasodepressor and vasodilator effects of isoproterenol and augment the pressor effects of epinephrine as a consequence of β-blocking activity. In contrast, the β-adrenergic blockade by propranolol does not inhibit the renal vasodilation induced by dopamine (because this effect is mediated by dopaminergic receptors). Vasodilation due to nitroglycerin and other direct-acting vasodilators is also unaffected by propranolol.

In the heart, most of the antiarrhythmic effects of propranolol are due to β-adrenergic blocking action: Although a resting heart rate is only slightly affected, the acceleration of sinus rate during exercise or as a result of S-A node disease can be significantly reduced.[332] Propranolol can also reduce automaticity in the Purkinje system. Excitability and threshold of the atria or ventricles are not significantly influenced by the drug, although it does reverse the action of catecholamines in lowering the threshold for fibrillation. Propranolol does cause a substantial increase in the effective refractory period of the A-V node owing to its β-blocking action; this action is the basis for its major use as an antiarrhythmic drug (see under Antiarrhythmic Agents).

The β blockers are widely used in adults to treat coronary artery disease. The reduction in ventricular contractivity and heart rate, in addition to a reduced afterload, increases coronary filling time (diastole). Redistribution of blood flow from normal to ischemic areas of the myocardium is also regarded as an important mechanism for the therapeutic employment of β receptor agonists for mid- and long-range cardioprotective therapy.[226] These beneficial aspects of β blockade are sometimes offset by the decrease in cardiac contractility, increased ventricular size, and filling pressure, wall tension, and end-diastolic pressure.

In the lung, adrenergic bronchodilation is mediated by β_2 receptors. As a consequence, propranolol consistently increases airway resistance. This effect is potentially dangerous in patients with hyperactive airways (e.g., asthmatics). Although propranolol has little effect on pulmonary vascular resistance under conditions of normoxia, it enhances hypoxic vasoconstriction, suggesting that enhanced β receptor responsiveness occurs during hypoxia and that the ratio of α to β activity in vivo participates in maintenance of pulmonary vascular homeostasis.[274]

Propranolol and other β-adrenergic blocking agents modify carbohydrate and lipid metabolism and inhibit glycogenolysis in the heart and skeletal muscle. The ability of sympathomimetic amines or of the sympathetic nervous system to increase plasma-free fatty acids or to mobilize fat from lipid tissue is inhibited by β-adrenergic blocking drugs. Although propranolol does not affect plasma glucose or insulin concentrations in normal individuals, it does slow the recovery of glucose concentration following insulin administration. These effects are due to the inhibition of glycogenolytic and lipolytic actions of endogenous catecholamines released as a consequence of the development of hypoglycemia. Therefore, β-adrenergic blocking agents must be used with care in patients susceptible to hypoglycemia, particularly patients receiving insulin. Patients with basal hyperinsulinemia due to insulinoma have shown a correction of insulin levels and a reduction in hypoglycemic attacks with propranolol therapy.[200] The in vitro inhibition of platelet aggregation and thromboxane B_2 formation by propranolol requires concentrations that are not achieved in vivo, thus explaining the absence of these effects in clinical use.[441]

Clinical Pharmacology. The half-life of propranolol in normal adults depends on the route and duration of drug administration but rarely exceeds 6 hours.[292] Values for plasma half-life of propranolol in neonates have not been re-

ported. In infants over 7 months of age the half-life of the drug appears to be similar to that in adults.[404] Half-life in adult patients with liver disease is variable, ranging from normal to as long as 35 hours in patients with cirrhosis, but is relatively unaffected by renal dysfunction. Serum concentrations of propranolol ranging from 50 to 100 ng/ml are associated with reduction of plasma renin activity, reduction of elevated blood pressure, and antiarrhythmic activity.[292] Shand and colleagues[322] observed plasma propranolol levels of approximately 25 ng/ml in four children (aged 8 wk–3 yr) 1 1/2 to 3 hours after a dose of 0.57 mg/kg PO. A dose of 25 mg/m² (of body surface) produced plasma levels of approximately 50 ng/ml. In infants, Ponce and coworkers[303] observed peak serum levels between 20 and 115 ng/ml 2 hours following a dose of 1 mg/kg given PO. Two infants with Down's syndrome had 2-hour values of 211 and 467 ng/ml, respectively, suggesting a genetically linked defect in propranolol degradation or excretion. Boerth[201] observed plasma propranolol levels between 40 and 310 ng/ml with doses of 1.8 to 16 mg/kg/day administered to infants and children (aged 7 mo–16 yr) with hypertension.

In Boerth's series,[201] blood pressure fell to less than 90 mm Hg in all 11 infants and children with hypertension (diastolic >98 mm Hg) following propranolol therapy (1.8–16 mg/kg/day, route and interval not specified). In the study by Potter and colleagues,[305] eight of 10 children with hypertension associated with a renal transplant and high plasma renin activity responded to propranolol therapy (0.25 to 2 mg/kg/dose q 6 hr, route not specified). Gillette and coworkers[240] used oral propranolol for treatment of idiopathic hypertrophic subaortic stenosis (IHSS), paroxysmal hypoxemic spells, or arrhythmias in 64 infants and children (aged 1 day–13.6 yr). Propranolol was considered successful in 47 of 64 subjects (doses ranged from 0.25 to 0.75 mg/kg q 6 hr). In IHSS, symptoms regressed in all six patients so affected. Paroxysmal hypoxemic spells were obliterated in 13 of 17 patients, and arrhythmias were controlled in 28 of 41 patients. Griswold and coauthors[246] reported successful treatment of hypertension in nine patients (aged 5–16 yr) by propranolol (0.15–1.6 mg/kg q 6 hr); no correlation was found between pretreatment plasma renin activity and dose of drug required to lower blood pressure. Adelman[184] employed propranolol alone or in combination with methyldopa or hydralazine in the treatment of three neonates with hypertension; good control of blood pressure was noted without complications.

Propranolol has also been widely used for the management of neonatal thyrotoxicosis. Most of the reports are individual cases managed with other agents in addition to propranolol.[296,298,326] Smith and Howard[326] employed an oral dose of propranolol (1 mg/kg/dose) and observed a significant reduction in heart and respiratory rate within 24 hours; gradual withdrawal of therapy was instituted at 4 weeks of age. Pemberton and colleagues[298] observed similar results in one infant treated at 3 weeks of age with 0.5 mg (2.7-kg birth weight) given PO 4 times daily; the dose was increased over a 2-week period to 8 mg given 4 times daily. Propranolol plasma level in this patient was 89 ng/ml 2 hours after an 8-mg dose. Pearl and Chambers[296] began with a 0.5-mg dose 3 times daily PO, increasing to 7 mg 4 times daily, to control signs and symptoms of thyrotoxicosis in a premature infant (1.6-kg birth weight, gestation 34 wk). The propranolol was discontinued at 53 days of age without complications.

Therapeutic Indications. One of the earliest uses of propranolol in pediatric patients was for *palliation of tetralogy of Fallot.*[216,217,332,249,303] Although some inconsistent results have been observed, overall frequency of hypoxic spells is reduced.[303] The use of propranolol for *treatment of hypertension* occurred later, primarily because of concern about reduction in cardiac contractility, the unclear mechanism of action, lack of immediate onset of action, and general increase in peripheral resistance subsequent to the antihypertensive effect.[306] Propranolol has also been utilized in infants and children for the *management of cardiac arrhythmias,*[350] and in *neonatal thyrotoxicosis.*[239,326]

Propranolol is used either alone as the sole antihypertensive drug or in combination with direct vasodilators (Fig. 7–13). Patients with high-renin hypertension are most likely to respond to propranolol.[308] The drug is equally effective whether given IV or PO; however, marked differences in dose requirements exist for these administration routes (see Table 7–18). The initial oral dose should be 0.25 mg/kg given every 6 to 8 hours, with frequent observation of blood pressure and heart rate response to this initial dosing; subsequent doses can be increased as needed on a daily basis up to a maximum of 1 to 4 mg/kg per dose. The IV dose is 0.01–0.15 mg/kg, given every 6 hours. Owing to slow rates of hepatic metabolism, some patients require dosing only once or twice daily. Monitoring of blood pressure is helpful in establishing the appropriate dosing interval. Caution must be exercised with the initiation of therapy, as the most dramatic change in the sympathetic environment of the heart takes place when treatment is started. Therefore, the initial starting dose should be small, with subsequent increases in dose as necessary for control of the hypertension. Dosage adjustment does not appear to be necessary with renal insufficiency.[233]

The antiarrhythmic properties of propranolol have lead to its use in a wide variety of cardiac arrhythmias. Its greatest success appears to be in the treatment of digitalis-resistant supraventricular tachycardia.[363] The oral dose requirements may be as high as 3 to 4 mg/kg per dose given every 6 hours; see Antiarrhythmic Agents later in the chapter for additional details.

The use of propranolol in the management of neonatal thyrotoxicosis remains controversial.[239] There is little question that propranolol should not be used alone in the treatment of neonatal thyrotoxicosis. Whether controlling the β-adrenergic related effects of thyrotoxicosis results in benefit to the neonate remains unestablished. The dose requirements for control of symptoms of thyrotoxicosis appear to vary widely among patients. The recommended initial oral dose is 0.25 mg/kg given every 6 hours, increasing daily to a maximum of 1 mg/kg per dose. Newman and coauthors[291] appropriately comment that propranolol may merely control the signs and symptoms of hyperthyroidism (tachycardia), leaving the patient with inadequate circulatory support (nutrition) to meet the hypermetabolic demands, which go on unaltered. Other signs and symptoms of hypermetabolism and hypertension are controlled only with the addition of iodides and propylthiouracil.[440] In all circumstances, continuous cardiac monitoring is mandatory.

Clinical Toxicology. Propranolol toxicity is an extension of the β-adrenergic blocking action. Episodes of bradycardia, increase in airway resistance, and augmentation of the hypoglycemic action of insulin have all been reported.[245,422] Two important adverse effects due to β-adrenergic blockade that can be avoided by careful attention to patient selection are heart failure and increase in airway resistance. Rarely, propranolol can significantly diminish cardiac output. Patients with left ventricular insufficiency should not be given β-blocking drugs without prior administration of digoxin and diuretics. If the heart failure is uncontrolled, β-blocking drugs should be avoided.[306]

There is no evidence that the direct membrane effects of the β blockers (Table 7-24) contribute significantly to the development of heart failure. The greatest danger for precipitation of heart failure appears at the start of therapy. The rationale for starting therapy with small doses is therefore obvious. All nonselective β-adrenergic receptor blocking drugs increase airway resistance, particularly in asthmatic patients. *Propranolol therapy is contraindicated in asthmatics.* Glycogenolysis is controlled in part by β-adrenergic receptors; therefore, β-adrenergic receptor blockade can interfere with this mechanism for increasing blood sugar. Hypoglycemia has been reported in infants born to mothers given propranolol during pregnancy (see Chapter 11) and in diabetics receiving insulin therapy.

A withdrawal syndrome has been associated with sudden cessation of propranolol therapy.[442] Patients receiving the drug for therapy of hypertension may have a life-threatening hypertensive crisis appearing within hours to 1 to 2 days after the drug is abruptly discontinued. Nervousness, sweating, and tachycardia may preceed the onset of acute hypertension. If hypertensive therapy with propranolol is to be discontinued, it should be done gradually.

Propranolol can cause A-V dissociation and cardiac arrest in patients with preexisting partial heart block due to digitalis or other factors. It is of note, however, that the inotropic action of digitalis is not prevented by propranolol.

CNS Sympathetic Antagonists

The central nervous system (CNS) plays an important role in regulating the activity of the peripheral sympathetic nervous system. This interaction is complex and incompletely understood. The cortex, as well as regions in the brain stem (hypothalamus, nucleus tractus solitarii), is involved in the central sympathetic regulation of cardiovascular activity and blood pressure. Clonidine and methyldopa are two antihypertensive agents whose activity is attributed to inhibition of the outflow of sympathetic activity from the CNS.

Clonidine

Pharmacology. Clonidine is closely related chemically to tolazoline. When clonidine is administered orally to adults, the bioavailability is about 75%. The maximum antihypertensive ef-

fect, occurring between 2 and 4 hours after oral dosing, correlates well with peak plasma levels at 1.5 to 5 hours.[250] The drug distributes widely to all tissues, the highest drug levels being reached in the liver, kidney, and spleen. About 40% to 60% of the drug is eliminated unchanged by the kidneys.[220] A late increase in declining plasma levels and a nonlinear relationship between dose and absolute plasma concentrations have been attributed to enterohepatic recirculation of clonidine.[190]

Clonidine has many diverse pharmacologic actions.[250] Its antihypertensive action is believed to originate from a stimulation of α-adrenergic receptors in the CNS, which results in diminished efferent sympathetic neuronal vasoconstrictor tone in the heart, kidneys, and peripheral vasculature.[250] The initial increase in blood pressure observed in some patients is believed to result from the peripheral α-adrenergic stimulation produced by the drug; this increase is seen only following IV administration, not after oral dosing. Other effects on the CNS resemble those produced by chlorpromazine (sedation, decreased spontaneous motor activity, reduction in body temperature). The central action of clonidine also results in suppression of the level of circulating plasma renin. Renal vascular resistance decreases, and renal blood flow is maintained despite lowered blood pressure.

Clinical Pharmacology. In adults the drug is rapidly distributed but slowly eliminated from the body. The average elimination half-life was originally reported to be 8 1/2 hours,[220] but new analytic methods indicate a plasma half-life of 20 to 24 hours.[190] Reduction in blood pressure by clonidine is sustained and correlates with decreases in circulating catecholamines and heart rate.[336] Cardiac output, renal blood flow, glomerular filtration rate, plasma renin activity, and plasma aldosterone generally remain unchanged. There are no reports dealing with the pharmacokinetics of clonidine in infants.

Therapeutic Indications. Clonidine is an effective *antihypertensive agent* that can be used alone or in combination with other therapy. Dosage recommendations are given in Table 7-18. In patients with renal failure, the dosing interval may need to be extended in order to prevent accumulation of toxic levels of drug and metabolites.[287] Its use in infants must be considered experimental.

Clonidine has recently been successfully employed in the management of major symptoms of *neonatal narcotic withdrawal.*[415] The effective dose was 0.5 μg/kg, given PO every 6 hours.

Additional discussion of this use can be found in Chapter 11.

Clinical Toxicology. The major side-effects associated with clonidine therapy are drowsiness and dry mucous membranes (incidence > 40%). A large number of other adverse effects have been reported, but the incidence of most is less than 1%.[250] Rebound hypertensive crisis has occurred with either gradual or abrupt withdrawal.[332]

Methyldopa

Pharmacology. About 25% of the administered dose of methyldopa is absorbed following PO administration, although considerable variability (9–50%) has been reported.[263] Methyldopa is less than 15% protein-bound, and the volume of distribution is 0.6 l/kg.[432] The rate of elimination of methyldopa from plasma in adults is about 2 hours, with about 50% of the clearance occurring by way of renal excretion. The major metabolite is a sulfate conjugate. There is no evidence that dosage regimens require adjustment with significant renal or hepatic dysfunction, although high serum levels of metabolites (methylnorepinephrine and methyldopamine) have been reported in patients with renal insufficiency.[287] Methyldopa and its metabolites can interfere with standard chemical analyses for catecholamines.

The major antihypertensive action of methyldopa is a result of effects in the CNS, although peripheral mechanisms may play a minor role. The earlier impressions regarding the mechanism of action of methyldopa have undergone considerable revision.[287] The major CNS effect of methyldopa occurs as a result of a metabolite of methyldopa, alpha-methylnorepinephrine, which stimulates central α-adrenergic receptors, resulting in inhibition of central sympathetic outflow. Alpha-methylnorepinephrine also is formed in the peripheral circulation, where it acts as a vasoconstrictor, weaker than norepinephrine, in the vascular bed. The hemodynamic effect of methyldopa is a reduction in blood pressure and total peripheral resistance; cardiac output and renal blood flow remain largely unchanged. Plasma renin activity decreases in hyperreninemic patients, although this action is not a major contributor to the antihypertensive action of methyldopa.

Clinical Pharmacology. The plasma half-life of methyldopa in adults (1–2 hr) is shorter than the duration of its antihypertensive action.[432] Reported half-life values in neonates exposed to methyldopa in utero range from 9 to 20 hours.[419] Although methyldopa has been used in pediatric patients, most of the published experience is anecdotal. Adelman[184] utilized methyldopa in combination with hydralazine for the management of hypertension in five neonates. Some of the infants were obviously sedated by the drug.

Therapeutic Indications. Methyldopa is used as an *adjunct to other antihypertensive agents* for chronic blood pressure control. The usual starting dose is 2 to 3 mg/kg given PO every 6 to 8 hours. The dose may be increased as required for blood pressure control to a maximum of 12 to 15 mg/kg per dose. The IV dose is 5 to 10 mg/kg given every 6 to 8 hours, as required for blood pressure control (Table 7–18). Patients with renal failure may require reduced dosage to prevent accumulation of toxic metabolites in the blood, which can lead to significant side-effects.[287]

Clinical Toxicology. The major adverse effect of methyldopa is sedation. In adults, other undesirable CNS side-effects include vertigo, extrapyramidal signs, nightmares, and psychic depression. Retention of water and salt with edema occur with methyldopa therapy, as with the use of many other antihypertensive agents. Methyldopa-induced bradycardia is apparently less pronounced than that caused by clonidine.

More unique side-effects attributed to methyldopa include drug fever, which can be severe and suggestive of sepsis. Elevation of hepatic enzymes and the appearance of jaundice have also been observed. Up to 25% of adult patients receiving large doses of methyldopa for prolonged periods (6 mo) may develop positive direct Coombs' test.[251] The drug should be discontinued if there is an associated hemolytic process. Sudden withdrawal of the drug has resulted in rebound hypertensive crisis; this phenomenon appears with less frequency than that observed with clonidine.

Calcium-Channel Blockers

Drugs that alter the rate of entry of calcium into cells are useful in a number of cardiovascular disorders. These drugs are called **calcium-channel blockers** (other terms used include calcium-entry blockers, calcium antagonists, and slow channel blockers). The mechanism of action of these drugs involves interruption of the role of calcium in muscle contraction and in electrical excitation; several recent articles review these subjects.[205,267,290,448] Basically, calcium plays a key role in generation of action potentials and in coupling of excitation and contraction. The action potential is initiated by a fast inward sodium current (depolarization), followed by a slower inward current (plateau phase) due largely to calcium influx. The inward current of calcium triggers the release of sequestered intracellular calcium, which binds to a regulatory protein, troponin. Troponin activates tropomyosin, thus allowing the force-generating interaction between actin and myosin to occur. There are differences between myocardium and vascular smooth muscle in the regulatory sequence, although the role of calcium influx is similar.

Figures 7–15 and 7–16 outline the role and regulation of calcium in vascular smooth muscle and in the myoplasma of the myocardium, respectively. Calcium channels consist of macromolecular proteins that transverse the lipid bilayer membrane of the sarcolemma (inner layer of the cell membrane). They selectively permit calcium ions to move from one side of the sarcolemma to the other. It is important to recognize that considerable controversy continues to exist with respect to regulation of calcium movement and the exact mechanism(s) of action of the calcium-channel blockers.[417,448] The fact that the molecular structures of the

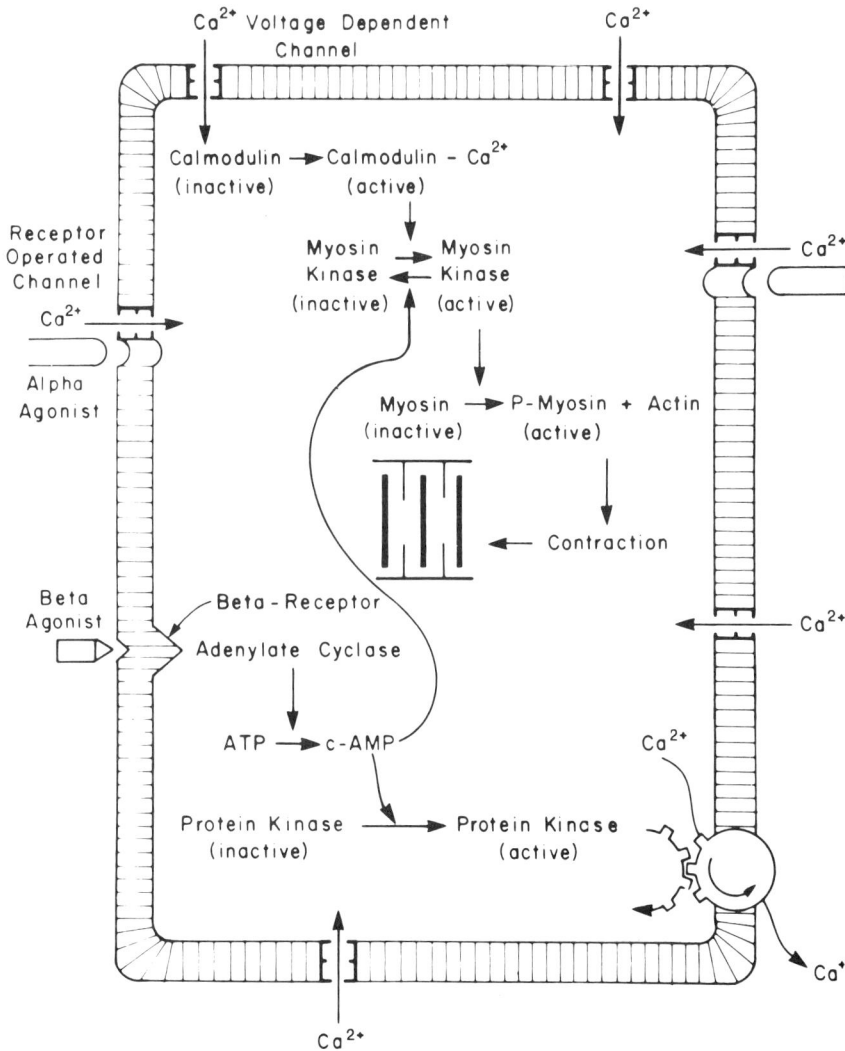

Figure 7–15. Schematic representation of the role of calcium in vascular smooth muscle. Calcium (Ca^{2+}) can enter the cell through voltage-dependent channels that are vulnerable to inhibition by the calcium-channel blockers. Additional receptor-operated Ca^{2+} channels are thought to be recruited as a consequence of activation of α-adrenergic receptors in the sarcolemma. Activation of β receptors results in a reduction of intracellular $[Ca^{2+}]$ through two possible mechanisms, both dependent on cyclic AMP. P = phosphorylated. (From Braunwald E: N Engl J Med 307:1618, 1982.)

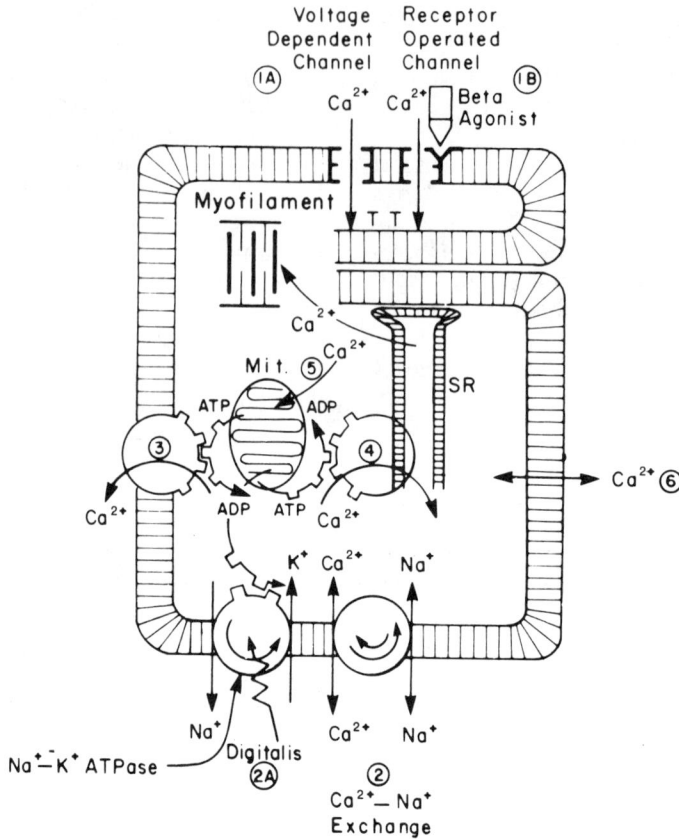

Figure 7-16. Proposed mechanisms for regulation of calcium concentration, [Ca^{2+}], in the myoplasm of the myocardium. TT = transverse tubule; SR = sarcoplasmic reticulum; Mit = mitochondrion.)
(1A) and (1B), Slow Ca^{2+} channels provide inward calcium movement; (2), Na$^+$–Ca^{2+} exchange system moves Ca^{2+} out of the cell after each contraction or inward if intracellular [Na$^+$] is elevated (inhibition of Na$^+$–K$^+$ ATPase by digoxin, (2A)); (3), Ca^{2+} extrusion from cell by ATPase-dependent system in the sarcolemma; (4), Ca^{2+}-stimulated magnesium ATPase in membrane of SR transports and sequesters Ca^{2+} into SR lumen (this accounts for the more rapid contraction and relaxation of cardiac muscle exposed to catecholamines); (5), uptake and release of Ca^{2+} by other intracellular structures such as mitochondria; (6), selective movement of Ca^{2+} along its concentration gradient, which can be affected by a variety of ionophores. Ca^{2+} can also be bound by intracellular proteins. The site of action of the calcium-channel blockers are the slow Ca^{2+} channels ((1A)), although other sites of action have been proposed. (From Braunwald E: N Engl J Med 307:1618, 1982.)

calcium-channel blockers differ (Fig. 7-17) is most consistent with differing modes and sites of action rather than a specific receptor site analogous to that for adrenergic blockers. With respect to vascular smooth muscle, the arteriolar bed is far more sensitive than the venous bed to the action of the calcium-channel blockers (Table 7-17). Therefore, the predominant effect is afterload reduction. The coronary arterial bed also appears to be particularly sensitive to the action of calcium-channel blockers. The pulmonary, hepatic, femoral, renal, cerebral, and superior mesenteric arterial beds are all responsive to the vasodilating properties of the calcium-channel blockers. Bronchial smooth muscle and esophageal muscle relaxation have been observed with administration of calcium channel blockers.[405] The cardiovascular effects

of these agents have been employed effectively in a variety of conditions (Table 7-25).

Nifedipine

Pharmacology. Orally administered nifedipine is nearly completely absorbed (90%) and undergoes extensive metabolism by the liver.[421] The metabolites exhibit no pharmacologic activity. The drug is 90% bound to albumin. Preparations of nifedipine for IV administration are not commercially available, and the drug is highly unstable when exposed to light. Rapid absorption from buccal mucosa has been found clinically useful. The drug appears in the plasma within 20 minutes, and peak concentrations in adults are reached by 1 to 2 hours. Urinary excretion accounts for 70% to 80% of

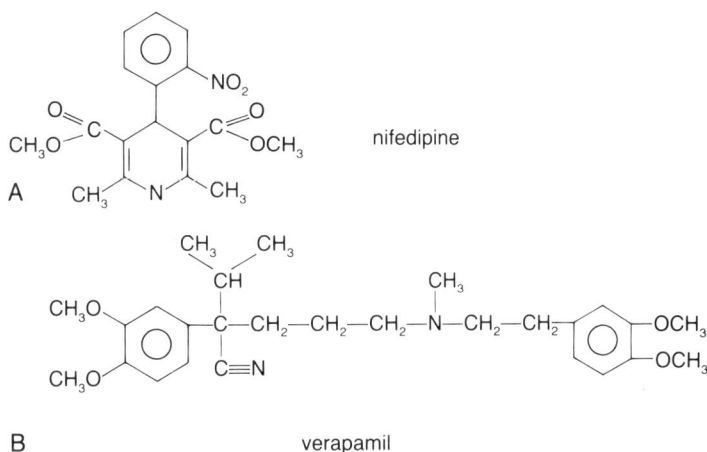

Figure 7-17. Chemical structures of calcium-channel blockers: nifedipine (*A*) and verapamil (*B*).

the drug elimination. The mechanism of action of nifedipine in vascular smooth muscle (Fig. 7-15) and in myocardium (Fig. 7-16) is believed to involve actual "plugging" of the Ca^{2+} channels,[205] although intracellular sites of effect may exist as well.

Clinical Pharmacology. There are no reports dealing with the use of nifedipine in infants. Dilmen and coworkers[407] studied the acute antihypertensive effect of nifedipine given sublingually (0.25-0.50 mg/kg) to 21 children (8 to 16 yr) with a variety of underlying illnesses. Systolic and diastolic blood pressure was reduced (28% and 23%, respectively) by 30 min and the antihypertensive effect persisted for 6 hr. Heart rate increased (108 ± 9 to 117 ± 9 beats/min), and cutaneous flushing was observed in 4 patients, but postural hypotension did not occur. In adults, the half-life after PO administration is 10 hours, and the disappearance pattern follows multicompartment pharmacokinetics. Maximum plasma concentrations range between 60 and 170 ng/ml with oral doses of 20 to 60 mg in adults.[400]

The major therapeutic use of nifedipine is for the treatment of angina, myocardial ischemia and infarction, and systemic and pulmonary hypertension. Its use in angina is based on an increase in myocardial oxygen supply via an increase in coronary blood flow along with a decrease in myocardial oxygen demand due to afterload reduction. Nifedipine has not demonstrated clinical usefulness as an antiarrhythmic, in contrast to verapamil. The potential advantages for the use of nifedipine in hypertension relate to the ability to induce coronary and cerebral artery dilation along with ventricular relaxation and improved subendocardial perfusion.[205] The potent afterload reduction makes nifedipine potentially useful in the treatment of congestive heart failure, particularly that related to hypertension and aortic or mitral regurgitation and in patients with congestive cardiomyopathy.[281] Camerini and coauthors[208] and De Feyter and colleagues[406] reported a significant fall in pulmonary and systemic vascular resistance in adult patients with severe pulmonary hypertension. Simonneau and coworkers[323] observed significant lessening of hypoxic pulmonary vasoconstriction in adult patients with chronic air flow obstruction and acute respiratory failure; they noted a significant reduction in pulmonary resistance without deleterious effects on arterial oxygenation. Similar findings have been reported in experimental studies in adult and neonatal animals.[402,436] Nifedipine has also been shown to inhibit exercise-induced and histamine-induced bronchospasm in children and adults.[401,434,447] No bronchodilator effect was observed to occur in nonstimulated asthmatic or normal subjects

Table 7-25. CURRENT THERAPEUTIC USES OF CALCIUM-CHANNEL BLOCKERS[a]

Clinical Problem	Drug(s) Employed
angina	nifedipine, verapamil
acute myocardial infarction	nifedipine, verapamil
myocardial injury (surgical)	nifedipine, verapamil
system hypertension (chronic, acute emergency)	nifedipine, verapamil
pulmonary hypertension	nifedipine
congestive heart failure	nifedipine
artrial arrhythmias	verapamil (only drug useful)
asthma (exercise-induced)	nifedipine, verapamil

[a] These therapeutic uses have been reported in studies in adults; some are considered experimental.

with the administration of nifedipine. The use of nifedipine for hypertensive emergencies appears to be successful, although still experimental.[213]

Therapeutic Indications. The use of nifedipine in neonates remains experimental. Nifedipine appears to be a promising agent for the *treatment of hypertension,* for *afterload reduction in myocardial failure,* and potentially for *reduction of elevated pulmonary resistance.* The capability of nifedipine to reduce bronchospasms induced by histamine, coupled with the interference with hypoxemia-induced pulmonary vasoconstriction, may prove useful in the management of chronic lung disease in infants. No dosing information is available for infants. In children doses of 0.25 to 0.50 mg/kg given sublingually have been successful in reducing blood pressure without significant complications.[407] In adults, the usual starting dose is 10 to 20 mg given 3 to 6 times daily.

Clinical Toxicology. Nifedipine has been well tolerated in adults. The overall incidence of side-effects is about 20%. The most frequent adverse effects include dizziness, edema, gastrointestinal distress, headache, flushing or paresthesias, palpitation, nervousness, and weakness.[425] Caution should be exercised in combining β blockers with nifedipine because of the possibility of acute congestive heart failure and serious hypotension.

Verapamil

Pharmacology. The chemical structure of verapamil differs strikingly from nifedipine; yet they both possess calcium-channel blocking activity (Fig. 7–17). Verapamil is nearly completely absorbed after PO administration (>90%) but undergoes extensive first-pass metabolism in the liver. The estimated bioavailability of an oral dose is 20% to 50%.[235,421] The metabolites of verapamil have little pharmacologic activity and are excreted by the kidneys (70% of dose); only 3% of the dose is excreted unchanged. Verapamil is extensively bound to albumin (90%). Approximately 70% of the administered dose is excreted in the urine. The onset of activity is observed within 20 to 30 minutes of PO administration, with the peak effect occurring at 1 to 2 hours.

Verapamil is similar in pharmacologic activity to nifedipine. In contrast to nifedipine, however, the calcium-blocking activity of verapamil is a function of the frequency of muscular contraction. Since both verapamil and β blockers exert a negative inotropic effect and depress automaticity and conduction, this combination may be hazardous in patients with preexisting left ventricular dysfunction and in those with impaired function of the S-A or A-V node.[205] Verapamil, in contrast to nifedipine, is useful in the control of arrhythmias associated with atrial disease, mitral valve prolapse, or certain forms of digitalis intoxication. The blocking effect of verapamil on A-V conduction is believed to be the mechanism through which it affects supraventricular tachycardia (nodal-reentrant tachycardia) and ventricular response in atrial flutter and fibrillation.

Clinical Pharmacology. Plasma disappearance after oral administration of verapamil shows a biexponential decline with an early distribution phase of approximately 30 minutes and an elimination-phase half-life of 3 to 8 hours.[421] The average half-life in adults is 6.3 ± 4 hours; clearance is 13.3 ± 7.7 mg/min/kg; and steady-state volume of distribution is 4.3 ± 1.3 l/kg.[267] In patients with cirrhosis, the elimination half-life increases to approximately 14 hours (twice that of normal patients).[327]

Therapeutic Indications. The use of verapamil in infants is experimental. The therapeutic indications for verapamil in adults are similar to those of nifedipine. The use of verapamil as an *antiarrhythmic agent* for atrial fibrillation and flutter, and for paroxysmal supraventricular tachycardia (recurrent A-V nodal–reentrant tachycardia) is reviewed under Antiarrhythmic Agents later in the chapter.

The recommended dose is 0.1 to 0.2 mg/kg given IV over 2 minutes; this dose can be repeated for control of the arrhythmia (Table 7–18). Verapamil has been used for the treatment of supraventricular tachycardia in pediatric patients.[367] Normal sinus rhythm is established following a dose of 0.25 mg/kg given IV over a 10-minute period, followed by oral therapy, 3 mg/kg every 8 hours. It is recommended that in patients with liver disease, IV doses be reduced to one half the usual dose, and that the oral dose be decreased to one fifth the usual dose.[327] Dosage adjustments for chronic renal failure have apparently not been determined.

Clinical Toxicology. The incidence of side-effects of verapamil in adult patients is approximately 10%, with 1% of the patients requiring discontinuation of the drug.[425] With IV administration, headache, dizziness, and hypotension were among the more common complaints. Life-threatening bradycardia and hypotension have been reported in neonates receiving intravenous verapamil (0.1 mg/kg).[437] Complete heart block and ventricular asystole have been reported with concomitant use of verapamil and IV β blockers; their negative inotropic effects evidently are not merely additive but are mutually enhancing.[368] Verapamil should not be used in patients with hypotension, low cardiac output, or second- or third-degree A-V block.[304] Intravenous calcium has been effective in reversing toxic cardiovascular reactions to verapamil therapy[431] (see Antiarrhythmia section).

Renin – Angiotensin System Inhibitors

The importance of the renin–angiotensin system in the regulation of circulation and blood pressure has been under investigation for a number of years. In summary, renin, a proteolytic enzyme secreted by the juxtaglomerular (J-G) apparatus of the kidney, acts on the renin substrate that is produced by the liver to form angiotensin I. Angiotensin-converting enzyme (ACE) catalyzes the conversion of the inactive angiotensin I to angiotensin II. Angiotensin II has several very important actions: It causes contraction of vascular smooth muscle, which raises blood pressure; stimulates aldosterone production, which causes sodium and water

retention and potassium excretion; and acts directly on the kidney to cause sodium and water retention.[186] The actions of angiotensin II are blocked by inhibition of ACE activity, which prevents the conversion of angiotensin I to angiotensin II (Fig. 7–18).

Captopril

Pharmacology. Captopril is a potent, relatively specific competitive inhibitor of ACE. Captopril is rapidly absorbed after PO administration, with peak blood levels occurring within 30 to 90 minutes. Approximately 75% of the administered dose is absorbed, but food in the gastrointestinal tract reduces absorption by 30% to 40%. The drug distributes rapidly to most tissues, with the exception of the CNS; about 30% in blood is protein bound.[338]

Captopril is rapidly metabolized, with about 60% of administered dose appearing in the urine as metabolites within 24 hours; the remaining 40% is excreted in the urine unchanged. The plasma concentration of captopril correlates closely with endogenous creatinine clearance. Therefore, the dose must be reduced in patients with renal impairment.

The inhibition of ACE not only results in a

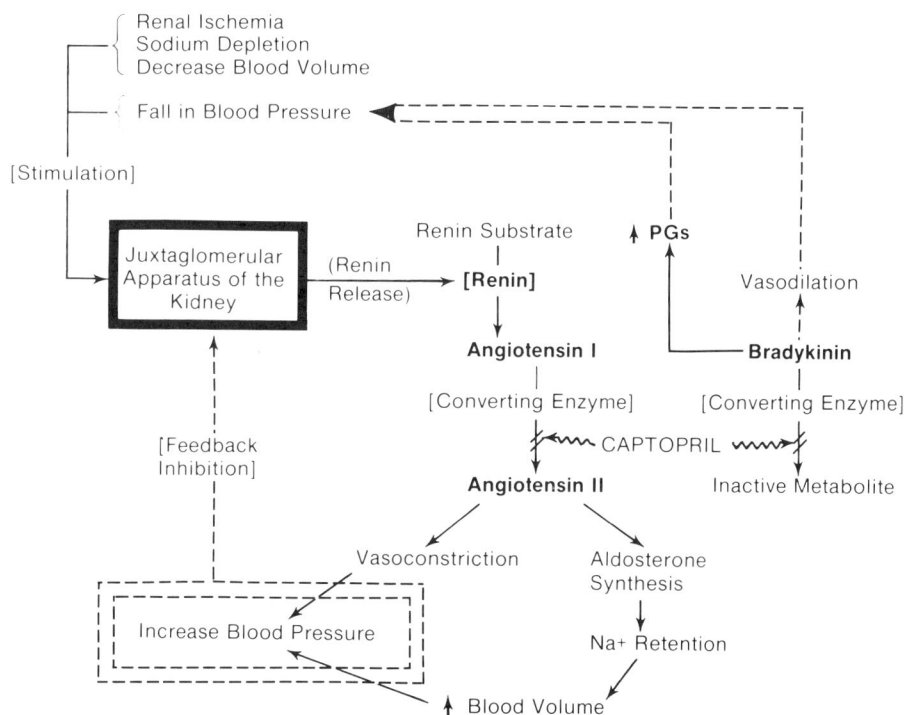

Figure 7–18. Schematic diagram of the renin–angiotensin system, illustrating the factors controlling renin release, angiotensin II formation (vasoconstriction), and bradykinin (vasodilator) inactivation. Also depicted are the consequences of converting-enzyme inhibition by captopril.

decrease in production of vasoconstrictor substances (angiotensin II) but also causes a rise in levels of bradykinin, a vasodilator (see Fig. 7-18). Bradykinin causes the release of prostaglandins, which possibly contributes further to the antihypertensive effects of captopril. Although the antihypertensive action of captopril does involve enhanced production of vasodilators such as bradykinin, there is evidence that the antihypertensive effect is largely the result of inhibition of angiotensin II generation.[338,445]

Captopril lowers total peripheral vascular resistance and causes little change in cardiac output, heart rate, or pulmonary wedge pressure.[310] However, in patients with congestive heart failure due to primary myocardial disease, cardiac output may increase, with moderate to excellent clinical improvement. Although numerous reports have identified a relationship between acute response of blood pressure and initial plasma renin activity, long-term blood pressure control by captopril does not appear to be dependent on or related to a high level of renin activity.[338]

Clinical Pharmacology. Oberfield and co-workers[293] used captopril for the treatment of malignant hypertension in a 10-year-old child who had failed to respond to a variety of other antihypertensive drugs. Captopril (initial dose 0.4 mg/kg, increased to 2 mg/kg q 6 hr) was effective in controlling systemic blood pressure in this patient. The response followed a triphasic pattern as noted previously in adults: an initial decrease, subsequent rise to pretreatment levels, and a final decrease in blood pressure. No untoward effects were noted with chronic administration. Rosendahl and Hayduk[438] employed captopril in two infants (4 and 20 months old) with renin-induced hypertension. Blood pressure control had been unsatisfactory with other agents. Individual doses of captopril ranged from a high of 10 mg/kg PO required for initial control of blood pressure to a maintenance dose of 3 mg/kg PO given every 8 hours. Water retention was the only noted side-effect. Bifano and colleagues[197] used captopril therapy in three neonates with severe (high-renin) hypertension. The infants, ranging in weight from 1.8 to 3.6 kg, had all failed to respond to other antihypertensive drugs. Captopril reduced systemic blood pressure in all three infants at doses ranging from 0.3 to 0.7 mg/kg given PO every 6 hours. These investigators recommend an initial dose of 0.1 to 0.4 mg/kg given 1 to 4 times per day as required for blood pressure control. There was no evidence of hematologic or renal side-effects. Captropril successfully controlled

blood pressure in a 2-week-old premature infant with renovascular hypertension.[446] The dose ranged from 0.25 to 1 mg/kg PO given every 6 hours. After an oral dose of 1 mg/kg, captopril plasma levels ranged between 50 and 100 ng/ml. Severe neutropenia developed after 2 weeks of therapy, requiring discontinuation of the drug. In older children, doses of 0.8 to 2.3 mg/kg PO given every 8 hours produced blood concentrations of captopril ranging between 100 and 700 ng/ml.[443] The clearance of captopril ranged from 14.1 to 18.8 ml/min/kg. Blood pressure control was achieved with chronic therapy in 9 of the 10 children.

Studies in adults have indicated that captopril is useful in patients with various forms of hypertension and congestive heart failure.[218,223,339,423] Beneficial effects include increased cardiac output, decreased left ventricular end-diastolic pressure, increased exercise capacity, and decreased peripheral and pulmonary vascular resistance. Captopril had no effect on primary pulmonary hypertension in adult patients.[424]

Therapeutic Indications. Captopril appears to be an effective antihypertensive agent for the control of *hypertension associated with renovascular abnormalities and hyperreninemia*.[413,443,445,446] Until such time that its effectiveness and safety can be thoroughly evaluated, captopril should be reserved for infants whose hypertension fails to respond to more conventional therapy. The recommended initial PO dose is 0.5 mg/kg. The usual PO maintenance dose will vary from 0.1 to 1.0 mg/kg, given every 6 to 12 hr as required for control of hypertension (Table 7-18). The maximum single PO dose should not exceed 2 mg/kg. The drug is contraindicated in infants with bilateral renal artery thrombosis (see Clinical Toxicology section).

Clinical Toxicology. Clinical trials with captopril have demonstrated a low incidence of serious side-effects. The various side-effects reported include rash or pruritus with fever and/or eosinophilia (in 14% of patients), taste impairment (6%), proteinuria (1%), neutropenia (0.3%), hypotension (1-2%), gastrointestinal tract disturbances (2-4%),[310] and azotemia.[403,445] It has been suggested that the serious side-effects of captopril therapy (hematologic and renal) are similar to those reported for penicillamine; severe neutropenia has been reported in infants and children.[443,446] Certain chemical similarities of the two drugs reinforce this hypothesis. Captopril should be used with extreme caution in patients with low renal perfusion pressure,[218] such as those with bilateral renal artery stenosis or thrombosis, or stenosis or thrombosis of a solitary kidney.

ANTIARRHYTHMIC AGENTS

A great deal of information exists regarding cardiac conduction and rhythm in both normal and abnormal hearts. This information has been combined with a greater understanding of the pharmacology and pharmacokinetics of antiarrhythmic drugs to allow more effective treatment of cardiac arrhythmias. Several excellent review articles and texts are available that deal comprehensively with the details of electrophysiologic abnormalities involved in cardiac arrhythmias.[345,350,353,355,356,369]

Drug therapy of cardiac arrhythmias in infants should be conditioned on the fact that many of the cardiac arrhythmias are relatively benign in nature, particularly when the inherent toxicity of many of the antiarrhythmic drugs is considered.[353] The rational choice of the proper antiarrhythmic agent must be based on (1) an accurate diagnosis naming the specific cardiac arrhythmia and excluding secondary etiologies as the cause (e.g., sepsis, electrolyte abnormalities, drug toxicity); (2) understanding of the electrophysiologic basis for the initiation and maintenance of the arrhythmia; (3) coordination of this information with the pharmacologic properties of the antiarrhythmic drugs; and (4) identification of any contraindications for use of the antiarrhythmic drug(s) selected.

Antiarrhythmic drugs have been classified by actions on cardiac impulse formation or propagation, or by mechanism of action. No proposed system of classification is totally satisfactory because of the incomplete knowledge about both drug action and the mechanics of cardiac arrhythmias. The pharmacologic actions of the antiarrhythmic drugs on electrophysiologic, electrocardiographic, and hemodynamic functions are summarized in Table 7–26. Note that all decrease automaticity and would therefore be expected to suppress arrhythmias resulting from enhanced pacemaker activity. Another common feature of these drugs is that they prolong the **effective refractory period (ERP)** relative to the effect on the **action potential duration (APD),** so that protection of the myocardium against propagation of early ectopic depolarizations is enhanced.

The differences in the electrophysiologic effects of the antiarrhythmic drugs confer certain advantages or disadvantages in effectiveness against specific cardiac arrhythmias. Table 7–27 presents the anticipated clinical effectiveness of the various antiarrhythmic drugs in the treatment of selected cardiac arrhythmias in pediatric patients.

Amiodarone

Pharmacology. Amiodarone, an iodinated benzofuran derivative, is an effective agent for treatment of angina and a variety of cardiac arrhythmias.[458] The drug is structurally related to thyroxine, unlike other available antiarrhythmic drugs. The drug is effective after oral or IV administration. It is capable of decreasing

Table 7–26. ELECTROPHYSIOLOGIC, ELECTROCARDIOGRAPHIC, AND HEMODYNAMIC EFFECTS OF ANTIARRHYTHMIC DRUGS

Drug	Electrophysiologic Effects					ECG Effects			Hemodynamic Effects		
	Automaticity	Conduction	ERP	APD	ERP/APD	P–R	QRS	Q–T	BP	CO	LVEDP
amiodarone	0	↓ A,V	↑	↑	0	↑	0	0	↓	0,↑	↑
digoxin	↓ A ↑ V	↑ A ↓ A-V	↓ A, V ↓ A-V	↓ A, V		↑	0	↓	0,↑	↑	0,↓
lidocaine	↓	variable	↓	↓	↑	0,↓	0	0,↓	0,↓	0,↓	0,↑
phenytoin	↓	variable	↓	↓	↑	0,↓	0	↓	0,↓	0,↓	0,↑
procainamide	↓	↓ A, A-V, V	↑	↑	↑	0,↑	↑	↑	↓	↓	↑
propranolol	↓	↓ A-V	↓	↓	↑	0,↑	0	0,↓	0,↓	↓	↑
quinidine	↓	↓ A, A-V, V	↑	↑	↑	0,↑	↑	↑	↓	↓	↑
verapamil	↓, 0	↓ A-V	↑ A-V	↑ A-V	↑,0	↑	0	0	↓	0,↓	↑

↑ = increase or lengthen; ↓ = decrease or shorten; 0 = no effect. ERP = effective refractory period (minimal interval between two propagating responses); APD = action potential duration; A = atrial; V = ventricular; A-V = atrioventricular node. BP = blood pressure; CO = cardiac output; LVEDP = left ventricular end-diastolic pressure.

Table 7-27. CLINICAL EFFECTIVENESS OF ANTIARRHYTHMIC DRUGS

Arrhythmia	Amiodarone	Digoxin	Lidocaine	Phenytoin	Procainamide	Propranolol	Quinidine	Verapamil
Supraventricular								
atrial premature extrasystole		4	2	2	4	2	(3)	
paroxysmal atrial tachycardia		4	2	2	3	3	3	3
atrial flutter	4 (WPW)	4 (Not WPW)	0	0	1	2	2	2
atrial fibrillation	4 (WPW)	4 (Not WPW)	0	0	3	2	(3)	2
Ventricular								
ventricular premature extrasystole	4	0	4	2	3	2	3	0
ventricular tachycardia	4	0	4	2	3	2	2	0
Digitalis-induced								
atrial arrhythmia			3	4	0	2	0	0
ventricular arrhythmia			3	4	0	2	0	0

4 = drug of choice; 3, 2 = effective; 1 = poor; 0 = no effect; WPW = Wolff-Parkinson-White syndrome; ( ) = should not be administered until ventricular rate has been controlled with digoxin.

Data from studies by Hernandez et al,[354] Gelband and Rosen,[350] Radford and Izukawa,[366] Guntheroth,[353] Pickoff et al,[363] Sapire et al,[367] Stevens et al,[370] Bigger and Hoffman,[345] Martin and Hernandez,[361] and Pratt and Lichstein.[365]

peripheral vascular resistance and increasing cardiac output and coronary blood flow. Atropine-resistant bradycardia and noncompetitive inhibition of both α- and β-adrenergic receptors are additional pharmacologic effects of amiodarone. Myocardial contractility remains unchanged.

The antiarrhythmic actions of amiodarone are believed to involve reduction of the outward potassium current as well as the rapid inward sodium current.[450] There is no effect on the slow calcium channel. The major electrophysiologic effects are to depress sinus, atrial, and A-V nodal function by increasing S-A conduction and recovery time; increasing the refractory period of atrial, A-V node, and ventricular function; and slowing conduction in the A-V node and specialized conduction system. Other electrophysiologic effects are summarized in Table 7–26. A single mechanism of action seems unlikely considering the drug's widespread effectiveness in treatment of a great many different arrhythmias.

Clinical Pharmacology. There is little information on the pharmacokinetics of amiodarone. On the basis of clinical experience, it appears that the drug has a half-life in adults of 5 to 7 days,[458] although children are believed to metabolize the drug faster.[450] Although rapid onset of antiarrhythmic effect is frequently noted, the full therapeutic response may not be evident for 1 week or more. The duration of action after cessation of drug therapy is less than a few weeks in children as opposed to 1 to 2 months in adults.

Amiodarone has been effective in controlling a wide variety of cardiac arrhythmias in children. Coumel and Fidelle[450] reported experience in 135 infants and children ranging in age from 1 day to 15 years. The arrhythmias included atrial, junctional, and ventricular; those associated with congenital cardiopathies, valvular disease, cardiomyopathies, and Wolff-Parkinson-White syndrome; and those that were idiopathic in nature. The ECG and clinical outcome were totally or partially improved in 90% of the cases. The onset of drug effect averaged 4.1 days after oral therapy was instituted. Shahar and colleagues[466] reported the successful employment of amiodarone in treatment of 10 children (3 months to 15 years old) with recurrent SVT associated with the Wolff-Parkinson-White syndrome. Each patient received an oral loading dose of 10 to 15 mg/kg, followed by a 5 mg/kg daily oral dose. All children became asymptomatic of tachyarrhythmias within 5 days of therapy and remained asymptomatic for

5 to 36 months. Pickoff et al.[467] treated 4 children (11 to 14 years old) with primary ventricular arrhythmias with amiodarone. All responded to oral therapy (10 mg/kg/day). Hesslein[454] used amidarone in 13 children (6 months to 17 years old) with a variety of cardiac arrhythmias. Among those who responded to amiodarone were two patients with Wolff-Parkinson-White syndrome. A serious interaction with ongoing digoxin therapy (increased digoxin serum levels) was observed in 6 of 9 patients. In general, the therapeutic experience with amiodarone in infants and children is comparable to the reported experience in adults.[455,459,464,465,471,472]

Therapeutic Indications. Amiodarone is a versatile and highly effective antiarrhythmic agent to be used in carefully selected situations. It would appear to be the drug treatment of choice for Wolff-Parkinson-White syndrome when surgical treatment is not feasible.[351,454,466] The drug also appears to be highly successful in controlling most of the supraventricular as well as ventricular tachyarrhythmias that fail to respond to various conventional drugs.[450,459,464,465,471,472] Additional positive features of the drug include single daily dosing (occasional missed doses are probably inconsequential), lack of myocardial depressant effects, and reasonable safety (see Clinical Toxicology section). However, the use of amiodarone must still be considered experimental because of the relatively brief experience with the drug in infants.

The recommended dose for infants and children is a loading dose of 10 to 15 mg/kg PO or 5 mg/kg IV, followed 24 hours later by a maintenance dose of 5 mg/kg given PO once daily.

Clinical Toxicology. The incidence of adverse reactions to amiodarone varies with dose and duration of therapy.[453,459] The most common adverse effect is corneal microdeposits (lysosomal inclusions of a lipofuscin-like substance in the cytoplasm of the basal and intermediary cells of the cornea), which occur in virtually every patient treated for a 2-week period or longer.[458,469] This effect is rarely symptomatic and resolves when the drug is discontinued. Among the serious complications reported with amiodarone is alteration of thyroid function. Both hyper- and hypothyroidism have been reported; the incidence is between 2% and 6%.[450,454,458,459] Several mechanisms for the disturbance in thyroid function have been postulated, including the organic iodine load from amiodarone, direct effect of amiodarone on the thyroid gland, and amiodarone inhibition of conversion of T_4 to T_3.[453] Spontaneous recovery occurs with discontinuation of amiodarone therapy, although some investigators have continued the drug while treating with thyroxine or propranolol for hypothyroidism or hyperthyroidism, respectively. Another serious complication of amiodarone therapy is the development of pneumonitis and pulmonary fibrosis.[457,459,469] The incidence of occurrence (up to 6%) is dose-related, with an average onset of 5 months in adults.[457,459] Corticosteroid therapy appears to be useful in reversing amiodarone-induced pneumonitis, supporting a role of immunomediated mechanisms in the pathogenesis.[451,459] Cutaneous photosensitivity, which is both dose- and duration-dependent, may appear in 3% to 57% of patients during therapy. Up to 14% complain of gastrointestinal upset. Neurologic complications have included tremor and ataxia (up to 35% incidence), peripheral neuropathy (proximal weakness, stocking and glove sensorimotor deficits), headaches, nightmares, hallucinations, and personality problems. Elevation of hepatic enzymes is a dose-related effect that appears to be transient and not progressive.[453] A-V block and sinus bradycardia have also been noted, prompting the recommendation by some that amiodarone not be used in patients with intraventricular or A-V block.[458]

Digoxin

Digoxin is the drug of choice for paroxysmal atrial tachycardia. The primary actions of digoxin that render it effective are (1) prolongation of A-V nodal conduction and (2) reduction of the refractory period of the circus movement[353] (the mechanism for atrial flutter). The increase in vagal activity (the indirect effect of digoxin) increases the likelihood of conversion to sinus rhythm. The clinical features, response to treatment, and findings in long-term follow-up studies in patients with supraventricular tachycardia have been reviewed by Garson and colleagues.[349] The response to initial treatment in this series is shown in Figure 7–19. IV digoxin therapy (40–50 μg/kg total digitalizing dose) was the most frequent treatment used and was successful in 68% of the patients. Intrauterine supraventricular tachycardia (defined as a constant and regular rate between 180 and 360 beats per minute) is commonly treated with digoxin.[461] Maternal digoxin therapy should be guided by frequent serum level determinations. Treatment of newborns with edema and ascites must take the excess weight into consideration in digoxin dose calculation to avoid overdosing. Digoxin should be used with caution in infants with pre-excitation and atrial fibrillation. Atrial flutter in infancy and its treatment has been

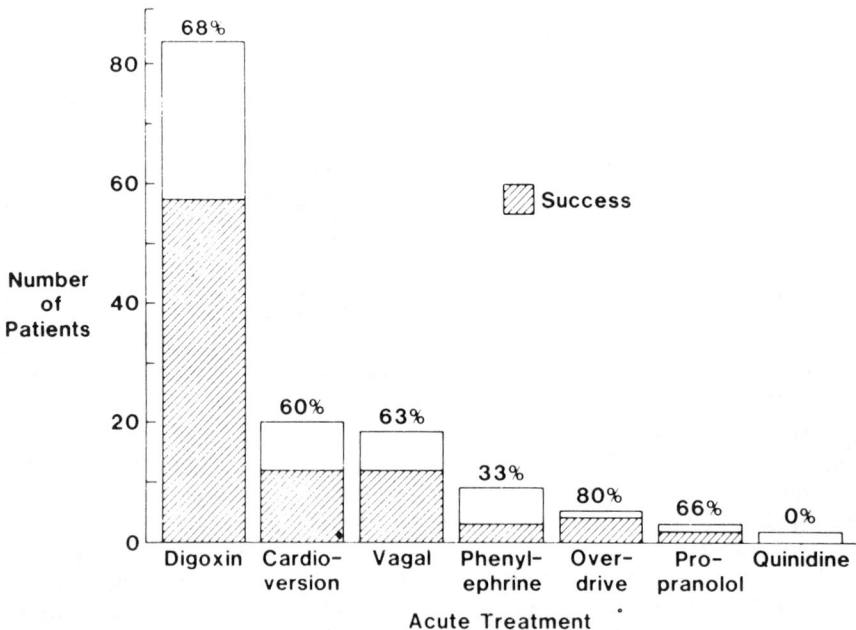

Figure 7–19. Initial treatment of superventricular tachycardia and response. Patients in this series ranged in age from newborn through 17 years, with the < 1-month-old neonates comprising the largest single age group. The percent value above each treatment bar represents success rate in the number of patients treated. (From Garson A Jr et al: J Pediatr 98:875, 1981.)

reviewed by Margin and Hernandez;[361] atrial fibrillation in children and its treatment has been examined by Radford and Iukawa.[366] Symptomatic infants with supraventricular arrhythmias may be candidates for immediate DC cardioversion rather than drug therapy.[351]

The pharmacology of digoxin is presented under Inotropic Agents earlier in this chapter. Table 7–28 reviews some of the more critical aspects of pharmacology and dosage recommendations for digoxin and other antiarrhythmic drugs.

Lidocaine

Pharmacology. The IV route is used for lidocaine administration because effective plasma levels cannot be achieved when the drug is given PO, owing to rapid metabolism by the liver coupled with a comparatively slow rate of absorption in the gastrointestinal tract. In addition, side-effects appear to be exaggerated with PO administration. A bolus IV dose is required to achieve therapeutic serum concentrations prior to continuous infusion. About 50% of lidocaine in plasma is protein bound at therapeutic concentrations. In keeping with the extensive metabolism by the liver, severe liver disease or decreased hepatic blood flow can significantly alter the plasma clearance of lidocaine and thus reduce the dosage requirements.[345] The plasma half-life for lidocaine in neonates is about 3 hours, compared with 1.8 hours in adults.[362] In neonates, about 30% of the administered lidocaine is excreted unchanged in the urine, compared with less than 5% in adults.[362]

In contrast to quinidine and procainamide, lidocaine acts directly on the heart, the effects being directed primarily to disturbances of ventricular origin. It has a narrow spectrum of antiarrhythmic activity (Table 7–27). Ordinarily, lidocaine has no effect on the automaticity of the S-A node (except with preexisting disease of the S-A node) or on conduction velocity in the His-Purkinje system or ventricular muscle. The duration of the action potential (APD) is decreased in the Purkinje fibers and ventricular muscle but not in the atrial muscle or conduction system. Although the effective refractory period (ERP) is also reduced, the effect of lidocaine on the APD is more pronounced (Table 7–26). The result of these electrophysiologic effects is the capacity to abolish ventricular reentry, but little effect on atrial arrhythmias is seen. The electrocardiographic effects of lidocaine are quite different from those of quinidine

and procainamide (Table 7–26). The QRS complex remains unchanged, and the effects on the P–R and Q–T intervals are variable.

Alterations in hemodynamics due to lidocaine depend on the status of the patient and on the dose administered. In contrast to quinidine, procainamide, and propranolol, lidocaine has little effect on the autonomic nervous system: Myocardial contractility and vascular tone are depressed only slightly, if at all, by therapeutic doses but may be adversely affected by higher doses or by blood concentrations above the therapeutic level (1–6 μg/ml; see Table 7–28).

Therapeutic Indications. The use of lidocaine is limited to short-term control of *ventricular arrhythmias,* including ventricular tachycardia, premature ventricular beats, and arrhythmias due to digitalis intoxication (Table 7–27). The appropriate loading dose is 1 to 5 mg/kg given IV as 1-mg/kg bolus doses, followed by a constant infusion of 10 to 50 μg/kg/min. Plasma drug levels must be monitored carefully and the infant observed for signs of toxicity.

The major contraindication to the use of lidocaine is presence of complete heart block, since lidocaine suppresses ventricular pacemakers and would result in ventricular standstill.

Clinical Toxicology. The major adverse effects of lidocaine are on the CNS. These effects are seen with serum levels above 5 μg/ml and include drowsiness, agitation, dissociation, hearing loss, disorientation, muscle twitching, convulsions, and respiratory arrest.[345]

Phenytoin

Pharmacology. The pharmacology and toxicology of phenytoin are presented in Chapter 5. With respect to electrophysiologic effects, phenytoin is very similar to lidocaine: There is little effect on the S-A node or other atrial tissues. The effects on ventricular tissue include an increase in threshold, but no alteration of conduction velocity occurs except in ischemic tissue, where conduction is usually decreased. Ventricular reentry arrhythmias can be abolished either by improving conduction or by producing a two-way block. Phenytoin produces minimal effects in the atria; its effect on certain digitalis-induced arrhythmias is related to abolishing abnormal automaticity in Purkinje fibers. The electrocardiographic effects of phenytoin are summarized in Table 7–26.

Therapeutic Indications. Phenytoin, like lidocaine, has been found more effective in the treatment of ventricular than supraventricular

Table 7–28. DOSAGE RECOMMENDATIONS AND PHARMACOKINETICS OF THE ANTIARRHYTHMIC DRUGS[a]

Drug	Initial Dose	Maintenance Dose	Effective Plasma Concentration	Serum Half-life ($T\frac{1}{2}$)	Gastrointestinal Absorption (%)	Protein Binding (%)	Metabolism	Renal Excretion (% unchanged)
amiodarone	10–15 mg/kg PO or 5 mg/kg IV over 10 min	5 mg/kg PO once daily	?	days	—	—	—	—
digoxin	See Table 7–4		1–2 ng/ml	15–72 hr (range of means, Table 7–3)	70	20	liver, gastro-intestinal tract	60
lidocaine	1–5 mg/kg IV	10–50 µg/kg/min IV	1–6 µg/ml	15–30 min	<35	10–50	liver	<10
phenytoin	2–5 mg/kg IV over 5–10 min; repeat up to 20 mg/kg	2–8 mg/kg q 8–12 hr PO (see Table 5–5)	5–18 µg/ml	8–197 hr (range of means, Table 5–6)	>80	>70	liver	<10
procainamide	1 mg/kg IV q 5 min to maximum 10 mg/kg	20–50 µg/kg/min IV, or 5–15 mg/kg q 4–6 hr PO	3–10 µg/ml NAPA: 5–30 µg/ml	2–4 hr	>75	15	liver	50–60
propranolol	0.01–0.2 mg/kg IV over 10 min	0.05–2 mg/kg q 6 hr PO	20–100 ng/ml	3–6 hr	>90 (<30 bioavailable)	90	liver	5
quinidine	not recommended	5–15 mg/kg q 6 hr PO	2–6 µg/ml	6–7 hr	>90	60–80	liver	20–50
verapamil	0.1–0.2 mg/kg IV over 2 min, repeat dose × 1		0.1–0.5 µg/ml	3–7 hr	>90 (20 bioavailable)	90	liver	>70

a Portions of this information were derived from adult patients. Data from studies by Gelband and Rosen,[350] Guntheroth,[353] Somogyi et al,[327] Brown and Shand,[449] and Follath et al.[452]

arrhythmias. It is effective in treating *ventricular arrhythmias* associated with digitalis toxicity, acute myocardial infarction, open-heart surgery, and cardiac catheterization.[360] Phenytoin is particularly useful in digoxin toxicity manifested by both ectopic beats and partial A-V block because phenytoin tends to decrease A-V conduction time, in addition to suppressing ectopic beats. The drug can also increase ventricular rate in the presence of atrial flutter or fibrillation by virtue of its ability to enhance A-V conduction.

The recommended dose is 2 to 5 mg/kg given IV over 5 to 10 minutes (maximum rate 0.5 mg/kg/min);[345] the maximum loading dose is 20 mg/kg. The maintenance dose is 2 to 8 mg/kg given PO every 8 to 12 hours. Chronic therapy with phenytoin requires periodic monitoring of serum levels to assure maintenance of therapeutic concentrations (Table 7–28). Bigger and coworkers[344] studied the relationship between plasma levels of phenytoin and antiarrhythmic effects; three fourths of the responsive arrhythmias were abolished at plasma levels between 10 and 18 μg/ml (Table 7–28).

Procainamide

Pharmacology. Procainamide is well absorbed from the gastrointestinal tract, with peak plasma levels achieved in 40 to 90 minutes. PO and IV doses of procainamide produce very similar plasma levels. About 15% to 20% of the drug in plasma is protein bound at therapeutic concentrations.

The metabolism of procainamide has been investigated extensively in adults. There is a bimodal genetic variation in the *N*-acetyl transferase conversion of procainamide to *N*-acetylprocainamide (NAPA), similar to that seen for isoniazid;[359] NAPA is an active antiarrhythmic agent. Renal excretion, which is much slower for NAPA than for procainamide, is the primary mechanism of elimination. Up to 60% of administered procainamide is eliminated unchanged in the urine; all the NAPA is excreted in the urine except for a small percentage (<3%) metabolized back to procainamide. Renal or hepatic dysfunction requires monitoring of drug levels in serum (for both procainamide and *N*-acetylprocainamide) so that appropriate dosage adjustments can be made.

Information on the metabolism of procainamide in pediatric patients is limited. Singh and coworkers[467] examined procainamide kinetics in six children (7 to 12 years old) after a single IV dose (5.5 ± 0.9 mg/kg). The elimination half-life of 1.7 ± 0.1 hr observed in this study is considerably shorter than the reported values for adults (2.5–4.7 hr). The plasma clearance of procainamide observed in children (19.4 ± 2.0 ml/min/kg) is higher than reported values in adults (8–10 ml/min/kg). Peak NAPA levels were observed in serum samples collected from the children 1 to 2 hours after dosing. A half-life of 13.5 hours for procainamide and 19.5 hours for NAPA was reported in one neonate born to a mother treated with procainamide prior to birth.[456]

The electrophysiologic effects of procainamide are virtually the same as those of quinidine. There is little effect on the S-A node automaticity except in patients with abnormal S-A node activity. The automaticity of the Purkinje system is suppressed, accounting for the antiarrhythmic activity of procainamide, and also the hazard of its use in the presence of A-V block. Threshold in atrial and ventricular tissue is increased, and the responsiveness of conduction is decreased; a greater increase in ERP than in ADP explains these effects (Table 7–26). Other electrocardiographic effects include an increase in P–R, QRS, and Q–T intervals.

The hemodynamic effects of procainamide are the same as those of quinidine. Depression of myocardial contractility and hypotension associated with procainamide use, as reported in earlier studies, are now known to be due to excessive dosage or rate of administration.[357]

Therapeutic Indications. Procainamide is effective in treating *premature atrial contractions, paroxysmal atrial tachycardia,* and *atrial fibrillations* (Table 7–27). In addition, a large percentage of patients with ventricular premature contractions and ventricular tachycardia respond to procainamide.[354]

Quinidine is usually more satisfactory than procainamide for long-term therapy, because it has greater efficacy and has significantly less toxicity. The contraindications for the use of procainamide are similar to those of quinidine. Because of its effects on A-V nodal and His-Purkinje conduction, procainamide should be administered with caution in the presence of second-degree A-V block and bundle-branch block.

The recommended initial dose of procainamide is 1 mg/kg IV repeated every 5 minutes as required to a maximum of 10 to 15 mg/kg, not to exceed 100 mg total dose. For maintenance therapy, a constant IV infusion of 20 to 50 μg/kg/min, or a dose of 5 to 15 mg/kg given PO every 4 to 6 hours, is recommended. Monitoring of procainamide serum levels is important with IV or long-term therapy. Since the major metabolite of procainamide, N-acetylprocainamide (NAPA), is active (and toxic), its plasma levels should be monitored as well, especially in cases of renal dysfunction. Therapeutic serum levels of procainamide are 3 to 10 μg/ml and 5 to 30 μg/ml for NAPA. Because NAPA has one third the potency by weight and lesser effects than procainamide on conduction regardless of dose, plasma levels of these two components must not be simply added in interpretations of efficacy or toxicity.

Clinical Toxicology. Procainamide has electrophysiologic toxicities similar to those of quinidine, but the extracardiac adverse effects are different. Gastrointestinal disturbances, agranulocytosis, and occasionally hepatic toxicity have occurred with procainamide therapy.[358] Lupus erythematosus is a well-recognized adverse reaction to long-term therapy with procainamide. A positive antinuclear antibody (ANA) develops in 50% to 80% of adult patients on long-term therapy.[345] The lupus syndrome develops in about 20% of those who develop a positive ANA. Cardiac toxicity correlates with plasma levels; therapeutic levels are 3 to 10 μg/ml.

Propranolol

Pharmacology. Propranolol has two separate actions on the heart: One involves the consequences of β-adrenergic blockade and the removal of adrenergic influences, and the other involves direct myocardial effects, which account for its antiarrhythmic actions. The electrophysiologic and electrocardiographic effects of propranolol are outlined in Table 7–26. Depending on the clinical circumstance in which the drug is used, either the antiadrenergic or the direct-membrane effects can be of importance. Other pharmacologic details and the hemodynamic effects of propranolol are reviewed under β-Adrenergic Blockers earlier in this chapter.

Therapeutic Indications. Propranolol has been employed for a variety of cardiac rhythm abnormalities. Selected cases of *sinus tachycardia* have been treated with propranolol, including that associated with *thyrotoxicosis*. Propranolol alone or in conjunction with digoxin has been used to control ventricular rate in patients with *atrial flutter* or *atrial fibrillation*. Tachyarrhythmias associated with digitalis toxicity (including supraventricular and ventricular extrasystoles and tachycardia, as well as ventricular fibrillation) have been suppressed by propranolol administered IV or PO. However,

phenytoin and lidocaine remain the drugs of choice for treatment of digitalis-induced arrhythmias (Table 7–27).

The recommended initial dose of propranolol is 0.01 to 0.2 mg/kg given IV over 10 minutes. For maintenance or non-emergency situations a dose of 0.05 to 2 mg/kg given PO every 6 hours is recommended (Table 7–28).

Quinidine

Pharmacology. Quinidine is a naturally occurring alkaloid that retains a primary role as a maintenance therapy antiarrhythmic agent despite the development of several new drugs. The drug is rapidly and completely absorbed following PO administration. Nearly 80% of drug in plasma is bound to albumin. Peak plasma levels are reached within 1 to 4 hours of PO administration, depending on the pharmaceutical preparation employed. The majority of the drug is metabolized by the liver. Renal excretion accounts for 10% to 30% of the elimination of quinidine from the body. The elimination half-life of quinidine in infants and children is about 4 hours compared with 6 hours in adults.[470] The effect of renal and heart failure on quinidine plasma levels is controversial, but care should be used in administering the drug in these circumstances. Increases in urine pH from a range of 6–7 to 7–8 will decrease renal clearance by as much as 50% in adults.[346]

Quinidine produces significant changes in automaticity, excitability, and conduction. It has little effect on the atria or S-A node but has direct and indirect effects on the A-V junction at therapeutic plasma concentrations. The early anticholinergic or indirect properties may facilitate A-V transmission and present a hazard when quinidine is given as the initial drug in the presence of atrial flutter.[360] The important therapeutic action of quinidine is the depression of the automaticity of ventricular pacemakers with prolongation of the QRS complex. Quinidine causes an increase in the P–R, QRS, and Q–T intervals (Table 7–26).

Quinidine can depress myocardial contractility and decrease peripheral vascular resistance. Although mild, these effects can become significant in patients with compromised cardiovascular status and are exaggerated on IV administration of the drug, a route that is not recommended.

Therapeutic Indications. Quinidine has been effectively employed for abolishing and preventing recurrences of *premature contraction* of atrial, A-V junctional, or ventricular origin

(Table 7–27). It is useful as an adjunct to digoxin for restoring sinus rhythm in atrial flutter and fibrillation but should not be given until the ventricular rate has been controlled. Quinidine is not primarily indicated for either prophylaxis or active treatment of ventricular flutter or ventricular fibrillation since such therapy requires use of the IV route. One absolute contraindication for the use of quinidine is complete A-V block. Its depressant actions on the myocardium and peripheral vasodilating effects limit its use in congestive heart failure and hypotensive states. Quinidine may aggravate the arrhythmias associated with digoxin toxicity.

The recommended maintenance dose of quinidine is 5 to 15 mg/kg given PO every 6 hours. Quinidine plasma levels should be monitored and maintained in the therapeutic range (2–6 μg/ml). The QRS interval may be used to monitor therapy because it correlates with plasma concentrations; an increase of 25% or less in the QRS interval is expected, but a 50% increase requires a reduction in the dosage.

Clinical Toxicology. Acute adverse drug reactions occur in 30% of all patients receiving quinidine and in about 14% of those maintained on chronic therapy.[346] Nausea, vomiting, and especially diarrhea often require termination of therapy. Febrile reactions may occur within 1 to 2 weeks of initial quinidine therapy. Cardiac and hematologic reactions are the most serious. Quinidine may cause A-V block or asystole in patients with a preexisting A-V block and ventricular escape rhythm. Short bursts of ventricular tachycardia or fibrillation may develop with quinidine therapy, causing syncope or sudden death even with nontoxic plasma levels (quinidine syncope). Hypotension is a problem with IV administration. Life-threatening thrombocytopenia, agranulocytosis, hemolytic anemia, and hypoplastic anemia have also been reported. Cinchonism (tinnitus, auditory and visual impairment, nausea, headache, photophobia, flushing, vomiting, abdominal pain, and CNS symptoms ranging from confusion to psychosis) may also occur.

Verapamil

Pharmacology. The pharmacology of verapamil is reviewed under Calcium-channel Blockers earlier in this chapter.

Verapamil directly suppresses sinus node pacemaker activity and is one of the most potent inhibitors of A-V nodal conduction.[364] Usually, depression of the S-A node is not evident because the hypotensive action of the drug

leads to reflex (baroreceptor-initiated) changes of autonomic tone in the sinus node (sympathetic stimulation and parasympathetic withdrawal). Although this reflex mechanism minimizes sinus slowing of the heart, mild bradycardia is usually observed. Rarely, sinus arrest appears in patients with underlying abnormalities of sinus node pacemaker activity. The first sign of verapamil action is prolongation of the P–R interval, caused by the slowing of conduction through the A-V node. Verapamil has no effect on the QRS and Q–T intervals of the electrocardiogram.

Verapamil can also produce a negative inotropic effect on the heart as well as arteriolar vasodilation. Conflicting observations with respect to the negative inotropic action of verapamil may be due to different drug doses, different experimental models, or differences in the relative contribution of its direct and indirect actions.[348,364] Marked vasodilation occurs in most peripheral vascular beds, including mesenteric and coronary arteries. Overall, the negative inotropic effects of verapamil are minimized by the reduction in afterload, so that the cardiac index is unchanged.

Therapeutic Indications. Verapamil has been demonstrated to have efficacy in the treatment of a relatively narrow spectrum of arrhythmias including *supraventricular tachycardia, atrial flutter,* and *fibrillation.*[467] The drug does not appear to be very effective against ventricular arrhythmias (Table 7–27).

Verapamil blocks the slow inward calcium current in cardiac fibers, thereby limiting the ability of ectopic pacemakers to discharge prematurely. Sapire and coauthors[367] reported the successful control of ectopic supraventricular tachycardia in a 2 1/2-year old-child with verapamil after failure with other antiarrhythmic therapy. Greco and coworkers[352] compared therapeutic benefits of digitalis, adenosine-5′-triphosphate (ATP), and verapamil in 62 infants and children (aged 4 days–12 yr) with paroxysmal supraventricular tachycardia. Success rate was 90% with verapamil and ATP and 61% to 71% with digitalis (Lantoside C). The effect of verapamil in converting 80% to 100% of cases of supraventricular tachycardia after IV administration of the drug appears to be the most clinically significant antiarrhythmic action.

The recommended initial dose is 0.1 to 0.2 mg/kg given IV over 1 to 2 minutes under ECG and blood pressure monitoring. The maximum cumulative dose should be no greater than 0.3 mg/kg.[364] No information is available on maintenance therapy in infants or children. In adults the oral tablet formulation is administered at an interval of every 8 hours for treatment of angina.[368] The safety and value of verapamil in infants less than 6 months old has been seriously questioned.[364]

Clinical Toxicology. Of adult patients given verapamil, 9% will manifest toxicity; about 1% of all patients treated will require discontinuation of therapy. Side-effects include systemic hypotension, bradycardia, seizures, headache, nausea, and vomiting. Orally administered verapamil appears to be well tolerated, although there are occasional complaints of gastric pain and constipation. IV administration commonly produces transient and mild falls in blood pressure. Epstein and Rosing[348] have reported an increased incidence of bradycardia, second-degree A-V block, and sinus arrest among patients with hypertrophic cardiomyopathy receiving verapamil. Worsening outflow obstruction, related to a marked drop in blood pressure, and development of pulmonary edema and deterioration of left ventricular function were also described.

Contraindications to the use of verapamil include severe hypotension, A-V block, sick sinus syndrome, and severe congestive heart failure. Complete heart block and ventricular asystole have been reported with the concomitant use of verapamil and IV β blockers.[368] Greco and colleagues[352] reported cardiac arrest in two infants given an initial dose of 0.125 to 0.175 mg/kg of verapamil; one infant had a low serum calcium, and the other had been on maintenance therapy with a β blocker. The occurrence of life-threatening bradycardia and hypotension following intravenous administration of verapamil (0.1 mg/kg) in 2 neonates has prompted the recommendation that intravenous verapamil not be given to infants.[463]

Serious toxic effects of verapamil (hypotension, bradycardia) can be treated with 10 to 20 mg/kg of elemental **calcium** (Ca^{++}) IV over 30 min, along with volume expansion.[460] **Atropine** (10 μg/kg) and **isoproterenol** (0.05–0.1 μg/kg/min) can also be used in patients unresponsive to calcium therapy.

References

Digoxin

1. Andersson KE, Bertler A, Wettrell G: Post-mortem distribution and tissue concentrations of digoxin in infants and adults. Acta Paediatr Scand 64:497, 1975.

2. Aperia A, Broberger O, Elinder G, et al: Postnatal development of renal function in pre-term and full-term infants. Acta Paediatr Scand 70:183, 1981.
3. Berman W Jr, Dubynsky O, Whitman V, et al: Digoxin therapy in low-birth-weight infants with patent ductus arteriosus. J Pediatr 93:652, 1978.
4. Berman W Jr, Musselman J, Shortencarrier R: The physiologic effects of digoxin under steady-state drug conditions in newborn and adult sheep. Circulation 62:1165, 1980.
5. Berman W Jr, Musselman J, Shortencarrier R: Localization of digoxin in sheep myocardium by immunofluorescent microscopy. Biol Neonate 40:295, 1981.
6. Berman W Jr, Yabel SM, Dillon T, et al: Effects of digoxin in infants with a congested circulatory state due to a ventricular septal defect. N Engl J Med 308:363, 1983.
7. Brown DD, Spector R, Juhl RP: Drug interactions with digoxin. Drugs 20:198, 1980.
8. Caldwell JH, Cline CT: Biliary excretion of digoxin in man. Clin Pharmacol Ther 19:410, 1976.
9. Collins-Nakai RL, Ng PK, Beaudry MA, Ocejo-Moreno R, et al: Total body digoxin clearance and steady-state concentrations in low birth weight infants. Dev Pharmacol Ther 4:61, 1982.
10. Collins-Nakai RL, Schiff, D, Ng PK: Pharmacokinetics of digoxin in low-birth-weight infants. Dev Pharmacol Ther 5:86, 1982.
11. Coltart J, Howard M, Chamberlain D: Myocardial and skeletal muscle concentrations of digoxin in patients on long-term therapy. Br Med J 2:318, 1972.
12. Cree JE, Coltart DJ, Howard MR: Plasma digoxin concentration in children with heart failure. Br Med J 1:443, 1973.
13. Deutscher RN, Harrison DC, Goldman RH: The relation between myocardial ³H-digoxin concentration and its hemodynamic effects. Am J Cardiol 29:47, 1972.
14. Dohlemann C, Buhlmeyer K: Ergebnisse vergleichender oraler und intravenoser digitalis-therapie bie sauglingen. Monatsschr Kinderheilkd 120:458, 1972.
15. Dungan WT, Doherty JE, Harvey C, et al: Titrated digoxin XVIII. Studies in infants and children. Circulation 46:983, 1972.
16. Ekins BR, Watanabe AS: Acute digoxin poisonings: review of therapy. Am J Hosp Pharm 35:268, 1978.
17. Finley JP, Howman-Giles RB, Gilday DL, et al: Transient myocardial ischemia of the newborn infant demonstrated by thallium myocardial imaging. J Pediatr 94:263, 1979.
18. Gazes PC, Holmes CR, Moseley V, Pratt-Thomas HR: Acute hemorrhage and necrosis of the intestines associated with digitalization. Circulation 23:358, 1961.
19. Gibson TP, Quintanilla AP: Effect of volume expansion and furosemide diuresis on the renal clearance of digoxin. J Pharmacol Exp Ther 219:54, 1981.
20. Gibson TP, Nelson HA: The question of cumulation of digoxin metabolites in renal failure. Clin Pharmacol Ther 27:219, 1980.
21. Gorodischer R, Krasner J, Yaffe SJ: Serum protein binding of digoxin in newborn infants. Res Commun Chem Pathol Pharmacol 9:387, 1974.
22. Gorodischer R, Jusko WJ, Yaffe SJ: Tissue and erythrocyte distribution of digoxin in infants. Clin Pharmacol Ther 19:256, 1976.

23. Gorodischer R, Jusko WJ, Yaffe SJ: Renal clearance of digoxin in young infants. Res Commun Chem Pathol Pharmacol 16:363, 1977.

24. Greenblatt DJ, Duhme DW, Koch-Weser J: Pain and CPK elevation after intramuscular digoxin. N Engl J Med 288:689, 1973.

25. Halkin H, Radomsky M, Millman P, et al: Steady state serum concentrations and renal clearance of digoxin in neonates, infants, and children. Eur J Clin Pharmacol 13:113, 1978.

26. Halkin H, Radomsky M, Blieden L, et al: Steady state serum digoxin concentration in relation to digitalis toxicity in neonates and infants. Pediatrics 61:184, 1978.

27. Hartel G, Kyllonen K, Merikallio E, et al: Human serum and myocardial digoxin. Clin Pharmacol Ther 19:153, 1976.

28. Hastreiter AR, Simonton RL, van der Horst RL, et al: Digoxin pharmacokinetics in premature infants. Pediatr Pharmacol 2:23, 1982.

29. Hayes CJ, Butler VP Jr, Gersony WM: Serum digoxin studies in infants and children. Pediatrics 52:561, 1973.

30. Hernandez A, Burton RM, Pagtakhan RD, Goldring D: Pharmacodynamics of H-digoxin in infants. Pediatrics 44:418, 1969.

31. Hoffman BF, Bigger JT Jr: Digitalis and allied cardiac glycosides. In Gilman AG, Goodman LS, Gilman A (eds): The Pharmacological Basis of Therapeutics, 6th ed. Chap 30. New York, Macmillan 1980.

32. Hofstetter R, Lang D, von Bernuth G: Effect of digoxin on left ventricular contractility in newborns and infants estimated by echocardiography. Eur J Cardiol 9:1, 1979.

33. Horwitz LD, Atkins JM, Saito M: Effect of digitalis on left ventricular function in exercising dogs. Circ Res 41:744, 1977.

34. Iisalo E, Dahl M: Serum levels and renal excretion of digoxin during maintenance therapy in children. Acta Paediatr Scand 63:699, 1974.

35. Johnson GL, Desai NS, Pauly TH, Cunningham MD: Complications associated with digoxin therapy in low-birth-weight infants. Pediatrics 69:463, 1982.

36. Joos HA, Johnson JL: Digitalis intoxication in infancy and childhood. Pediatrics 20:866, 1957.

37. Jusko WJ, Weintraub M: Myocardial distribution of digoxin and renal function. Clin Pharmacol Ther 16:449, 1974.

38. Karjalainen J, Ojala K, Reissell P: Tissue concentrations of digoxin in an autopsy material. Acta Pharmacol Toxicol 34:385, 1974.

39. Kearin M, Kelly JG, O'Malley K: Digoxin "receptors" in neonates: An explanation of less sensitivity to digoxin than in adults. Clin Pharmacol Ther 28:346, 1980.

40. Kim, PW, Krasula RW, Soyka LF, Hastreiter AR: Postmortem tissue digoxin concentrations in infants and children. Circulation 52:1128, 1975.

41. Koup JR, Jusko WJ, Elwood CM, Kohli RK: Digoxin pharmacokinetics: Role of renal failure in dosage regimen design. Clin Pharmacol Ther 18:9, 1975.

42. Kramer WG, Bathala MS, Reuning RH: Specificity of the digoxin radioimmunoassay with respect to dihydrodigoxin. Res Commun Chem Pathol Pharmacol 14:83, 1976.

43. Krasula RW, Pellegrino PA, Hastreiter AR, Soyka LF: Serum levels of digoxin in infants and children. J Pediatr 81:566, 1972.

44. Krasula RW, Hastreiter AR, Levitsky S, et al: Serum, atrial, and urinary digoxin levels during cardiopulmonary bypass in children. Circulation 49:1047, 1974.

45. Krasula R, Yanagi R, Hastreiter AR, et al: Digoxin intoxication in infants and children: Correlation with serum levels. Pediatr Pharmacol Ther 84:265, 1974.

46. Krivoy N, Rogin N, Greif Z, et al: Relationship between digoxin concentration in serum and saliva in infants. J Pediatr 99:810, 1981.

47. Lang D, von Bernuth G: Serum concentration and serum half-life of digoxin in premature and mature newborns. Pediatrics 59:902, 1977.

48. Lang D, Hofstetter R, von Bernuth G: Postmortem tissue and plasma concentrations of digoxin in newborns and infants. Eur J Pediatr 128:151, 1978.

49. Langer GA: Mechanism of action of the cardiac glycosides on the heart. Biochem Pharmacol 30:3261, 1981.

50. Larese RJ, Mirkin BL: Kinetics of digoxin absorption and relation of serum levels to cardiac arrhythmias in children. Clin Pharmacol Ther 15:387, 1974.

51. Lathers CM, Roberts J: Digitalis cardiotoxicity revisited. Life Sci 27:1713, 1980.

52. Levine OR, Blumenthal S: Digoxin dosage in premature infants. Pediatrics 29:18, 1962.

53. Levy AM, Leaman DM, Hanson JS: Effects of digoxin on systolic time intervals of neonates and infants. Circulation 46:816, 1972.

54. Linday LA, Engle MA, Reidenberg MM: Maturation and renal digoxin clearance. Clin Pharmacol Ther 30:735, 1981.

55. Lindenbaum J, Rund DG, Butler VP Jr, et al: Inactivation of digoxin by the gut flora: Reversal by antibiotic therapy. N Engl J Med 305:789, 1981.

56. Lindenbaum J, Tse-Eng D, Butler VP Jr, Rund DG: Urinary excretion of reduced metabolites of digoxin. Am J Med 71:67, 1981.

57. Lloyd BL, Greenblatt DJ, Allen MD, Harmatz JS, Smith TW: Pharmacokinetics and bioavailability of digoxin capsules, solution, and tablets after single and multiple doses. Am J Cardiol 42:129, 1978.

58. Marvin WJ, Spratt JL, Schieken M: Echocardiographic changes during digitalization in infancy. Pediatr Res 10:314, 1976.

59. Mason DT, Spann JF Jr, Zeis R: New developments in the understanding of the actions of the digitalis glycosides. Prog Cardiovasc Dis 11:443, 1969.

60. Mason DT: Regulation of cardiac performance in clinical heart disease: Interactions between contractile state mechanical abnormalities and ventricular compensatory mechanisms. Am J Cardiol 32:437, 1973.

61. Mason DT: Digitalis pharmacology and therapeutics: Recent advances. Ann Intern Med 80:520, 1974.

62. Milstein JM, Goetzman BW, Bennett SH: Pulmonary vascular response to digoxin. Pediatr Res 15:468, 1981.

63. Mintz GS, Bharadwaja K: Clinical pharmacology of digoxin. Drug Ther 1:15, 1976.

64. Morselli PL, Assael BM, Gomeni R, et al: Digoxin pharmacokinetics during human development. In Morselli PL, Garattini S, Sereni F (eds): Basic and Therapeutic Aspects of Perinatal Pharmacology, New York, Raven Press, 1975.

65. Neblett CR, McNeel DP, Waltz TA Jr, Harrison GM: Effect of cardiac glycosides on human cerebrospinal-fluid production. Lancet II:1008, 1972.

66. Neutze JM, Rutherford JD, Hurley PJ: Serum digoxin

levels in neonates, infants, and children with heart disease. N Z Med J 86:7, 1977.

67. Ng PK, Cote J, Schiff D, Collins-Nakai RL: Renal clearance of digoxin in premature neonates. Res Commun Chem Pathol Pharmacol 34:207, 1981.

68. Nyberg L, Wettrell G: Digoxin dosage schedules for neonates and infants based on pharmacokinetic considerations. Clin Pharmacol 3:453, 1978.

69. Nyberg L, Wettrell G: Pharmacokinetics and dosage of digoxin in neonates and infants. Eur J Clin Pharmacol 18:69, 1980.

70. Ochs HR, Greenblatt DJ, Grube E, Boden G: Pharmacokinetics and pharmacodynamics of intravenous digoxin in humans. Clin Pharmacol Ther 27:276, 1980.

71. O'Malley K, Coleman EN, Doig WB, Stevenson IH: Plasma digoxin levels in infants. Arch Dis Child 48:55, 1973.

72. Park MK, Ludden T, Arom KV, et al: Myocardial vs serum digoxin concentrations in infants and adults. Am J Dis Child 136:418, 1982.

73. Peters U, Falk LC, Kaman SM: Digoxin metabolism in patients. Arch Intern Med 138:1074, 1978.

74. Pinsky WW, Jacobsen JR, Gillette PC, et al: Dosage of digoxin in premature infants. J Pediatr 96:639, 1979.

75. Pudek MR, Seccombe DW, Whitfield MF, Ling E: Digoxin-like immunoreactivity in premature and full-term infants not receiving digoxin therapy. N Engl J Med 308:904, 1983.

76. Rogers MC, Willerson JT, Goldblatt A, Smith TW: Serum digoxin concentrations in the human fetus, neonate, and infant. N Engl J Med 287:1010, 1972.

77. Rosen MR, Wit AL, Hoffman BF: Electrophysiology and pharmacology of cardiac arrhythmias. IV. Cardiac antiarrhythmic and toxic effects of digitalis. Am Heart J 89:391, 1975.

78. Sahn DJ, Vaucher Y, Williams DE, et al: Echocardiographic detection of large left to right shunts and cardiomyopathies in infants and children. Am J Cardiol 73:73, 1976.

79. Sandor GGS, Bloom KR, Izukawa T, et al: Noninvasive assessment of left ventricular function related to serum digoxin levels in neonates. Pediatrics 65:541, 1980.

80. Schwartz A, Lindenmayer GE, Allen JC: The sodium–potassium adenosine triphosphatase: Pharmacological, physiological, and biochemical aspects. Pharmacol Rev 27:3, 1975.

81. Smith TW, Haber E: Digitalis (second of four parts). N Engl J Med 289:1010, 1973.

82. Smith TW, Haber E: Digitalis (fourth of four parts). N Engl J Med 289:1125, 1973.

83. Sodums MT, Walsh RA, O'Rourke RA: Digitalis in heart failure: Farewell to the foxglove? JAMA 246:158, 1981.

84. Spector R: Digitalis therapy in heart failure: A rational approach. J Clin Pharmacol 19:692, 1979.

85. Steiness E: Renal tubular secretion of digoxin. Circulation 50:103, 1974.

86. Steiness E, Svendsen O, Rasmussen F: Plasma digoxin after parenteral administration: Local reaction after intramuscular injection. Clin Pharmacol Ther 16:430, 1974.

87. Szefler SJ, Koup JR, Giacoia GP: Paradoxical behavior of serum digoxin concentrations in an anuric neonate. J Pediatr 91:487, 1977.

88. Viana AP: Respiratory effects of digoxin and ouabain in the dog. Arch Int Pharmacodyn 203:130, 1973.

89. Warburton D, Bell EF, Oh W: Pharmacokinetics and echocardiographic effects of digoxin in low-birth-weight infants with left-to-right shunting due to patent ductus arteriosus. Dev Pharmacol Ther 1:189, 1980.

90. Wettrell G, Andersson KE, Bertler A, Lundstrom NR: Concentrations of digoxin in plasma and urine in neonates, infants, and children with heart disease. Acta Paediatr Scand 63:705, 1974.

91. Wettrell G, Andersson KE: Absorption of digoxin in infants. Eur J Clin Pharmacol 9:49, 1975.

92. Wettrell G: Digoxin therapy in infants: A clinical pharmacokinetic study. Acta Paediatr Scand 257(Suppl):7, 1976.

93. Wettrell G: Distribution and elimination of digoxin in infants. Eur J Clin Pharmacol 11:329, 1977.

94. Wettrell G, Andersson KE: Clinical pharmacokinetics of digoxin in infants. Clin Pharmacol 2:17, 1977.

95. White RD, Clark EB, Varghese PJ, et al: Echocardiographic left ventricular function in infants with congestive heart failure. Pediatr Res 10:319, 1976.

96. White RD, Lietman PS: Commentary: A reappraisal of digitalis for infants with left-to-right shunts and "heart failure." J Pediatr 92:867, 1978.

97. Zannad F, Marchal F, Royer RJ, et al: Study of the sensitivity of neonates to digoxin: Contribution of erythrocyte [86]Rubidium uptake test. Pediatr Pharmacol 1:221, 1981.

Sympathomimetics

98. Arant BS Jr: Nonrenal factors influencing renal function during the perinatal period. Clin Perinatol 8:225, 1981.

99. Barcroft H, Starr I: Comparison of the actions of adrenaline and noradrenaline on the cardiac output in man. Clin Sci 10:295, 1951.

100. Beregovitch J, Bianchi C, Rubler S, et al: Dose-related hemodynamic and renal effects of dopamine in congestive heart failure. Am Heart J 87:550, 1974.

101. Bohn DJ, Poirier CS, Edmonds JF, Barker GA: Hemodynamic effects of dobutamine after cardiopulmonary bypass in children. Crit Care Med 8:367, 1980.

102. Brodde O: Vascular dopamine receptors: Demonstration and characterization by *in vitro* studies. Life Sci 31:289, 1982.

103. Bucciarelli RL, Nelson RM, Egan EA II, et al: Transient tricuspid insufficiency of the newborn: A form of myocardial dysfunction in stressed newborns. Pediatrics 59:330, 1977.

104. Cabel LA, Devaskar U, Siassi B, et al: Cardiogenic shock associated with perinatal asphyxia in preterm infants. J Pediatr 96:705, 1980.

105. Crone RK: Acute circulatory failure in children. Pediatr Clin North Am 27:525, 1980.

106. Daoud FS, Reeves JT, Kelly DB: Isoproterenol as a potential pulmonary vasodilator in primary pulmonary hypotension. Am J Cardiol 42:817, 1978.

107. DiSessa TG, Leitner M, Ti CC, et al: The cardiovascular effects of dopamine in the severely asphyxiated neonate. J Pediatr 99:772, 1981.

108. Driscoll DJ, Gillette PC, McNamara DG: The use of dopamine in children. J Pediatr 92:309, 1978.

109. Driscoll DJ, Gillette PC, Duff DF, et al: Hemodynamic effects of dobutamine in children. Am J Cardiol 43:581, 1979.

110. Driscoll DJ, Gillette PC, Lewis RM, et al: Comparative hemodynamic effects of isoproterenol, dopa-

mine, and dobutamine in the newborn dog. Pediatr Res 13:1006, 1979.

111. Driscoll DJ, Pinsky WW, Entman ML: How to use inotropic drugs in children. Drug Ther (Hosp) 4:39, 1979.

112. Driscoll DJ, Gillette PC, Fukushige J, et al: Comparison of the cardiovascular action of isoproterenol, dopamine, and dobutamine in the neonatal and mature dog. Pediatr Cardiol 1:307, 1980.

113. Driscoll DJ, Fukushige J, Hartley CJ, et al: The comparative hemodynamic effects of isoproterenol in chronically instrumented puppies and adult dogs. Dev Pharmacol Ther 2:91, 1981.

114. Drummond WH, Webb IB, Purcell KA: Cardiopulmonary response to dopamine in chronically catheterized neonatal lambs. Pediatr Pharmacol 1:347, 1981.

115. Drummond WH, Gregory GA, Heymann MA, Phibbs RA: The independent effects of hyperventilation, tolazoline, and dopamine on infants with persistent pulmonary hypertension. J Pediatr 98:603, 1981.

116. Fiddler GI, Chatrath R, Williams GJ, et al: Dopamine infusion for the treatment of myocardial dysfunction associated with a persistent transitional circulation. Arch Dis Child 55:194, 1980.

117. Friedman WF: The intrinsic physiologic properties of the developing heart. In Friedman WF, Lesch M, Sonnenblick EM (eds): Neonatal Heart Disease. New York, Grune and Stratton, 1973, p 21.

118. Goldberg LI, Blodwell RD, Braunwald E, Morrow AG: The direct effects of norepinephrine, epinephrine, and methoxamine on myocardial contractile force in man. Circulation 22:1125, 1960.

119. Goldberg LI: Dopamine—clinical uses of an endogenous catecholamine. N Engl J Med 291:391, 1974.

120. Goldberg LI, Hsieh YY, Resnekov L: Newer catecholamines for treatment of heart failure and shock: An update on dopamine and a first look at dobutamine. Prog Cardiovasc Dis 19:327, 1977.

121. Goldenberg M, Pines KL, Baldwin EF, et al: The hemodynamic response to man to norepinephrine and epinephrine and its relation to the problem of hypertension. Am J Med 5:792, 1948.

122. Gootman N, Buckley BJ, Gootman PM, et al: Maturation-related differences in regional circulatory effects of dopamine infusion in swine. Dev Pharmacol Ther 6:9, 1983.

123. Greenberg MI, Roberts JR, Baskin SI, Wagner DK: The use of endotracheal medication for cardiac arrest. Top Emerg Med 1:29, 1979.

124. Gunnar RM, Loeb HS, Pietras RJ, Tobin JR Jr: Ineffectiveness of isoproterenol in shock due to acute myocardial infarction. JAMA 202:64, 1967.

125. Guntheroth WG: Neonatal and pediatric cardiovascular crises. JAMA 232:168, 1975.

126. Hardaker WT Jr, Wechsler AS: Redistribution of renal intracortical blood flow during dopamine infusion in dogs. Circ Res 33:437, 1973.

127. Hoffman BB, Lefkowitz RJ: Adrenergic receptors in the heart. Ann Rev Physiol 44:475, 1982.

128. Holloway EL, Stinson EB, Derby GC, Harrison DC: Action of drugs in patients early after cardiac surgery. I. Comparison of isoproterenol and dopamine. Am J Cardiol 35:656, 1975.

129. Huckauf H, Ramdohr B, Schroder R: Dopamine-induced hypoxemia in patients with left heart failure. Int J Clin Pharmacol 14:217, 1976.

130. Insel PA, Snavely MD: Catecholamines and the kidney: Receptors and renal function. Annu Rev Physiol 43:625, 1981.

131. Jardin F, Sportiche M, Bazin M, et al: Dobutamine: A hemodynamic evaluation in human septic shock. Crit Care Med 9:329, 1981.

131a. Kirsh MM, Bove E, Detmer M, et al: The use of levarterenol and phentolamine in patients with low cardiac output following open-heart surgery. Ann Thorac Surg 29:26, 1980.

132. Kliegman R, Fanaroff AA: Caution in the use of dopamine in the neonate. J Pediatr 93:540, 1978.

133. Lang P, Williams RG, Norwood WI, Castaneda AR: The hemodynamic effects of dopamine in infants after corrective cardiac surgery. J Pediatr 96:630, 1980.

134. LeBlanc H, Lachelin GCL, Abu-Fadil S, Yen SSC: Effects of dopamine infusion on pituitary hormone secretion in humans. J Clin Endocrinol Metab 43:668, 1976.

135. LeBlanc H, Lachelin GCL, Abu-Fadil S, Yen SSC: The effect of dopamine infusion on insulin and glucagon secretion in man. J Clin Endocrinol Metab 44:196, 1977.

136. Lee MH: Perinatal asphyxia and the myocardium. J Pediatr 96:675, 1980.

137. Lefer AM, Spath JA Jr: Pharmacologic basis of the treatment of circulatory shock. In Antonaccio M (ed): Cardiovascular Pharmacology. P 377. New York, Raven Press, 1977.

138. Lefkowitz RJ: Beta-adrenergic receptors: recognition and regulation. N Engl J Med 295:323, 1976.

139. Leier CV, Heban PT, Huss P, et al: Comparative systemic and regional hemodynamic effects of dopamine and dobutamine in patients with cardiomyopathic heart failure. Circulation 58:466, 1978.

140. Loeb HS, Bredakis J, Gunnar RM: Superiority of dobutamine over dopamine for augmentation of cardiac output in patients with chronic low output cardiac failure. Circulation 55:375, 1977.

141. Lorenzi M, Karam JH, Tsalikian E, et al: Dopamine during alpha- or beta-adrenergic blockade in man. J Clin Invest 63:310, 1979.

142. Lucchesi BR: Inotropic agents and drugs used to support the failing heart. In Antonaccio M (ed): Cardiovascular Pharmacology. P 337. New York, Raven Press, 1977.

143. Lupi-Herrera E, Bialostozky D, Sobrino A: The role of isoproterenol pulmonary artery hypertension of unknown etiology (primary). Chest 79:292, 1981.

144. MacCannell KL, Giraud GD, Hamilton PL, Groves G: Haemodynamic responses to dopamine and dobutamine infusions as a function of duration of infusion. Pharmacology 26:29, 1983.

145. Maggi JC, Angelats J, Scott JP: Gangrene in a neonate following dopamine therapy. J Pediatr 100:323, 1982.

146. Manders WT, Pagani M, Vatner SF: Depressed responsiveness to vasoconstrictor and dilator agents and baroreflex sensitivity in conscious, newborn lambs. Circulation 60:945, 1979.

147. Maroko PR, Kjekshus JK, Sobel BE, et al: Factors influencing infarct size following experimental coronary artery occlusions. Circulation 63:67, 1971.

148. Mayer SE: Neurohumoral transmission and the autonomic nervous system. In Gilman AG, Goodman LS. Gilman A (eds): The Pharmacological Basis of Therapeutics. Chap 4. New York, Macmillan, 1980.

149. McNay JL, Goldberg LI: Comparison of the effects of

dopamine, isoproterenol, norepinephrine, and bradykinin on canine renal and femoral blood flow. J Pharmacol Exp Ther 151:23, 1966.

150. Mentzer RM Jr, Alegre CA, Nolan SP: The effects of dopamine and isoproterenol on the pulmonary circulation. J Thorac Cardiovasc Surg 71:807, 1976.

151. Motulsky HJ, Insel PA: Adrenergic receptors in man: Direct identification, physiologic regulation, and clinical alterations. N Engl J Med 307:18, 1982.

152. Otto CW, Yakaitis RW, Redding JS, Blitt CD: Comparison of dopamine, dobutamine, and epinephrine in CPR. Crit Care Med 9:640, 1981.

153. Park MK, Sheridan PH, Morgan WW, Beck N: Comparative inotropic response of newborn and adult rabbit papillary muscles to isoproterenol and calcium. Dev Pharmacol Ther 1:70, 1980.

154. Perkin RM, Levin DL: Shock in the pediatric patient. Part I. J Pediatr 101:163, 1982.

155. Perkin RM, Levin DL: Shock in the pediatric patient. Part II. Therapy. J Pediatr 101:319, 1982.

156. Perkin RM, Levin DL, Webb R, et al: Dobutamine: A hemodynamic evaluation in children with shock. J Pediatr 100:977, 1982.

157. Polumbo RA, Harrison DC: Response of the pulmonary circulation to dopamine infusion in man. Circulation 46(Suppl II):56, 1972.

158. Redding JS, Pearson JW: Evaluation of drugs for cardiac resuscitation. Anesthesiology 24:203, 1963.

159. Reid PR, Thompson WL: The clinical use of dopamine in the treatment of shock. Johns Hopkins Med J 137:276, 1975.

160. Riemenschneider TA, Nielsen HC, Ruttenberg HD, Jaffe RB: Disturbances of the transitional circulation: Spectrum of pulmonary hypertension and myocardial dysfunction. J Pediatr 89:622, 1976.

161. Rigaud M, Boschat J, Rocha P, et al: Comparative haemodynamic effects of dobutamine and isoproterenol in man. Intensive Care Med 3:57, 1977.

162. Roberts JR, Greenberg MI, Knaub M, Baskin SI: Comparison of the pharmacological effects of epinephrine administered by the intravenous and endotracheal routes. JACEP 7:260, 1978.

163. Roberts JR, Greenberg MI, Knaub MA, et al: Blood levels following intravenous and endothelial epinephrine administration. JACEP 8:53, 1979.

164. Robie NW, Nutter DO, Moody C, McNay JL: In vivo analysis of adrenergic receptor activity of dobutamine. Circ Res 34:663, 1974.

165. Rosenblum R, Berkowitz WD, Lawson D: Effect of acute intravenous administration of isoproterenol on cardiorenal hemodynamics in man. Circulation 38:158, 1968.

166. Rudolph AM, Mesel E, Levy JM: Epinephrine in the treatment of cardiac failure due to shunts. Circulation 28:3, 1963.

167. Schoeppe W: Effect of dopamine on kidney function. Proc Roy Soc Med 70(Suppl 2):36, 1977.

168. Schranz D, Stopfkuchen H, Jungst BK, et al: Hemodynamic effects of dobutamine in children with cardiovascular failure. Eur J Pediatr 139:4, 1982.

169. Shahar E, Lotan D, Barzilay Z: Dopamine-induced paroxysmal supraventricular tachicardia in an infant. Clin Pediatr 20:541, 1981.

170. Shettigar UR, Hultgren HN, Specter M, et al: Primary pulmonary hypertension: Favorable effect of isoproterenol. N Engl J Med 295:1414, 1976.

171. Smith HJ, Driol A, Morch J, McGregor M: Hemodynamic studies in cardiogenic shock. Treatment with isoproterenol and metaraminol. Circulation 35:1084, 1967.

172. Somani P, Rojas-Vigo AE: Dopamine interactions. Drug Ther (Hosp) 2:31, 1977.

173. Sonnenblick EH, Frishman WH, LeJemtel TH: Dobutamine: A new synthetic cardioactive sympathetic amine. N Engl J Med 300:17, 1979.

174. Steen PA, Tinker JH, Pluth JR, et al: Efficacy of dopamine, dobutamine, and epinephrine during emergence from cardiopulmonary bypass in man. Circulation 57:378, 1978.

175. Talley RC, Goldberg LI, Johnson CE, McNay JL: A hemodynamic comparison of dopamine and isoproterenol in patients in shock. Circulation 39:361, 1969.

176. Tarazi RC: Sympathomimetic agents in the treatment of shock. Ann Intern Med 81:364, 1974.

177. Tuttle RR, Mills J: Development of a new catecholamine to selectively increase cardiac contractility. Circ Res 36:185, 1975.

178. Volkman PH: Use of dopamine for shock in neonates. J Pediatr 94: 852, 1979.

179. Weiner N: Norepinephrine, epinephrine, and the sympathomimetic amines. In Gilman AG, Goodman LS, Gilman A (eds): The Pharmacological Basis of Therapeutics, 6th ed. P 138. New York, Macmillan, 1980.

180. Whitsett JA, Noguchi A, Moore JJ: Developmental aspects of alpha and beta-adrenergic receptors. Semin Perinatol 6:125, 1982.

181. Yeager SB, Horbar J, Lucey JF: Sympathomimetic drugs in the neonate. N Engl J Med 303:1122, 1980.

Antihypertensives and Vasodilators

182. Abbott TR, Rees GJ, Dickinson D, et al: Sodium nitroprusside in idiopathic respiratory distress syndrome. Br Med J 1:1113, 1978.

183. Abrams J: Nitrate tolerance and dependence. Am Heart J 99:113, 1980.

184. Adelman RD: Neonatal hypertension. Pediatr Clin North Am 25:99, 1978.

185. Altszuler N, Hampshire J, Moraru E: On the mechanism of diazoxide-induced hyperglycemia. Diabetes 26:931, 1977.

186. Antonaccio MJ: Angiotensin converting enzyme (ACE) inhibitors. Annu Rev Pharmacol Toxicol 22:57, 1982.

187. Appelbaum A, Blackstone EH, Kouchoukos NT, Kirklin JW: Afterload reduction and cardiac output in infants early after intracardiac surgery. Am J Cardiol 39:445, 1977.

188. Armstrong PW, Walker DC, Burton JR, Parker JO: Vasodilator therapy in acute myocardial infarction: A comparison of sodium nitroprusside and nitroglycerin. Circulation 52:1118, 1975.

189. Armstrong PW, Armstrong JA, Marks GS: Pharmacokinetic–hemodynamic studies of intravenous nitroglycerine in congestive cardiac failure. Circulation 62:160, 1980.

190. Arndts D, Doevendans J, Kirsten R, Heintz B: New aspects of the pharmacokinetics and pharmacodynamics of clonidine in man. Eur J Clin Pharmacol 24:21, 1983.

191. Atkins JM, Mitchell HC, Pettinger WA: Increased pulmonary vascular resistance with systemic hypertension: Effect of minoxidil and other antihypertensive agents. Am J Cardiol 39:802, 1977.

192. Baaske DM, Amann AH, Wagenknecht DM, et al: Nitroglycerin compatibility with intravenous fluid filters, containers, and administration sets. Am J Hosp Pharm 37:201, 1980.

193. Bailie MD, Mattioli LF: Hypertension: Relationships between pathophysiology and therapy. J Pediatr 96:789, 1980.

194. Beekman RH, Rocchini AP, Rosenthal A: Hemodynamic effects of hydralazine in infants with a large ventricular septal defect. Circulation 65:523, 1982.

195. Benson LN, Bohn D, Edmonds JF, et al: Nitroglycerin therapy in children with low cardiac index after heart surgery. Cardiovasc Med 4:207, 1979.

196. Benzing G III, Helmsworth JA, Schrieber JT, et al: Nitroprusside after open-heart surgery. Circulation 54:467, 1976.

197. Bifano E, Post EM, Springer J, et al: Treatment of neonatal hypertension with captopril. J Pediatr 100:143, 1982.

198. Blaschke TF, Melmon KL: Antihypertensive agents and the drug therapy of hypertension. In Gilman AG, Goodman LS, Gilman A (eds): The Pharmacological Basis of Therapeutics, 6th ed. P 793. New York, Macmillan, 1980.

199. Bloss RS, Turmen T, Beardmore HE, Aranda JV: Tolazoline therapy for persistent pulmonary hypertension after congenital diaphragmatic hernia repair. J Pediatr 97:984, 1980.

200. Blum I, Doron M, Laron Z, Atsmon A: Prevention of Hypoglycemic attacks by propranolol in a patient suffering from insulinoma. Diabetes 24:535, 1975.

201. Boerth RC: Effect of propranolol in the treatment of hypertension in children. Pediatr Res 10:328, 1976.

202. Boerth RC, Long WR: Dose–response relation of diazoxide in children with hypertension. Circulation 56:1062, 1977.

203. Borman JB, Merin G, Majblum S, et al: The beneficial effects of chlorpromazine on pulmonary hemodynamics after cardiopulmonary bypass. Ann Thorac Surg 11:570, 1971.

204. Boucek MM, Chang R, Synhorst DP: Effects of prazosin (P) and hydralazine (H) on the hemodynamics of chronically instrumented lambs with ventricular septal defect. Circulation 62 (Suppl II):115, 1980.

205. Braunwald E: Mechanism of action of calcium-channel-blocking agents. N Engl J Med 307: 1618, 1982.

206. Brodie BB, Aronow L, Axelrod J: The fate of benzazoline (Priscoline) in dog and man and a method for its estimation in biological material. J Exp Pharmacol Ther 106:200, 1952.

207. Brogden RN, Heel RC, Speight TM, Avery GS: Prazosin: A review of its pharmacological properties and therapeutic efficacy in hypertension. Drugs 14:163, 1977.

208. Camerini F, Alberti E, Klugmann S, Salvi A: Primary pulmonary hypertension: Effects of nifedipine. Br Heart J 44:352, 1980.

209. Chatterjee K, Parmley WW: Vasodilator therapy for chronic heart failure. Annu Rev Pharmacol Toxicol 20:475, 1980.

210. Chatterjee K, Ports TA: Physiologic and pharmacologic basis for the use of vasodilators in heart failure. In Wilkerson RD (ed): Cardiac Pharmacology. Chap 8, P 150. New York, Academic Press, 1981.

211. Cohen RS, Stevenson DK, Malachowski N, et al: Late morbidity among survivors of respiratory failure treated with tolazoline. J Pediatr 97:644, 1980.

212. Colucci WS, Williams GH, Alexander RW, Braunwald E: Mechanisms and implications of vasodilator tolerance in the treatment of congestive heart failure. Am J Med 71:89, 1981.

213. Conen D, Bertel O, Dubach UC: An oral calcium antagonist for treatment of hypertensive emergencies. J Cardiovasc Pharmacol 4:S378, 1982.

214. Conolly ME, Kersting F, Dollergy CT: The clinical pharmacology of beta-adrenoceptor-blocking drugs. Prog Cardiovasc Dis 19:203, 1976.

215. Cotton EK: The use of Priscoline in the treatment of the hypoperfusion syndrome. Pediatrics 36:149, 1965.

216. Cumming GR, Carr W: Hemodynamic effects of propranolol in patients with Fallot's tetralogy. Am Heart J 74:29, 1967.

217. Cumming GR: Propranolol in tetralogy of Fallot. Circulation 44:13, 1970.

218. Curtis JJ, Luke RG, Whelchel JD, et al: Inhibition of angiotensin-converting enzyme in renal-transplant recipients with hypertension. N Engl J Med 308:377, 1983.

219. Dargie HJ, Dollery CT, Daniel J: Minoxidil in resistant hypertension. Lancet 2:515, 1977.

220. Davies DS, Wing LMH, Reid JL, et al: Pharmacokinetics and concentration-effect relationships of intravenous and oral clonidine. Clin Pharmacol Ther 21: 593, 1977.

221. Davies DW, Greiss L, Kadar D, Steward DJ: Sodium nitroprusside in children: Observations on metabolism during normal and abnormal responses. Can Anaesth Soc J 22:553, 1975.

222. Davis BA, Crook JE, Vestal RE, Oates JA: Prevalence of renovascular hypertension in patients with grade III or IV hypertensive retinopathy. N Engl J Med 301:1273, 1979.

223. deBruyn JHB, Man in't Veld AJ, Wenting GJ, et al: Haemodynamic profile of captopril treatment in various forms of hypertension. Eur J Clin Pharmacol 20:163, 1981.

224. deSwiet M, Fayers P, Shinebourne EA: Systolic blood pressure in a population of infants in the first year of life. The Brompton study. Pediatrics 65:1028, 1980.

225. Dillon TR, Janos GG, Meyer RA, et al: Vasodilator therapy for congestive heart failure. J Pediatr 96:623, 1980.

226. Dobbs W, Povalski JH: Coronary circulation, angina pectoris, and antianginal agents. In Antonacci M (ed): Cardiovascular Pharmacology. P 461. New York, Raven Press, 1977.

227. Drew JH, Arroyave CM: Histamine: Serum concentrations in respiratory disorders of the newborn infant. Acta Paediatr Scand 71:663, 1982.

228. Drummond WH, Gregory GA, Heymann MA, Phibbs RA: The independent effects of hyperventilation, tolazoline, and dopamine on infants with persistent pulmonary hypertension. J Pediatr 98:603, 1981.

229. Earley A, Fayers P, Ng S, et al: Blood pressure in the first 6 weeks of life. Arch Dis Child 55:755, 1980.

230. Ein SH, Barker G, Olley P, et al: The pharmacologic treatment of newborn diaphragmatic hernia—a 2-year evaluation. J Pediatr Surg 15:384, 1980.

231. Elkayam U, Mathur M, Frishman W, et al: Dynamic responses to continuous use of prazosin and hydralazine in patients with refractory heart failure. Clin Pharmacol Ther 30:23, 1981.

232. Eriksson BO, Thoren C, Zetterqvist P: Long-term treatment with propranolol in selected cases of Fallot's tetralogy. Br Heart J 31:37, 1969.

233. Fabre J, Fox HM, Dayer P, Balant L: Differences in kinetic properties of drugs: Implications as to the selection of a particular drug for use in patients with renal failure with special emphasis on antibiotics and beta-adrenoceptor blocking agents. Clin Pharmacol 5:441, 1980.

234. Ferrer MI, Bradley SE, Wheeler HO, et al: Some

effects of nitroglycerin upon the splanchnic, pulmonary, and systemic circulations. Circulation 33:357, 1966.

235. Flaim SF, Zelis R: Clinical use of calcium entry blockers. Fed Proc 40:2877, 1981.

236. Franciosa JA, Cohn JN: Hemodynamic responsiveness to short- and long-acting vasodilators in left ventricular failure. Am J Med 65:126, 1978.

237. Frank MJ, Johnson JB, Rubin SH: Spectrophotometric determination of sodium nitroprusside and its photodegradation products. J Pharm Sci 65:44, 1976.

238. Fried R, Steinherz LJ, Levin AR, et al: Use of hydralazine for intractable cardiac failure in childhood. J Pediatr 97:1009, 1980.

239. Gardner LI: Is propranolol alone really beneficial in neonatal thyrotoxicosis? Am J Dis Child 134:819, 1980.

240. Gillette P, Garson A Jr, Eterovic E, et al: Oral propranolol treatment in infants and children. J Pediatr 92:141, 1978.

241. Goetzman BW, Sunshine P, Johnson JD, et al: Neonatal hypoxia and pulmonary vasospasm: Response to tolazoline. J Pediatr 89:617, 1976.

242. Goetzman BW, Milstein JM: Pulmonary vasodilator action of tolazoline. Pediatr Res 13:942, 1979.

243. Gordillo-Paniagua G, Velasquez-Jones L, Martini R, Valdez-Bolanos E: Sodium nitroprusside treatment of severe arterial hypertension in children. J Pediatr 87:799, 1975.

244. Graham RM, Pettinger WA: Prazosin. N Engl J Med 300:232, 1979.

245. Greenblatt DJ, Koch-Weser J: Adverse reactions to beta-adrenergic receptor blocking drugs: A report from the Boston Collaborative Drug Surveillance Program. Drugs 7:118, 1974.

246. Griswold WR, McNeal R, Mendoza SA, et al: Propranolol as an antihypertensive agent in children. Arch Dis Child 53:594, 1978.

247. Grover RI, Reeves JT, Blount SG Jr: Tolazoline hydrochloride (Priscoline): An effective pulmonary vasodilator. Am Heart J 61:5, 1961.

248. Hill NS, Antman EM, Green LH, Alpert JS: Intravenous nitroglycerin: A review of pharmacology, indications, therapeutic effects, and complications. Chest 79:69, 1981.

249. Honey M, Chamberlain DA, Howard J: The effect of beta-sympathetic blockade on arterial oxygen saturation in Fallot's tetralogy. Circulation 30:501, 1964.

250. Houston MC: Clonidine hydrochloride: Review of pharmacologic and clinical aspects. Prog Cardiovasc Dis 23:337, 1981.

251. Hunter E, Raik E, Gordon S, Taylor KB: Incidence of positive Coombs' test, LE cells and antinuclear factor in patients on alpha-methyldopa ("Aldomet") therapy. Med J Aust 2:810, 1971.

252. Inselman LS, Mellins RB: Growth and development of the lung. J Pediatr 98:1, 1981.

253. Johnson BF: Diozoxide and renal function in man. Clin Pharmacol Ther 12:815, 1971.

254. Johnson GL, Cunningham MD, Desai NS, et al: Echocardiography in hypoxemic neonatal pulmonary disease. J Pediatr 96:716, 1980.

255. Jones ODH, Shore DF, Rigby ML, et al: The use of tolazoline hydrochloride as a pulmonary vasodilator in potentially fatal episodes of pulmonary vasoconstriction after cardiac surgery in children. Circulation 64(Suppl II):134, 1981.

256. Khatri I, Uemura N, Notargiacomo A, Freis ED: Direct and reflex cardiostimulating effects of hydralazine. Am J Cardiol 40:38, 1977.

257. Kirkland RT, Kirkland JL: Systolic blood pressure measurement in the newborn infant with the transcutaneous Doppler method. J Pediatr 80:52, 1972.

258. Kitterman JA, Phibbs RH, Tooley WH: Aortic blood pressure in normal newborn infants during the first 12 hours of life. Pediatrics 44:959, 1969.

259. Klinke WP, Gilbert JAL: Diazoxide in primary pulmonary hypertension. N Engl J Med 302:91, 1980.

260. Koch-Weser J: Hydralazine. N Engl J Med 295:320, 1976.

261. Korones SB, Eyal FG: Successful treatment of "persistent fetal circulation" with tolazoline. Pediatr Res 9:367, 1975.

262. Kramer RS, Mason DT, Braunwald E: Augmented sympathetic neurotransmitter activity in the peripheral vascular bed of patients with congestive heart failure and cardiac norepinephrine depletion. Circulation 38:629, 1968.

263. Kwan KC, Foltz EL, Breault GO, et al: Pharmacokinetics of methyldopa in man. J Pharmacol Exp Ther 198:264, 1976.

264. Lakier JB, Khaja F, Stein PD: Rationale and use of vasodilators in the management of congestive heart failure. Am Heart J 97:519, 1979.

265. Larsson LE, Ekstrom-Jodal B, Hjalmarson O: The effect of chlorpromazine in severe hypoxia in newborn infants. Acta Paediatr Scand 71:399, 1982.

266. Laux BE, Raichle ME: The effect of acetazolamide on cerebral blood flow and oxygen utilization in the rhesus monkey. J Clin Invest 62:585, 1978.

267. Leonard RG, Talbert RL: Calcium-channel blocking agents. Clin Pharm 1:17, 1982.

268. Levin DL, Heymann MA, Kitterman JA, et al: Persistent pulmonary hypertension of the newborn infant. J Pediatr 89:626, 1976.

269. Levison H, Kidd SL, Gemmell PA, Swyer RP: Blood pressure in normal full-term and premature infants. Am J Dis Child 3:374, 1966.

270. Linday LA, Levin AR, Klein AA, et al: Acute effects of vasodilators on left-to-right shunts in infants and children. Pediatr Pharmacol 1:267, 1981.

271. Little RC, Little WC: Cardiac preload, afterload, and heart failure. Arch Intern Med 142:819, 1982.

272. Lock JE, Coceani F, Olley PM: Direct and indirect pulmonary vascular effects of tolazoline in the newborn lamb. J Pediatr 95:600, 1979.

273. Lock JE, Hamilton F, Luide H, et al: Direct pulmonary vascular responses in the conscious newborn lamb. J Appl Physiol 48:188, 1980.

274. Lock JE, Olley PM, Coceani F: Enhanced beta-adrenergic-receptor responsiveness in hypoxic neonatal pulmonary circulation. Am J Physiol 240:H697, 1981.

275. Loggie JMH, New MI, Robson AM: Hypertension in the pediatric patient: A reappraisal. J Pediatr 94:685, 1979.

276. Lowenthal DT, Affrime MB: Pharmacology and pharmacokinetics of minoxidil. J Cardiovasc Pharmacol 2(Suppl 2):S93, 1980.

277. Lupi-Herrera E, Sandoval J, Seoane M, Bialostozky D: The role of hydralazine therapy for pulmonary arterial hypertension of unknown cause. Circulation 65:645, 1982.

278. Makker SP, Moorthy B: Rebound hypertension following minoxidil withdrawal. J Pediatr 96:762, 1980.

279. Mason DT: Afterload reduction and cardiac performance: Physiologic basis of systemic vasodilators as a new approach in treatment of congestive heart failure. Am J Med 65:106, 1978.

280. Matsuo M, Aida M, Yamada T, et al: Duodenal perforation with tolazoline therapy. J Pediatr 100:1005, 1982.

281. Matsumoto S, Ito T, Sada T, et al: Hemodynamic effects of nifedipine in congestive heart failure. Am J Cardiol 46:476, 1980.

282. McCrory WW, Kohaut EC, Lewy JE, et al: Safety of intravenous diazoxide in children with severe hypertension. Clin Pediatr 18:661, 1979.

283. McGrath JC: Vascular adrenergic receptors. In Vanhoutte PM, Leusen I (eds): Vasodilation. P 97. New York, Raven Press, 1981.

284. McIntosh N, Walters RO: Effect of tolazoline in severe hyaline membrane disease. Arch Dis Child 54:105, 1979.

285. McLaine PN, Drummond KN: Intravenous diazoxide for severe hypertension in childhood. J Pediatr 79:829, 1971.

286. Miller RR, Fennell WH, Young JB, et al: Differential systemic arterial and venous actions and consequent cardiac effects of vasodilator drugs. Prog Cardiovasc Dis 24:353, 1982.

287. Mirkin BL, Green TP, O'Dea RF: Disposition and pharmacodynamics of diuretics and antihypertensive agents in renal disease. Eur J Clin Pharmacol 18:109, 1980.

288. Monin P, Vert P, Morselli PL: A pharmacodynamic and pharmacokinetic study of tolazoline in the neonate. Dev Pharmacol Ther 4(Suppl 1):124, 1982.

289. Moodie DS, Kleinberg F, Telander RL, et al: Tolazoline as adjuvant therapy for III neonates with pulmonary hypoperfusion. Chest 74:604, 1978.

290. Moore PB, Dedman JR: Minireview: Calcium binding proteins and cellular regulation. Life Sci 31:2937, 1982.

291. Newman TJ, Virnig NL, Athinarayana PR: Complications of propranolol use in neonatal thyrotoxicosis. Am J Dis Child 134:707, 1980.

292. Nies AS, Shand DG: Clinical pharmacology of propranolol. Circulation 52:6, 1975.

293. Oberfield SE, Case DB, Levine LS, et al: Use of the oral antiotensin I–converting enzyme inhibitor (captopril) in childhood against malignant hypertension. J Pediatr 95:641, 1979.

294. Packer M, Le Jemtel TH: Physiologic and pharmacologic determinants of vasodilator response: A conceptual framework for rational drug therapy for chronic heart failure. Prog Cardiovasc Dis 24:275, 1982.

295. Palmer RF, Lasseter KC: Sodium nitroprusside. N Engl J Med 292:294, 1975.

296. Pearl KN, Chambers TL: Propranolol treatment of thyrotoxicosis in a premature infant. Br Med J 2:738, 1977.

297. Peckham GJ, Fox WW: Physiologic factors affecting pulmonary artery pressure in infants with persistent pulmonary hypertension. J Pediatr 93:1005, 1978.

298. Pemberton PJ, McConnell B, Shanks RG: Neonatal thyrotoxicosis treated with propranolol. Arch Dis Child 49:813, 1974.

299. Pennisi AJ, Takahashi M, Bernstein BH, et al: Minoxidil therapy in children with severe hypertension. J Pediatr 90:813, 1977.

300. Pettinger WA: Minoxidil and the treatment of severe hypertension. N Engl J Med 303:922, 1980.

301. Pierpont G, Hale KA, Franciosa JA, et al: Effects of vasodilators on pulmonary hemodynamics and gas exchange in left ventricular failure. Am Heart J 99:208, 1980.

302. Plumer LB, Kaplan GW, Mendoza SA: Hypertension in infants—a complication of umbilical arterial catheterization. J Pediatr 89:802, 1976.

303. Ponce FE, Williams LC, Webb HM, et al: Propranolol palliation of tetralogy of Fallot: Experience with long-term drug treatment in pediatric patients. Pediatrics 52:100, 1973.

304. Porter CJ, Garson A, Gillette PC: Verapamil: An effective calcium blocking agent for pediatric patients. Pediatrics 71:748, 1983.

305. Potter DE, Schamberlan M, Salvatierra O Jr, et al: Treatment of high-renin hypertension with propranolol in children after renal transplantation. J Pediatr 90:307, 1977.

306. Prichard BNC: Beta-adrenergic receptor blockade in hypertension, past, present and future. Br J Clin Pharmacol 5:379, 1978.

307. Pruitt AW, Dayton PG, Patterson JH: Disposition of diazoxide in children. Clin Pharmacol Ther 14:73, 1973.

308. Pruitt AW: Pharmacologic approach to the management of childhood hypertension. Pediatr Clin North Am 28:135, 1981

309. Purohit DM, Pai S, Levkoff AH: Effect of tolazoline on persistent hypoxemia in neonatal respiratory distress. Crit Care Med 6:14, 1978.

310. Ram CVS: Captopril. Arch Intern Med 142:914, 1982.

311. Reid LM: The pulmonary circulation: Remodeling in growth and disease. Am Rev Resp Dis 119:531, 1979.

312. Reidenberg MM, Drayer D, DeMarco AL, Bello CT: Hydralazine elimination in man. Clin Pharmacol Ther 14:970, 1973.

313. Robin ED: Some basic and clinical challenges in the pulmonary circulation. Chest 81:357, 1982

314. Ross J Jr: Effects of afterload or impedance on the heart: Afterload reduction in the treatment of cardiac failure. Cardiovasc Med 2:1115, 1977.

315. Rubin LJ, Peter RH: Oral hydralazine therapy for primary pulmonary hypertension. N Engl J Med 302:69, 1980.

316. Rubis LJ, Stephenson LW, Johnston MR, et al: Comparison of effects of prostaglandin E1 and nitroprusside on pulmonary vascular resistance in children after open-heart surgery. Ann Thorac Surg 32:563, 1981.

317. Rubin LJ, Handel F, Peter RH: The effects of oral hydralazine on right ventricular end-diastolic pressure in patients with right ventricular failure. Circulation 65:1369, 1982.

318. Rudolph AM: High pulmonary vascular resistance after birth. I. Pathophysiologic considerations and etiologic classification. Clin Pediatr 19:585, 1980.

319. Schwartz JF, Zwiren GT: Islet cell adenomatosis and adenoma in an infant. J Pediatr 79:232, 1971.

320. Scriabine A: Beta-adrenergic blocking drugs in hypertension. Ann Rev Pharmacol Toxicol 19:269, 1979.

321. Sellers EM, Koch-Weser J: Influence of intravenous injection rate on protein binding and vascular activity of diazoxide. Ann NY Acad Sci 226:319, 1973.

322. Shand DG, Nuckolls EM, Oates JA: Plasma propranolol levels in adults with observations in four children. Clin Pharmacol Ther 11:112, 1970.

323. Simonneau G, Escourrou P, Duroux P, Lockhart A:

Inhibition of hypoxic pulmonary vasoconstriction by nifedipine. N Engl J Med 304:1582, 1981.

324. Sinaiko AR, Mirkin BL: Management of severe childhood hypertension with minoxidil: A controlled clinical study. J Pediatr 91:138, 1977.

325. Sinaiko AR, O'Dea RF, Mirkin BL: Clinical response of hypertensive children to long-term minoxidil therapy. J Cardiovasc Pharmacol 2(Suppl 2):S181, 1980.

326. Smith CS, Howard NJ: Propranolol in treatment of neonatal thyrotoxicosis. J Pediatr 83:1046, 1973.

327. Somogyi A, Albrecht M, Kliems G, et al: Pharmacokinetics, bioavailability, and ECG response of verapamil in patients with liver cirrhosis. Br. J Clin Pharmacol 12:51, 1981.

328. Stephenson LW, Edmunds LH Jr, Raphaely R et al: Effect of nitroprusside and dopamine on pulmonary arterial vasculature in children after cardiac surgery. Circulation 60(Suppl 1):I-104, 1979.

329. Stevens DC, Schreiner RL, Bull MJ, et al: An analysis of tolazoline therapy in the critically ill neonate. J Pediatr Surg 15:964, 1980.

330. Stevenson DK, Kasting DS, Darnall RA Jr, et al: Refractory hypoxemia associated with neonatal pulmonary disease: The use and limitations of tolazoline. J Pediatr 95:595, 1979.

331. Strauer BE, Scherpe A: Ventricular function and coronary hemodynamics after intravenous nitroglycerin in coronary artery disease. Am Heart J 95:210, 1978.

332. Strauss FG, Franklin SS, Lewin AJ, Maxwell MH: Withdrawal of antihypertensive therapy. Hypertensive crisis in renovascular hypertension. JAMA 238:1734, 1977.

333. Subramanyam R, Tandon R, Shrivastava S: Hemodynamic effects of sodium nitroprusside in patients with ventricular septal defect. Eur J Pediatr 138:307, 1982.

334. Sumner E, Frank JD: Tolazoline in the treatment of congenital diaphragmatic hernias. Arch Dis Child 56:350, 1981.

335. Synhorst DP, Lauer RM, Doty DB, Brody MJ: Hemodynamic effects of vasodilator agents in dogs with experimental ventricular septal defects. Circulation 54:472, 1976.

336. Thananopavarn C, Golub MS, Eggena P, et al: Clonidine, a centrally acting sympathetic inhibitor, as monotherapy for mild to moderate hypertension. Am J Cardiol 49:153, 1982.

337. Versmold HT, Kitterman JA, Phibbs RH, et al: Aortic blood pressure during the first 12 hours of life in infants with birth weight 610 to 4,220 grams. Pediatrics 67:607, 1981.

338. Vidt DG, Bravo EL, Fouad FM: Captopril. N Engl J Med 306:214, 1982.

339. Walter NMA, Whitworth JA, Kincaid-Smith P: Clinical experience with the angiotensin-converting enzyme inhibitor captopril. Clin Exp Pharmacol Physiol 7(Suppl):117, 1982.

340. Wilkinson R: Beta-blockers and renal function. Drugs 23:195, 1982.

341. Yellin TO, Sperow JW, Buck SH: Antagonism of tolazoline by histamine H$_2$-receptor blockers. Nature 253:561, 1975.

342. Zavecz JH, Yellin TO: Interaction of alpha-adrenergic imidazolines with cardiac histamine H$_2$-receptors. Eur J Pharmacol 71:297, 1981.

343. Zelis R, Flaim SF: Alterations in vasomotor tone in congestive heart failure. Prog Cardiovasc Dis 24:437, 1982.

Antiarrhythmics

344. Bigger JT Jr, Schmidt DH, Kutt H: Relationship between the plasma level of diphenylhydantoin sodium and its cardiac antiarrhythmic effects. Circulation 38:363, 1968.

345. Bigger JT Jr, Hoffman BF: Antiarrhythmic drugs. In Gilman AG, Goodman LS, Gilman A (eds): The Pharmacological Basis of Therapeutics. Chap 77, p 761. New York, Macmillan, 1980.

346. Cohen IS, Jick H, Cohen SI: Adverse reactions to quinidine in hospitalized patients: Findings based on data from the Boston Collaborative Drug Surveillance Program. Prog Cardiovasc Dis 20:151, 1977.

347. Earnest MP, Marx JA, Drury LR: Complications of intravenous phenytoin for acute treatment of seizures. JAMA 249:762, 1983.

348. Epstein SE, Rosing DR: Verapamil: Its potential for causing serious complications in patients with hypertrophic cardiomyopathy. Circulation 64:437, 1981.

349. Garson A Jr, Gillette PC, McNamara DG: Supraventricular tachycardia in children: Clinical features, response to treatment, and long-term follow-up in 217 patients. J Pediatr 98:875, 1981.

350. Gelband H, Rosen MR: Pharmacologic basis for the treatment of cardiac arrhythmias. Pediatrics 55:59, 1975.

351. Gillette PC, Garson A Jr, Kugler JD, et al: Surgical treatment of supraventricular tachycardia in infants and children. Am J Cardiol 46:281, 1980.

352. Greco R, Musto B, Arienzo V, et al: Treatment of paroxysmal supraventricular tachycardia in infancy with digitalis, adenosine-5'-triphosphate, and verapamil: A comparative study. Circulation 66:504, 1982.

353. Guntheroth WG: Disorders of heart rate and rhythm. Pediatr Clin North Am 25:869, 1978.

354. Hernandez A, Strauss A, Kleiger RE, Goldring D: Idiopathic paroxysmal ventricular tachycardia in infants and children. J Pediatr 86:182, 1975.

355. Hoffman BF, Cranefield PF: Electrophysiology of the Heart. New York, McGraw-Hill, 1960.

356. Hoffman BF, Cranefield PF: The physiological basis of cardiac arrhthmias. Am J Med 37:670, 1964.

357. Koch-Weser J, Klein SW: Procainamide dosage schedules, plasma concentrations, and clinical effects. JAMA 215:1454, 1971.

358. Lawson DH, Jick H: Adverse reactions to procainamide. Br J Clin Pharmacol 4:507, 1977.

359. Lima JJ, Jusko WJ: Determination of procainamide acetylator status. Clin Pharmacol Ther 23:25, 1978.

360. Lucchesi BR: Antiarrhythmic drugs. In Antonaccio M (ed): Cardiovascular Pharmacology. P 269. New York, Raven Press, 1977.

361. Martin TC, Hernandez A: Atrial flutter in infancy. J Pediatr 100:239, 1982.

362. Mihaly GW, Moore G, Thomas J, et al: The pharmacokinetics and metabolism of the anilide local anesthetics in neonates. Eur J Clin Pharmacol 13:143, 1978.

363. Pickoff AS, Zies L, Ferrer PL, et al: High-dose propranolol therapy in the management of supraventricular tachycardia. J Pediatr 94:144, 1979.

364. Porter CJ, Garson A, Gillette PC: Verapamil: An effective calcium blocking agent for pediatric patients. Pediatrics 71:748, 1983.

365. Pratt C, Lichstein E: Ventricular antiarrhythmic effects of beta-adrenergic blocking drugs: A review of

mechanism and clinical studies. J Clin Pharmacol 22:335, 1982.

366. Radford DJ, Izukawa T: Atrial fibrillation in children. Pediatrics 59:250, 1977.
367. Sapire DW, Mongkolsmai C, O'Riordan AC: Control of chronic ectopic supraventricular tachycardia and verapamil. J Pediatr 94:312, 1979.
368. Singh BN, Ellrodt G, Peter CT: Verapamil: A review of its pharmacological properties and therapeutic use. Drugs 15:169, 1978.
369. Spear JF, Moore EN: Mechanisms of cardiac arrhythmias. Ann Rev Physiol 44:485, 1982.
370. Stevens DC, Schreiner RL, Hurwitz RA, Gresham EL: Fetal and neonatal ventricular arrhythmia. Pediatrics 63:771, 1979.

Additional References

Digoxin

371. Bendayan R, McKenzie MW: Digoxin pharmacokinetics and dosage requirements in pediatric patients. Clin Pharm 2:224, 1983.
372. Cogan JJ, Humphreys MH, Carlson CJ, Benowitz NL, Rapaport E: Acute vasodilator therapy increases renal clearance of digoxin in patients with congestive heart failure. Circulation 64:973, 1981.
373. Cohen L, Kitzes R: Magnesium sulfate and digitalis-toxic arrhythmias. JAMA 249:2808, 1983.
374. Dobkin JF, Saha JR, Butler VP, Neu HC, Lindenbaum J: Digoxin-inactivating bacteria: Identification in human gut flora. Science 220:325, 1983.
375. Fleg JL, Gottlieb SH, Lakatta EG: Is digoxin really important in treatment of compensated heart failure? A placebo-controlled crossover study in patients with sinus rhythm. Am J Med 73:244, 1982.
376. Godfraind T, De Pover A, Hernandez GC, Fagoo M: Cardiodigin: Endogenous digitalis-like material from mammalian heart. Arch Int Pharmacodyn Ther 258:165, 1982.
377. Graves SW, Brown B, Valdes R Jr: An endogenous digoxin-like substance in patients with renal impairment. Ann Int Med 99:604, 1983.
378. Gruber KA, Whitaker JM, Buckalew VM Jr: Endogenous digitalis-like substance in plasma of volume-expanded dogs. Nature 287:743, 1980.
379. Hastreiter AR, van der Horst RL: Postmortem digoxin tissue concentration and organ content in infancy and childhood. Am J Cardiol 52:330, 1983.
380. Lundell BPW, Boreus LO: Digoxin therapy and left ventricular performance in premature infants with patent ductus arteriosus. Acta Paediatr Scand 72:339, 1983.
381. Ochs HR, Greenblatt DJ, Bodem G, Dengler HJ: Disease-related alterations in cardiac glycoside disposition. Clin Pharmacokinet 7:434, 1982.
382. Patterson MWH, Reid G, Sandor GGS: Serum digoxin levels in neonates whose weights are less than 1,500 grams. Pediatr Pharmacol 2:217, 1982.
383. Valdes R Jr, Graves SW, Brown BA, Landt M: Endogenous substance in newborn infants causing false positive digoxin measurements. J Pediatr 102:947, 1983.
384. Wagner JG, Dick M II, Behrendt DM, Lockwood GF, Sakmar E, Hees P: Determination of myocardial and serum digoxin concentrations in children by specific and nonspecific assay methods. Clin Pharmacol Ther 33:577, 1983.

Sympathomimetics

385. Baim DS, McDowell AV, Cherniles J, Monrad ES, Parker AJ, Edelson J, Braunwald E, Grossman W: Evaluation of a new bipyridine inotropic agent—milrinone—in patients with severe congestive heart failure. New Engl J Med 309:748, 1983.
386. Brown MJ, Brown DC, Murphy MB: Hypokalemia from beta$_2$-receptor stimulation by circulating epinephrine. New Engl J Med 309:1414, 1983.
387. Edelson J, LeJemtel TH, Alousi AA, Biddlecome CE, Maskin CS, Sonnenblick EH: Relationship between amrinone plasma concentration and cardiac index. Clin Pharmacol Ther 29:723, 1981.
388. Hoshino K: Clinical usefulness of dopamine in the shock state of neonates. Jpn J Anesth 25:11, 1976.
389. Klein NA, Siskind SJ, Frishman WH, Sonnenblick EH, LeJemtel TH: Hemodynamic comparison of intravenous amrinone and dobutamine in patients with chronic congestive heart failure. Am J Cardiol 48:170, 1981.
390. Leier CV, Unverferth DV: Dobutamine. Ann Intern Med 99:490, 1983.
391. Lindemann R: Endotracheal administration of epinephrine during cardiopulmonary resuscitation. Am J Dis Child 136:753, 1982.
392. Lokhandwala MF, Barrett RJ: Dopamine receptor agonists in cardiovascular therapy. Drug Develop Res 3:299, 1983.
393. Maskin CS, Sinoway L, Chadwick B, Sonnenblick EH, LeJemtel TH: Sustained hemodynamic and clinical effects of a new cardiotonic agent, WIN 47203, in patients with severe congestive heart failure. Circulation 67:1065, 1983.
394. Park GB, Kershner RP, Angellotti J, Williams RL, Benet LZ, Edelson J: Oral bioavailability and intravenous pharmacokinetics of amrinone in humans. J Pharm Sci 72:817, 1983.
395. Siskind SJ, Sonnenblick EH, Forman R, Scheuer J, LeJemtel TH: Acute substantial benefit of inotropic therapy with amrinone on exercise hemodynamics and metabolism in severe congestive heart failure. Circulation 64:966, 1981.
396. Unverferth DV, Blanford M, Kates RE, Leier CV: Tolerance to dobutamine after a 72 hour continuous infusion. Am J Med 69:262, 1980.
397. Weber KT, Andrews V, Janicki JS, Wilson JR, Fishman AP: Amrinone and exercise performance in patients with chronic heart failure. Am J Cardiol 48:164, 1981.
398. Wynne J, Malacoff RF, Benotti JR, Curfman GD, Grossman W, Holman BL, Smith TW, Braunwald E: Oral amrinone in refractory congestive heart failure. Am J Cardiol 45:1245, 1980.

Antihypertensives and Vasodilators

399. Aynsley-Green A, Polak JM, Bloom SR, et al: Nesidioblastosis of the pancreas: Definition of the syndrome and the management of severe neonatal hyperinsulinaemic hypoglycaemia. Arch Dis Child 56:496, 1981.
400. Banzet O, Colin JN, Thibonnier M, Singlas E, Alexandre JM, Corvol P: Acute antihypertensive effect and pharmacokinetics of a tablet preparation of nifedipine. Eur J Clin Pharmacol 24:145, 1983.
401. Barnes PJ, Wilson NM, Brown MJ: A calcium antagonist, nifedipine, modifies exercise-induced asthma. Thorax 36:726, 1981.
402. Bishop MJ, Cheney FW: Comparison of the effects of

minoxidil and nifedipine on hypoxic pulmonary vasoconstriction in dogs. J Cardiovasc Pharmacol 5:184, 1983.

403. Chrysant SG, Dunn M, Marples D, DeMasters K: Severe reversible azotemia from captopril therapy: Report of three cases and review of the literature. Arch Intern Med 143:437, 1983.

404. Cottrill CM, McAllister RG, Noonan JA: Propranolol administration in infancy. Pediatr Res 11:415, 1977.

405. Council on Scientific Affairs: Calcium channel blocking agents. JAMA 250:2522, 1983.

406. De Feyter PJ, Kerkkamp HJJ, de Jong JP: Sustained beneficial effect of nifedipine in primary pulmonary hypertension. Am Heart J 105:333, 1983.

407. Dilmen U, Cağlar MK, Senses A, Kinik E: Nifedipine in hypertensive emergencies of children. Am J Dis Child 137:1162, 1983.

408. Drew RH: The use of hydroxocobalamin in the prophylaxis and treatment of nitroprusside-induced cyanide toxicity. Vet Hum Toxicol 25:342, 1983.

409. Drummond WH, Williams BJ: Effect of continuous tolazoline infusion on cardiopulmonary response to dopamine in unanesthetized newborn lambs. J Pediatr 103:278, 1983.

410. Eklund B, Hjemdahl P, Seideman P, Atterhog JH: Effects of prazosin on hemodynamics and sympatho-adrenal activity in hypertensive patients. J Cardiovasc Pharmacol 5:384, 1983.

411. Fitchett DH, Neto JAM, Oakley CM, Goodwin JF: Hydralazine in the management of left ventricular failure. Am J Cardiol 44:303, 1979.

412. Franciosa JA, Weber KT, Levine TB, Kinasewitz GT, Janicki JS, West J, Henis MMJ, Cohn JN: Hydralazine in the long-term treatment of chronic heart failure: Lack of difference from placebo. Am Heart J 104:587, 1982.

413. Friedman AL, Chesney RW: Effect of captopril on the renin-angiotensin system in hypertensive children. J Pediatr 103:806, 1983.

414. Garrett BN, Kaplan NM: Efficacy of slow infusion of diazoxide in the treatment of severe hypertension without organ hypoperfusion. Am Heart J 103:390, 1982.

415. Hoder EL, Leckman JF, Ehrenkranz R, Kleber H, Cohen DJ, Poulsen JA: Clonidine in neonatal narcotic-abstinence syndrome. New Engl J Med 305:1284, 1981.

416. Jaffe AS, Roberts R: The use of intravenous nitroglycerin in cardiovascular disease. Pharmacotherapeutica 2:273, 1982.

417. Janis RA, Triggle DJ: New developments in CA^{2+} channel antagonists. J Med Chem 26:775, 1983.

418. Johnson BF, Kapur M: The influences of rate of injection upon the effects of diazoxide. Am J Med Sci 263:481, 1972.

419. Jones HMR, Cummings AJ, Setchell KDR, Lawson AM: A study of the disposition of alpha-methyldopa in newborn infants following its administration to the mother for the treatment of hypertension during pregnancy. Br J Clin Pharmacol 8:433, 1979.

420. Kashani IA, Swensson RE: Pulmonary vasodilators in postoperative pulmonary hypertension. Am Heart J 106:778, 1983.

421. Kates RE: Calcium antagonists: Pharmacokinetic properties. Drugs 25:113, 1983.

422. Kendall MJ, Beeley L: Beta-adrenoceptor blocking drugs: Adverse reactions and drug interactions. Pharmacol Ther 21:351, 1983.

423. Kramer BL, Massie BM, Topic N: Controlled trial of captopril in chronic heart failure: A rest and exercise hemodynamic study. Circulation 67:807, 1983.

424. Leier CV, Bambach D, Nelson S, Hermiller JB, Huss P, Magorien RD, Unverferth DV: Captopril in primary pulmonary hypertension. Circulation 67:155, 1983.

425. Lewis JG: Adverse reactions to calcium antagonists. Drugs 25:196, 1983.

426. Ludden TM, McNay JL Jr, Shepherd AMM, Lin MS: Clinical pharmacokinetics of hydralazine. Clin Pharmacokinet 7:185, 1982.

427. Man in 't Veld AJ, Schalekamp MADH: Effects of 10 different beta-adrenoceptor antagonists on hemodyanamics, plasma renin activity, and plasma norepinephrine in hypertension: The key role of vascular resistance changes in relation to partial agonist activity. J Cardiovasc Pharmacol 5:S30, 1983.

428. Markham RV Jr, Corbett JR, Gilmore A, Pettinger WA, Firth BG: Efficacy of prazosin in the management of chronic congestive heart failure: A 6-month randomized, double-blind, placebo-controlled study. Am J Cardiol 51:1346, 1983.

429. Massie B, Ports T, Chatterjee K, Parmley W, Ostland J, O'Young J, Haughom F: Long-term vasodilator therapy for heart failure: Clinical response and its relationship to hemodynamic measurements. Circulation 63:269, 1981.

430. McNair A, Andreasen F, Nielsen PE: Antihypertensive effect of diazoxide given intravenously in small repeated doses. Eur J Clin Pharmacol 24:151, 1983.

431. Morris DL, Goldschlager N: Calcium infusion for reversal of adverse effects of intravenous verapamil. JAMA 249:3212, 1983.

432. Myhre E, Rugstad HE, Hansen T: Clinical pharmacokinetics of methyldopa. Clin Pharmacokinet 7:221, 1982.

433. Pasch T, Schulz V, Hoppelshauser G: Nitroprusside-induced formation of cyanide and its detoxication with thiosulfate during deliberate hypotension. J Cardiovasc Pharmacol 5:77, 1983.

434. Patel KR: The effect of calcium antagonist, nifedipine in exercise-induced asthma. Clin Allergy 11:429, 1981.

435. Pearl RG, Rosenthal MH, Schroeder JS, Ashton JPA: Acute hemodynamic effects of nitroglycerin in pulmonary hypertension. Ann Intern Med 99:9, 1983.

436. Philips JB, Lyrene RK, Leslie GI, McDevitt M, Cassady G: Cardiopulmonary effects of nifedipine in normoxic and hypoxic newborn lambs. Circulation 66(Suppl II):111, 1982.

437. Radford D: Side effects of verapamil in infants. Arch Dis Child 58:465, 1983.

438. Rosendahl W, Hayduk K: Successful acute and long-term treatment of renin-induced hypertension in two infants with captopril. Eur J Pediatr 136:161, 1980.

439. Rubin LJ, Lazar JD: Influence of prostaglandin synthesis inhibitors on pulmonary vasodilatory effects of hydralazine in dogs with hypoxic pulmonary vasoconstriction. J Clin Invest 67:193, 1981.

440. Schonwetter BS, Libber SM, Jones MD Jr, Park KJ, Plotnick LP: Hypertension in neonatal hyperthyroidism. Am J Dis Child 137:954, 1983.

441. Siess W, Lorenz R, Roth P, Weber PC: Effects of propranolol in vitro and in vivo on platelet function and thromboxane formation in normal volunteers. Agents Actions 13:29, 1983.

442. Silber BM, Holford NHG, Riegelman S: Dose-dependent elimination of propranolol and its major metabolites in humans. J Pharm Sci 72:725, 1983.

443. Sinaiko AR, Mirkin BL, Hendrick DA, Green TP,

O'Dea RF: Antihypertensive effect and elimination kinetics of captopril in hypertensive children with renal disease. J Pediatr 103:799, 1983.

444. Tinker JH, Michenfelder JD: Sodium nitroprusside: Pharmacology, toxicology and therapeutics. Anesthesiology 45:340, 1976.

445. Vlasses PH, Ferguson RK, Chatterjee K: Captopril: Clinical pharmacology and benefit-to-risk ratio in hypertension and congestive heart failure. Pharmacotherapy 2:1, 1982.

446. Weismann D, Erenberg A, Robillard J, Wispe J: Accumulative plasma drug levels and neutropenia in a hypertensive neonate treated with captopril. Am J Dis Child 137:917, 1938.

447. Williams DO, Barnes PJ, Vickers HP, Rudolf M: Effect of nifedipine on bronchomotor tone and histamine reactivity in asthma. Br Med J 283:348, 1981.

448. Zsoter TT, Church JG: Calcium antagonists: Pharmacodynamic effects and mechanism of action. Drugs 25:93, 1983.

Antiarrhythmics

449. Brown JE, Shand DG: Therapeutic drug monitoring of antiarrhythmic agents. Clin Pharmacokinet 7:125, 1982.

450. Coumel P, Fidelle J: Amiodarone in the treatment of cardiac arrhythmias in children: One hundred thirty-five cases. Am Heart J 100:1063, 1980.

451. Dan M, Greif J: Amiodarone and pneumonitis. Ann Int Med 99:732, 1983.

452. Follath F, Ganzinger U, Schuetz E: Reliability of antiarrhythmic drug plasma concentration monitoring. Clin Pharmacokinet 8:63, 1983.

453. Harris L, McKenna WJ, Rowland E, et al: Side effects of long-term amiodarone therapy. Circulation 67:45, 1983.

454. Hesslein PS: Amiodarone therapy in children: A cautionary comment. Pediatrics 72:817, 1983.

455. Leak D, Eydt JN: Control of refractory cardiac arrhythmias with amiodarone. Arch Intern Med 139:425, 1979.

456. Lima JJ, Kuritzky PM, Schentag JJ, Jusko WJ: Fetal uptake and neonatal disposition of procainamide and its acetylated metabolite: A case report. Pediatrics 61:491, 1978.

457. Marchlinski FE, Gansler TS, Waxman HL, Josephson ME: Amiodarone pulmonary toxicity. Ann Intern Med 97:839, 1982.

458. Marcus FI, Fontaine GH, Frank R, Grosgogeat Y: Clinical pharmacology and therapeutic applications of the antiarrhythmic agent, amiodarone. Am Heart J 101:480, 1981.

459. Morady F, Sauve MJ, Malone P, et al: Long-term efficacy and toxicity of high-dose amiodarone therapy for ventricular tachycardia or ventricular fibrillation. Am J Cardiol 52:975, 1983.

460. Morris DL, Goldschlager N: Calcium infusion for reversal of adverse effects of intravenous verapamil. JAMA 249:3212, 1983.

461. Newburger JW, Keane JF: Intrauterine supraventricular tachycardia. J Pediatr 95:780, 1979.

462. Pickoff AS, Singh S, Flinn CJ, Wolff GS, Gelband H: Use of amiodarone in the therapy of primary ventricular arrhythmias in children. Dev Pharmacol Ther 6:73, 1983.

463. Radford D: Side effects of verapamil in infants. Arch Dis Child 58:465, 1983.

464. Rosenbaum MB, Chiale PA, Halpern MS, Nau SJ, Przyblyski J, Levi RJ, Lazzari JO, Elizari MV: Clinical efficacy of amiodarone as an antiarrhythmic agent. Am J Cardiol 38:934, 1976.

465. Rowland E, Krikler DM: Electrophysiological assessment of amiodarone in treatment of resistant supraventricular arrhythmias. Br Heart J 44:82, 1980.

466. Shahar E, Barzilay Z, Frand M, Feigl A: Amiodarone in control of sustained tachyarrhythmias in children with Wolff-Parkinson-White syndrome. Pediatrics 72:813, 1983.

467. Singh S, Gelband H, Mehta AV, Kessler K, Casta A, Pickoff AS: Procainamide elimination kinetics in pediatric patients. Clin Pharmacol Ther 32:607, 1982.

468. Singh BN, Nademanee K, Baky SH: Calcium Antagonists: Clinical use in the treatment of arrhythmias. Drugs 25:125, 1983.

469. Sobol SM, Rakita L: Pneumonitis and pulmonary fibrosis associated with amiodarone treatment: A possible complication of a new antiarrhythmic drug. Circulation 65:819, 1982.

470. Szefler SJ, Shen D, Gingell RL: Quinidine elimination in pediatric patients. Pediatr Res 14:473, 1980.

471. Ward DE, Camm AJ, Spurrell RAJ: Clinical antiarrhythmic effects of amiodarone in patients with resistant paroxysmal tachycardias. Br Heart J 44:91, 1980.

472. Wellens HJJ, Lie KI, Bar FW, Wesdorp JC, Dohmen HJ, Duren DR, Durrer D: Effect of amiodarone in the Wolff-Parkinson-White syndrome. Am J Cardiol 38:189, 1976.

EIGHT

Diuretics

Diuretics are an extremely useful and effective group of drugs for removing excess extracellular fluid in a wide variety of pathophysiologic states. Some diuretic agents are very effective in the management of hypertension as well. Rational use of this class of drugs in infants requires a basic understanding of renal physiology and of the mechanism of action and clinical pharmacology of the various diuretics.

FUNCTIONAL ANATOMY OF THE NEPHRON

It is important to understand the functional aspects of the various anatomic segments of the nephron before beginning a discussion of the mechanisms of action of the various diuretic drugs. (Renal physiology and its developmental aspects are the subject of several excellent reviews[8,50,62] and a comprehensive text.[95])

In the newborn, glomerular filtration rate (GFR) is about 30% of that in the adult (per unit surface area) but reaches adult levels within the first two years of life. Of the filtered sodium and chloride, about 70% is reabsorbed in the proximal tubule in both the immature and mature kidney. Bicarbonate and phosphate also have major transport loci in the proximal tubule, where approximately 80% to 90% of these ions are reabsorbed in the adult kidney; less reabsorption occurs in the immature kidney. Water and sodium are transported isoosmotically in the proximal portion of the nephron.

Chloride is actively transported in the ascending limb of the loop of Henle, with sodium following passively. About 20% to 25% of the filtered load of sodium chloride is reabsorbed in this segment. The epithelium of the ascending limb of the loop of Henle is essentially impermeable to water. In the distal segments (distal convoluted tubule and collecting tubule), about

5% to 10% of filtered sodium is reabsorbed. Sodium reabsorption occurs with chloride or in exchange for potassium or hydrogen ions. The tubular function in the loop of Henle and in the distal segment is less in the immature kidney than in the kidney of the adult.

The exchange of sodium for hydrogen and potassium, which occurs in the distal segments, is regulated by the mineralocorticoid system, principally aldosterone, and by the amount of filtered sodium present in the distal segments, which is independent of hormonal control. No more than 2% to 5% of the filtered sodium is ordinarily reabsorbed by these distal-segment exchange mechanisms. Filtered potassium is reabsorbed almost completely in the proximal nephron; therefore, any potassium in the urine ordinarily represents only the fraction excreted distally by the exchange mechanisms. The transport of water beyond the loop of Henle depends upon the action of antidiuretic hormone on the distal convoluted tubule and collecting ducts. Acid excretion occurs primarily by three mechanisms: the regeneration of bicarbonate (reabsorption); the excretion of hydrogen ion by means of phosphate; and excretion of ammonium ion. The functions of the various portions of the nephron are illustrated in Figure 8–1.

MECHANISMS OF DIURETIC EFFECT

The mechanisms responsible for renal regulation of fluid and electrolyte movement provide the basis for explaining the mode of action of various diuretic drugs (Fig. 8–1). Increases in GFR can produce diuresis by exceeding the reabsorptive capability of the tubule. Although none of the currently employed diuretics have a major or primary effect on GFR, any drug that improves cardiac output in a patient with signif-

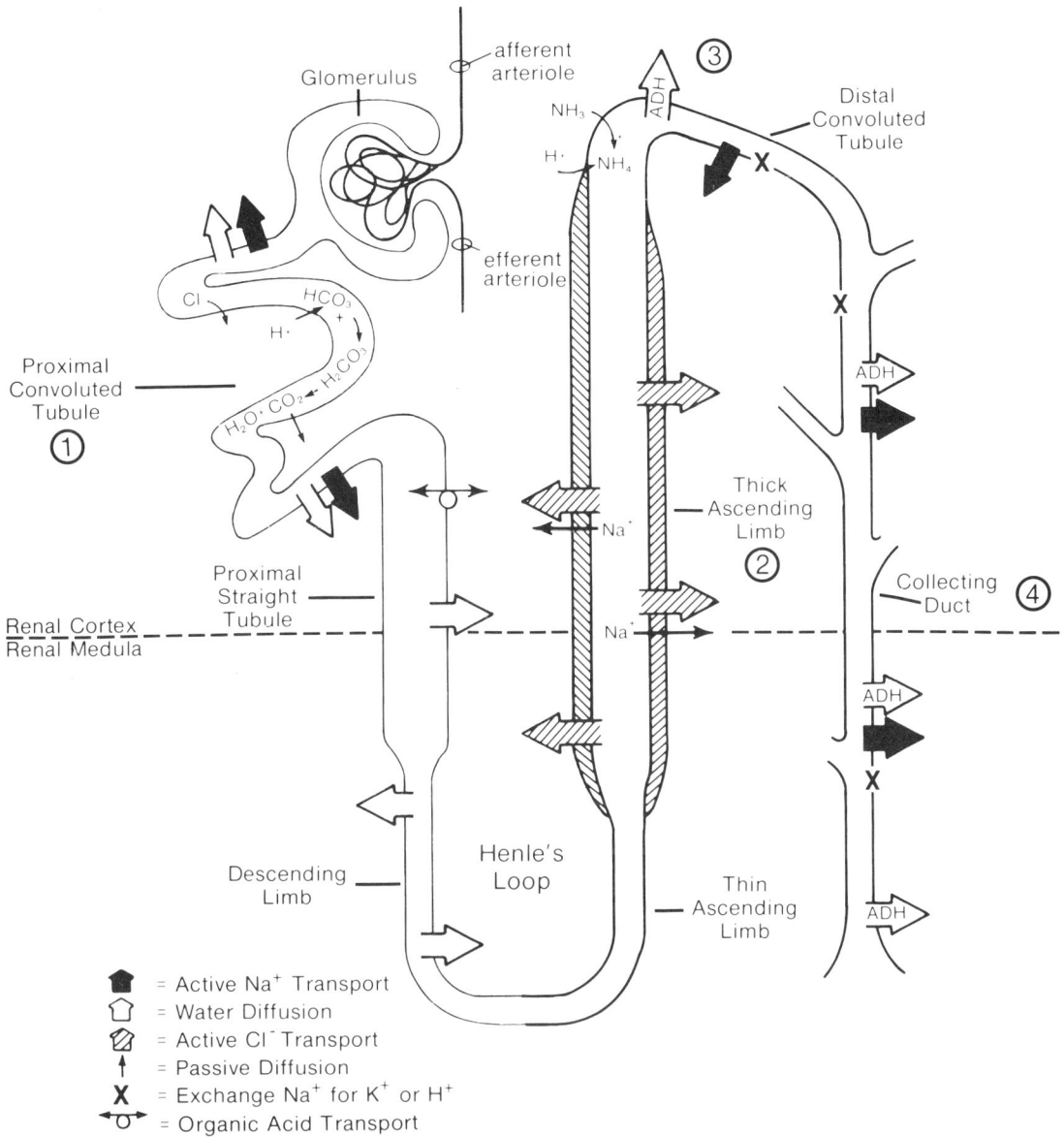

Figure 8-1. Functional organization of the nephron, showing sites of reabsorption of sodium, chloride, and bicarbonate; exchange of hydrogen and potassium; and the accompanying movement of water with and without the influence of antidiuretic hormone (ADH). Also illustrated are the sites of action of the various diuretic drugs (see Table 8-1).

icant congestive heart failure can produce a diuresis by this mechanism.

Interference with proximal tubular reabsorption of ions can result in fluid volume loss unless more distal tubular mechanisms are able to compensate. Generally, diuretics that inhibit sodium chloride transport proximally will not produce potent natriuretic and diuretic effects because of the compensatory ability of the more distal segments of the nephron. For example, acetazolamide, a carbonic anhydrase inhibitor (CAI), produces a diuretic effect via the proxi-

mal tubular mechanism by inhibiting the enzyme carbonic anhydrase; this causes decreased reabsorption of bicarbonate ion in the proximal tubules. The bicarbonate ion retains sodium or potassium as well as water in the tubule. However, much of the sodium and water is subsequently absorbed in more distal segments.

In the thick ascending limb of the loop of Henle, only solute is reabsorbed. Currently, chloride is believed to be the major ion actively reabsorbed. Because only salt, not water, is reabsorbed, a dilute tubular fluid is formed.

Table 8-1. SITE OF ACTION AND EFFECT ON URINARY EXCRETION OF ELECTROLYTES AND SELECTED IONS FOR VARIOUS DIURETICS

Drug	Major Site of Action[a]	RBF[b]	Fraction of Filtered Sodium Excreted (%)	Urinary Excretion of Electrolytes and Selected Ions[c]					
				Cl^-	K^+	HCO_3^-	$H_2PO_4^-$	Ca^{2+}	Mg^{2+}
acetazolamide	proximal tubule ①	↓, redis	3–5	0	↑↑↑	↑↑↑	↑↑	0, ↑	0, ↑
ethacrynic acid	ascending limb, loop of Henle ②	↑, redis	20–25	↑↑↑	↑↑	0	0, ↑	↑↑	↑↑
furosemide	ascending limb, loop of Henle ②	↑, redis	20–25	↑↑↑	↑↑	↑	↑	↑↑	↑↑
metolazone	distal segment ③	0	5–8	↑↑	↑	0	↑	0	↑
spironolactone	distal segment ④	0	2–3	↑	↓	0	0	↑	↑
thiazides	distal segment ③	0	5–8	↑↑	↑↑	↑↑	↑	0, ↓	↑

[a] Circled numbers refer to sites illustrated in Figure 8–1.

[b] Renal blood flow; ↓, ↑, 0 = effect of drug on total (absolute) RBF; redis = redistribution of RBF within the kidney. See under specific agents for details.

[c] ↑ = increase; ↓ = decrease; 0 = no change. Increases or decreases are in *quantity* excreted in the urine, not concentrations.

Both furosemide and ethacrynic acid inhibit the active reabsorption of chloride in this segment of the ascending loop of Henle, causing a chloruresis. The probability that a substantial proportion of the inhibited ions will appear in the final urine is much greater, because there are fewer, more distal transport sites available for compensating and because these sites have only a small transport capability. Thus, furosemide and ethacrynic acid produce a potent diuresis compared to diuretics that affect more proximal sites.

In the distal segments (distal convoluted tubule and collecting tubule), sodium is actively reabsorbed, carrying with it chloride and water, or undergoes exchange for potassium or hydrogen ions. The reabsorption is partially under the control of aldosterone and is also linked to the excretion of potassium. Spironolactone interferes with the aldosterone-controlled sodium reabsorption and potassium secretion, resulting in sodium loss and potassium retention. A summary of the major sites of action of the various diuretics, along with their effects on electrolytes, can be found in Table 8–1.

The thiazide diuretics are believed to have their major effect on the distal segment, causing an inhibition of sodium reabsorption and its attendant anion, chloride. The diuretic potency of agents with this more distal effect would be expected to be less that that of agents affecting the ascending limb of the loop of Henle. Potassium excretion is also increased by thiazides as a result of the increased sodium in the distal segment, which stimulates the exchange.

The pharmacologic response to a diuretic agent is inherently dependent upon the level of renal function present and the ability of the drug to reach and perturb this function.[75] Access of diuretics to their renal tubular sites of action is determined by factors such as plasma protein binding, active tubular secretion, nonionic diffusion, and intrarenal metabolism. For example, furosemide and the thiazides are transported across the proximal tubule; their diuretic effect is dependent upon reaching the tubular lumen (concentration in tubular fluid), not on the plasma drug concentration. Ethacrynic acid is also secreted but in addition is metabolized to a cysteine adduct, which is the active form of the drug. Unless the drugs are effectively transported by the kidney, little or no diuretic response can be expected.

Electrolyte and water excretion induced by potent diuretics such as ethacrynic acid or furosemide is greatest during the first few days of therapy. Factors leading to a decreased diuretic response include decreased GFR and hyperaldosteronism resulting from hypovolemia.[63] Enhanced proximal tubular reabsorption of sodium may also occur during prolonged diuretic therapy, which will reduce electrolyte and water excretion; the mechanism for the adaptation is unknown.

Tubular function is related to both gestational and postnatal age. GFR as well as tubular reabsorption is lower in infants born before 34 weeks' gestation than in infants born at term.[3,47] A nonlinear increase in GFR occurs in full-term infants after birth (rapid increase in GFR over the first 4 days of life followed by a slower but progressive increase over the next 3 to 5 weeks). This is greater than the increase in GFR observed over the same period in pre-term infants.[3] Thus, the response to diuretic agents may be significantly different in premature compared with full-term neonates. Clinical and experimental evidence, however, suggests a surprising lack of age-related differences in diuretic responsiveness.[50,74]

SPECIFIC DIURETIC AGENTS

There is no question that infants are responsive to the diuretic action of a number of drugs. The following sections review the pharmacology of the diuretic drugs and related clinical experience. Table 8–2 lists the recommended dosages and signs of toxicity for the specific agents; Table 8–3 gives the commercial preparations and their available forms for use in infants.

Acetazolamide

Pharmacology. Acetazolamide is the prototype of the carbonic anhydrase inhibitor (CAI) diuretics. The chemical structure is illustrated in Figure 8–2. A sulfonamide moiety ($-SO_2NH_2$) has been determined to be a requisite for carbonic anhydrase activity.[80] Acetazolamide, furosemide, and chlorothiazide all contain this moiety and therefore are CAIs, whereas ethacrynic acid, which lacks the sulfonamide group, is not.

Acetazolamide is readily absorbed from the gastrointestinal tract, with peak plasma concentrations reached within 2 hours of PO administration. The drug is not believed to be metabolized but does bind avidly to carbonic anhydrase. Acetazolamide is excreted by the kidney via active tubular secretion in the proximal tubule. In adults, virtually all of an administered dose is excreted within 24 hours.

The major pharmacologic action of acetazolamide is the noncompetitive inhibition of carbonic anhydrase activity (Fig. 8–3). Carbonic anhydrase catalyzes the hydration of carbon dioxide in the tubular cells,[65] which in turn facilitates the secretion of hydrogen ions in exchange for sodium ions. These secreted hydro-

Table 8–2. DOSAGE RECOMMENDATIONS AND SIGNS OF TOXICITY FOR DIURETIC AGENTS IN INFANTS

Drug	Recommended Dosage	Signs of Toxicity
acetazolamide (Diamox)	5 mg/kg q 6–8 hr PO; increase as required to 25 mg/kg/dose	metabolic acidosis, hypokalemia, drowsiness, paresthesias, rare allergic reaction
ethacrynic acid (Edecrin)	same as furosemide	dehydration and electrolyte (Na, Cl, K) imbalances, gastrointestinal bleeding, ototoxicity
furosemide (Lasix)	initial dose: 1 mg/kg IV, IM, or PO; increase as required to maximum of 2 mg/kg IV or IM and 6 mg/kg PO; repeat as required, but no more often than q 12 hr (full-term) or 24 hr (premature); > 1 mo old may tolerate dosing as often as q 6 hr (see text)[a]	dehydration and electrolyte (Na, Cl, K) imbalances, ototoxicity, metabolic alkalosis
metolazone (Diulo)	not established	dehydration and electrolyte (Na, Cl, K) imbalances
spironolactone (Aldactone)	1–3 mg/kg q 24 hr PO	hyperkalemia, drowsiness, gastrointestinal upset, rash
chlorothiazide (Diuril)	10–20 mg/kg q 12 hr PO[b]	dehydration and electrolyte (Na, Cl, K) imbalances, hyperglycemia, hypercalcemia, liver and renal disease, metabolic alkalosis, hyperuricemia
hydrochlorothiazide (Esidrix, HydroDiuril, Oretic)	1–2 mg/kg q 12 hr PO[b]	same as chlorothiazide

[a] The plasma clearance of furosemide varies considerably in infants. Since the diuretic effect occurs subsequent to renal tubular secretion, excessive plasma concentrations are more likely to result in displacement of bilirubin or ototoxicity than enhanced diuretic effect. Avoiding excessive plasma concentrations of drug by appropriate dose and dosing intervals is prudent. Attention to the duration of diuretic response along with frequent assessment of diuretic needs (particularly when initiating therapy) will assist in determining the appropriate dose and dosing interval (as opposed to an arbitrary 12- or 24-hr routine).[100]

[b] The thiazides have a relatively flat dose–response curve, indicating that significant increases in dose are not associated with comparable increases in diuretic or antihypertensive effects. Because of the dependence of diuretic effect on renal elimination, an increase in dosing interval is recommended with renal failure (give every 24 hr with 50% or less of normal creatinine clearance).

Table 8–3. PHARMACEUTICAL PREPARATIONS OF DIURETICS COMMERCIALLY AVAILABLE FOR USE IN INFANTS

Drug	Available Preparations		Comments
	Form	Concentration	
acetazolamide	capsules	500 mg	solution stable for 1 wk
(Diamox)	tablets	125, 250 mg	
	injection	500-mg vial (powder for reconstitution)	
ethacrynic acid	tablets	25, 50 mg	use of solution not recommended
(Edecrin)	injection	50-mg vial (powder for reconstitution)	after 24 hr following reconstitution
furosemide	tablets	20, 40, 80 mg	
(Lasix)	solution	10 mg/ml	
	injection	10 mg/ml	
metolazone	tablets	2.5, 5, 10 mg	
(Diulo)			
spironolactone	tablets	25 mg	suspension in cherry syrup; stable
(Aldactone)			for 1 mo
chlorothiazide	tablets	250, 500 mg	
(Diuril)	suspension	250 mg/5 ml	
	injection	500 mg/20 ml	
hydrochlorothiazide	tablets	25, 50, 100 mg	
(Esidrix, HydroDiuril, Oretic)			

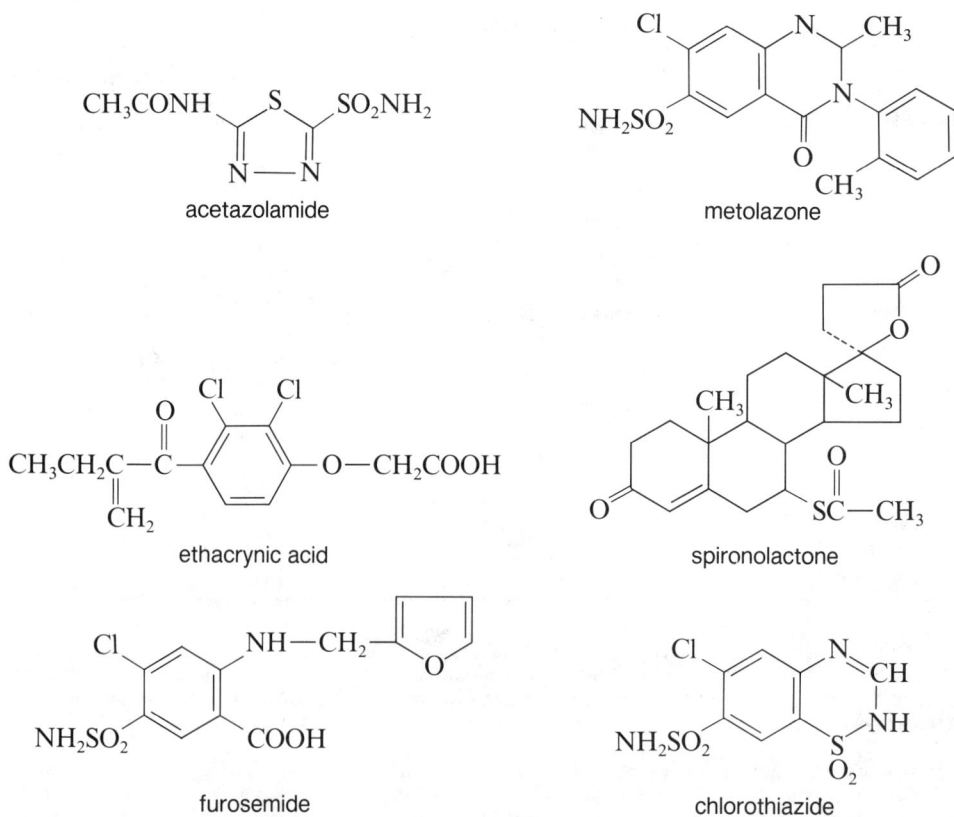

Figure 8–2. Structural formulas of diuretic drugs.

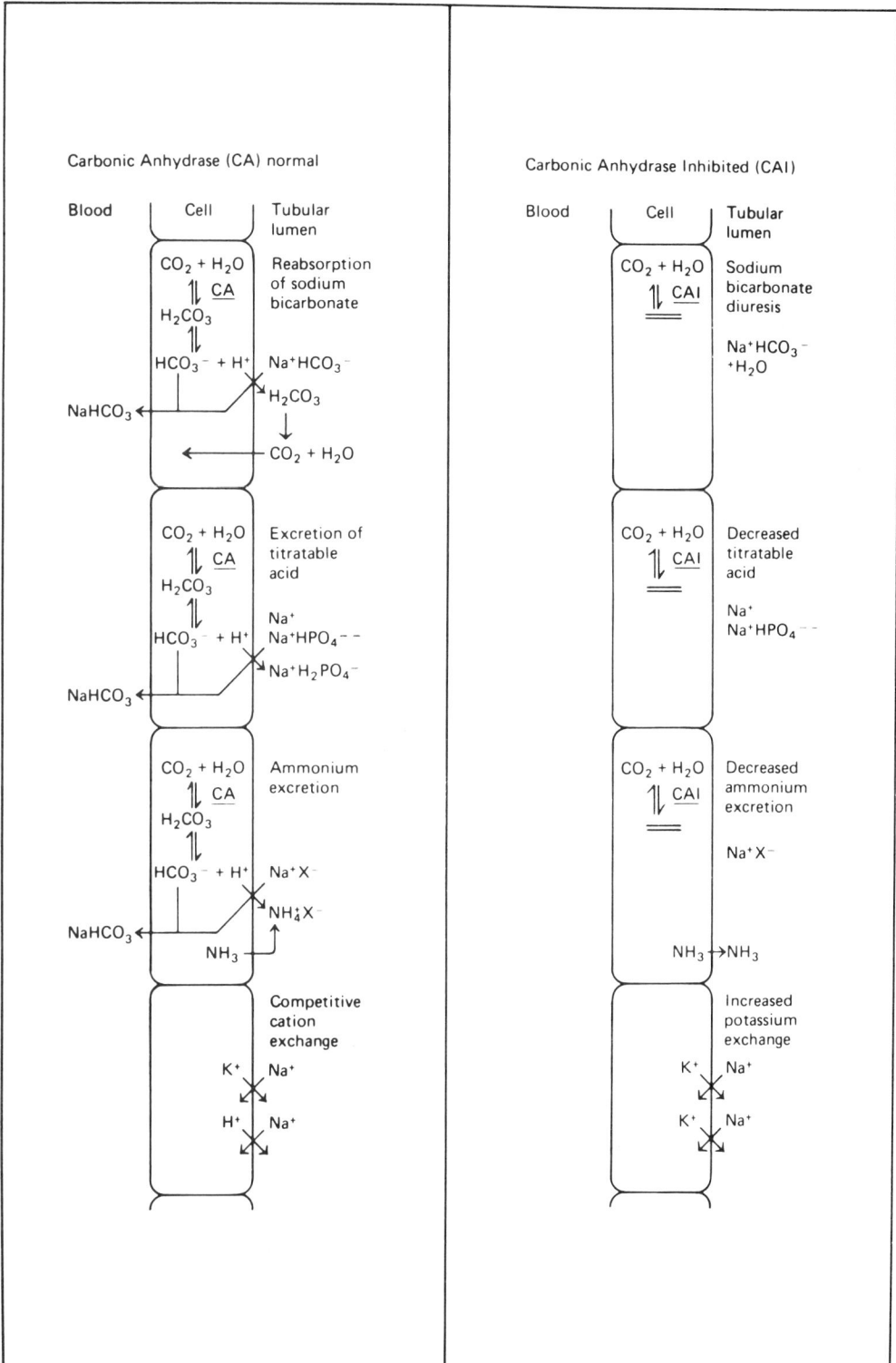

Figure 8–3. *Left,* Normal renal mechanisms for reabsorption of sodium bicarbonate and the excretion of titratable acid, ammonium, and potassium, in the presence of carbonic anhydrase (CA). *Right,* The disruption of these processes in the presence of a carbonic anhydrase inhibitor (CAI) such as acetazolamide. (From Anderton JL, Kincaid-Smith P: Drugs 1:54, 1971.)

gen ions provide for the excretion of titratable acid and ammonium ions and for the reabsorption of filtered bicarbonate ions. Inhibition of carbonic anhydrase, therefore, decreases the supply of hydrogen ions, causing sodium and bicarbonate to remain in the tubule (alkaline diuresis). Titratable acid and ammonium excretion also falls, and the lack of a competitive cation (H⁺) for exchange with sodium results in an increase in potassium exchange and excretion. Over 99% of the carbonic anhydrase enzyme activity must be inhibited in the kidney before the pharmacologic effects of acetazolamide become apparent.[2,73] In newborn infants, carbonic anhydrase activity in the kidneys is known to be diminished compared with that in adults,[63,113] so that a bicarbonate diuresis may be more readily achieved.

In general, the increase in bicarbonate anion in the urine is matched by sodium and substantial amounts of potassium, but the urinary concentration of chloride falls. As the amount of bicarbonate excreted increases, the extracellular body fluid concentration of bicarbonate decreases, and metabolic acidosis results. With metabolic acidosis, the renal response to acetazolamide is greatly reduced. Although this reduced diuretic activity is primarily a consequence of less substrate upon which acetazolamide can act (bicarbonate), potassium depletion also decreases the diuretic response to acetazolamide. The effects of acetazolamide on electrolyte excretion are summarized in Table 8–1.

Because the dynamic state of carbon dioxide is related to carbonic anhydrase activity, acetazolamide may create a disequilibrium in the carbon dioxide transport system, giving rise to increased CO_2 tensions in the tissues and a decreased CO_2 tension in the expired gas.

Acetazolamide reduces total renal blood flow and causes a redistribution of blood flow to the superficial cortex. However, because of the magnitude of renal blood flow reduction, even this area of redistributed blood flow has a reduced total flow.[79]

Other tissues affected by acetazolamide include the eye and the CNS. Acetazolamide reduces the rate of aqueous humor formation as a consequence of its CAI activity in the ciliary processes; this effect makes the drug a useful agent for reducing intraocular pressure in patients with glaucoma. In the CNS, acetazolamide has been observed to inhibit seizure activity and to decrease the rate of formation of CSF.[67,84] The development of systemic acidosis has been linked to the ability of acetazolamide

to diminish certain seizure disorders, although a more direct action on the CNS appears to be the major mechanism.[73] Inhibition of carbonic anhydrase in the choroid plexus by acetazolamide may be associated with a decrease in CSF production;[67] however, there may be a transient elevation of CSF pressure as a result of an increase in intracranial blood flow.[61]

Clinical Pharmacology. There are no published pharmacokinetic studies of acetazolamide in infants. Tudvad and colleagues[99] utilized acetazolamide in studies of bicarbonate and potassium excretion in seven healthy premature infants. IV injections (5 or 10 mg/kg) increased the excretion of bicarbonate and potassium, the onset occurring by about 2 to 3 hours; no change in GFR was observed. Walker and Cumming[101] administered 50 mg of acetazolamide to six normal infants (aged 6–47 days) and demonstrated an increase in urine flow and total sodium and potassium excretion. A large increase in urinary pH occurred and persisted for the entire 8-hour observation period. One infant given a single dose of 25 mg PO did not demonstrate diuresis.

Huttenlocher[53] studied the effect of acetazolamide on unselected types of hydrocephalus. The children in this series were given doses of 40 to 100 mg/kg PO per day in 2 to 4 divided doses. Doses above 50 mg/kg per day produced signs of significant metabolic acidosis. In addition, a weight loss was noted in some children during the initial period of therapy; this was thought to be related to a transient diuretic effect. Studies of serum and ventricular fluid electrolytes showed a reduction of potassium and an elevation of chloride; blood CO_2 concentration was also reduced. Hydrocephalus was arrested in 8 of the 15 children studied.

Other reports dealing with the use of acetazolamide in hydrocephalus in infants have demonstrated mixed success.[69,86] Mealy and Barker[69] conducted a double-blind clinical study in 32 neonates with myelomeningocele and found that acetazolamide given PO (12.5 mg/kg q 6 hr for 3 days, then 25 mg/kg q 6 hr) had no significant influence on the course of the hydrocephalus. Schain[86] used acetazolamide (20–55 mg/kg PO in 2 or 3 divided doses) in four children (aged 2–4 yr) with chronic infantile hydrocephalus; no change or a only small decrease in CSF pressure was noted. Donat[37] reported the use of acetazolamide (100 mg/kg q 24 hr in divided doses) in an 11-day-old full-term male infant with moderate dilation of the lateral and third ventricles. Computed tomography (CT) of the brain showed reduction in the size of the ventricular system subsequent to acetazolamide therapy. Marked increase in hydrocephalus occurred 1 month following discontinuation of therapy. This author concluded that acetazolamide may be useful in the temporary control of hydrocephalus in patients who cannot be immediately brought to surgery. Chaplin and coworkers[28] used acetazolamide and furosemide as well as repeated lumbar puncture in the management of posthemorrhagic hydrocephalus in the pre-term infant. The doses of acetazolamide ranged from 15 to 50 mg/kg per day given in 3 divided doses. Although the contribution of the drug therapy to control of the disorder is unclear, progression of hydrocephalus was successfully interrupted in seven of the ten infants studied. The resulting hyperchloremic metabolic acidosis was controlled with approximately 3 mEq/kg of potassium bicarbonate given PO.

Therapeutic Indications. Acetazolamide is rarely indicated as a diuretic, and its use in the *management of hydrocephalus* in the neonate remains investigational. There is apparently some justification for use of the drug as a temporary means of controlling the progression of hydrocephalus in certain patients who are not good surgical candidates (such as prematures or patients in precarious clinical condition). The doses employed have ranged from 15 to 100 mg/kg per day given PO. The recommended starting dose is 5 mg/kg given PO every 6 to 8 hours; the dose may be increased to up to 25 mg/kg (Table 8–2).

Clinical Toxicology. The most frequent side-effects associated with acetazolamide are those related to the development of metabolic acidosis and hypokalemia. With large doses, drowsiness and paresthesias have been reported. Hypersensitivity-type reactions (fever, skin reactions, bone marrow depression, and renal toxicity) are rare.

Ethacrynic Acid

Pharmacology. The structure of ethacrynic acid is shown in Figure 8–2. Ethacrynic acid is well absorbed from the gastrointestinal tract and is largely bound to plasma protein. Following IV administration, about one third of the dose is excreted by the liver, and the remaining two thirds, by the kidney. Approximately equal portions of two different metabolites and the parent compound can be recovered from the urine. Ethacrynic acid is secreted by the organic acid secretory system in the proximal tubule

(Fig. 8–1). Metabolism to a cysteine adduct, which is believed to be the active form of the drug, also occurs.

The major site of action of ethacrynic acid is in the ascending limb of the loop of Henle (Fig. 8–1), where it inhibits the chloride transport system.[24] Proximal and more distal sites of action have been identified, but their contribution to the drug's diuretic effects remains unclear.[25]

Ethacrynic acid does not inhibit carbonic anhydrase activity nor alter the excretion of bicarbonate.[80] The diuretic response to ethacrynic acid is independent of acid–base balance. An increase in potassium excretion is a consequence of the increased exchange with sodium in the distal segment and the increased rate of urine flow in this segment of the nephron. The excretion of magnesium and calcium is increased in proportion to the percentage increase in sodium excretion. The effects of ethacrynic acid on urine electrolyte excretion are summarized in Table 8–1.

The biochemical mechanism of action of ethacrynic acid on the renal tubule remains unclear.[75] The coadministration of ethacrynic acid and furosemide does not result in additive diuretic effects, although minor changes can be demonstrated, perhaps related to different effects of the two drugs on more proximal or distal mechanisms.

Ethacrynic acid has been shown to increase renal blood flow and to cause redistribution of blood flow away from the superficial cortex; these effects are similar to those of furosemide.[79] If hypovolemia results from administration of ethacrynic acid, a decrease in GFR can result. In contrast to furosemide, ethacrynic acid does not appear to have a direct effect on the pulmonary vasculature. Adult patients with congestive heart failure subsequent to myocardial infarction show no response following ethacrynic acid administration, whereas patients given furosemide show a prompt decrease in pulmonary artery diastolic pressure.[87]

Clinical Pharmacology. Following PO administration of ethacrynic acid to adults, diuresis begins in approximately 30 minutes and peaks at 2 hours; on average, this effect continues for 6 to 8 hours.[39] With the IV route, the time of onset, time of peak effect, and duration of action are about half that observed with the PO route.

James[55] administered ethacrynic acid to seven edematous children with acute nephritis, ten children with the nephrotic syndrome, and one with chronic congestive heart failure (aged 2–12 yr). The doses employed ranged from 0.5

to 2.5 mg/kg PO every 6 hours. Weight loss, associated with increased excretion of sodium and chloride, was observed in almost all children receiving the drug. Sparrow and coworkers[94] studied the effects of IV doses of ethacrynic acid (1 mg/kg) in 22 infants and children (aged 6 days–17 yr) with congestive heart failure. The onset of diuresis occurred within 30 minutes, with peak water, chloride, sodium, potassium, magnesium, and calcium excretion occurring by 60 minutes. In nearly all cases, clinical improvement was noted within a few hours.

Therapeutic Indications. Ethacrynic acid may be utilized when prompt diuresis is mandatory in situations in which refractoriness to other diuretics has been demonstrated. It has proved useful as a diuretic in severe edema, in acute left ventricular failure, and in chronic renal failure resistant to furosemide therapy. However, Bailie and coworkers[8] recommend that ethacrynic acid not be used in children because of its toxicity. The usual dose of ethacrynic acid is 1 mg/kg administered PO or IV as clinically indicated but no more often than every 12 hours in full-term neonates or 24 hours in prematures. The maximum recommended dose is 2 mg/kg for the IV or IM route and 6 mg/kg for the PO route. Infants over 1 month of age may tolerate more frequent dosing than neonates (Table 8–2).

Clinical Toxicology. Fluid and electrolyte imbalances make up the majority of the adverse effects of ethacrynic acid. Gastrointestinal side-effects are much more common with ethacrynic acid than with furosemide;[91] those reported for ethacrynic acid include nausea, epigastric pain, vomiting, and diarrhea. Gastric hemorrhage following IV administration has also been reported.[91] The development of deafness, though rare, has been described with use of ethacrynic acid; a possible mechanism for the ototoxicity is a change in the electrolyte composition in the endolymph consistent with the diuretic action of the drug. These ototoxic effects can be potentiated by factors such as noise or the use of other ototoxic drugs. The use of furosemide rather than ethacrynic acid as the diuretic of choice appears to be justified on the basis of the greater toxicity of ethacrynic acid.

Furosemide

Pharmacology. Furosemide, an anthranilic acid derivative (Fig. 8–2), is one of the most widely employed diuretic agents. The bioavail-ability of furosemide following PO administration is 60% to 70% in healthy adults and in patients with cardiac or liver failure but is only 43% to 46% in patients with end-stage renal disease.[33] Peak serum levels are reached between 1 and 2 hours following PO administration (10–30 μg/ml). Delay in absorption can occur when furosemide is given PO too soon after meals, although total bioavailability remains unaffected. The principal difference between the IV and PO routes of administration is the rapid onset of diuretic response seen with the former. Noteworthy is the fact that total fluid and electrolyte excretion with IV administration is no different from that with an equal dose given PO when measured over a 24-hour period.[18,59]

Because furosemide is extensively bound to plasma proteins (95%),[5] there is some concern regarding the drug's potential to displace bilirubin from albumin.[89,103] Aranda and colleagues[4] and Cashore and colleagues[109] found no significant difference in bilirubin binding capacity (using different analytical methods) within 1 hour after an IV dose of furosemide in neonates. These investigators, as well as Wennberg and coworkers,[103] concluded that a single dose of furosemide (1 mg/kg IV) does not significantly displace bilirubin from albumin binding sites; however, doses greater than 2 mg/kg or repeated dosing can generate plasma drug concentrations sufficient to cause a bilirubin–furosemide interaction at the albumin–bilirubin binding sites. The reported values for volume of distribution of furosemide range from 0.2 to 0.3 l/kg.[108]

Investigation of the metabolism of furosemide has been fraught with technical difficulties.[12] The metabolism of furosemide to an acid metabolite (2-amino-4-chloro-5-sulfamoyl anthranilic acid) is now believed by some to represent an analytic artifact.[12] Glucuronide conjugation of the drug ranges from 3% to 44% in various reports, but again technical difficulties appear to be responsible for this variability. Newer analytic techniques suggest that 10% to 20% of the available dose of drug undergoes glucuronide conjugation in adults. Neonates are believed to excrete the majority of an administered dose as unchanged drug in the urine, the remainder being excreted as the glucuronide and acid metabolite. Aranda and coworkers[6] observed about 23% of the dose of furosemide excreted as the glucuronide and a similar amount as the acid metabolite. Tuck and associates[118] found virtually the entire dose of furosemide excreted in the urine unchanged.

The tubular secretion of furosemide has been investigated experimentally in isolated perfused kidney.[16] Tubular drug clearance was found to be increased by six- to 20-fold when the concentration of albumin was decreased in the perfusate, suggesting that the renal secretory process is dependent on the concentration of unbound drug. This finding raises serious questions regarding the practice of the administration of albumin immediately prior to the administration of potent diuretics such as furosemide, particularly in patients with normal levels of plasma proteins: Not only does it add considerably to the cost of the diuretic therapy, but the diuretic response to furosemide may be blunted.

Although the major route of elimination of furosemide is by renal mechanisms, nonrenal routes of elimination (hepatic and intestinal) can account for a considerable portion of the total fraction eliminated, especially in the presence of renal failure.[19,51] In healthy adults, between 6% and 18% of an IV dose is found in the feces; in severe renal failure, however, up to 60% of the injected dose is eliminated by this route.[33] The relevance of these observations in the neonate with abnormal renal function is unknown.

The major pharmacologic actions of furosemide are renal (tubular function and renin release) and hemodynamic (renal and extrarenal). The major mechanism of its diuretic effect is blocking of chloride transport in the thick ascending limb of the nephron (Fig. 8–1); the precise cellular mechanism of this action is not known.[24,25] Sodium transport systems located in the proximal and more distal segments of the nephron may also be partially inhibited;[25] as a consequence of these tubular effects, a major loss in chloride and sodium occurs. The transport systems for potassium excretion are not directly affected. However, increases in potassium loss are to be expected because of the increased load of sodium presented to the distal segments. As a weak CAI, furosemide increases urinary pH (i.e., the urine becomes more alkaline), in contrast to ethacrynic acid, which is not a CAI and tends to cause the excretion of a more acidic urine. Furosemide has been shown to decrease CSF production in experimental animals[67] and to lower intracranial pressure in human adults.[31] These effects may be related to inhibition of carbonic anhydrase activity, although additional mechanisms may be involved.

Furosemide therapy results in a significant increase in urine calcium excretion.[52,119] The major portion of filtered calcium is resorbed in the proximal tubule, and in the loop of Henle, it is linked to sodium reabsorption.[96] Furosemide-induced decrease in sodium reabsorption secondary to chloride transport inhibition in the loop of Henle results in increased urinary loss of calcium. Chlorothiazide has been shown to reduce furosemide-induced hypercalciuria.[52] In large doses, furosemide increases the excretion of phosphate (Table 8–1).

The role of prostaglandins in the tubular effects of furosemide is unclear at present (see Chapter 9, Prostaglandins). Furosemide-induced diuresis and saliuresis is associated with an increase in urinary prostaglandins. The mechanism for the increase has been proposed to involve a furosemide-induced decrease in degradation of prostaglandins or in stimulation of prostaglandin synthesis.[7,41] The weight of evidence appears to favor furosemide-induced release of the rate-limiting prostaglandin precursor, arachidonic acid. However, the critical link between prostaglandins, furosemide, and renal tubular transport remains controversial.[30]

The effects of furosemide on renal hemodynamics (vasodilation with an increase in renal blood flow[79]) appear to be mediated by one of the prostaglandins (PGE_2, PGI_2, or PGD_2), but changes in hemodynamics account for only a small fraction of the drug's diuretic effects. Indomethacin inhibits the renal vasodilation caused by furosemide and also diminishes a portion of the overall diuresis and natriuresis caused by furosemide.[41,93] The effects of indomethacin evidently are related not to changes in furosemide disposition but to inhibition of furosemide-induced increase in prostaglandin release.[20] The possible direct effects of prostaglandins on tubular function remain to be resolved. Furosemide-induced increase in renin release, by direct activation of macula densa chemoreceptors, also appears to be prostaglandin-mediated. The ability of furosemide to elevate plasma renin activity is also blocked by indomethacin.

In order for furosemide to produce its competitive inhibition of the chloride transport system in the lumen of the ascending limb of the loop of Henle,[64] the drug must be present at this site.[16] Therefore, plasma drug concentration does not represent the critical determinant for diuretic response; instead, the concentration of furosemide in the tubular lumen appears to be rate-limiting.[92] Plasma concentrations of furosemide do not correlate consistently with the diuretic response.[21,76] The action of furosemide on the transport system appears to involve free

Table 8–4. STUDIES OF PHARMACOKINETICS AND PHARMACODYNAMICS OF FUROSEMIDE IN INFANTS AND CHILDREN

Author(s) of Published Study[a]	No. of Patients[b]	Study Group Diagnosis[c]	Dose Employed	Plasma Concentration ($\mu g/ml$)	Serum Half-life ($T\frac{1}{2}:hr$)	Peak Onset	Duration (hr)	Clinical Response[d]
Richardson[82]	11 infants (3 days–6 mo)	CHF, PDA	1.0–1.25 mg/kg IM			20–40 min	<12–24	8/16 improved
Krongrad and Joos[60]	16 children (35 days–12 yr)	8: renal dis. / 6: CHF / 2: LF	PO: 1–3 mg/kg; IM: 1–3 mg/kg; IV: 1–1.5 mg/kg				>6	13/16 improved
Repetto et al[81]	5 infants / 5 children	AGN / CHF	1 mg/kg IV over 5–10 min			30 min	<4	10/10 improved
Moylan et al[72]	6 newborns (2–14 days) / 4 children (9 wk–15 yr)	RDS / misc.	1–2 mg/kg IV			<2 hr		10/10 improved ($\uparrow PaO_2$)
Savage et al[85]	7 newborns (1.2–4 kg)	RDS	1.5 mg/kg IV at 2.6 and 12 hr of age					no effect on PaO_2 or $PaCO_2$
Aranda et al[4]	8 neonates (26–40 wk at 1–40 days)	3: RDS / 7: CHF, PDA / 2: apnea	1.0–1.5 mg/kg IV	1.7 ± 0.3 (range 0.9–3.2)	7.7 ± 1.0 (range 4.5–12)			pharmacokinetic study: $V_d = 0.83 \pm 0.12$ l/kg; $Cl = 81.6 \pm 15.0$ ml/kg/hr
Ross et al[83]	6 prematures (26–35 wk at 10–57 days)	RDS, CHF	1.0 mg/kg IV			1–3 hr	<6	6/6 improved
Engle et al[38]	28 infants (1 day–3 mo)	CHD	1–2 mg/kg IV; 1–6 mg/kg PO			<3 hr		efficacy and safety study
Friedman et al[140]	7 prematures (28–36 wk at 2–23 days)	4: HMD / 1: BPD / 2: PDA	2 mg/kg IV over 3–5 min					3/5 improved
Woo et al[106]	9 infants (30–40 wk at 1–68 days)	fluid overload (RDS, CHF, PDA, misc.)	1 mg/kg IV or IM			1–2 hr	<5	significant effects but wide variability
Marks et al[66]	12 newborns (31 wk at 30–40 hr of life)	5: HMD (controls) / 7: HMD (furosemide)	2 mg/kg IV				<6	5/5 improved; diuresis but no change in blood gases, pH, or LA/AO ratio
Baylen et al[10]	15 infants (1 wk–9 mo)	11: CHF / 4: BPD	2.5 mg/kg q 24 hr PO or IM					7/13 improved; response correlated with aldosterone levels

Reference	Patients[b]	Indication[c]	Dose			Comments[d]
Peterson et al[76]	26 infants (26–36 wk at 1–20 days); (1–4 mo)	14: PDA, CHF; 12: BPD	1 mg/kg IV over 2 min	4.9 ± 0.5 (range 1.9–10.2)	19.9 ± 3 (range 8.7–46)	pharmacokinetic study: $V_d = 0.24 \pm 0.03$ l/kg; $Cl = 10.6 \pm 2.1$ ml/kg/hr
Sulyok et al[97]	19 neonates (30–41 wk at 4–7 days)	moderate edema	1 mg/kg IM			increase in urine volume, Na, K, Cl, aldosterone, PGE, $PGF_{2\alpha}$, plasma aldosterone and renin activity
Aranda et al[6]	7 neonates (26–40 wk at 2–40 days)	PDA, CHF, BPD	1 mg/kg IV			urine metabolites detected (84% of dose by 24 hr)
Vert et al[100]	21 neonates (27–34 wk at 2–69 days; 37–41 wk at 1–18 days)	PDA, CHF, misc.	0.3–1.1 mg/kg IV		prematures: 27 ± 12 (range 8–44) full-term: 13.9 ± 9 (range 4–29) chronic dosing: 15 ± 15 (range 5–55)	prematures: $V_d = 0.2 \pm 0.08$ l/kg $Cl = 6.9 \pm 5$ ml/kg/hr full-term: $V_d = 0.5 \pm 0.4$ l/kg $Cl = 12 \pm 9$ ml/kg/hr
Green et al[46]	99 prematures (mean 31 wk, at <2 wk of life)	PDA	1 mg/kg IV			significant increase in urine volume and PGE and sodium excretion; incidence of PDA greater with furosemide treatment vs. chlorothiazide or controls
Tuck et al[117]	6 neonates (29–40 wk, at 3–32 days)	fluid overload	1 mg/kg IV		9.5 ± 4.4 (urine 9.6 ± 4.5)	$Cl = 15.3 \pm 8.4$ ml/kg/hr

a Listed in order of publication; see References at end of chapter.
b Age or weight at time of study is given if available in parentheses; gestational age (wk) is given for prematures.
c CHF = congestive heart failure; PDA = patent ductus arteriosus; AGN = acute glomerular nephritis; LF = liver failure; RDS = respiratory distress syndrome; misc. = miscellaneous; HMD = hyaline membrane disease; BPD = bronchopulmonary dysplasia; LA/AO = left atrial to aortic root ratio.
d V_d = volume of distribution; Cl = rate of clearance from body.

(unbound) drug. Furosemide has been shown to bind not only to proteins in plasma but also to protein present in urine.[71] It has been proposed that if a significant portion of furosemide is present as a protein-bound complex in the tubular lumen, the diuretic response will be reduced; this phenomenon has been demonstrated to occur in nephrotic animals.[43]

Although the beneficial effects of furosemide in relieving cardiac failure and pulmonary congestion and edema can be attributed to its diuretic properties,[105] the drug does appear to have important hemodynamic effects that are independent of its diuretic effects.[36,54] Dikshit[36] and Ikram[54] and their colleagues demonstrated in adults with heart failure that furosemide produced a reduction in left ventricular filling pressure, a decrease in pulmonary artery pressure, and an increase in venous capacitance within 5 minutes of administration; these effects preceded the onset of diuresis. In the series of Dikshit and colleagues,[36] three anuric patients also showed responses to furosemide similar to those seen in patients with functioning kidneys.

From experimental studies in animals, Bourland and coworkers[17] concluded that furosemide does not act directly but rather elicits the release of substances from the kidney, possibly prostaglandins, which then mediate the vascular action. In their studies, nephrectomy and indomethacin abolished the ability of furosemide to decrease left atrial pressure in the hypervolemic dog. Other studies in experimental lambs suggest the major action of furosemide is its diuretic effect, which decreases lung vascular hydraulic pressure, increases the transvascular gradient for protein osmotic pressure, and thereby diminishes the net transvascular filtration of fluid in the lung.[15]

In normal volunteers, indomethacin inhibited furosemide-induced increase in venous capacitance.[41] Furosemide does not have any direct effect on myocardial contractility by which to explain the systemic hemodynamic effects.[105] Thus, the systemic venous effects of furosemide appear to somehow be dependent upon renal prostaglandin generation. The effect of furosemide on the ductus arteriosus is discussed subsequently under Therapeutic Indications.

Clinical Pharmacology. Furosemide has been extensively studied in infants (Table 8–4). In general, doses of 1 mg/kg given IV have produced a significant increase in urine output and in renal excretion of chloride, sodium, bicarbonate, phosphate, calcium, magnesium, aldosterone, and PGE and $PGF_{2\alpha}$ (Table 8–4).[25,38,40,46,66,97,106] Diuretic activity begins

within 1 hour of parenteral administration and is generally completed by 6 hours, although more prolonged effects have been reported.[82] Duration of these pharmacodynamic effects in infants is considerably shorter than the mean plasma half-life for the drug (7.7–27 hr; Table 8–4). Repetitive furosemide dosing increases the plasma drug concentration and decreases the apparent volume of distribution.[5] These observations suggest that distribution sites (e.g., tissue proteins) or elimination mechanisms become saturated with repeated dosing. Vert and colleagues[100] studied six premature infants who had received more than 3 doses of furosemide. The plasma clearance values in most cases were consistently higher than those in infants receiving only a single dose of the drug. The mean volume of distribution, however, was not different. Phenobarbital treatment did not affect furosemide plasma clearance or half-life.

No consistent relationship has been found between gestational age, birth weight, and postnatal age and the rate of elimination of furosemide.[6,76,117] A significant difference in the elimination rate between pre-term ($Cl = 6.9 \pm 5$ ml/kg/hr) and full-term infants (12 ± 9 ml/kg/hr) has been observed.[100] Dosage recommendations cautioning against more than one daily dose of furosemide in the premature or renal-impaired infant are consistent with these pharmacokinetic observations.[6,100] On the other hand, plasma clearance data from infants 1 to 4 months of age indicate a much more rapid rate of furosemide elimination (> 80 ml/kg/hr) compared with that in neonates less than 20 days of age.[76] Infants 1 to 36 months of age have been found to have a plasma half-life of 1.8 hours, similar to that found in adults with normal renal function.[45]

The reported plasma concentration values for furosemide in infants range from 0.9 to 10.2 μg/ml following IV doses of 1 mg/kg.[4,76] The volume of distribution values reported for infants ranges between 0.2 and 0.8 l/kg.[4,76,100,118]

The slow plasma clearance of furosemide in neonates compared with that in adults is apparently related primarily to the low tubular secretion rate and possibly deficient conjugative and oxidative metabolism compounded by an absence of nonrenal elimination.[5] In neonates, about 34% of an administered dose of drug is found in the urine by 6 hours, whereas adults excrete 37% by 1 hour.[6] This major elimination period of 6 hours correlates with the onset and duration of diuretic response to furosemide in neonates (Fig. 8–4). The time of peak onset (20 min–3 hr) and duration of diuretic action (4–

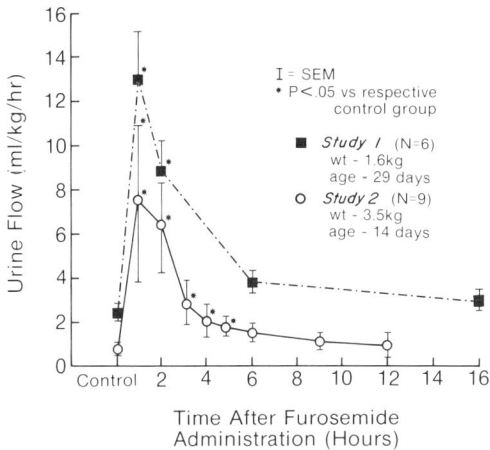

Figure 8-4. Effect of furosemide on urine flow in neonates treated with 1 mg/kg intravenously in two different studies. Weights and ages given are averages for the infant populations studied. Note the higher rate of urine flow for Study 1 during the control period; such apparent differences in response are not significant, reflecting only the variation to be expected with different populations. (Values have been recalculated from original data to ml/kg/hr. Study 1 data, from Ross BS et al: J Pediatr 92:149, 1978; Study 2 data, from Woo WCR et al: Clin Pharmacol Ther 23:266, 1978.)

6 hr) and pharmacokinetic values ($T\frac{1}{2}$ = 8 – 27 hr) for furosemide are considerably longer in neonates than those reported for adults (Table 8 – 4). Tuck and colleagues[118] observed similar plasma and renal clearances of furosemide (15.3 ± 8.4 versus 14.9 ± 7.7 ml/kg per hr, respectively) in newborn infants which are markedly less than those in adults (171 ± 23 versus 85 ± 21 ml/kg per hr). In adults, the onset of action following IV administration occurs within 5 minutes, the peak effect occurs in 30 to 60 minutes, and the usual duration of action is 2 to 4 hours.[39,59] The half-life of the drug in adults also shows wide variation but is generally between 20 and 90 minutes.[33]

It has been proposed that the diuretic response to furosemide is associated with the intraluminal concentration of the drug rather than the concentration of drug in the plasma.[21,92] Observed rates of furosemide excretion suggest that onset will be more rapid and diuretic response will probably be greater in the adult than in the neonate. Dependency on intraluminal concentrations of furosemide may also explain the discrepancies observed between the blood drug level and the diuretic response in clinical and experimental studies.[21,76] Possibly, plasma concentrations correlate with diuretic response to furosemide only when parallel changes are occurring in urine drug concentration. A parallel relationship between plasma

and urine concentration may be susceptible to a variety of disruptive insults, particularly renal dysfunction. Smith and Benet[92] have demonstrated in experimental animals that furosemide inhibits its own renal elimination at higher plasma concentrations; they propose that this dose-dependent phenomenon may in part be responsible for previously reported discrepancies in the relation between plasma levels and diuretic response. Such a phenomenon would argue against the use of increasing doses of furosemide to further increase the diuretic response, since an increase in dose may inhibit access of the additional drug to the intraluminal site of action. However, dose-dependent self-inhibition of furosemide tubular excretion has not been substantiated in humans.

The route of administration of furosemide has been the subject of several studies. Peterson and coworkers[76] estimated bioavailability of the drug given PO in one infant at 20% of the IV dose. Diuresis followed the parenteral dose but not the oral dose. Pruitt and Boles[77] found that children with glomerulonephritis responded well to furosemide given IV (1 mg/kg) but that doses of less than 2 mg/kg given PO were often minimally effective. In carefully controlled studies in adults, Kelly[59] and Branch[18] and their colleagues found that the only difference between IV and PO administration of furosemide was a more rapid onset of diuretic response with the IV route. Studies designed to compare the effectiveness of PO and IV furosemide therapy in neonates have not been done. Investigations by Woo and coworkers[106] confirm that neonates with low GFR respond to furosemide, as do adults and older children with renal disease; infants with a history of asphyxia, however, appear to respond poorly.

Therapeutic Indications. Furosemide is effective in the treatment of *fluid overload* regardless of the etiology. The use of furosemide, however, should not circumvent rigorous attention to appropriate fluid and electrolyte management. The drug has been demonstrated to produce an increase in urine output and an increase in excretion of sodium, chloride, potassium, bicarbonate, phosphate, calcium, and magnesium (Table 8 – 1). Because furosemide is a very potent agent (its actions are not self-limiting), its use can result in serious depletion of these ions and water, leading to dehydration and circulatory collapse.

The use of furosemide for the treatment of *congestive heart failure* in infants has been demonstrated to be effective in a number of studies (Table 8 – 4). A wide variety of congenital heart abnormalities are represented in these clinical studies. In most patients, however, management also included digoxin therapy and fluid restriction, making the specific value of the diuretic difficult to establish. Of interest are the reports of hyperaldosteronism in infants with a wide variety of congenital and acquired cardiac lesions, including cor pulmonale secondary to chronic lung disease (bronchopulmonary dysplasia, BPD).[10] These observations are consistent with those in adults with heart failure, demonstrating the role of the renin–angiotensin–aldosterone system in the accumulation of fluid and sodium. It has been suggested that excessive circulating aldosterone may lead to a diminished response to diuretic drugs, because this hormone increases tubular reabsorption of sodium and water at a site distal to the action of diuretic agents such as furosemide and the thiazides. If cardiac output does not improve adequately with diuretic therapy or if effective systemic blood volume is reduced, there may be additional stimulation of aldosterone production. As a consequence, chronic diuretic therapy may result in no overall benefit. In these situations an aldosterone inhibitor (see under Spironolactone) may be beneficial.

More controversial is the use of diuretics in the management of *respiratory distress syndrome (RDS)*. Savage and coworkers[85] studied the effect of furosemide in seven infants randomly assigned to either control or diuretic therapy. Furosemide produced a fourfold increase in urinary volume and a tenfold increase in urinary sodium and calcium excretion but did not improve arterial oxygen or carbon dioxide tension. Unfortunately, the groups were not matched for severity of respiratory distress. Marks and colleagues[66] studied infants with RDS who were randomly assigned to treatment or placebo groups (blinded study design); their observations were similar to those of Savage. Moylan and coworkers[72] studied patients with various illnesses, including six infants with RDS. They observed a lessening of hypoxemia following furosemide treatment, which was believed to be due to a decrease in right-to-left shunting and subsequent development of a more normal ventilation/perfusion ratio. Najak and associates[114] observed improvement in alveolar to arterial oxygen gradient and pulmonary compliance shortly after furosemide-induced diuresis in 10 premature infants with RDS. Similiar changes were not observed in a comparable control population. Green and co-authors[111] concluded that the use of furosemide was statistically correlated with beneficial ef-

fects in premature infants with RDS when spontaneous diuresis did not occur. The routine employment of furosemide, particularly in the acute phase of RDS, cannot be supported by available data, especially in infants who are managed with conservative fluid therapy.

Furosemide has frequently been utilized in premature infants who are clinically deteriorating owing to a *patent ductus arteriosus (PDA)*. The rationale for use of the drug in such patients includes the association of PDA with fluid overload and the manifestations of congestive heart failure with pulmonary edema. A paradox to this use of furosemide is the evidence gathered by Green and coworkers[44,46] that the drug increases the incidence of PDA in premature infants with respiratory distress syndrome. Furosemide has been demonstrated to acutely lower pulmonary vascular resistance[36,54] and to decrease afterload, resulting in increased ventricular performance, in adult patients with heart failure.[105] The hemodynamic effects of chronic furosemide therapy appear to differ from the acute effects. A decrease in cardiac output and in activation of the renin–angiotensin system has been observed in adults after 8 to 10 days of therapy with furosemide.[54] Similar studies of the acute and chronic hemodynamic effects of furosemide have not been done in neonates. In premature infants with PDA and respiratory distress syndrome, the duration of mechanical ventilation and hospitalization and the incidence of complications were reported to be unaffected by furosemide therapy.[46] The lack of clear evidence of beneficial effects of furosemide in treatment of premature infants with PDA, the evidence for increased incidence of PDA in prematures given furosemide, and the drug's demonstrated effects on hemodynamics and circulating vasoactive substances (renin–angiotensin, prostaglandins) all delegate the assignment of furosemide in treatment of PDA to an experimental category. Of interest, however, is the demonstration with controlled studies that furosemide prevents the reduction in urine output, GFR, and fractional excretion of sodium and chloride seen in neonates receiving indomethacin for PDA.[107] The effectiveness of indomethacin in closing the PDA appeared to be unaffected by furosemide (PDA closure was achieved in seven of nine patients receiving indomethacin versus seven of ten patients receiving indomethacin plus furosemide).

Diuretic therapy in the management of more *chronic forms of lung disease* in the premature infant (e.g., bronchopulmonary dysplasia or

BPD) appears to be beneficial, particularly in periods of acute increase in pulmonary edema.[57,90,98] Furosemide has been reported to improve clinical respiratory scores,[117] decrease ventilator requirements, and improve dynamic pulmonary compliance[113] in infants with ventilatory dependent chronic lung disease (BPD). Kao and coworkers[57] observed a decrease in airway resistance and an increase in specific airway conductance and dynamic pulmonary compliance in 10 infants with BPD who did not require either mechanical ventilation or supplemental oxygen. These effects were only significant within one hour of furosemide administration. The beneficial effects of furosemide in chronic lung disease in infants may not develop solely as a consequence of diuretic response with secondary reduction in vascular afterload[105]; the mechanism may also involve a direct nondiuretic vascular action (see under Pharmacology). Long-term use of furosemide is not without complications (see Clinical Toxicology section); its use in chronic lung disease in infants must therefore be carefully monitored. Some regard this use of furosemide as still experimental.[110]

Furosemide has been employed in an attempt to arrest the progression of *posthemorrhagic hydrocephalus* in pre-term infants.[28] The drug was administered in conjunction with acetazolamide to 2 infants who failed to respond to repeated lumbar punctures. These infants eventually required placement of ventricular shunts. Furosemide has also been shown to inhibit CSF production in experimental animals[67] and to lower intracranial pressure in adult humans,[31] but its use to treat hydrocephalus in neonates must be considered experimental.

The *recommended initial dose* of furosemide is 1 mg/kg given IV, IM, or PO. The dose can thereafter be increased according to the duration and intensity of the diuretic response. The maximum recommended dose is 2 mg/kg for the IV or IM route and 6 mg/kg for the PO route (Table 8–2). This difference in maximum dose for the parenteral versus the oral route represents the difference in bioavailability for these two routes (the evidence for such a bioavailability difference in neonates is limited, however). One of the major advantages of furosemide is its ability to elicit a diuretic response even in patients with severe renal failure; clinical experience suggests that, at least in adults, larger doses are required in such cases.[11,59] However, the initial dose should still be 1 mg/kg in order to substantiate the need for larger doses. In the case of poor or no diuretic response within 3 to

6 hours, a second dose of 1 to 2 mg/kg can be administered.

The choice of administration route — PO versus IV — should be based on the clinical needs of the infant. The IV route would appear to be better for acute treatment of pulmonary edema in order to take advantage of the pulmonary hemodynamic effects of furosemide as well as the rapid onset of diuresis. Otherwise, the PO route should be considered adequate in infants unless proved otherwise. An additional consideration is the development of furosemide toxicity: With the PO route, the high peak plasma drug concentrations attained with bolus IV therapy do not develop, so that the risk of ototoxicity and degree of displacement of bilirubin bound to albumin are less. Kelly and coworkers[59] recommend IV therapy only when the PO route is not possible and diuresis is required, or when a rapid onset of diuresis is desirable and mild vasodilation is useful, as in acute pulmonary edema. The *frequency of administration* should be established by the clinical response to the initial dose and the subsequent clinical status of the patient. Because of the potency of furosemide, care must be exercised to avoid intravascular volume depletion and cardiovascular collapse. Once-daily dosing is usually adequate in the neonate. The need for routine daily dosing should be confirmed. Full-term neonates or older infants may be dosed every 12 hours with minimal danger of accumulation of toxic plasma drug levels. Infants over 1 month of age may tolerate dosing every 6 hours because of adult-like clearance of the drug.[45] Plasma levels of 25 μg/ml or greater are associated with ototoxicity and can cause the displacement of albumin-bound bilirubin, predisposing to kernicterus. The dosage recommendations are outlined in Table 8–2.

Clinical Toxicology. Many of the side-effects associated with the use of furosemide relate to its potent diuretic action with resulting abnormalities of fluid and electrolytes. Careful monitoring of electrolytes, especially potassium and chloride, is imperative. Potassium deficit is often of great concern because of the concomitant use of furosemide and digoxin in infants with cardiac abnormalities and fluid overload. Potassium deficiency markedly enhances the toxicity of digoxin (see Chap. 7).

Ototoxicity, including both transient and permanent hearing loss, is possible with furosemide use. This adverse effect is rare and is typically associated with excessive plasma drug levels (25 μg/ml). Of concern, however, are the potentiating effects of noise and other ototoxic drugs such as the aminoglycosides.[23] Bess and colleagues[14] studied the noise levels in infant incubators with and without additional life-support equipment. They concluded that the sick neonate is potentially at great risk for ototoxicity because of prolonged exposure to noise levels characteristic of intensive care equipment and infant incubators and the use of other ototoxic drugs. Reducing this risk by appropriate furosemide dosing programs is therefore of added importance in the neonate.[26,104]

The routine use of furosemide daily in infants with chronic lung disease (BPD) can result in significant accumulation of serum bicarbonate and carbon dioxide; this effect must not be misinterpreted as a worsening of pulmonary function (i.e., increased CO_2 retention). The serum abnormalities are caused by several mechanisms: reduction of the extracellular fluid volume, resulting in "contraction" alkalosis; increased reabsorption of bicarbonate due to H^+ and K^+ depletion; and massive chloride loss, resulting in compensatory retention of bicarbonate (HCO_3^- anion).[27]

Another problem associated with chronic furosemide therapy in infants is hypercalciuria. Hufnagle and coworkers[52] reported the development of renal calcifications in ten premature infants with chronic lung disease who were receiving long-term furosemide therapy. The authors concluded that the stone formation was precipitated by the hypercalciuria induced by furosemide. An important complication of the stone formation was sepsis secondary to urinary tract infections. These infants all received at least 2 mg/kg of furosemide daily for a minimum of 12 days. Venkataraman and colleagues[119] observed increased urinary calcium excretion (> 4.0 mg/kg/day) in four infants with chronic lung disease who were receiving long-term furosemide therapy (1.9 to 6.0 mg/kg/day). Serum parathyroid hormone concentrations were sharply elevated above normal in three infants who had urinary calcium losses > 14 mg/kg/day. Renal calcifications were identified by ultrasound in two infants. Bone demineralization was detected in three infants. All these effects were attributed to furosemide-induced calciuria.

In two different series,[26,104] cholelithiasis developed in premature infants undergoing prolonged furosemide therapy. All six infants, however, received total parenteral nutrition in addition to furosemide, so that it is difficult to ascertain the contribution of each or both to the development of the gallstones.

Other toxic effects of furosemide reported in adults include dehydration with circulatory collapse, vascular thrombosis and embolism, hyperuricemia, blood dyscrasia, liver damage, vomiting, diarrhea, and alterations in glucose tolerance test results. Various forms of dermatitis, including urticaria, exfoliative dermatitis, erythema multiforme, and bullous pemphigoid, have also been reported.[73] Studies in adults have not demonstrated any significant alteration of digoxin pharmacokinetics by furosemide.[22] See Pharmacology section for a discussion of furosemide displacement of bilirubin from albumin binding sites and Therapeutic Indications section for discussion of increased incidence of PDA associated with the use of furosemide in newborns with RDS.

Metolazone

Pharmacology. Metolazone is a long-acting diuretic and antihypertensive agent derived from quinethazone (Fig. 8–2). The drug is active when given orally or parenterally. Approximately 95% of the drug is bound to plasma protein, and excretion is primarily by a combination of glomerular filtration (minor) and tubular secretion. Only a small percentage of the dose is believed to be metabolized. Metolazone has a relatively prolonged duration of natriuresis and a half-life of about 8 hours in adults, making once-daily dosing feasible. The prolonged duration of action is believed to be related to protein binding and enterohepatic recycling.

The site of action of metolazone appears to be both in the proximal convoluted tubule and in either the late ascending limb of the loop of Henle or the early distal convoluted tubule.[13] Metolazone has been reported to have the least tendency of all the diuretic agents to induce urinary potassium loss.[78] Like ethacrynic acid, metolazone has minimal or no carbonic anhydrase inhibitory activity;[95b] it does not alter renal blood flow.[79] Table 8–1 summarizes the effects of metolazone on electrolyte excretion.

Clinical Pharmacology. There have been no reports dealing with pharmacokinetics of metolazone in infants or children. No effect on cardiac hemodynamics, total peripheral resistance, or blood volume occurred when metolazone was given IV to adult patients with severe renal failure.[88] These observations are in contrast to hemodynamic effects demonstrated with ethacrynic acid and furosemide. There is evidence that metolazone possesses a potent synergistic action with furosemide sufficient to require dose reductions.[1,9,42] In addition, metolazone has been reported to maintain or increase GFR, in contrast to the thiazide diuretics, which may decrease it.[32]

Therapeutic Indications. The major use of metolazone in adults has been for the management of fluid overload conditions refractory to thiazides or furosemide. The drug appears to possess both diuretic and antihypertensive properties.[56] Its use in neonates remains experimental. Doses used in adults have generally ranged from 5 to 20 mg IV or PO, with doses as high as 100 mg in certain patients otherwise unresponsive to diuretics.[35] A single daily dose is recommended owing to this agent's long duration of action (12 to 24 hr).

Clinical Toxicology. Side-effects associated with metolazone are consistent with other potent diuretics (fluid–electrolyte imbalance). Some controversy exists regarding its effect on potassium excretion, although hypokalemia is a known complication.[13]

Spironolactone

Pharmacology. Spironolactone is a competitive antagonist of mineralocorticoids such as aldosterone. The drug is effective when given PO. Spironolactone is rapidly and completely metabolized to a large number of metabolites, the major active metabolite being canrenone.[58] In adults, approximately 50% of a PO dose is excreted in the urine as canrenone and other metabolites. Between 5% and 35% of the administered dose can be recovered in the bile. The drug is extensively bound to protein (98%).

Spironolactone is particularly effective in situations of increased aldosterone secretion. By competitively binding to specific cellular macromolecules in the distal segment of the nephron (Fig. 8–1), spironolactone inhibits aldosterone's regulatory effect on electrolytes; this results in an increase in sodium excretion and a decrease in potassium excretion. Stimuli for the secretion of aldosterone include a reduction in effective blood volume, hyponatremia, and hyperkalemia. The production of aldosterone is also stimulated by angiotensin, which is increased as a consequence of renin release by the kidney (see Fig. 7–18). Many investigators have demonstrated the role of the renin–angiotensin–aldosterone system in the accumulation of fluid and sodium in patients with heart failure.[10] Elevated plasma concentrations of aldosterone have been observed in infants with congestive heart failure.[10]

As a consequence of interfering with aldosterone binding, spironolactone produces only a slight diuresis. The explanation for its low potency as a diuretic lies in the fact that aldosterone-dependent distal mechanisms for sodium excretion involve only a small fraction of excreted sodium ($< 2\%$). The effect of spironolactone is usually not evident until a few days after initiation of therapy. This delay is due to the fact that the effects of aldosterone involve the synthesis of protein or peptide subsequent to its combining with its receptor. The newly synthesized protein or peptide, as well as its associated activity, persists for 2 to 3 days. When spironolactone therapy is discontinued, resynthesis of adequate protein or peptide by aldosterone stimulation of mineralocorticoid receptors may be delayed for an equivalent period (2 to 3 days). Spironolactone also has an effect on tubular transport of calcium, resulting in an increase in calcium excretion.[73] The effects of spironolactone on electrolyte excretion are summarized in Table 8–1.

Clinical Pharmacology. In healthy adults, the half-life of spironolactone ranges from 10 to 35 hours.[58] Conflicting information exists regarding the influence of liver disease on the disposition and metabolism of spironolactone. Walker and Cumming[101] gave spironolactone (50 mg in divided doses) to three infants and noted a moderately large increase in urine volume and sodium excretion. Danks[34] noted the value of spironolactone in the treatment of fluid retention in infants and children with liver disease; the doses employed were 25 mg twice a day in infants under 12 months and 25 mg 3 times a day in infants between 12 months and 2 years of age. About 25% of the infants failed to demonstrate an adequate diuretic response. Baylen and colleagues[10] employed spironolactone in four infants with cor pulmonale secondary to bronchopulmonary dysplasia who had elevations of serum aldosterone and equivocal responses to furosemide. Treatment with spironolactone (1–2 mg/kg q 24 hr) resulted in an improved diuresis and a decrease in mean aldosterone levels from 426 to 139 ng/dl. Hobbins and coworkers,[49] utilizing random allocation of spironolactone, examined its effect in 11 infants with congestive heart failure secondary to congenital heart disease: All patients received digoxin and chlorothiazide with or without spironolactone (0.5–1 mg/kg q 12 hr PO). A significant reduction occurred in liver size and weight and in respiratory rate in the spironolactone-treated group. The authors concluded that in infants with congestive heart failure, the addition of spironolactone hastens and enhances the response to standard treatment with digoxin and chlorothiazide.

Therapeutic Indications. Spironolactone appears to be a valuable adjunct to therapy of congestive heart failure associated with hyperaldosteronism, including congenital heart disease and chronic lung disease (BPD). The recommended dose is 1 to 3 mg/kg administered PO once daily (Table 8–2).

Clinical Toxicology. Reported side-effects with spironolactone therapy include headache, drowsiness, rashes, nausea, vomiting, diarrhea, paresthesias, dose-dependent androgenic effects in females, and gynecomastia in males.[63] Monitoring of serum potassium is critically important during chronic therapy because of the danger of development of hyperkalemia.

Thiazides

Pharmacology. The thiazides represent a group of diuretics that were originally synthesized in an attempt to develop an inhibitor of carbonic anhydrase activity with ideal diuretic properties. All of the thiazides appear to have parallel dose–response curves and comparable saliuretic effects; they differ primarily in their duration of action. The structural formula of the thiazides includes a sulfonamide moiety ($-SO_2NH_2$) that has been determined to be a requisite for carbonic anhydrase activity;[80] this group is not essential for the saliuretic activity of the thiazides since substitution of the amino portion does not decrease the activity of these agents. (Acetazolamide and furosemide, which have carbonic anhydrase–inhibiting effects, also have the unsubstituted sulfonamide moiety; see Fig. 8–2.) The thiazides are rapidly but incompletely absorbed from the gastrointestinal tract, with an onset of action within 1 hour of administration. Gastrointestinal absorption is increased from an average of 65% of the dose to 75% by simultaneous administration with food.[108] The thiazides are distributed largely in the extracellular space and do not accumulate in tissues other than the kidney.[63,73] Most of the thiazides are rapidly excreted, largely unchanged (90%), by active secretion in the proximal renal tubule. The protein binding of hydrochlorothiazide is approximately 40%.

The thiazides exert their major diuretic effect by inhibiting sodium reabsorption in the distal nephron[63] (Fig. 8–1); the inhibitory mechanism is not clear, although some aspect of energy metabolism necessary for sodium transport appears to be involved.[96] The thiazides also inhibit carbonic anhydrase activity in the proximal tubule and thereby inhibit sodium reabsorption proximally; however, this effect is not thought to make a major contribution to the diuresis. The inhibition of sodium reabsorption in the distal segment causes more sodium to remain in the lumen of this segment and leads to an enhanced exchange of sodium for potassium. The consequence is an increased excretion of potassium, which may result in the development of hypokalemia. Chloride is lost in association with the inhibition of sodium reabsorption.

In contrast to other natriuretic agents, the thiazides decrease the renal excretion of calcium.[112] Although the thiazides may increase calcium excretion slightly on initial administration, the excretion of calcium is reduced on continued administration; the mechanism(s) involved is only partially understood. The bulk of calcium is reabsorbed in the proximal tubule and in the loop of Henle in association with sodium reabsorption. Calcium reabsorption also occurs in the distal nephron but is not associated with sodium reabsorption.[96] Thus, the thiazides act on distal reabsorptive sites for sodium that are not shared by calcium. (In contrast, the reabsorptive sites for sodium affected by the potent loop diuretics such as furosemide appear to be linked with calcium reabsorption.) Therefore, thiazides increase sodium excretion without markedly affecting calcium excretion. The loss of sodium leads to a small volume depletion, which results in increased proximal tubular reabsorption of sodium and, hence, also of calcium reabsorption. As long as the deficit in extracellular volume is maintained, enhanced calcium reabsorption in the proximal tubule will result in decreased renal excretion of this ion. Other proposed mechanisms for the retention of calcium include a stimulation of parathyroid secretion or potentiation of the action of parathyroid hormone on the renal tubule.[63]

Chronic administration of the thiazide diuretics can lead to significant urinary losses of magnesium that can precipitate symptoms of magnesium deficiency. Table 8–1 summarizes the spectrum of electrolyte effects of the thiazides.

The thiazides have a direct vasoconstricting effect on the renal vasculature following IV administration. The result is a reduction in GFR. It is to be expected that the therapeutic efficacy of the thiazide diuretics will diminish with reduced GFR. Although GFR is low in infants, thiazides do appear to be effective in this age group. As a consequence of their multiple actions on the kidney, the thiazides tend to produce less distortion in the composition of extracellular fluid than that caused by other diuretic agents. For example, with an excess of bicarbonate, thiazides tend to increase the excretion of bicarbonate rather than chloride; with an excess of chloride in the body, bicarbonate excretion is decreased and chloride excretion is enhanced.

The thiazides are also commonly employed in the management of hypertension. Although the diuretic and antihypertensive actions have a similar time course, the precise mechanism of action of the antihypertensive effect is unknown. An alteration of sodium balance appears to contribute. Clearly, the antihypertensive action of the thiazides depends upon the depletion of sodium as demonstrated in anephric animals and humans. Upon initiation of thiazide therapy, cardiac output is decreased as blood volume is diminished. With chronic therapy, cardiac output returns to normal, peripheral resistance falls, and there is a persistent small reduction in extracellular water and plasma volume. Reduction in peripheral vascular resistance produced by the thiazides is a consequence not of direct arteriolar smooth muscle effects but of an alteration of electrolyte levels in arteriolar smooth muscle. The mechanism of action of the thiazides is different from that of diazoxide, a close structural analog with direct vasodilator activity (see Diazoxide in Chap. 7).

Clinical Pharmacology. The thiazide diuretics are poorly metabolized in the human. The average elimination half-life of hydrochlorothiazide from the body is between 5 and 10 hours in normal adults following PO administration of a single dose.[71,108] In patients who have diminished renal function (decreased creatinine clearance), thiazides will have a substantially prolonged half-life. Mirkin and colleagues[71] have shown that only 9% of administered hydrochlorothiazide is excreted in an adult patient with a creatinine clearance of 38 ml/min per 1.73 m^2 (body surface), compared with 52% excretion in an adult with a creatinine clearance of 110 ml/min per 1.73 m^2. These same investigators have demonstrated extremely high serum concentrations of hydrochlorothiazide in children with impaired renal function; in children with normal renal function, serum concentrations ranged between 130 and 190 and 260 and 600 ng/ml with doses of 1 to 1.5 and 2 to 2.7 mg/kg, respectively. Serum concentrations of 1000 to 4000 ng/ml were observed in children with 50% of normal renal function.[70]

In one of the few reported clinical studies with thiazides in neonates, Walker and Cumming[101] administered chlorothiazide (75 mg PO) to seven normal infants. An increase in urine flow and sodium, chloride, and potassium excretion occurred during the subsequent 8 hours, with peak diuresis occurring between the second and sixth hours. A small diuresis was observed in two other infants receiving 5 mg PO twice daily. No significant clinical side-effects were noted. Hobbins and colleagues[49] employed digoxin and chlorothiazide (5–10 mg/kg q 12 hr) in 21 infants (aged 1–12 mo) with congestive heart failure secondary to congenital heart disease; hepatomegaly and respiratory rates decreased significantly within 24 hours of initiation of therapy. Green and co-workers[46] used hydrochlorothiazide (20 mg/kg) as a control treatment in their examination of the effect of furosemide on PDA in premature infants. Hydrochlorothiazide produced a diuretic response equivalent to that of furosemide in the doses employed but did not appear to enhance the incidence of PDA. These authors were careful to point out that their studies did not constitute an endorsement for using thiazides in the management of respiratory distress syndrome.

Therapeutic Indications. The thiazide diuretics are useful in the management of *mild to moderate edema* associated with cardiac failure, cirrhosis of the liver, and renal disease. All the thiazides are effective when given PO and appear to act independently of the acid–base status of the patient. Parenteral administration of the thiazides does not increase their efficacy as diuretics. The thiazides also are extremely useful in the management of *mild to moderate hypertension,* either alone or as an adjunct to other antihypertensive agents.

Combined therapy with loop diuretics such as furosemide has been very effective in patients with *refractory edema.*[116] The synergistic effect of combined use of thiazides and loop diuretics has resulted in fluid removal in adult patients with previously resistant severe sodium retention associated with congestive heart failure, hypertension, renal failure, hepatic cirrhosis, and nephrotic syndrome. The mechanism for the diuretic-diuretic potentiation is unknown. It has been postulated that the thiazide-type diuretic acts to counter the enhanced distal tubular sodium reabsorption that limits the natriuresis induced by the loop-active diuretics. Serious fluid and electrolyte deficits and death have resulted in cases in which the potent synergistic effects have not been anticipated and adequately monitored. Combined therapy should be restricted to carefully considered cases of refractory edema.

The oral dose is 10 to 20 mg/kg for chlorothiazide and 1 to 2 mg/kg for hydrochlorothiazide. The frequency of administration should be determined by clinical need, the usual dosing interval being no more often than every 12 hours (Table 8–2). Increases in dose are not likely to impart any additional therapeutic effect.[68] Other than the consideration of dosing frequency, there are no clear advantages to the use of one thiazide over another.

Clinical Toxicology. Thiazide-induced hypokalemia is one of the more common electrolyte disturbances associated with chronic therapy. A variety of other adverse effects have been reported. Borderline renal or hepatic insufficiency may be aggravated by thiazide therapy;[73] hypertensive patients with decreased renal reserve appear to be most susceptible. Patients with preexisting liver disease may manifest deterioration of mental function, including the onset of coma. Increased concentrations of ammonia in the blood and cholestatic hepatitis have also been reported.

The thiazides can produce impairment of glucose tolerance, which is reversible on discontinuation of the drug. Latent diabetes can be exacerbated by the thiazides in some pre-diabetic patients.[63] Hyperglycemia is believed to be due to an inhibition of pancreatic release of insulin in conjunction with blockage of peripheral glucose utilization.

Serum uric acid is frequently elevated by thiazide diuretics. The mechanism involved is believed to be secondary to vascular volume contraction.[95a,102] Hypercalcemia and hypophosphatemia, sometimes confused with primary hyperparathyroidism, have also been reported with prolonged thiazide therapy in adults.[29]

The effects of the thiazides on magnesium balance have led to manifestations of magnesium deficiency in patients on long-term therapy. Exacerbation of digoxin toxicity may occur as a consequence of depletion of magnesium as well as of potassium, leading to cardiac arrhythmias, nausea, and vomiting.

Hypersensitivity reactions including severe skin reactions, photosensitivity, and bone marrow depression have been reported. The thiazide-induced syndrome of inappropriate secretion of antidiuretic hormone (ADH) has

been described; the clinical presentation includes the classic sign of inappropriate secretion of ADH (i.e., hyponatremia) accompanied by hypokalemia and alkalosis. Withdrawal of the diuretic is associated with return of the serum sodium concentration to normal and with an appropriate excretion of water load within 10 days.[48]

References

1. Allen JM, Hind CRK, McMichael HB: Synergistic action of metolazone with "loop" diuretics. Br Med J 282:1873, 1981.
2. Anderton JL, Kincaid-Smith P: Diuretics. I. Physiological and pharmacological considerations. Drugs 1:54, 1971.
3. Aperia A, Broberger O, Elinder G, et al: Postnatal development of renal function in pre-term and full-term infants. Acta Paediatr Scand 70:183, 1981.
4. Aranda JV, Perez J, Sitar DS, et al: Pharmacokinetic disposition and protein binding of furosemide in newborn infants. J Pediatr 93:507, 1978.
5. Aranda JV, Turmen T, Sasyniuk BI: Pharmacokinetics of diuretics and methylxanthines in the neonate. Eur J Clin Pharmacol 18:55, 1980.
6. Aranda JV, Lambert C, Perez J, et al: Metabolism and renal elimination of furosemide in the newborn infant. J Pediatr 101:777, 1982.
7. Attallah AA: Interaction of prostaglandins along with diuretics. Prostaglandins 18:369, 1979.
8. Bailie MD, Linshaw MA, Stygles VG: Diuretic pharmacology in infants and children. Pediatr Clin North Am 28:217, 1981.
9. Bamford JM: Synergistic action of metolazone with "loop" diuretics. Br Med J 283:618, 1981.
10. Baylen BG, Johnson G, Tsang R, et al: The occurrence of hyperaldosteronism in infants with congestive heart failure. Am J Cardiol 45:305, 1980.
11. Benet LZ: Pharmacokinetics/pharmacodynamics of furosemide in man: A review. J Pharmacokinet Biopharm 7:1, 1979.
12. Benet LZ, Smith DE, Lin ET, et al: Furosemide assays and disposition in healthy volunteers and renal transplant patients. Fed Proc 42:1695, 1983.
13. Bennett WM, Porter GA: Efficacy and safety of metolazone in renal failure and the nephrotic syndrome. J Clin Pharmacol 13:357, 1973.
14. Bess FH, Finlayson B, Chapman JJ: Further observations on noise levels in infant incubators. Pediatrics 63:100, 1979.
15. Bland RD, McMillian DD, Bressack MA: Decreased pulmonary transvascular fluid filtration in awake newborn lambs after intravenous furosemide. J Clin Invest 62:601, 1978.
16. Bowman RH: Renal secretion of [^{35}S] furosemide and its depression by albumin binding. Am J Physiol 229:93, 1975.
17. Bourland WA, Kay DK, Williamson HE: The role of the kidney in the early nondiuretic action of furosemide to reduce elevated left atrial pressure in the hypervolemic dog. J Pharmacol Exp Ther 202:221, 1977.
18. Branch RA, Roberts CJC, Homeida M, Levine D: Determinants of response to furosemide in normal subjects. Br J Clin Pharmacol 4:121, 1977.
19. Branch RA: Role of binding in distribution of furose-

mide: Where is nonrenal clearance? Fed Proc 42:1699, 1983.

20. Brater DC: Resistance to diuretics: Emphasis on a pharmacological perspective. Drugs 22:477, 1981.

21. Brater DC: Determinants of the overall response to furosemide: Pharmacokinetics and pharmacodynamics. Fed Proc 42:1711, 1983.

22. Brown DD, Dormois JC, Abraham GN, et al: Effect of furosemide on the renal excretion of digoxin. Clin Pharmacol Ther 20:395, 1976.

23. Brummett RE, Traynor J, Brown R, Himes D: Cochlear damage resulting from kanamycin and furosemide. Acta Otolaryngol 80:86, 1975.

24. Burg MB: Tubular chloride transport and the mode of action of some diuretics. Kidney Int 9:189, 1976.

25. Cafruny EJ, Itskovitz HD: Sites of action of loop diuretics. J Pharmacol Exp Ther 223:105, 1982.

26. Callahan J, Haller JO, Cacciarelli AA, et al: Cholelithiasis in infants: Association with total parenteral nutrition and furosemide. Radiology 143:437, 1982.

27. Cannon PJ, Heinemann HO, Albert MS, et al: "Contraction" alkalosis after diuresis of edematous patients with ethacrynic acid. Ann Intern Med 62:979, 1965.

28. Chaplin ER, Goldstein GW, Myerberg DZ, et al: Posthemorrhagic hydrocephalus in the preterm infant. Pediatrics 65:901, 1980.

29. Christensson T, Hellstrom K, Wengle B: Hypercalcemia and primary hyperparathyroidism. Prevalence in patients receiving thiazides as detected in a health screen. Arch Intern Med 137:1138, 1977.

30. Chrysant SG, Baxter PR, Amonette RL: The mechanism for the renal hemodynamic and tubular action of furosemide. Arch Int Pharmacodyn 248:289, 1981.

31. Cottrell JE, Robustelli A, Post K, Turndorf H: Furosemide- and mannitol-induced changes in intracranial pressure and serum osmolality and electrolytes. Anesthesiology 47:28, 1977.

32. Craswell PW, Ezzat E, Kopstein J, et al: Use of metolazone, a new diuretic, in patients with renal disease. Nephron 12:63, 1973.

33. Cutler RE, Blair AD: Clinical pharmacokinetics of frusemide. Clin Pharmacokin 4:279, 1979.

34. Danks DM: Diuretic therapy in infants and children. J Pediatr 88:695, 1976.

35. Dargie HJ, Allison MEM, Kennedy AC, Gray MJB: High-dosage metolazone in chronic renal failure. Br Med J 4:196, 1972.

36. Dikshit K, Vyden JK, Forrester JS, et al: Renal and extrarenal hemodynamic effects of furosemide in congestive heart failure after acute myocardial infarction. N Engl J Med 288:1087, 1973.

37. Donat JF: Acetazolamide-induced improvement in hydrocephalus. Arch Neurol 37:376, 1980.

38. Engle MA, Lewy JE, Lewy PR, Metcoff J: The use of furosemide in the treatment of edema in infants and children. Pediatrics 62:811, 1978.

39. Frazier HS, Yager H: The clinical use of diuretics (first of two parts). N Engl J Med 288:246, 1973.

40. Friedman Z, Demers LM, Marks KH, et al: Urinary excretion of prostaglandin E following the administration of furosemide and indomethacin in sick low-birth-weight infants. J Pediatr 93:512, 1978.

41. Gerber JG: Role of prostaglandins in the hemodynamic and tubular effects of furosemide. Fed Proc 42:1707, 1983.

42. Ghose RR, Gupta SK: Synergistic action of metola-

43. Green TP, Mirkin BL: Resistance of proteinuric rats to furosemide: Urinary drug protein binding as a determinant of drug effect. Life Sci 26:623, 1980.

44. Green TP, Thompson TR, Johnson D, Lock JE: Furosemide use in premature infants and appearance of patent ductus arteriosus. Arch Dis Child 135:239, 1981.

45. Green TP: The use of diuretics in infants with the respiratory distress syndrome. Semin Perinatol 6:172, 1982.

46. Green TP, Thompson TR, Johnson DE, Lock JE: Furosemide promotes patent ductus arteriosus in premature infants with the respiratory distress syndrome. N Engl J Med 308:743, 1983.

47. Guignard JP: Renal function in the newborn infant. Pediatr Clin North Am 29:777, 1982.

48. Hamburger S, Koprivica B, Ellerbeck E, Covinsky JO: Thiazide-induced syndrome of inappropriate secretion of antidiuretic hormone. Time course of resolution. JAMA 246:1235, 1981.

49. Hobbins SM, Fowler RS, Rowe RD, Korey AG: Spironolactone therapy in infants with congestive heart failure secondary to congenital heart disease. Arch Dis Child 56:934, 1981.

50. Hook JB, Bailie MD: Perinatal renal pharmacology. Ann Rev Pharmacol Toxicol 19:491, 1979.

51. Huang CM, Atkinson AJ, Levin M, et al: Pharmacokinetics of furosemide in advanced renal failure. Clin Pharmacol Ther 16:659, 1974.

52. Hufnagle KG, Khan SN, Penn D, et al: Renal calcifications: A complication of long-term furosemide therapy in preterm infants. Pediatrics 70:360, 1982.

53. Huttenlocher PR: Treatment of hydrocephalus with acetazolamide. J Pediatr 66:1023, 1965.

54. Ikram H, Chan W, Espiner EA, Nicholls MG: Haemodynamic and hormone responses to acute and chronic frusemide therapy in congestive heart failure. Clin Sci 59:443, 1980.

55. James JA: Ethacrynic acid in edematous states in children. J Pediatr 71:881, 1967.

56. Johns CT: Metolazone: A convenient new long-acting diuretic/antihypertensive agent. Clin Ther 1:43, 1977.

57. Kao LC, Warburton D, Sargent CW, et al: Furosemide acutely decreases airways resistance in chronic bronchopulmonary dysplasia. J Pediatr 103:624, 1983.

58. Karim A: Spironolactone: Disposition, metabolism, pharmacodynamics, and bioavailability. Drug Metab Rev 8:151, 1978.

59. Kelly MR, Blair AD, Forrey AW, et al: A comparison of the diuretic response to oral and intravenous furosemide in "diuretic-resistant" patients. Curr Ther Res 21:1, 1977.

60. Krongrad E, Joos HA: Furosemide in treatment of edema in infants and children. NY State J Med, 71:2521, 1971.

61. Laux BE, Raichle ME: The effect of acetazolamide on cerebral blood flow and oxygen utilization in the rhesus monkey. J Clin Invest 62:585, 1978.

62. Loggie JMH, Kleinman LI, Van Maanen EF: Renal function and diuretic therapy in infants and children. Part I. J Pediatr 86:485, 1975.

63. Loggie JMH, Kleinman LI, Van Maanen EF: Renal function and diuretic therapy in infants and children. Part II. J Pediatr 86:657, 1975.

64. Ludens JH: Nature of the inhibition of Cl⁻ transport

by furosemide: Evidence for competitive inhibition of active transport in toad cornea. J Pharmacol Exp Ther 223:25, 1983.

65. Maren TH: Carbonic anhydrase: Chemistry, physiology, and inhibition. Physiol Rev 47:595, 1967.

66. Marks KH, Berman W Jr, Friedman Z, et al: Furosemide in hyaline membrane disease. Pediatrics 62:785, 1978.

67. McCarthy KD, Reed DJ: The effect of acetazolamide and furosemide on cerebrospinal fluid production and choroid plexus carbonic anhydrase activity. J Pharmacol Exp Ther 189:194, 1974.

68. McLeod PJ, Ogilvie RI, Ruedy J: Effects of large and small doses of hydrochlorothiazide in hypertensive patients. Clin Pharmacol Ther 11:733, 1970.

69. Mealey J Jr, Barker DT: Failure of oral acetazolamide to avert hydrocephalus in infants with myelomeningocele. J Pediatr 72:257, 1968.

70. Mirkin B, Sinaiko A, Cooper M, Anders M: Hydrochlorothiazide (HCT) therapy in hypertensive (HT) and renal insufficient (RI) children: Elimination kinetics and metabolic effects. Pediatr Res 11:418, 1977.

71. Mirkin B, Green TP, O'Dea RF: Disposition and pharmacodynamics of diuretics and antihypertensive agents in renal disease. Eur J Pharmacol 18:109, 1980.

72. Moylan FMB, O'Connell KC, Todres ID, Shannon DC: Edema of the pulmonary interstitium in infants and children. Pediatrics 55:783, 1975.

73. Mudge GH: Diuretics and other agents employed in the mobilization of edema fluid. In Gilman AG, Goodman LS, Gilman A (eds): The Pharmacological Basis of Therapeutics, 6th ed. p 892. New York, Macmillan, 1980.

74. Noordewier B, Bailie MD, Hook JB: Pharmacological analysis of the action of diuretics in the newborn pig. J Pharmacol Exp Ther 207:236, 1978.

75. Odlind B: Determinants of access of diuretics to their site of action. Fed Proc 42:1703, 1983.

76. Peterson RG, Simmons MA, Rumack BH, et al: Pharmacology of furosemide in the premature newborn infant. J Pediatr 97:139, 1980.

77. Pruitt AW, Boles A: Diuretic effects of furosemide in acute glomerulonephritis. J Pediatr 89:306, 1976.

78. Puschett JB, Rastegar A: Comparative study of the effects of metolazone and other diuretics on potassium excretion. Clin Pharmacol Ther 15:397, 1973.

79. Puschett JB, Kuhrman MA: Differential effects of diuretic agents on electrolyte excretion in the dog. Nephron 23:38, 1979.

80. Puschett JB: Sites and mechanisms of action of diuretics in the kidney. J Clin Pharmacol 21:564, 1981.

81. Repetto HA, Lewy JE, Braudo JL, Metcoff J: The renal functional response to furosemide in children with acute glomerulonephritis. J Pediatr 80:660, 1972.

82. Richardson H: Frusemide in heart failure of infancy. Arch Dis Child 46:520, 1971.

83. Ross BS, Pollak A, Oh W: The pharmacologic effects of furosemide therapy in the low-birth-weight infant. J Pediatr 92:149, 1978.

84. Rubin RC, Henderson ES, Ommaya AK, et al: The production of cerebrospinal fluid in man and its modification by acetazolamide. J Neurosurg 25:430, 1966.

85. Savage MO, Wilkinson AR, Baum JD, Roberton NRC: Frusemide in respiratory distress syndrome. Arch Dis Child 50:709, 1975.

86. Schain RJ: Carbonic anhydrase inhibitors in chronic infantile hydrocephalus. Am J Dis Child 117:621, 1969.

87. Schenk KE, Biamino G, Schroder R: Vergleichende hamodynamische untersuchangen uber die extrarenale Wirkung von furosemide und ethacrynasaure. Klin Wochenschr 2:1133, 1975.

88. Schoonees R, Mostert JW, Moore RH, et al: Evaluation of metolazone. New diuretic in chronic renal disease. NY State J Med, 71:566, 1971.

89. Shankaran S, Poland RL: The displacement of bilirubin from albumin by furosemide. J Pediatr 90:642, 1977.

90. Singhal N, McMillian DD, Rademaker AW: Furosemide improves lung compliance in infants with bronchopulmonary dysplasia. Pediatr Res 17:336A, 1983.

91. Slone D, Jick H, Lewis GP, et al: Intravenously given ethacrynic acid and gastrointestinal bleeding. JAMA 209:1668, 1969.

92. Smith DE, Benet LZ: Relationship between urinary excretion rate, steady-state plasma levels and diuretic response of furosemide in the rat. Pharmacology 19:301, 1979.

93. Smith DE, Brater DC, Lin ET, Benet LZ: Attenuation of furosemide's diuretic effect by indomethacin: Pharmacokinetic evaluation. J Pharmacokin Biopharm 7:265, 1979.

94. Sparrow AW, Friedberg DZ, Nadas AS: The use of ethacrynic acid in infants and children with congestive heart failure. Pediatrics 42:291, 1968.

95. Spitzer A (ed): The Kidney During Development: Morphology and Function. New York, Masson Publishing USA, 1982.

95a. Steele TH, Oppenheimer S: Factors affecting urate excretion following diuretic administration in man. Am J Med 47:564, 1969.

95b. Steinmuller SR, Puschett JB: Effects of metolazone in man. Comparison with chlorothiazide. Kidney Int 1:169, 1972.

96. Suki WN, Eknoyan G, Martinez-Maldonado M: Tubular sites and mechanisms of diuretic action. Ann Rev Pharmacol 13:91, 1973.

97. Sulyok E, Varga F, Nemeth M, et al: Furosemide-induced alterations in the electrolyte status, the function of renin–angiotensin–aldosterone system, and the urinary excretion of prostaglandins in newborn infants. Pediatr Res 14:765, 1980.

98. Tapia JL, Gerhardt T, Goldberg RN, et al: Furosemide and lung function in neonates with chronic lung disease (CLD). Pediatr Res 17:338A, 1983.

99. Tudvad F, McNamara H, Barnett HL: Renal response of premature infants to administration of bicarbonate and potassium. Pediatrics 13:4, 1954.

100. Vert P, Broquaire M, Legagneur M, Morselli PL: Pharmacokinetics of furosemide in neonates. Eur J Clin Pharmacol 22:39, 1982.

101. Walker RD, Cumming GR: Response of the infant kidney to diuretic drugs. Can Med Assoc J 91:1149, 1964.

102. Weinman EJ, Eknoyan G, Suki WN: The influence of extracellular fluid volume on the tubular reabsorption of uric acid. J Clin Invest 55:283, 1975.

103. Wennberg RP, Rasmussen LF, Ahlfors CE: Displacement of bilirubin from human albumin by three diuretics. J Pediatr 90:647, 1977.

104. Whitington PF, Black DD: Cholelithiasis in premature infants treated with parenteral nutrition and furosemide. J Pediatr 97:647, 1980.

105. Wilson JR, Reichek N, Dunkman WB, Goldberg S:

Effect of diuresis on the performance of the failing left ventricle in man. Am J Med 70:234, 1981.

106. Woo WCR, Dupont C, Collinge J, Aranda JV: Effects of furosemide in the newborn. Clin Pharmacol Ther 23:266, 1978.

107. Yeh TF, Wilks A, Singh J, et al: Furosemide prevents the renal side effects of indomethacin therapy in premature infants with patent ductus arteriosus. J Pediatr 101:433, 1982.

108. Beerman B, Groschinsky-Grind M: Clinical pharmacokinetics of diuretics. Clin Pharmacokin 5:221, 1980.

109. Cashore WJ, Oh W, Brodersen R: Bilirubin-displacing effect of furosemide and sulfisoxazole. An *in vitro* and *in vivo* study in neonatal serum. Dev Pharmacol Ther 6:230, 1983.

110. Finberg L: Furosemide — uses, abuses, and unsolved puzzles. Am J Dis Child 137:1145, 1983.

111. Green TP, Thompson TR, Johnson DE, Lock JE: Diuresis and pulmonary function in premature infants with respiratory distress syndrome. J Pediatr 103:618, 1983.

112. Jørgensen FS: Effect of thiazide diuretics upon calcium metabolism. Danish Med Bull 23:223, 1976.

113. Lönnerholm G, Wistrand PJ: Carbonic anhydrase in the human fetal kidney. Ped Res 17:390, 1983.

114. McCann EM, Deming DD, Brady JP: Lasix improves lung function in infants with chronic lung disease. Clin Res 31:141A, 1983.

115. Najak Z, Harris EM, Lazzara A, Pruitt AW: Pulmonary effects of furosemide in premature infants with lung disease. Ped Res 15:674, 1981.

116. Oster JR, Epstein M, Smoller S: Combined therapy with thiazide-type and loop diuretic agents for resistant sodium retention. Ann Int Med 99:405, 1983.

117. Sniderman S, Chung M, Roth R, Ballard R: Treatment of neonatal chronic lung disease with furosemide. Clin Res 26:201A, 1978.

118. Tuck S, Morselli P, Broquaire M, Vert P: Plasma and urinary kinetics of furosemide in newborn infants. J Pediatr 103:481, 1983.

119. Venkataraman PS, Han BK, Tsang RC, Daugherty CC: Secondary hyperparathyroidism and bone disease in infants receiving long-term furosemide therapy. Am J Dis Child 137:1157, 1983.

NINE

Prostaglandins, Prostaglandin Inhibitors, and Vitamin E

PROSTAGLANDINS

The extensive research effort over recent years in areas related to the prostaglandins has resulted in their use in the treatment of several diseases in neonates. Information about the physiologic effects of the various prostaglandins continues to emerge. Originally PGE_2 and $PGF_{2\alpha}$ were believed to be the most important prostaglandins. Currently, it is recognized that these "classic" prostaglandins constitute only a small fraction of the physiologically active "eicosanoids." The intermediates of these and other newly discovered compounds (see Fig. 9–1) have extremely potent biologic activity.

Biosynthesis, Metabolism, and Physiologic Effects

Prostaglandins are 20-carbon unsaturated fatty acids whose basic structure consists of a cyclopentane ring with two aliphatic side chains (see Fig. 9–1). Each prostaglandin is denoted by an uppercase letter that represents its cyclopentane substituents and by a subscript number indicating the number of carbon–carbon double bonds present in the side chains.

Biosynthesis and Metabolism. Linoleic acid is the essential fatty acid of origin of the prostaglandins. The majority of the biologically important eicosanoids are synthesized from arachidonic acid via the cyclo-oxygenase or lipoxygenase pathways (Fig. 9–1). Prostaglandins are not stored in the body but are synthe-

sized rapidly and released as required. The basic process involves the mobilization of arachidonic acid from cell membrane phospholipids by the enzyme phospholipase A_2, with subsequent biotransformation via one of the three pathways indicated in Figure 9–1: Pathway I is the classical cyclo-oxygenase pathway that yields PGE_2, PGD_2, $PGF_{2\alpha}$, the thromboxanes (e.g., TXA_2), and prostacyclin (PGI_2). Pathways II and III are more recently discovered pathways that yield a host of hydroxy, hydroperoxy, and epoxy products. The substances in pathway II are called the **leukotrienes,** which contain three conjugated double bonds; leukotriene C is identical with slow-reacting substance A (SRS-A).[44a] The details of the biosynthesis of the various eicosanoids are the subject of many recent articles and reviews.[10,24,38] Difficulties in studying these substances are related to their chemical instability—that is, their short chemical half-life (PGG_2 and PGH_2, 5 min; TXA_2, 30 sec; PGI_2, 3 min); efficient mechanisms exist for inactivation of most prostaglandins in vivo.

The metabolism of prostaglandins, PGI_2, and TXA_2 is illustrated in Figure 9–2. Catabolism of the prostaglandins involves four reactions: oxidation of the hydroxyl group at C15 (carbon 15), resulting in formation of a ketone; reduction of the double bond between C13 and C14, resulting in a single bond; removal of two carbon units from the C1 side chain (beta-oxidation); and removal of two carbon units from the C20 side chain (omega-oxidation).[40] The rate of these reactions varies depending upon

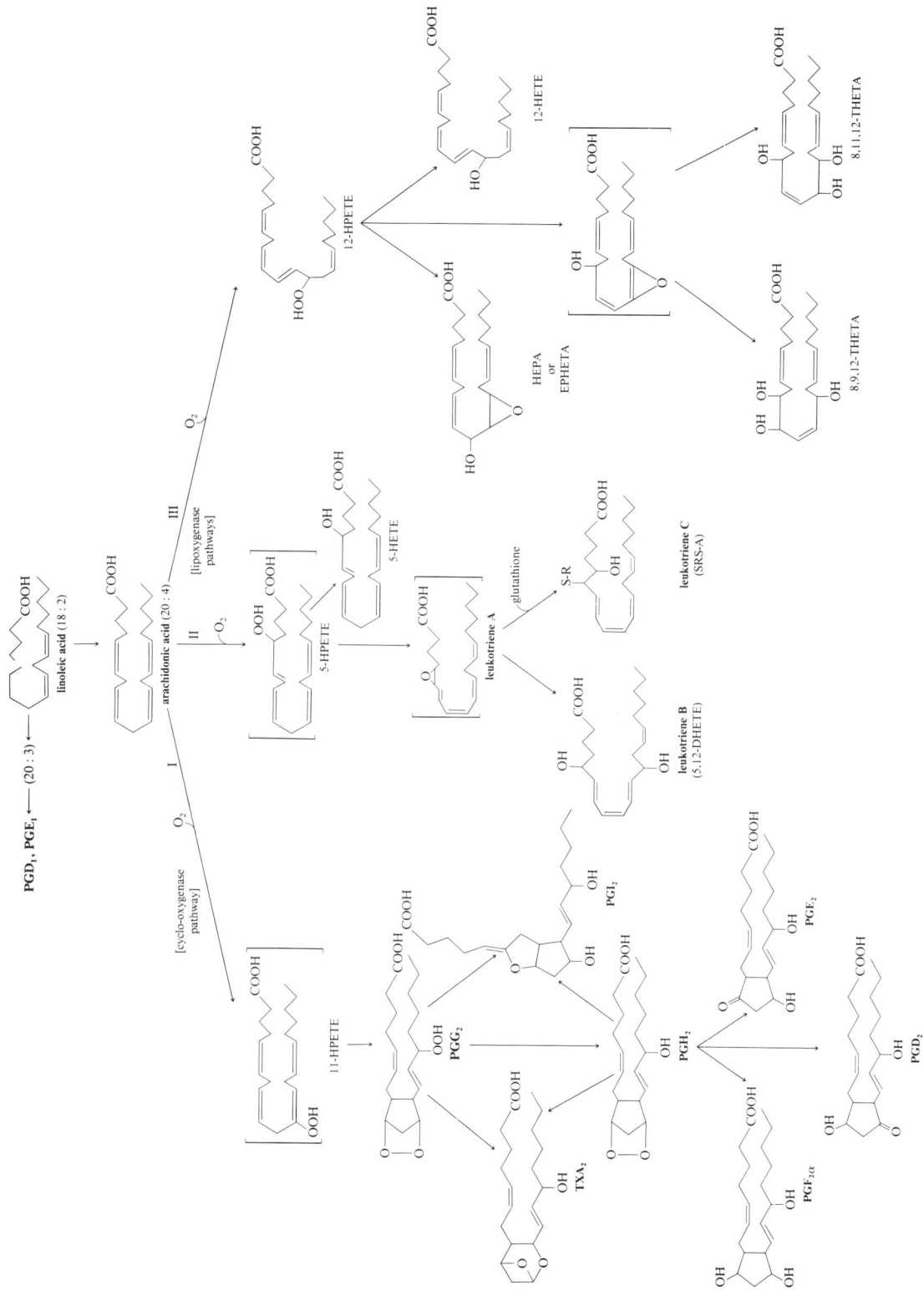

Figure 9–1. Prostaglandin synthesis: The pathways for biotransformation of linoleic acid (18:2) to various "eicosanoids," most of which involve metabolic transformation of arachidonic acid. *Pathway I,* The cyclo-oxygenase pathway; *Pathways II* and *III,* the noncyclized lipoxygenase pathways. (Adapted from Coceani F et al: Eur J Clin Pharmacol 18:75, 1980.)

active compound

major
blood metabolite

major
urinary metabolite

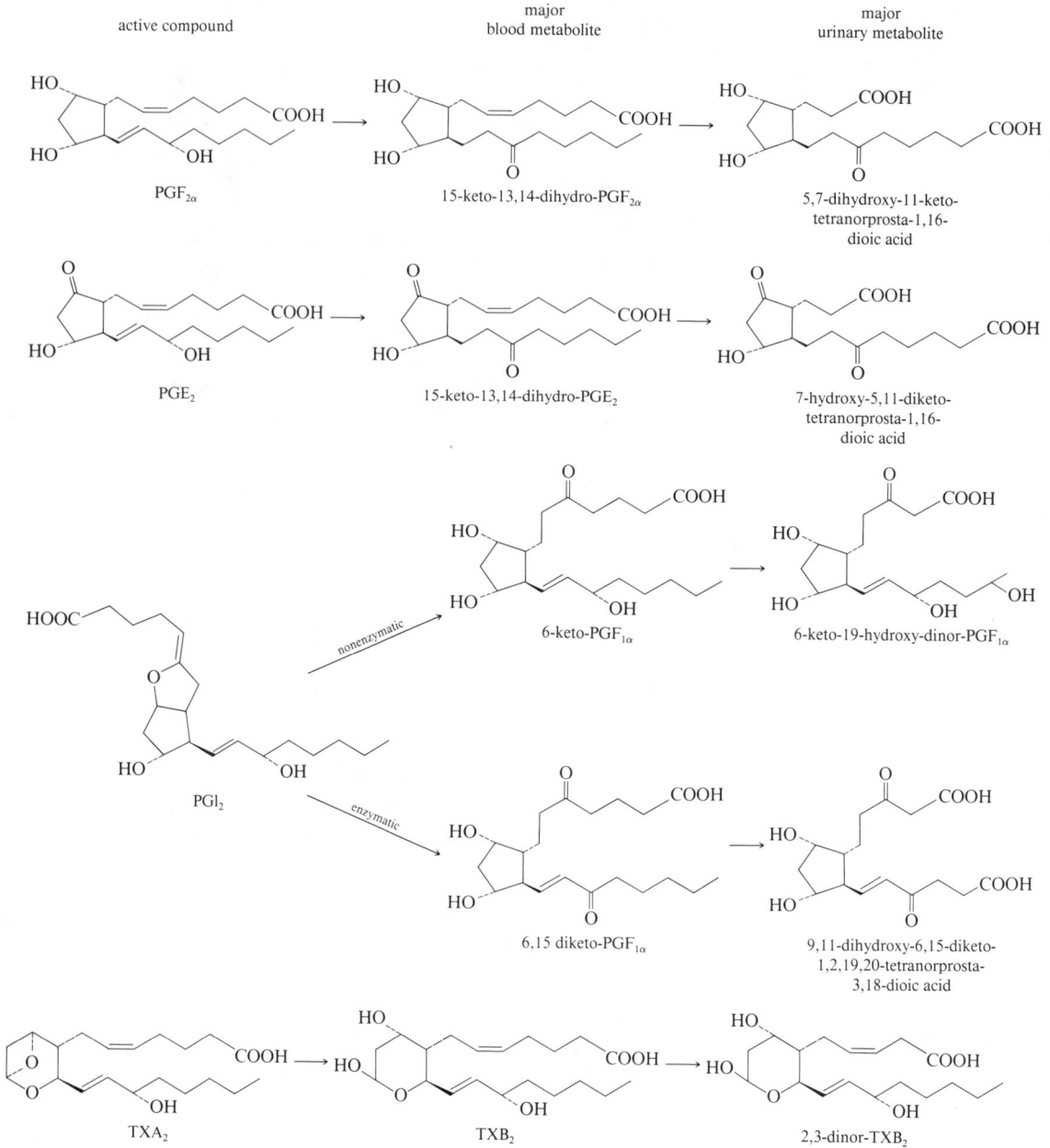

PGF$_{2\alpha}$

15-keto-13,14-dihydro-PGF$_{2\alpha}$

5,7-dihydroxy-11-keto-
tetranorprosta-1,16-
dioic acid

PGE$_2$

15-keto-13,14-dihydro-PGE$_2$

7-hydroxy-5,11-diketo-
tetranorprosta-1,16-
dioic acid

PGI$_2$

nonenzymatic

6-keto-PGF$_{1\alpha}$

6-keto-19-hydroxy-dinor-PGF$_{1\alpha}$

enzymatic

6,15 diketo-PGF$_{1\alpha}$

9,11-dihydroxy-6,15-diketo-
1,2,19,20-tetranorprosta-
3,18-dioic acid

TXA$_2$

TXB$_2$

2,3-dinor-TXB$_2$

Figure 9-2. Catabolism of prostaglandins (PGE$_2$, PGF$_{2\alpha}$), prostacyclin (PGI$_2$), and thromboxane A$_2$ (TXA$_2$). (From Ramwell PW et al: Semin Perinatol 4:3, 1980.)

the particular prostaglandin. Following IV administration of PGE$_2$, the rate of disappearance is equivalent to a half-life of about 2 hours, with recovery of about 70% of the administered dose in the urine (as metabolites) by 12 hours.[40] Initially there is a rapid loss of administered PGE$_2$ from the blood, with less than 1% remaining 4.5 minutes after injection. This rapid clearance of the prostaglandins is due to metabolism occurring primarily in the lungs, kidney,

and liver. The vascular bed of the lung can metabolize 95% of infused PGE$_2$ during a single pass through the pulmonary circulation. The pulmonary vascular bed is apparently an important mechanism for removing many but not all of the prostaglandins endogenously released from tissues into the venous circulation.

Prostaglandin 15-OH dehydrogenase (15-PGDH) is the enzyme responsible for the oxidation of the 15-OH group on the prostaglandins to the corresponding ketone (Fig. 9–2). The highest activities of 15-PGDH are located in the kidney and spleen. PGE_1 is the most reactive 15-PGDH substrate, followed by PGE_2, $PGF_{1\alpha}$, and $PGF_{2\alpha}$, respectively.

There appear to be two major catabolic pathways for PGI_2: one nonenzymatic and the other an enzymatic dehydrogenation. Approximately 35% of the metabolism is by the nonenzymatic breakdown of PGI_2 to the 6-keto-$PGF_{1\alpha}$ in experimental animals.

TXA_2 catabolism occurs rapidly, with less than 12% of the administered material remaining in the blood after 4 minutes. TXA_2 breaks down to form TXB_2, which is subsequently excreted in the urine along with other metabolites. Little is known about the catabolism of leukotrienes.

Physiologic Effects. Prostaglandins, prostacyclin (PGI_2), and thromboxanes are capable of producing numerous and diverse physiologic effects. Because of this, research efforts have focused on identifying agents that possess a high degree of specificity for certain desired effects. Although this effort has been challenging, several important therapeutic advances have evolved.

Cardiovascular effects of the prostaglandins observed in humans (unless otherwise noted) are outlined in Table 9–1. PGE_1, PGE_2, $PGF_{2\alpha}$, and PGI_2 are all potent vasodilators of the peripheral vascular bed.[12,23,41] The vasodilation involves arterioles, precapillaries, sphincters, and post-capillary venules. Certain vasoconstrictor responses to PGEs have been noted as well. Endogenous prostaglandins may also be the mediators of the vasodilating activity of certain drugs. Studies in fetal and newborn animals have shown that the pulmonary vasodilation produced by oxygen and by initiation of breathing at birth is primarily mediated through prostaglandins.[53,162] The pulmonary vasodilating effects of hydralazine also appear to be prostaglandin-mediated.[42]

Because of its instability, few clinical studies on TXA_2 have been accomplished; it has been shown to produce vasoconstriction of peripheral vascular beds in experimental animals.[44] PGI_2 is about five times more potent than PGE_2 in producing vasodilation and hypotension. PGI_2 causes dilation in every vascular bed examined, including the coronary, renal, mesentery, and pulmonary beds and that of skeletal muscle. Because it is not inactivated by the pulmonary vasculature, PGI_2 produces vasodilation when it is administered either intra-arterially or IV.[49]

The effects of PGD_2 are more complicated. Most studies have demonstrated a smooth-muscle stimulatory activity of PGD_2 in a variety of species.[5] In fetal and newborn animals, however, PGD_2 has been shown to decrease pulmonary vascular resistance and have minimal or no effect on peripheral vascular resistance.[5,47,165] Unlike the E and F series prostaglandins, PGD_2 is not metabolized by the lungs, but conversion to $PGF_{2\alpha}$ in the peripheral circulation has been noted in adult animals. Cassin and colleagues[5] have speculated that the different responses observed in the newborn and in the adult (vasodilation and vasoconstriction, respectively) may relate to greater peripheral conversion of PGD_2 (a vasodilator) to $PGF_{2\alpha}$ (a vasoconstrictor) in the adult. Another possible consideration they proposed is the presence of vasodilator-specific receptors having an affinity for PGD_2 greater than that of vasoconstrictor receptors. Thus, at low concentrations of PGD_2, the dilator receptors would bind the drug to a greater extent than the constrictor receptors, resulting in a predominant vasodilating effect; with increasing concentrations of PGD_2, the vasoconstrictor receptors would become occupied and thus predominate. Since PGE_2 has also been reported to be a pulmonary vasoconstrictor in adults and a vasodilator in newborn animals, similar mechanisms can be hypothesized. These mechanisms may also in part explain the conflicting data regarding the effects of PGD_2 on the pulmonary vascular bed.[4,10] Leukotrienes, C_4 and D_4, have been identified in lung lavage fluids of neonates with hypoxemia and pulmonary hypertension.[166] Leukotrienes were not demonstrated in lavage fluids obtained from neonates with requirements for ventilation and hyperoxia but without pulmonary hypertension. Leukotrienes were proposed as a possible mechanism for persistant pulmonary hypertension in the newborn. Age-dependent differences in effects of leukotrienes on the pulmonary vascular bed were not discussed.

$PGF_{2\alpha}$ has been shown to be a vasodilator and vasoconstrictor in various peripheral vascular beds. It produces vasoconstriction of the pulmonary vascular bed in both neonates and adults.[37]

Increased understanding of the role of prostaglandins, PGI_2, and the thromboxanes in the control of patency and postnatal closure of the ductus arteriosus has lead to effective management of neonates with patent ductus arteriosus (PDA) and ductus-dependent cyanotic congenital heart disease. A number of factors other

Table 9–1. PHYSIOLOGIC EFFECTS OF PROSTAGLANDINS, PGI$_2$, AND TXA$_2$ IN NEONATES

	Cardiac Output[a]	Peripheral Vascular	Pulmonary Vascular	Ductus Arteriosus	Platelet Aggregation	Bronchial Muscle	Kidney	Gastrointestinal Tract
PGE$_1$	increase	dilate	dilate	dilate	inhibit	relax	increase diuresis, natriuresis, renal blood flow, and renin release	delay gastric emptying; decrease acid secretion; increase intestinal motility
PGE$_2$ PGD$_2$	increase	dilate minimal	dilate[b] dilate[b] (constrict with large doses)	dilate dilate	variable inhibit	relax	same as PGE$_1$ same as PGEs except no effect on renin	same as PGE$_1$
PGF$_{2\alpha}$	variable	constrict and dilate	constrict	constrict		constrict	inhibit release of renin	no effect on gastric acid secretion
PGI$_2$		dilate	dilate	dilate	inhibit	no effect to mild relax	same as PGEs	decrease gastric acid secretion
TXA$_2$		constrict		constrict	induce	constrict		

a Increase in cardiac output is largely a reflex sympathetic effect in response to the hypotensive actions.
b Effects in experimental newborn animals; older animals show pulmonary vasoconstriction.

254

than products of arachidonic acid metabolism can affect the ductus arteriosus.[8,9] This has lead to confusion about controlling factors in abnormal patency of the ductus arteriosus. Both PGE_1 and PGE_2 are dilators of the ductus arteriosus (Table 9–1). PGE_2 is the most potent relaxing agent known, its effect exceeding by several orders of magnitude that of PGI_2. Both $PGF_{2\alpha}$ and TXA_2 are constrictors of the ductus arteriosus. The role of the prostaglandins with respect to the ductus arteriosus is discussed further under Indomethacin later in this chapter.

Platelet function is markedly influenced by the metabolites of arachidonic acid.[15] PGE_1 and PGD_2 are inhibitors of aggregation of human platelets. However, PGI_2 is 30 to 50 times more potent than either. The potency of PGI_2, plus the fact that it is generated in the endothelium of the vascular wall, has lead to the hypothesis that PGI_2 controls the aggregation of platelets in vivo.[32] PGE_2 exerts variable effects on platelets. TXA_2 is a powerful inducer of platelet aggregation and release. The generation of TXA_2 by platelets is very sensitive to the action of aspirin and azoprostanoids.[17]

Prostaglandins contribute significantly to inflammatory reactions in conjunction with *polymorphonuclear leukocytes (PMNLs), macrophages,* and *lymphocytes* as well as with various other vasoactive substances.[15,37] The E-type prostaglandins are the most powerful pyretics known, producing a dose-dependent febrile reaction. PMNLs have been shown to release PGE_1 following stimulation of these cells during phagocytosis. The synthesis and release of prostaglandins by PMNLs at sites of inflammation may be under total or partial control of lysosomal enzyme released from invading cells. Macrophages have been shown to release PGE_2-like material during in vitro culture.[3] In lymphocytes the formation and release of antibodies from B cells is suppressed, and the functions of T suppressor cells are modulated by prostaglandins.

The *kidney* is capable of synthesizing a variety of prostaglandins including PGE_2, $PGF_{2\alpha}$, PGD_2, and PGI_2.[11,48,52] PGE_2, PGD_2, and PGI_2 all produce renal vasodilation. $PGF_{2\alpha}$ does not appear to affect renal vasculature but does inhibit the release of renin. The role of TXA_2 in renal physiology is unclear (see Table 9–1). Exogenous administration of PGE_2, PGD_2, or PGI_2 produces an increase in total renal blood flow by a direct vasodilation (decrease in renal vascular resistance), as well as a redistribution of blood flow from the outer cortex to the juxtamedullary cortex.[16] These effects

are seen with doses that do not alter systemic blood pressure or glomerular filtration rate (GFR). $PGF_{2\alpha}$ does not appear to affect renal blood flow, intrarenal blood flow distribution, renal vascular resistance, or GFR.[6,50] PGE_2, PGD_2, and PGI_2 produce diuresis, natriuresis, and an increased urine flow, all of which occur without changes in GFR.[14] Infusion of these prostaglandins has demonstrated variable effects on potassium excretion (increase or no effect). These effects on tubular function by the various prostaglandins may or may not be related to the vasodilation and intrarenal blood flow redistribution produced by these substances.[6,52]

Both PGE_2 and PGI_2 increase the release of renin from the juxtaglomerular apparatus of the kidney, resulting in increased synthesis of angiotensin II (see Table 7–16). PGD_2 does not affect renin release.[16] Paradoxically, the vasopressor actions of angiotensin II can be blunted by the vasodilatory actions of PGE_2 and PGI_2. There is evidence as well that angiotensin II may stimulate the intrarenal production of PGE_2, which then attenuates the angiotensin-induced renal vasoconstriction.[31] An interaction between the kallikrein–kinin system and renal prostaglandins to maintain normal blood pressure has also been proposed.[14] The complex and sometimes conflicting literature on prostaglandins and the renin–angiotensin–aldosterone system has been reviewed by Overturf and colleagues.[39]

Many aspects of *gastrointestinal tract* physiology and function are influenced by the prostaglandins.[1,14] Effects include alterations in motility, secretion, mucosal blood flow, and mucus production. The oral or parenteral administration of PGE_2 produces relaxation of the circular muscle in the stomach, resulting in a flaccid gastric antrum and prolonged gastric emptying. In the gastrointestinal tract, PGE_2 produces contraction of longitudinal smooth muscle and inhibitory effects on the circular smooth muscle, which promotes shortened transit times. Diarrhea, cramps, and reflux of bile have been noted with PO administration of PGEs. Exogenous PGE_2 causes a dose-related suppression of basal gastric acid secretion. PGI_2 also is a potent inhibitor of gastric acid secretion, but $PGF_{2\alpha}$ has no effect (see Table 9–1). The usefulness of these antisecretory effects is limited by the large doses required, which produce cardiovascular side-effects, abdominal cramping, and diarrhea.[14]

Several other effects of the prostaglandins have been noted, including stimulation of the release of ACTH by PGE_1 and $PGF_{2\alpha}$ and enhanced release of growth hormone by PGEs. Various effects of PGEs on lipolysis have also been described.[32]

The effects of the prostaglandins reported to date have largely been observed in adult human and animal studies, and their relevance in the infant remains to be explored.

PGE_1, PGE_2, and PGI_2

Clinical Pharmacology. Insights gained by basic research on the prostaglandins have afforded the opportunity to explore their use in the management of several circulatory disorders affecting neonates. Elliott and coworkers[11] and Christensen and Fabricus[7] demonstrated a clinical improvement during PGE_1 infusion in neonates in whom patency of the ductus arteriosus was necessary to maintain arterial oxygen saturation. These early reports were followed by efforts to explore the value of PGEs in a variety of congenital heart lesions. Neutz and colleagues[35] observed improvement in 10 of 11 infants; these authors noted the potential value of pulmonary vasodilating effects of PGEs in clinical situations where relatively high pulmonary flow is necessary for optimal intracardiac mixing, such as in transposition of the great vessels. Lewis and coworkers[27] administered PGE_1 by the IV route in half the patients and by the intra-aortic route in the remainder. This was the first effort to clarify the relation between route of administration and physiologic effects. This study and others[19] established that intra-aortic and IV routes of prostaglandin administration produce the same effects. Heyman and coworkers[19] noted that in infants with aortic arch abnormalities, failure of PGE_1 therapy was associated with preexisting closure of the ductus arteriosus. The importance of the pulmonary vasodilating effect of PGE_1 in the management of transposition of the great arteries was demonstrated in a study of ten newborn infants by Benson and colleagues.[2]

A collaborative study involving 492 infants examined the effect of PGE_1 infusion of infants with cyanotic congenital heart disease as well as in those with reduced systemic blood flow due to coarctation of the aorta (juxtaductal), interrupted aortic arch, hypoplastic left-heart syndrome, and various other lesions.[13] PGE_1 doses employed ranged from 0.002 to 0.5 μg/kg/min, with the majority of patients receiving 0.1 μg/kg/min. In infants with cyanotic congenital heart disease, significant improvements in PaO_2 occurred; these effects could be correlated with age at time of initiation of the infusion and with pre-infusion PaO_2 values (Fig. 9–3). There was no correlation found between the response in PaO_2 and route of administration, gender, maternal age, or $PaCO_2$. PGE_1 therapy produced improvement in 19 out of 25 acyanotic infants with interruption of the aortic arch and in 24 of 30 with juxtaductal coarctation of the aorta. When the ductus was observed to be closed during cardiac catheterization before the start

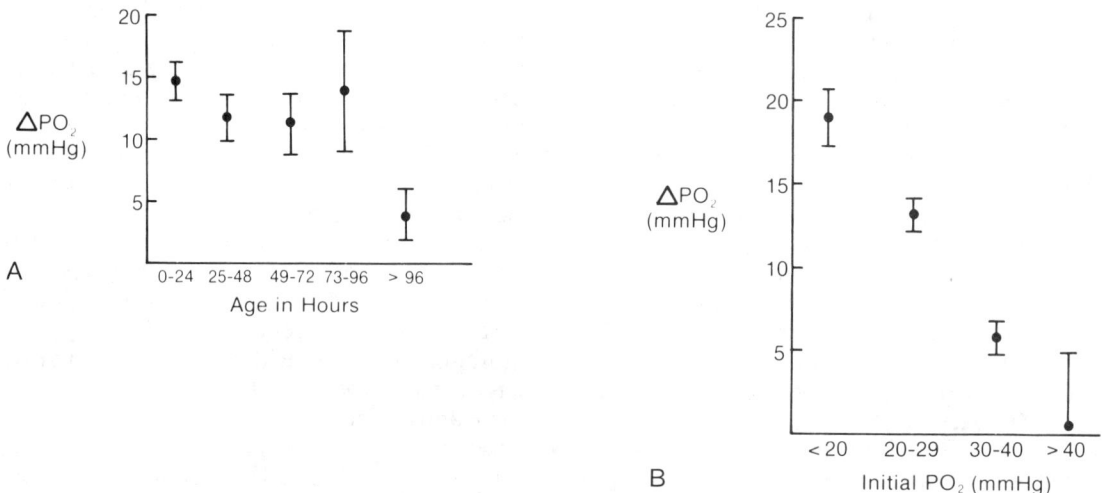

Figure 9–3. Changes in arterial oxygenation during infusion of PGE_1 in neonates with pulmonary stenosis or atresia or with tricuspid atresia. *A,* The influence of age at the start of infusion; *B,* the relationship of PaO_2 response to the initial PaO_2 before starting the PGE_1 infusion. The values are means ± SEM. (Adapted from Freed MD et al: Circulation 64:899, 1981.)

of PGE$_1$ infusion, reopening could not be accomplished regardless of age. The lack of response to PGE$_1$ in infants weighing more than 4 kg at birth was highly significant but could not be explained. Decreased response of the ductus arteriosus to PGE$_1$ infusion after 96 hours of age (Fig. 9–3) suggests either that anatomic closure is nearly complete by this time or that there is irreversible functional closure due to a lack of responsiveness of prostaglandin receptors. The improvement in infants with transposition was associated with an increase in obligatory shunt from the high-pressure aorta to the lower-pressure pulmonary artery, thus increasing the effective pulmonary flow and arterial saturation. The maximal improvement in PaO$_2$ in cyanotic infants occurred within 30 minutes, in contrast to 1.5 hours in acyanotic infants with interruption of the aortic arch or 3 hours with coarctation of the aorta. Continuing the infusion of PGE$_1$ for at least 3 hours in acyanotic infants is, therefore, necessary before deciding on its effectiveness.

Oral PGE$_2$ has been employed in ductus-dependent heart disease in neonates. Silove and coworkers[45] treated various lesions in 12 infants (9 with pulmonary atresia, 2 with tricuspid atresia, and 1 with transposition of the great arteries) with 12 to 65 μg/kg of PGE$_2$ given PO. The initial dosing interval was 1 hour; this was increased to up to 4 hours. Therapy was continued for as long as 130 days in some infants. Within 15 minutes of an oral dose, the mean plasma concentration of PGE$_2$ was 77 pg/ml and reached a maximum mean value of 130 pg/ml between 45 and 60 minutes. A mean plasma PGE$_2$ concentration of 95 pg/ml was obtained with constant IV infusion at 0.002 to 0.006 μg/kg/min. During the first few weeks of PO therapy, acceptable PGE$_2$ plasma levels could not be maintained and clinical deterioration occurred with dosing intervals longer than every 2 hours. In eight infants whose condition had been stable for a period of 1 to 10 weeks on IV or PO PGE$_2$ therapy, arterial oxygen saturations decreased between 2 and 5 hours after the last dose given (75 ± 7% to 57 ± 10% saturation). Reinstitution of PO therapy restabilized the oxygen saturation within 1 hour, but delay of reinstitution of therapy beyond 2 hours required several hourly doses before full recovery occurred.

Prostacyclin (PGI$_2$) was first reported useful in the treatment of pulmonary vasoconstriction in the newborn by Lock and colleagues.[29] Bolus doses of 0.3 to 0.5 μg/kg administered IV every 10 to 15 minutes resulted in improvement in arterial oxygenation. Tolerance did not occur, nor did systemic hypotension or metabolic alkalosis. A continuous infusion of 0.07 μg/kg/min was subsequently utilized with maintenance of satisfactory PaO$_2$ (Table 9–2). Rubin and coworkers[43] employed PGI$_2$ for treatment of primary pulmonary hypertension in 7 adult patients; doses of 0.002 to 0.012 μg/kg/min (mean 0.0057 μg/kg/min) increased cardiac output and reduced pulmonary artery pressure and resistance. These hemodynamic effects persisted during a continuous 24- to 48-hour infusion.

Murphy and colleagues[34] observed no therapeutic benefit following PGE$_1$ administration in four of five neonates critically ill with persistent fetal circulation. PGE$_1$ was infused into the pulmonary artery at a dose of 0.1 to 0.4 μg/kg/min. One infant demonstrated a rise in PaO$_2$ that lasted less than 48 hours despite continuous infusion.

Therapeutic Indications. PGE$_1$ is used to *maintain blood flow through the ductus arteriosus* when this is essential for sustaining either pulmonary or systemic circulation (Table 9–3). Among these conditions, obstructive right heart lesions are most commonly treated with PGE$_1$.[10] In general, PGE$_1$ infusion should follow diagnosis based on invasive or noninvasive techniques (echocardiography, cardiac catheterization, and cineangiography). However, the demonstrated beneficial effects and reasonable safety justify the initiation of PGE$_1$ therapy in life-threatening situations where dependency on ductal patency is suspected on clinical grounds.[20,161]

The recommended initial dose of PGE$_1$ is 0.05 μg/kg/min given IV (Table 9–4). There is no difference in response between intra-arterial and IV routes of administration.[13] In general, neonates with cyanotic heart disease responsive to PGE$_1$ will show improvement within 30 minutes. Response in neonates with acyanotic heart disease is more delayed; as long as 11 hours may be required before maximum response is observed. Once the maximum or desired response to PGE$_1$ has been obtained, the rate of infusion should be reduced to deliver the minimal dose necessary. One half or less of the initial effective dose is usually required for maintenance of the desired effect (Table 9–4).

Olley and Coceani[38] support the use of PGE$_1$ in delineating the pulmonary arterial anatomy prior to surgical systemic-to-pulmonary arterial anastomosis. Following such surgery, intractable pulmonary edema and death can ensue if obstructive total anomalous pulmonary venous

Table 9–2. SUMMARY OF CLINICAL STUDIES OF PGE$_1$, PGE$_2$, AND PGI$_2$ IN NEONATES

Authors of Published Study[a]	Study Group		Treatment	Clinical Response
	No. of Infants[b]	Diagnosis[c]		
Elliott et al[11]	2	1: PA 1: TGA	PGE$_1$: 0.1 μg/kg/min IV	increased PaO$_2$
Christensen and Fabricus[7]	1 (4 day)	PA	PGE$_1$: 0.1 μg/kg/min IV	improved
Neutze et al[35]	11 (1–99 days)	4: TGA 4: PA 2: PS 1: EA	PGE$_1$, PGE$_2$: 0.1–0.75 μg/kg/min IV	10/11: improvement in O$_2$ saturation (PA + TGA: no response)
Lang et al[25]	1 (17 days)	IAA	PGE$_1$: 0.1 μg/kg/min (via main pulmonary artery)	improved
Heyman and Rudolph[18]	10 full-term (<3 days)	PA	PGE$_1$: 0.05–0.1 μg/kg/min (via thoracic aorta)	10/10: improved PaO$_2$
Lewis et al[27]	12 (1 day–9 wk)	3: PA 2: TF 2: TA 3: CA 1: complex	PGE$_1$: 0.1 μg/kg/min (intra-aortic or IV)	9/12: improved PaO$_2$ (all 3 treatment failures > 10 days old)
Olley et al[36] Lang et al[26]	5 (<5 days)	D-transposition	PGE$_1$: 0.002–0.1 μg/kg/min (arterial or IV)	3/5 improved
Heymann et al[19]	15 full-term (1–150 days)	IAA CA	PGE$_1$: 0.025–0.1 μg/kg/min (via thoracic aorta, pulmonary artery, or IV)	13/15 improved
Murphy et al[34]	5 newborns	PPH	PGE$_1$: 0.1–0.4 μg/kg/min (via pulmonary artery)	1/5 improved transiently with increase in PaO$_2$; 5/5 died
Pitlick et al[163]	2 newborns (12 hr, 16 days)	1:TF 1:TGA	PGE$_1$: 0.05–0.1 μg/kg IV initial; maintenance dose 0.004–0.01 μg/kg/min	increase in PaO$_2$ sustained until surgical shunt procedure (24 days and 4.5 months, respectively)
Freed et al[13]	492 (1 day–5 mo)	125: PA + VSD 106: PA 47: PS 23: TA 21: TGA 46: CA 34: IAA 19: HLH	PGE$_1$: 0.002–0.5 μg/kg/min (intra-arterial or IV)	cyanotic population: significant increase in PaO$_2$: greatest response if <96 hr old, improvement inversely related to initial PaO$_2$ acyanotic population: IAA: 19/25 improved CA: 24/30 improved
Silove et al[45]	12 (1–60 days)	9: PA 2: TA 1: TGA	PGE$_2$: 12–65 μg/kg PO q 1–4 hr	12/12 improved and were maintained for 5 days–4 mo on oral PGE$_2$
Coe et al[159]	1 (newborn)	TA	PGE$_2$: 25 μg/kg PO q 1 to 3 hr	marked clinical improvement, maintained on PO therapy for 8 months
Lock et al[29]	1 (newborn)	PPH	PGI$_2$: 0.26–0.5 μg/kg bolus IV q 10–15 min, then 0.01–0.07 μg/kg/min IV infusion	pulmonary pressure reduced without systemic hypotension, PaO$_2$ improved

[a] Listed in order of publication; see References at end of chapter.

[b] If available, age at time of study is given in parentheses.

[c] PA, pulmonary atresia; TGA, transposition of the great arteries; PS, pulmonary stenosis; EA, Ebstein's anomaly; IAA, interrupted aortic arch; TF, tetralogy of Fallot; TA, tricuspid atresia; CA, coarctation of aorta; PPH, persistent pulmonary hypertension; VSD, ventricular septal defect; HLH, hypoplastic left heart.

Table 9 – 3. NEONATAL CONGENITAL HEART DISEASE POTENTIALLY RESPONSIVE TO PGE₁ THERAPY

Ductus-dependent pulmonary blood flow
  pulmonary atresia (with or without intact interventricular system)
  severe tetralogy of Fallot
  critical pulmonary stenosis
  tricuspid atresia

ductus-dependent systemic blood flow
  aortic arch interruption
  juxtaductal coarctation of the aorta
  hypoplastic left heart syndrome[a]

transposition of the great arteries

tricuspid valve anomalies
  tricuspid insufficiency
  Ebstein's anomaly

[a] Judicious use of PGE₁ therapy precludes employment in noncorrectable, terminal heart lesions.

Table 9 – 4. RECOMMENDED PROTOCOL FOR USE OF PGE₁ IN NEONATES

Patient Selection Criteria (A or B)
A. Treatable heart lesion diagnosed by cardiac catheterization (Table 9 – 3).
B. Clinical diagnosis of treatable cyanotic and acyanotic lesions (Table 9 – 3); prior to initiation of PGE₁ therapy; document in neonates with *cyanosis:*
    right radial arterial blood gas values following hyperoxic challenge test (20-minute exposure to FiO₂ of 1.0): Positive test is $PaO_2 < 50 - 60$ torr; $PaCO_2 < 40$ torr.
    chest film findings: decreased pulmonary vascularity with otherwise normal lung parenchyma.
    laboratory values: normal blood glucose, hematocrit <60%.

Therapeutic Regimen
Dissolve 500 μg of PGE₁ in 500 ml of 5% dextrose in water (1 μg/ml) (solution stable for 24 hr).
initial dose
  0.05 μg/kg/min given IV[a] (3 ml/kg/hr of 1 μg/ml concentration)
  maximal effect:
    cyanotic lesions <30 min
    acyanotic average <3 hr
  dosage: >0.1 μg/kg/min is rarely more effective and causes serious adverse reactions
maintenance dose
  Once stable improvement achieved, adequate response can be maintained with one half or less of the initial effective dose (as low as 0.002 μg/kg/min). Original infusion solution (1 μg/ml) may need to be diluted to accurately deliver the lower maintenance doses.

[a] The IV route of administration is preferred, although therapy has been effective with intra-arterial infusions. The duration of PGE₁ effect is short (1 – 2 hr after stopping the constant infusion). Therefore, precautions should be taken to ensure reliable IV access for continuous uninterrupted infusion of PGE₁.

return exists. Neonates in whom this anatomic arrangement is suspected may be "challenged" by an infusion of PGE₁; a resulting increase in pulmonary blood flow via the ductus arteriosus, with consequent clinical and radiographic deterioration (pulmonary edema), will identify patients with the abnormality, so that nonbeneficial surgical intervention can be avoided. The use of prostaglandins for *treatment of pulmonary disease* is experimental.[22]

The use of the prostaglandins requires appreciation of their chemical instability. PGE₁ appears to be stable for periods of 24 hours in dextrose solution (5% in water). PGI₂ is extremely labile in aqueous medium at physiologic pH and must be kept in ice until administration. Some of this instability can be overcome by dissolving the PGI₂ in a glycine buffer at pH 10.4.[38] Administration of this solution at a rate of 0.05 ml/min will not induce alkalosis in the infant. The clinical use of PGI₂ is experimental,[21] and commercial preparations are not available.

Clinical Toxicology. The reported side-effects of PGE₁ are summarized in Table 9 – 5. The information on toxicity was gathered in a collaborative study involving case reports of 492 infants with critical congenital cardiac disease treated with PGE₁.[28] Approximately 20% of infants were determined to have intercurrent medical events related to PGE₁ therapy. Cardiovascular abnormalities were the most common (18% incidence), with cutaneous vasodilation and edema occurring more frequently during intra-aortic infusion than during IV infusion. Respiratory depression or apnea was particularly common in infants weighing less than 2 kg. The etiology of the respiratory depression is believed to be related to the action of PGE₁ on the CNS. This side-effect reinforces the importance of the use of PGE₁ in a clinical environment where assisted ventilation is immediately available. The relationship between infection and PGE₁ therapy remains controversial. The majority of the side-effects appear comparatively minor relative to the clinical status of the neonates.

Prolonged PGE₁ infusion has been associated with evidence of morphologic disruption in the ductal and juxtaductal structures.[160] The histologic findings and intraoperative experience indicate the risk of spontaneous or surgically related rupture of the ductus arteriosus after prolonged infusion of PGE₁.

Ueda and coworkers[51] reported cortical hyperostosis following long-term administration of PGE₁. In their series, two full-term infants received PGE₁ (0.01 μg/kg/min) for periods in

Table 9–5. INCIDENCE OF SIDE-EFFECTS ASSOCIATED WITH USE OF PGE_1 IN NEONATES

Side-effect	Incidence (%)
cardiovascular	18
cutaneous vasodilation	
edema	
rhythm or conduction	
disturbance	
hypotension	
CNS	16
seizure-like activity	
temperature elevation	
irritability	
lethargy	
respiratory	12
apnea	
hypoventilation	
metabolic	2
hypoglycemia	
hypocalcemia	
infections	2
gastrointestinal	2
diarrhea	
necrotizing enterocolitis (rare)	
hyperbilirubinemia (rare)	
hematologic	2
hemorrhage	
disseminated intravascular	
coagulation (DIC)	
thrombocytopenia	
renal failure or insufficiency	2

Adapted from Lewis AB et al: Circulation 64:893, 1981.

excess of 3 months. Radiographs demonstrated bone lesions resembling infantile cortical hyperostosis. Improvement occurred on cessation of PGE_1 therapy. Subtle roentgenographic signs of periostitis with irregular and asymmetric distribution have been observed in neonates infused with PGE_1 for periods ranging from 9 to 205 hours.[164] Prostaglandin-induced periostitis appears to be a benign, self-limited process with no effect on subsequent bone growth and development.

PROSTAGLANDIN INHIBITORS: INDOMETHACIN

The use of indomethacin for closure of the ductus arteriosus is an outgrowth of understanding of the basic physiology of the ductus arteriosus.[56] Closure of the ductus after birth is believed to occur in two stages:[63] The initial stage is represented by functional closure brought about by contraction of the smooth muscle in the ductal wall. This is followed by permanent closure produced by destruction of the endothelium, proliferation of subintimal layers, connective tissue formation, and eventual obliteration of the lumen.[46]

Understanding the role of the prostaglandins in patency of the ductus arteriosus is fundamental to the understanding of the actions of indomethacin. Recent investigations have concluded that the patency of the ductus arteriosus in the fetus is not a passive condition established by hemodynamic factors but is instead an active process sustained by prostaglandins.[64] Figure 9–4 summarizes the factors operating to maintain ductal patency. PGE_2 and PGI_2 are the prostaglandins thought to be important in this regard. Although PGI_2 appears to be produced in greater amounts than PGE_2 by the ductus arteriosus itself, the vasodilating actions of PGE_2 are greater than those of PGI_2.[63] Circulating levels of PGE_2 may also participate in maintenance of the ductus arteriosus in a dilated state during normal fetal life. In addition, there is a gestational age dependency in the response of the ductus arteriosus to PGE_2 and PGI_2. The most active response of the ductus arteriosus to the prostaglandins occurs at about 24 to 28 weeks of gestation and abates thereafter.[64]

Figure 9–4 also shows the factors known to initiate ductal closure after birth. The triggering mechanism is the increase in oxygen tension that occurs with breathing and a simultaneous decrease in pulmonary artery pressure associated with the increase in vascular perfusion of the lung. This increase in lung perfusion provides the opportunity for increased catabolism of circulating prostaglandins by the lung. In addition, there is evidence that the increased oxygen tension diminishes the response of the ductus arteriosus to PGE_2's dilating action.[64] Oxygen tension, therefore, is obviously a key component because of its direct constricting activity as well as its role in reducing the response of the ductus to circulating and locally produced prostaglandins. Circulating PGE_2 and $PGF_{2\alpha}$ levels, although elevated in infants compared with adults, are no different in infants with persistant patency of the ductus arteriosus compared with matched normal infants.[168,172] Additional details regarding the role of prostaglandins and closure of the ductus arteriosus can be found in recent reviews.[62–65]

Pharmacology. Indomethacin is an indole derivative that was synthesized specifically for anti-inflammatory effects. It is one of the most potent inhibitors of the cyclo-oxygenase pathway (see Fig. 9–1). The oral absorption of indomethacin has been reported to range from 10% to over 90%.[67,89] Indomethacin is unusually sus-

Ductus Arteriosus

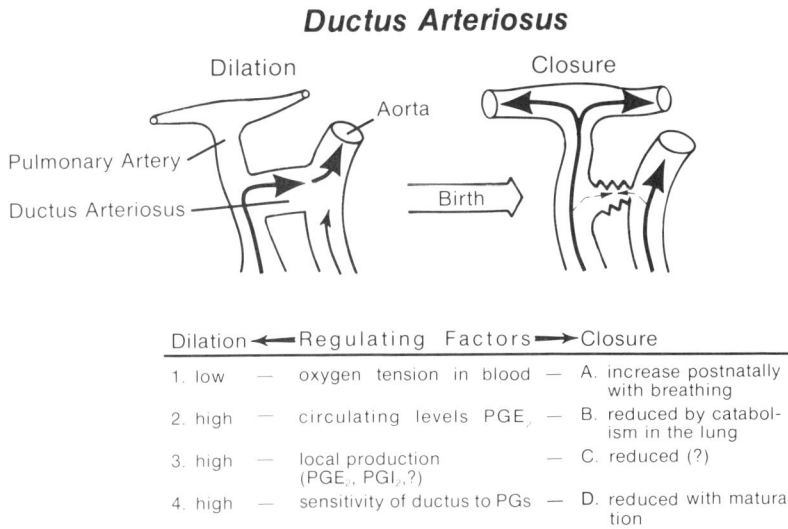

Figure 9-4. The major factors believed to determine the patency of the ductus arteriosus. Factors operating to maintain patency include low oxygen tensions in the blood (*1*); high circulating (*2*) and local (*3*) levels of PGE_2 and PGI_2; and high sensitivity of the ductus arteriosus to the dilating actions of PGE_2 and PGI_2 (*4*). Factors initiating closure following birth include an increase in oxygen tension (*A*), which directly triggers contraction of the ductus; subsequent reduction in the levels of circulating PGE_2 (*B*) as a consequence of catabolism by the lung, which is now being fully perfused by blood, as well as decreased local production of prostaglandins (*C*); and, with maturation, decreased sensitivity of the ductus arteriosus to the dilating actions of PGE_2 (*D*).

ceptible to chemical decomposition, particularly in alkaline solutions.[66] The lack of availability of commercial preparations suitable for use in neonates, coupled with the chemical instability in certain solutions, undoubtedly explains some if not all of the discrepancies in bioavailability data. Evans and coworkers[67] administered indomethacin PO as a suspension in saline and reported very low bioavailabilities (10 to 20%). In contrast, Alpert and colleagues[54] administered indomethacin PO dissolved in 0.2 M phosphate buffer, pH 7.2, and observed it to be well absorbed. Seyberth et al.[173] dissolved a lyophilized preparation of indomethacin in 0.9% NaCl solution just prior to IM injection. According to the authors, therapeutic levels were achieved, and the variability of indomethacin bioavailability was reduced by IM administration. Very careful attention to the stability of indomethacin solutions is of the utmost importance in both investigative and therapeutic use (see under Therapeutic Indications).

Peak plasma concentrations are observed within 1 to 3 hours after PO administration in neonates. Because indomethacin is highly protein-bound (95%), its use has been considered to be contraindicated in neonates with bilirubin levels greater than 10 mg/dl. However, no displacement of bilirubin from albumin occurs at usual therapeutic drug levels.[96,100,169] Therefore, jaundice should not be considered a contra-

indication for the use of indomethacin. Plasma levels of 10 to 40 μg/ml of indomethacin, achievable with a 2 mg/kg dose (10 times the recommended dose), have been shown to significantly reduce bilirubin binding to albumin.[100]

Indomethacin has been shown to undergo *O*-desmethylation and *N*-deacylation as well as conjugation with glucuronic acid in adults.[78] About 60% of a PO dose is excreted in the urine as a glucuronide derivative; the remainder is excreted in the feces following biliary secretion. A large portion of this dose may undergo biliary recirculation. Although variability in hepatic drug metabolism or renal excretion could be a major contributing factor to the observed pharmacokinetic differences among neonates (Table 9-6), enterohepatic recirculation could also be a major mechanism. Kwan and coworkers[81] found that an average of 50% of an IV, PO, or rectal dose of indomethacin undergoes such circulation. Serum concentration time curves for adult patients with severely impaired renal function are no different from those for patients with normal renal function.[101] Decreased renal excretion of the drug appears to be paralleled by a corresponding increase in the fecal excretion rate of indomethacin and its metabolites. Severe liver disease may alter the metabolism of indomethacin, and therefore its rate of elimination, and may diminish plasma

Table 9–6. SUMMARY OF CLINICAL INDOMETHACIN STUDIES IN NEONATES

Author(s) of Published Study[a]	Study Group[b]	Dose Employed	Peak Plasma Concentration (μg/ml)	T½ (hr)	Clinical Response: Closure of PDA (% of Patients) Initial	Final	Other Data[c]
Friedman et al[70]	6 prematures (29–36 wk)	2.5–5.0 mg/kg rectally or PO			100	100	
Neal et al[77]	11 prematures (27–33 wk)	0.26–1.1 mg/kg PO			88	18	
Friedman et al[72]	4 prematures (26–30 wk)	0.2–0.3 mg/kg PO	0.07–0.4	21–24		85	
McCarthy et al[84]	18 prematures (27–36 wk)	0.1–0.3 mg/kg PO (×1–3)				44	age-related response (>33 wk: poor or no response)
Merritt et al[86]	65 prematures (28–30 wk mean)	0.2 mg/kg PO or IV			85	80	mortality: 11.1% in indomethacin group vs. 6.5% in surgical ligation group (NS)
Heymann[79]	60 prematures (24–35 wk)	0.2 mg/kg PO q 8–12 hr (×3 max.)			65	50	
Alpert et al[54]	50 prematures (32–33 wk mean)	0.1–0.3 mg/kg PO or rectally q 8–12 hr (×3 max.)	0.72 (0.1 mg/kg) 1.01 (0.2 mg/kg)			44	
Bhat et al[55]	9 prematures (28–34 wk)	0.1–0.3 mg/kg PO q 8 hr	0.08 (range 0.03–0.3)	mean 16 (range 11–20) <1.5 kg: 19 >1.5 kg: 13		67	98% protein binding
Cifuentes et al[61]	12 prematures (27–35 wk)	0.1 mg/kg PO or rectally q 8 hr (×2)				50	decrease in urine volume, GFR, Na, Cl, K excretion
Halliday et al[76]	36 prematures (25–32 wk)	0.2–0.9 mg/kg PO or rectally total dose (1–3 doses q 8 hr)				67	
Bianchetti et al[57]	6 prematures (28–34 wk)	0.2 mg/kg PO or rectally q 24 hr (×3 max.)	0.4–1.6 (3rd dose)	30–90 (mean 40 ±12)		66	$V_d = 0.6–1.5$ l/kg $Cl = 0.076–0.335$ ml/min/kg
Nestrud et al[93]	15 prematures (28 ± 2 wk)	0.2 mg/kg PO q 12 hr (×3 max.)	0.1–3.1	1–>24	58 (placebo: 18)		double-blind control trial
Obeyesekere et al[95]	16 prematures (24–28 wk)	0.3 mg/kg PO q 24 hr (×3 max.)				56	
Procianoy et al[97]	15 prematures (28 ± 2 wk)	0.1 mg/kg PO q 8 hr (×?)				60	study of retinopathy

Reference	Patients	Dose	Plasma level	Half-life (hr)			Comments
Thalji et al[102]	17 prematures (31 ± 2 wk)	0.3 mg/kg IV q 24 hr (×3 max.)	1.16 ± 0.37	<1 wk old: 27.6 ± 8.3 >1 wk old: 18.5 ± 6.8	94	60	possible enterohepatic reentry effect on pharmacokinetics: $V_d = 0.35$ l/kg; $Cl = 13 \pm 9.5$ ml/kg/hr
Vert et al[103]	18 prematures (mean 29 wk)	PO or rectally: 0.2 mg/kg q 24 hr (×3 max.); IV: 0.2 mg/kg q 24 hr (×3 max.)	0.69 ± 0.39; 2.27 ± 0.79	40 ± 12; 34 ± 12		57; 82	$V_d = 0.35–0.88$ l/kg; $Cl = 0.13–0.25$ mg/kg/hr
Yaffe et al[104]	37 prematures	0.2 mg/kg IV q 12 hr (×3 max.)	0.8 (1st dose)	12–21 (mean 17.3 ± 2.8)			study of birth weight, age, and sex vs. $T_{1/2}$
Brash et al[58]	35 prematures (26–34 wk)	0.2 mg/kg IV (repeat if nec. after 24 hr)	0.24–1.10 (6-hr level)	32 (median)	90	86	plasma indomethacin level vs. ductal response
Evans et al[67]	18 neonates (28–40 wk)	PO: 0.1–0.3 mg/kg q 12 hr ×3; IV: 0.2 mg/kg q 12 hr ×3	0.05–0.07	12–20 (range)		66	$Cl = 7$ ml/kg/hr oral bioavailability: 10–20% (see text)
			1st dose: 1–2; 3rd dose: 4	10–25 (range)		78	$V_d = 0.36$ l/kg; $Cl = 10–25$ ml/kg/hr
Merritt et al[87]	24 neonates (<1.35 kg)	0.2 mg/kg IV q 24 hr (×3 max.)				early intervention: 83; late intervention: 85	
Petersen et al[96]	6 prematures (29–34 wk)	0.2 mg/kg IV q 24 hr (×3 max.)	1.3 ± 0.3	20 (range 9–50)		66	double-blind cross-over study
Neu et al[94]	15 prematures (29 wk)	0.25 mg/kg PO q 24 hr × 2				80	
Yanagi et al[105]	17 prematures (28–32 wk) 9: placebo 8: indomethacin	0.2 mg/kg PO q 24 hr (×3 max.)				75 (placebo: 44) (NS)	double-blind control study
	22 prematures (28–32 wk) 9: placebo 13: indomethacin	0.2 mg/kg PO q 8 hr (×3 max.)				85 (placebo: 11) ($p < .01$)	
Yeh et al[106]	27: placebo 28: Indo (30 ± 2 wk)	0.3 mg/kg IV q 24 hr (×3 max.)				89 (placebo: 22)	double-blind control trial
Friedman et al[69]	9 prematures (26–31 wk)	0.1 mg/kg PO, then 0.2 mg/kg q 12 hr, 0.3 mg/kg q 24 hr (max. 0.6 mg/kg)	responders: 0.93 ± 0.16 partial or nonresponders: 0.57 ± 0.08	19 ± 3.8 (range 14–24)	22	33	relationship between indo. plasma conc. and PDA closure

Table continued on following page

Table 9–6. SUMMARY OF CLINICAL INDOMETHACIN STUDIES IN NEONATES *(Continued)*

Author(s) of Published Study[a]	Study Group[b]	Dose Employed	Peak Plasma Concentration (μg/ml)	T½ (hr)	Clinical Response: Closure of PDA (% of Patients) Initial	Final	Other Data[c]
Harris et al[77]	67 prematures (29 wk)	0.2 mg/kg IV q 24 hr (×3 max.)			92	91	incidence of intraventricular hemorrhage, RLF, necrotizing enterocolitis unchanged; BPD reduced
Lindemann et al[82]	16 prematures (25–35 wk)	0.1–1.2 mg/kg PO or IV q 12 hr (×3 max.)				31	3/16 developed RLF
Mahony et al[83]	47 neonates (<1.7 kg)	0.2 mg/kg IV, then 0.1 mg 12 hr and 36 hr later				>1 kg: 82 (control: 79) <1 kg: 100 (control: 33)	randomized placebo-controlled, early prophylactic therapy
Mrongovius et al[89]	15 prematures (27–32 wk)	IV: 0.2 mg/kg q 12 hr (×3 max.) PO: 0.2 mg/kg q 12 hr (×3 max.)	1st, 2nd, 3rd dose: 0.6, 1.06, 1.33 0.8, 1.26, 1.57		100 86	30 57	bioavailability study: IV versus PO
Mullett et al[90]	47 neonates (<1.75 kg)	0.2 mg/kg PO q 24 hr ×2				57 (control: 17)	controlled, blinded placebo study
Seyberth et al[99]	8 prematures (25–35 wk)	0.2 mg/kg IV q 12 hr (×3 max.)	1.08 ± 0.12	28 (range 15–52)	100	62	controlled study of PG plasma levels and excretion

Reference	Patients	Dose	Plasma levels/V_d				Comments
Gersony et al[74]	405 neonates (<1.75 kg)	0.2 mg/kg IV, then 0.1–0.2 mg/kg q 12 hr (×2)	2 hr (1 dose): 0.61 ± 0.22 12 hr (1 dose): 0.43 ± 0.20 14 hr (2 doses): 1.04 ± 0.47		79 (placebo: 28)	79 (placebo: 35)	multicenter double-blind controlled, placebo study
Mehta and Calvert[85]	5 prematures (26–30 wk)	0.14–0.24 mg/kg IV	0.63–0.23	30 ± 14 (range 18–51)			
Kääpä et al[80]	37 prematures (33 ± 3 wk)	0.2 mg/kg PO, repeat at 24 hr if nec.			(27% early spontaneous closure) 54 (control: 30)	92 (control: 50)	study of effects of early closure of PDA
Seyberth et al[173]	11 treated (30 ± 2 wk) 9 control (33 ± 2 wk)	0.2 mg/kg IM then 0.1 to 0.4 mg/kg IM q 12 to 24 hr for 7 days	days 1–5: 0.47–1.52 µg/ml day 7: 0.14–0.77 µ/ml				37% decrease in creatinine clearance. No progressive deterioration in renal function during therapy
Yeh et al[178]	22 (26–35 wk)	0.3 mg/kg IV q 24 hr as required for PDA	<1 kg 0.97 ± 0.31 µg/ml >1 kg 1.31 ± 0.18 µg/ml		<1 kg 20 >1 kg 75	80 100	<1 kg infants received 2 ± 0.6 doses; >1 kg infants 1.2 ± 0.4 doses
Rudd et al[171]	30 (29 ± 1 wk)	0.2 mg/kg PO daily ×3 if required for PDA			87 placebo 20	47 13	

a Listed in order of publication; see References at end of chapter.
b If available, mean or range values for gestational age or birth weight are given in parentheses.
c V_d = volume of distribution; Cl = clearance; NS = not statistically significant.

protein, which may also affect disposition of the highly protein-bound drug.[78] Very little work has been published on indomethacin metabolism and excretion in neonates.[88] Analysis of urine in four infants revealed less than 1% of the dose of indomethacin recovered by 12 hours.[69]

The metabolites of indomethacin are inactive as inhibitors of the prostaglandin-forming cyclo-oxygenase enzyme. The effects of indomethacin on prostaglandin synthesis are nonspecific, diminishing the production of all of the prostaglandins (see Fig. 9–1); this decrease will occur in all tissues where indomethacin achieves inhibitory levels. Elevated plasma prostaglandin levels noted in preterm neonates with PDA showed a significant decline following indomethacin-induced PDA closure.[30] Seyberth and colleagues[99] have demonstrated a reduction in the renal excretion of PGE-M, a product of PGE_2 metabolism, following indomethacin therapy in premature infants with PDA; the decrease in PGE-M levels presumably reflects the diminished PGE_2 synthesis subsequent to indomethacin inhibition of cyclo-oxygenase.

Besides the anti-inflammatory and ductus arteriosus-related effects associated with indomethacin-induced inhibition of prostaglandin synthesis, cardiovascular effects of indomethacin have been demonstrated (see additional discussion in Clinical Toxicology section). Indomethacin can increase pulmonary vascular resistance in newborn animals by diminishing the presence of prostaglandin-related vasodilator influences.[170,174] Indomethacin has been shown to inhibit the pulmonary vasodilating effects of oxygen in newborn pigs[53] and to augment the increase in pulmonary vascular resistance induced by alveolar hypoxia.[174] Reduction in blood flow to the brain but not to the gastrointestinal tract or kidneys has been observed in newborn dogs.[167] However, a decrease in blood flow to the gastrointestinal tract has been observed in adult dogs,[73] and a decrease in renal blood flow has been reported in newborn lambs following indomethacin administration.[175] Similar studies of cardiovascular effects of indomethacin in human infants have not been reported.

Clinical Pharmacology. Indomethacin has been the subject of numerous clinical studies in neonates, many of which are summarized in Table 9–6. Since the early report by Friedman and coworkers,[70] various efforts have been made to describe the pharmacokinetics and pharmacodynamics of indomethacin in infants with patent ductus arteriosus (PDA). The most

frequently employed dose (0.2 mg/kg) when given IV produces peak plasma concentrations of around 1 μg/ml, although reported individual variations have been striking. The plasma levels resulting from PO or rectal dosing have in general been lower than those following dosing by the IV route. As mentioned previously, the chemical instability of indomethacin may in part explain its apparent poor bioavailability. Bioavailability studies by Mrongovius and colleagues[89] demonstrated equivalent plasma levels for both the IV and PO routes of administration (Table 9–6).

The plasma half-life values show considerable variability, ranging from a few up to 90 hours (Table 9–6). The most frequently reported half-life is between 15 and 30 hours. As noted by Thalji and coworkers,[102] enterohepatic recirculation of indomethacin can cause the calculated half-life of elimination to be longer than it would be if renal and biliary excretion were not complicated by intestinal reabsorption. Accordingly, individual differences in rate of absorption from the gastrointestinal tract, drug metabolism, rate of renal and biliary excretion, and reentry of drug into the circulation by enterohepatic recirculation will all contribute to the variability in half-life.

The mass of data collected on the effect of indomethacin on ductal patency clearly illustrates its effectiveness (Table 9–6). Neonates of less than 30 weeks' gestational age appear to be most responsive to indomethacin therapy.[74] Differences in response related to body weight have also been reported: Infants weighing less than 1 kg respond significantly to indomethacin therapy; spontaneous closure reduces the significance of indomethacin-induced closure in infants weighing more than 1 kg.[83] Yeh and coauthors[178] found that infants <1 kg required repeated doses of indomethacin compared with infants >1 kg for closure of the ductus. The importance of double-blind controlled studies has been illustrated by Yanagi,[105] Yeh,[106] Mahony,[83] Mullet,[90] Gersony,[74] Kääpä,[80] and Rudd[171] and their respective coworkers; in these studies, 17% to 79% of patients in placebo groups had spontaneous ductal closure (Table 9–6). There are conflicting observations on the incidence of recurrence of ductal patency after indomethacin therapy. Brash and colleagues[58] found a greater recurrence in infants of over 30 weeks' gestation at birth, while Rudd and associates[171] could not identify any factor contributing to relapse. The plasma concentrations associated with ductal closure have ranged from 0.25 μg/ml to more than 0.6 μg/ml.[69] Seyberth and coworkers[173] proposed prolonged indomethacin therapy for prevention of relapse of ductal patency. Indomethacin therapy consisted of an initial dose of 0.2 mg/kg IM, with subsequent doses of 0.1 to 0.4 mg/kg repeated every 12 to 24 hours for 7 days. Dosing was adjusted to maintain plasma levels of 0.5 to 1.5 μg/ml for the first 2 days and 0.15 to 0.75 μg/ml for the remainder of the 7-day therapy period. Other studies suggest that the plasma concentration time interval (area under the curve, AUC) demonstrates a better correlation with closure of the ductus than plasma drug levels alone.[58,102,103]

There is some evidence that the rate of elimination of indomethacin is inversely related to postnatal age.[58,102,103,178] Vert and coworkers[103] reported a significant correlation coefficient between gestational age and indomethacin half-life. However, variability in pharmacokinetics makes it impractical to apply these average values ($T\frac{1}{2}$, Cl) in the treatment of individual infants.

Therapeutic Indications. The major therapeutic indication for indomethacin in neonates is for *closure of PDA.* Indomethacin should not be used to the exclusion of other medical management modalities. The effectiveness of indomethacin is variable, as can be appreciated by examination of Table 9–6; the greatest success can be expected in low-birth-weight infants (<1.5 kg). Data from a large multicenter study indicate that the highest final closure rates occur in infants who are older than 5 days of life when treatment is given.[74] However, the findings did not support other reports that birth weight, gestational age, or age at administration significantly modifies the efficacy of indomethacin for ductal closure. Indomethacin has been employed on a prophylactic basis in premature infants, but this use should be considered experimental.[83]

Of the variety of initial doses employed, the most common has been 0.2 to 0.3 mg/kg given PO or IV. Subsequent doses have generally been given at 8- to 24-hour intervals if evidence of ductal patency persists. The maximum total dosage used in a course of therapy has usually been 0.7 mg/kg or less. Studies employing these dosages have consistently reported decreases in renal function, although these were generally transient and reversible. As mentioned under Clinical Pharmacology, adequate blood levels of indomethacin as reflected in both concentration and duration (AUC values) will be a function of both individual dose and interval of dosing. Achievement of an adequate concentration as quickly as possible for closure of the ductus, while avoiding concentrations that will result in renal toxicity, should be the goal of therapy. Petersen and colleagues[96] have suggested an initial dose of 0.2 mg/kg, followed by a second dose as early as 6 hours if no evidence of clinical effect is observed. A third dose of 0.1 mg/kg 24 hours after the first dose is administered to those still having evidence of PDA. Other investigators, however, have suggested use of a 24-hour dosing interval in all patients;[58,89,102] the half-life of indomethacin as reported in neonates is most consistent with the 24-hour dosing interval, although Vert and colleagues[103] suggest a dosing interval of every 36 hours if more than one dose is needed.

A large multicenter study employed a dosage schedule of 3 doses at 12-hour intervals (IV administration), with the second and third doses based on postnatal age:[74] Infants less than 48 hours of age received 0.1 mg/kg as the second and third doses; infants 2 to 7 days old, 0.2 mg/kg; and infants aged 8 days and older, 0.25 mg/kg. All infants received 0.2 mg/kg as the initial dose.

The lack of a commercially available IV indomethacin preparation is a serious deficiency. Any formulation of indomethacin, whether for PO or IV administration, requires strict attention to the chemical instability of the molecule. Curry and coworkers[66] emphasized the importance of pH on indomethacin stability. A preparation stable for 24 hours can be prepared by adding indomethacin to 0.9% NaCl, followed by the addition of a sodium carbonate solution to achieve no more than a 7.5% molar excess of sodium carbonate in the indomethacin solution. The sodium carbonate must be added slowly to the indomethacin slurry to avoid the creation of an alkaline pH. Another stable parenteral preparation involves adding indomethacin to a 0.1 M sodium bicarbonate solution and adjusting the pH to 7.4 as quickly as possible with HCl. Seyberth and colleagues[173] dissolved a lyophilized sodium salt of indomethacin in 0.9% sodium chloride (1 mg/ml) to prepare an IM injection. Although stability studies were not done, the preparation was used immediately, and therapeutic plasma indomethacin levels were observed. A suspension for enteral administration can be prepared using polyethylene glycol (PEG-400).

As outlined by Brash and colleagues,[58] the optimal therapeutic approach involves measurement of the concentration of indomethacin in plasma during the 6- to 24-hour period after the initial dose. This measurement serves as a basis for determining the adequacy of the dose and the subsequent dose and dosing intervals. Such an approach to dosage determination was successfully employed by Seyberth and colleagues.[173] Data from the multicenter study[74] indicate very little change in indomethacin blood levels between 2 and 12 hours (0.6 and 0.4 μg/ml, respectively) after the initial dose (0.2 mg/kg IV); a second dose at 12 hours doubled the blood levels of indomethacin (1.0 μg/ml).

Dose Recommendation. The recommended dosage for indomethacin for ductal closure is based on the following: (1) a dose of 0.2 mg/kg results in serum indomethacin levels of approximately 0.4 to 0.6 mg/ml (Table 9–6), while a dose of 0.3 mg/kg results in a therapeutic serum level of 0.6 μg/ml.[69,178] Therefore, the initial recommended dose is 0.3 mg/kg given PO or IV. (2) Provided adequate serum levels are reached with this initial dose (>0.6 μg/ml), constriction of the ductus will develop at 6 to 24 hours after administration.[58] Subsequent dosing with indomethacin should be based on persistence of PDA and determination of plasma indomethacin levels, which should be maintained between 0.2 and 0.8 μg/ml;[173] therefore, a second dose (0.2 mg/kg) need not be given before 24 hours. A third dose of 0.2 mg/kg can be given if necessary 48 hours after the initial dose. (3) The half-life of indomethacin is in the range of 10 to 30 hours (Table 9–6); therefore to minimize toxic effects, the total dose of indomethacin in a 36-hour period should not exceed 0.6 mg/kg (Table 9–7). If the infant responds to the initial dose but develops a recurrence after 48 hours, a second course of therapy identical with the above can be employed. Prolonged indomethacin therapy for 7 days (initial dose 0.2 mg/kg IM, followed by maintenance doses of 0.1 to 0.4 mg/kg IM q 12 to 24 hours as determined from plasma indomethacin level determinations) has been successfully employed without exaggeration of renal dysfunction.[173] Further studies of this approach are indicated before it can be endorsed.

It is important to note that a target serum concentration of indomethacin that provides optimal closure of the ductus arteriosus with minimal risk of toxicity is difficult to determine for all neonates. Individual differences in hemodynamics, prostaglandin synthesis, and other factors influence the likelihood of ductal closure as well as the disposition of indomethacin. Accordingly, a more realistic approach than the achievement of a target serum drug concentration is the careful selection of dose and dosing

Table 9–7. RECOMMENDED DOSE OF INDOMETHACIN FOR CLOSURE OF THE DUCTUS ARTERIOSUS IN NEONATES[a]

Initial Dose:	0.3 mg/kg given PO or IV[b]
Subsequent Dose(s):	If ductal closure fails to develop by 24 hr, a dose of 0.2 mg/kg is given. A third dose of 0.2 mg/kg can be given 48 hr after the initial dose. Although repeated courses of therapy can be employed, the total dose should not exceed 0.6 mg/kg in any given 36-hr period.

[a] A wide variety of dosages have been employed (see Table 9–6). The dosage recommendation in this table is based on the best information available on expectations for time of ductal closure and indomethacin pharmacokinetics. Critical comparisons of indomethacin dosing recommendations in neonates remain to be accomplished.

[b] No suitable preparations are commercially available in the U.S. for enteral or parenteral administration of indomethacin to neonates. Formulations can be prepared from indomethacin tablets if care is exercised to avoid alkaline pH (see text).

interval for each patient, so that drug accumulation in the serum is avoided (Table 9–7).

Clinical Toxicology. The use of indomethacin has been associated with serious complications in neonates. Whether the drug is solely responsible for the various complications is unclear (Table 9–8). The most frequent adverse effect that is clearly due to indomethacin is renal dysfunction, as evidenced by the following: oliguria; increase in blood urea nitrogen; decreased urinary sodium, chloride, and potassium; and increased serum creatinine concentration associated with a fall in GFR.[61] These complications are dose-related (>0.2 mg/kg) and appear to be reversible. Friedman and Fitzpatrick[71] reviewed their clinical experience with indomethacin use in 35 pre-term infants. Although doses of 0.2 mg/kg given 3 times at minimum intervals of 24 hours did not change blood urea nitrogen, creatinine, or salt excretion, a mild transient decrease in urine output (never <1 ml/kg/hr) developed for a 24- to 48-hour period. Furosemide has been shown to prevent the reduction in urine output caused by indomethacin without altering the efficacy in closure of the ductus arteriosus.[107] Since there is no evidence of permanent renal injury following indomethacin therapy, the use of furosemide in combination is not recomended. Catteron and coworkers[60] proposed that decreased GFR is a reflection of decreased renal blood flow induced by indomethacin inhibition of prostaglandin synthesis. These authors also in-

Table 9-8. REPORTED TOXICITY OF INDOMETHACIN IN NEONATES

Toxic Effect	Reporting Authors[a]

renal
  oliguria
  decreased excretion of
    Na, Cl, K
  increased serum
    creatinine, blood
    urea nitrogen,
    decreased creatinine
    clearance, GFR
	Friedman et al,[70] Neal et al,[92]
	Cifuentes et al,[61] Halliday
	et al,[76] Catterton et al,[60]
	Friedman and Fitzpatrick,[71]
	Gersony et al,[74] Seyberth et
	al[173]

gastrointestinal
  abdominal distension
  gastrointestinal
    bleeding
  necrotizing enteroco-
    litis (?)
  gastric perforation
  gastric ulceration
	Gray and Pemberton,[75]
	Friedman and Fitzpatrick,[71]
	Nagaraj et al,[91] Campbell et
	al[59]

miscellaneous
  increased incidence of
    RLF (?)
  platelet dysfunction
    and bleeding
    tendency
  lowering of plasma
    glucose
	Procianoy et al,[97] Lindemann
	et al,[82] Friedman et al,[72]
	Gersony et al,[74] Yeh et al[177]

[a] Listed in order of published study; see References.

dicate that serum creatine or blood urea nitrogen values may go unchanged in the face of significant decreases in GFR. Whether decreased GFR is due to a change in renal plasma flow, in intrarenal permeability, or a combination of these effects is unknown. Hyponatremia reported with indomethacin may reflect augmentation of ADH action.[68,100]

Seyberth and colleagues[173] found that a 7-day course of therapy with indomethacin did not exaggerate renal dysfunction experienced in premature infants being treated for symptomatic PDA. In fact, a tendency for recovery of renal function was observed. The authors theorized that closure of the ductus resulted in establishment of effective circulatory volume, improved renal vascular perfusion, and normalization of plasma renin activity and sympathetic nervous system activity. These effects would maintain renal function in spite of continued indomethacin administration.

Gastrointestinal complications associated with the use of indomethacin have also been reported in infants (Table 9-7). The most serious are perforation and necrotizing enterocolitis. Since both lesions are also known to occur in premature infants who have not been exposed to indomethacin, a cause-and-effect rela-

tionship remains to be established. A variety of other factors have been proposed as causes of perforation and necrotizing enterocolitis, including birth trauma, gastric distention, and stress (gastric perforation) and intestinal ischemia and infection. Thus, the complicated clinical situation in the sick infant makes it difficult to incriminate indomethacin as the sole perpetrator of these complications.[74,108] Nevertheless, there are pharmacologic actions of indomethacin consistent with these toxicities.[91] Intestinal blood flow has been shown to be reduced by indomethacin in some animal studies.[73] A compromise in mesenteric blood flow, possibly by inhibition of prostaglandin vasodilators (PGE_2 and PGI_2), could secondarily lead to diminution in the synthesis of gastrointestinal tract protective mucous material.[71] Further studies are needed to clarify the contribution of indomethacin therapy to gastrointestinal complications in infants.

There are conflicting reports regarding the development of retinopathy in premature infants given indomethacin. Procianoy and colleagues[97] observed no change in the incidence of retrolental fibroplasia (RLF) in very-low-birth-weight infants who received indomethacin, but Lindemann and coworkers[82] reported an increased incidence of RLF in their premature infant population given indomethacin.

Platelet aggregation was grossly abnormal for 2 to 4 days in four premature infants following administration of indomethacin.[72] Plasma glucose levels were observed to be less in indomethacin-treated infants than in a placebo control population, but the magnitude of the effect does not appear to be clinically significant.[177] The drug's effect on bilirubin-albumin binding has been demonstrated to be insignificant with therapeutic doses of 0.6 mg/kg.[169] In addition, indomethacin primary binding sites on albumin are remote from those of bilirubin.[98]

In a one-year follow-up study, growth and development were no different in control and indomethacin-treated infants.[108]

VITAMIN E

Since its discovery in the 1920s, alpha-tocopherol, commonly referred to as vitamin E, has been of interest as a nutrient. Recently, its use as a drug in pharmacologic doses has attracted considerable attention.[120]

Much of the research on vitamin E has focused on its antioxidant action in controlling or regulating events associated with lipid peroxi-

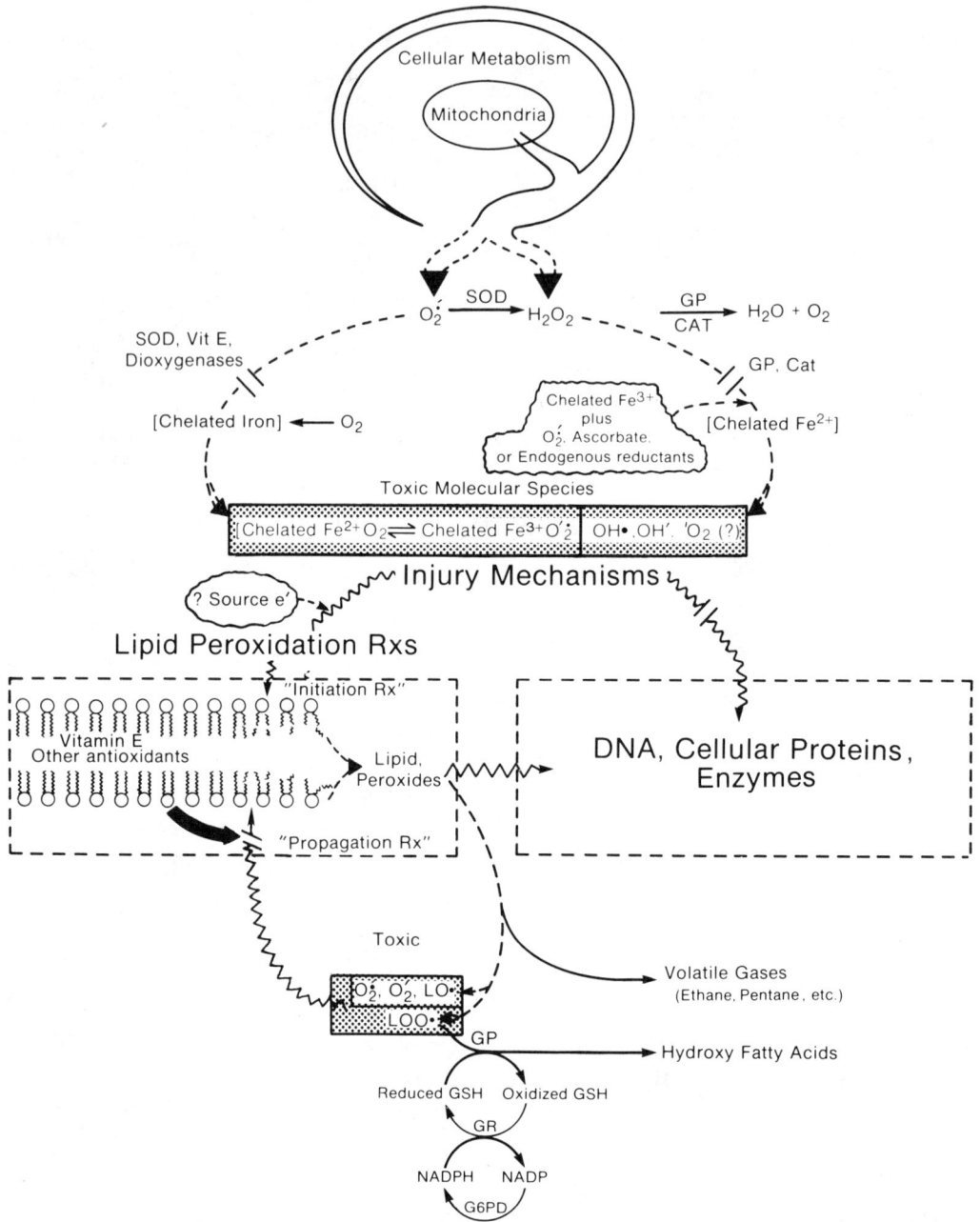

Figure 9-5. The source and generation of free radicals and reactive intermediates, and the role of cellular protective systems (enzymatic and nonenzymatic). These protective systems, including vitamin E, are believed to provide a protective environment for the cellular constituents by capturing or quenching the high energy state of the toxic reactive molecular species.

dation and perhaps other oxidative reactions. Figure 9-5 represents a general overview of lipid peroxidation reactions, including the proposed site(s) of vitamin E activity. This schematic representation also depicts the biochemical origin of adverse oxidative reactions that can give rise to membrane injury and subcellular dysfunction.

Several reactive molecular species can cause disruption or destruction of membrane systems and cellular metabolism. These reactive molecular species include superoxide radical, hydrogen peroxide, hydroxyl radical, peroxy radical, and singlet oxygen. These molecular species are unstable, high-energy molecules, some of which are believed to be critical components of "normal" cellular reactions that perform specific and important functional duties (e.g., killing of bacteria by granulocytes, synthesis of prostaglandins). Overproduction of these reactive molecular species relative to the protective systems available to the cell results in biochemical and cellular injury. The mechanisms involved in formation of the various reactive species are poorly understood. Protection of the cell from these reactive molecules is derived from nonenzyme and enzyme systems, including vitamin E, superoxide dismutase, catalase, and the glutathione enzyme systems. The protective mechanism is strongly influenced by cellular and subcellular compartmentalization of the reactions involved: Proximity of the protective system to its respective substrate (e.g., in vitamin E and lipid peroxidation reactions) allows the greatest efficiency in trapping or capturing the free energy of the toxic reactive species.

The role of oxidative injury and vitamin E in neonatal disease, including hemolytic anemia, hyperbilirubinemia, retrolental fibroplasia (RLF), acute and chronic lung disease, necrotizing enterocolitis, and intraventricular hemorrhage, is of great interest. Although the biochemical reactions depicted in Figure 9-5 provide a rational basis for the therapeutic use of vitamin E, the results of clinical trials in infants have been both encouraging and disappointing.[120] Although vitamin E is the only one of the protective substances employed extensively in a variety of clinical studies in infants, preliminary investigations have been conducted with other protective substances, including superoxide dismutase.[154]

Pharmacology. Vitamin E comprises a family of tocopherols, each of which has a different amount of antioxidant activity. The antioxidant activities of the various tocopherols have been determined by means of bioassays based on a variety of biologic responses (e.g., fetal resorption in rats, erythrocyte hemolysis).[117,179] The biologic significance and relevance of the bioassay findings have not been systematically examined; data from similar bioassays performed in vitro, however, are known to reflect not simply the intrinsic antioxidant activity of the compound examined but the source or nature of the oxidant challenge as well as the disposition characteristics of the antioxidant. The structures and metabolism of the naturally occurring tocopherols are shown in Figure 9-6. Although many different tocopherols with antioxidant activity have been found to occur naturally, alpha-tocopherol is considered to be the most important and accounts for approximately 90% of all tocopherols in animal tissue.[127] The standard unit of vitamin E activity is based on *dl*-alpha-tocopheryl acetate (1 mg = 1 IU). Alpha-tocopherol can be prepared by isolation from vegetable oils (natural) or synthesized from phytol. Pharmaceutical preparations of vitamin E are usually the synthetic form, which actually consists of several isomers of alpha-tocopherol in unspecified proportions.[138] The acetate ester of alpha-tocopherol is much more stable than the free alcohol in atmospheric oxygen under most conditions. The following discussion on vitamin E relates to *dl*-alpha-tocopherol and *dl*-alpha-tocopheryl acetate, which are the two primary pharmaceutical preparations available (Table 9-9).

Only limited information is available on the mechanism of gastrointestinal absorption of vitamin E in humans.[118] The actual intestinal site of absorption of tocopherol is unknown. Muller and colleagues[146] found that duodenal esterase is the principal hydrolytic enzyme responsible for conversion of tocopherol esters to free tocopherol. Melhorn and coworkers[144] concluded that premature infants have incompetent intestinal absorption of vitamin E, the degree of incompetence reflecting the relative gestational immaturity. This conclusion was based on studies of serum vitamin E levels following PO administration of alpha-tocopheryl acetate in neonates grouped according to gestational age (Table 9-10). Equivalent plasma vitamin E levels have been reported to result following PO administration of *dl*-alpha-tocopherol and *dl*-alpha-tocopheryl acetate in low-birth-weight infants.[115,129] In studies in adults, Baker and coworkers[113] observed that the increase in plasma tocopherol following PO administration is greater for *dl*-alpha-tocopherol than for *dl*-alpha-tocopheryl acetate. A dose response in plasma vitamin E levels was noted with the use

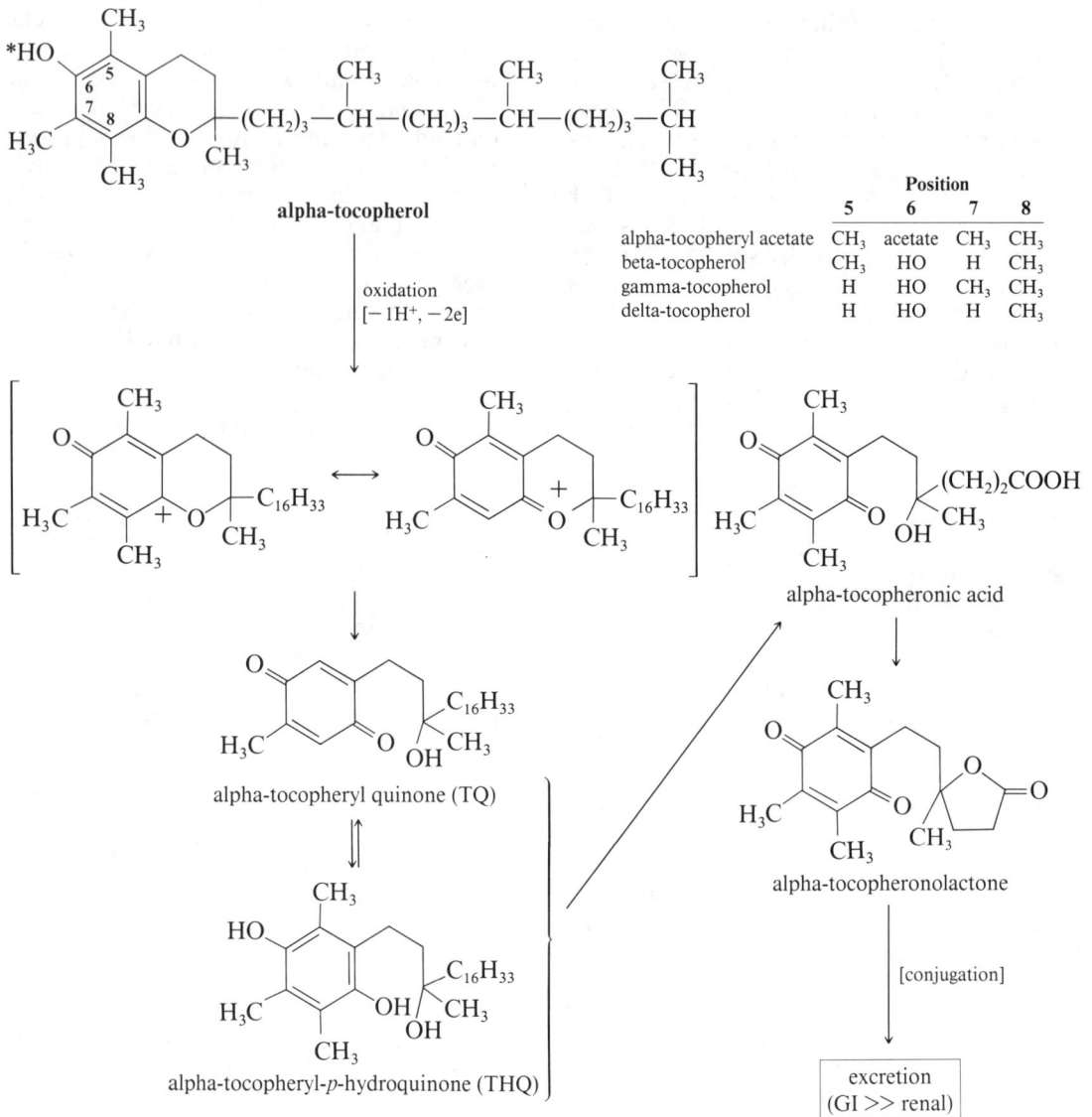

Figure 9-6. Proposed pathways for the metabolism of alpha-tocopherol. Chemical structures of other tocopherols differ as shown in the table.

Table 9-9. COMMERCIAL VITAMIN E PREPARATIONS COMMONLY USED IN INFANTS[a]

Commercial Preparation	Tocopherol Form	Administration Route	Concentration
Aquasol E	*dl*-alpha-tocopheryl acetate	PO	100, 400 IU capsule
		PO	500 IU/ml
Eferol Injectable	*dl*-alpha-tocopheryl acetate	IM	200 mg/ml
MVI, MVI-12, Multi-Vitamin Infusion	*dl*-alpha-tocopheryl acetate (many other vitamins included)	IV	5 IU/10 ml ampule 5 IU/5 ml concentrate 2 IU/ml (MVI-12)
Vi-Penta Infant Drops	*dl*-alpha-tocopherol (many other vitamins included)	PO	2 IU/0.6 ml

[a] Based on information available in the 1983 Physicians' Desk Reference (PDR) or official product labeling. This is not an exhaustive list of available vitamin E preparations.

of 400, 800, or 1600 mg of tocopherol (free or acetylated forms). It has been speculated that pancreatic insufficiency may result in incomplete gastrointestinal absorption of esterified tocopherols because of the lack of hydrolysis, whereas patients with biliary disease may manifest difficulty in absorption of free tocopherol.[113]

Reported values on the efficiency of absorption of alpha-tocopherol or its ester (e.g., acetate) from the gastrointestinal tract have ranged from 10% to over 80%.[118] The average fraction of dose of alpha-tocopherol or its ester absorbed from the gastrointestinal tract as alpha-tocopherol is believed to be about 55%, with the remainder excreted as degraded products in the feces.

Several studies in which vitamin E was administered parenterally document associated increases in plasma vitamin E levels (Tables 9–10 and 9–11). There are no published studies comparing the bioavailability of orally and parenterally administered vitamin E in neonates, although the results of Finer and coworkers[182] indicate greater serum tocopherol levels with daily 25 mg IM doses of alpha-tocopherol acetate than with daily PO doses of 200 mg (Table 9–10). The assay employed was a nonspecific colorimetric assay, and steady state levels of alpha-tocopherol may not have been reached. The use of more specific and sensitive techniques for analysis of tocopherols may assist in resolving the question of bioavailability of pharmacologic doses of vitamin E in neonates.

The concentration of vitamin E in plasma depends upon a number of factors, including extent of vitamin E and lipid absorption, total plasma lipid, triglyceride, and lipoprotein concentrations, and uptake and retention of vitamin E by nonvascular tissues.[138] Vitamin E appears to be associated with lipoproteins in plasma, but there is no evidence for a specific lipoprotein carrier.[114] Experimentally, it has been demonstrated that plasma vitamin E concentration does not consistently reflect vitamin E content in other tissues.[122] Tissue level following pharmacologic doses has not been determined in neonates, although a good correlation has been observed between lung alpha-tocopherol levels and vitamin E intake. Animal studies indicate extensive distribution of administered alpha-tocopherol, with the liver, spleen, adrenals, kidneys, and lungs showing the higher concentrations.[131,139,142] Alpha-tocopherol is distributed to tissues unchanged. Small amounts of metabolites,

including tocopheryl quinone, tocopheryl hydroquinine, and dimers, trimers, and more polar metabolites, have been found in tissue.

Excretion of administered vitamin E occurs predominantly via the gastrointestinal tract (10–75%), renal excretion being quantitatively unimportant. Fecal elimination of alpha-tocopherol appears to arise from incomplete absorption, secretion from the intestinal mucosa, and biliary excretion.[132] Urinary and biliary metabolites of tocopherol include tocopheronic acid and tocopheronolactone, excreted as either mono- or di-conjugates of glucuronic acid or sulfuric acid (see Fig. 9–6).

As illustrated in Figure 9–5, vitamin E is an antioxidant participating in the control of reactions associated with peroxidation of membrane lipids. Several mechanisms have been proposed to explain the antioxidant protective properties of vitamin E. Vitamin E may facilitate a closer physical "packing" of phospholipids in membranes, thus reducing exposure of unsaturated lipid components to free radicals. A biochemical mechanism proposed involves hydrogen "donation" by the tocopherol molecule; however, there is some evidence for the formation of hydrogen bond complexes between alpha-tocopherol, unsaturated phospholipids, and hydroperoxides without a change in the structure of alpha-tocopherol.[147] The donation of hydrogen by the tocopherol molecule would result in the formation of a metabolite, possibly tocopheryl quinone, which has been found in tissues; in some studies, however, it is notably absent.[119,126] Mechanisms have been proposed for the regeneration of vitamin E following hydrogen donation; these proposed regeneration pathways involve the glutathione system and the effects of vitamin C.[151]

Lucy[141] has proposed that vitamin E is an integral component of biologic membranes, interacting with the phospholipid components to ensure membrane structural stability. Molecular models of this membrane relationship designate vitamin E as the molecule with the responsibility of protecting the double-bond structures of linoleic, linolenic, and arachidonic acids. This relationship between polyunsaturated fatty acids (PUFAs) and vitamin E is consistent with the concept of a biologic requirement for vitamin E levels sufficient to maintain a critical concentration in membrane lipids (E:PUFA ratio). A change in PUFA dietary intake would necessitate a comparable change in requirement of vitamin E.

Clinical Pharmacology. Available studies with pharmacologic doses of vitamin E in neo-

Table 9–10. SUMMARY OF CLINICAL STUDIES ON VITAMIN E DOSE, GESTATIONAL AGE, CHRONOLOGIC AGE, AND SERUM VITAMIN E LEVELS IN NEONATES[a]

Author(s) of Published Study[b]	Study Group	Dose Employed	Serum or Plasma Vitamin E Levels (mg/dl) Premature	Full-term	Other data
Filer et al[129]	prematures (1.2–2.5 kg)	20 mg/kg PO × 1 alpha-tocopherol alpha-tocopheryl succinate	1 wk old: 1.9, 3.2; 2–4 wk old: 2.0–3.0, 2.2–2.6	2.5, 2.2	all values are 9-hr serum levels after 1 dose
Melhorn et al[144]	prematures (1.0–2.4 kg)	100 IU PO × 1, alpha-tocopheryl acetate	1–1.5 kg: 0.6, 6 wk: 1.3, 10 wk: 2.9; 1.5–2.0 kg: 3.2		peak serum levels after 1 dose at 3 wk of age (unless otherwise indicated)
Abrams et al[110]	full-term infants	100 mg PO q 24 hr from birth, alpha-tocopheryl acetate	0.7		mean plasma levels determined at 1 wk of age
Gross and Melhorn[134]	prematures (<2 kg); full-term infants	25 IU PO q 24 hr (×2–6 wk) alpha-tocopheryl polyethylene glycol succinate alpha-tocopheryl acetate	average: 1.0–1.4, peak: 3.7	peak: 2.4	average levels determined over duration of dosing; peak levels, at 8–10 hr after 1 dose: for prematures, at 3 wk of age; for full-terms, on day 3 of life
Graeber et al[133]	prematures (<1.5 kg)	125 mg/kg IM total, alpha-tocopheryl acetate, given in 4 divided doses on days 1, 2, 7, and 8 of life	0.5–0.8, 3.7; 1.6–1.9 (range of means)	0.9	range of mean serum levels between 4–6 wk of age; last dose given at day 8 of life
Bell et al[115]	prematures (<1.5 kg)	25 IU PO q 24 hr, alpha-tocopherol	2.1 ± 0.3 (mean ± SE)		determinations done at 2 wk of age
Gross[135]	prematures (1.0–2.0 kg)	50 mg/kg IM in 6 divided doses on days 1, 2, and 3 of life, alpha-tocopherol	1.0–1.5 kg: 3.0 ± 1.0; 1.5 ± 2.0 kg: 3.9 ± 1.1		determinations done on day 8 of life
Saldanha et al[155]	prematures (1.5 kg, mean)	25 mg IM q 24 hr, alpha-tocopherol, 4–10 doses	5 ± 1 (mean ± SE)		4–10 doses given
Chiswick et al[124]	prematures (0.6–1.7 kg)	20 mg/kg IM q 24 hr × 4 from birth, alpha-tocopherol	5		estimate (from data provided) on day 3 of life
Ehrenkranz et al[128]	prematures (1.5 kg, mean)	20 mg/kg IM on admission and 24, 48, and 168 hr later, alpha-tocopherol	after 3 doses: 5.5 ± 0.6; at 168 hr: 3.9 ± 0.2		
Colburn and Ehrenkranz[125]	prematures (1.5 kg)	20 mg/kg IM × 1, alpha-tocopherol	3.5–7 (peak)		pharmacokinetic study: $T\frac{1}{2}$ = 44 hr; peak conc. = 5 mg/dl reached at 4.3 hr; V_d = 0.4 l/kg
Finer et al[182]	prematures (<1.5 kg)	25 mg IM < 12 hr old, repeated dose in 12 hr, followed by 20 mg daily for 14 days. 50 mg PO q 6 hr, alpha-tocopheryl acetate	4.5 (IM dose); 3 (PO dose)		serum levels of Vitamin E estimated from data provided; after IM and PO dosing, serum levels significantly different.
Chiswick et al[180]	prematures (0.9–1.7 kg)	20 mg/kg IM daily × 3, alpha-tocopheryl acetate	3.0 ± 0.2		

a Additional studies are shown in Table 9–11.
b Listed in order of publications; see References at end of chapter.

Table 9–11. SUMMARY OF CLINICAL STUDIES OF VITAMIN E THERAPY IN NEONATES FOR PREVENTION OF RLF

Authors of Published Study[a]	Therapeutic Criteria	No. of Infants	Mean Birth Weight (g)	Total Mortality	Vitamin E Dosage	Mean Plasma Vitamin E Levels (mg/dl)	Results (No. Blind/Total No.) Vitamin E	Control
Hittner et al[136]†	<1500 g, O₂ required	150	1130	35% (53/150)	dl-alpha-tocopherol: 100 mg/kg PO q 24 hr for duration of hospitalization	1.0–1.2 (range)	0/50 (0%)	5/51 (9.8%)
Milner et al[145]‡	<1500 g (likely to live)	268	1158	12% (33/268)	?PO	(3 × control)	3/111 (2.7%)	5/114 (4.3%)
Puklin et al[150]‡	premature, RDS, O₂ required	100	1426	26% (26/100)	dl-alpha-tocopherol: 20 mg/kg IM on admission and 24, 48, and 168 hr later, then ×2 weekly	2.2–2.5 (range)	0/37 (0%)	0/37 (0%)
Finer et al[130]‡	750–1500 g	126	1202	21% (27/126)	vitamin E?: 25 mg IM at 12 and 24 hr of age, then 20 mg IM q 24 hr ×14, then 20 mg q 3 days ×5 (or 100 U PO q 24 hr)	2.9–5.7 (range)	0/48 (0%)	3/51 (5.9%)
Hittner et al[137]†	<1500 g, O₂ required, <24 hr old	100	1091	31% (31/100)	dl-alpha-tocopheryl acetate: 100 mg/kg PO q 24 hr (×8 wk min.)	1.6–2.0 (range)	2/69 (2.9%)	5/51 (9.8%) same control group as 1981 study

[a] Listed in order of publications; see References at end of chapter. †: authors found a statistically significant difference between the incidence of RLF in control group and in vitamin E–treated group; ‡: authors found no statistically significant effect of vitamin E therapy; ?: Insufficient information provided in original article to determine route of administration or dosage form of vitamin E employed.

275

nates that include a determination of vitamin E serum or plasma levels subsequent to oral and parenteral administration are summarized in Tables 9–10 and 9–11. Examination of these tables indicates that a wide range of vitamin E doses have been employed, but a clear dose–plasma level relationship is not apparent. A number of variables may be responsible for the discrepancy, including differences in dose, route of administration, dosage form, and differences in gestational and chronologic age of the patients. The analytic techniques employed in these studies differ in specificity and sensitivity.

Whether the differing serum vitamin E levels relate to differences in pharmacologic activity is controversial. Numerous studies have attempted to correlate pharmacologic doses of vitamin E with therapeutic effects.[120] There is no convincing evidence that vitamin E supplementation influences hemolytic anemia in premature infants given adequate nutritional sources of vitamin E. Abrams and coworkers[110] administered 100 mg of alpha-tocopheryl acetate PO to infants daily from birth to examine the impact on red blood cell survival times. Although plasma vitamin E levels increased, no significant effect on hemoglobin or plasma bilirubin concentration was noted during the first week of life. Gross[135] administered alpha-tocopherol to neonates during the first 3 days of life (50 mg/kg IM total) and observed a significant decrease in serum bilirubin concentration and in the duration of phototherapy required in infants weighing less than 1.5 kg. Chiswick and colleagues[180] found reduced hydrogen peroxide–induced red blood cell hemolysis in premature infants given 20 mg/kg of alpha-tocopheryl acetate IM daily for 3 days. The plasma vitamin E level after 3 days of treatment was 3.0 ± 0.2 mg/dl. The magnitude of the observed effect on red blood cell hemolysis, however, does not warrant the routine use of vitamin E for this purpose.

Vitamin E can affect platelet and polymorphonuclear leukocyte function.[112,140,156] In pharmacologic doses, it has also been shown to produce a significant depression in bactericidal activity of leukocytes in older children and adults[149] and in experimental weanling animals.[121] In vitro studies with human platelets have demonstrated a time-dependent, irreversible inhibition of platelet cyclo-oxygenase, with a resulting reduction in TXB_2 and PGD_2 synthesis. These effects on prostaglandin formation are consistent with the known ability of alpha-tocopherol to inhibit platelet aggregation.[111,156]

Stuart and Oski[157] demonstrated inhibitory effects of vitamin E (1600 IU/day for 2 wk) on platelet malonyldialdehyde (MDA) formation. Zipursky and colleagues[158] examined the effect of vitamin E therapy (25 mg q 24 hr PO for first 6 wk of life) on coagulation tests in newborn infants; none of the coagulation factors in infants receiving vitamin E differed significantly from those in controls. These studies were done to examine the clinical relevance of reports that vitamin E therapy can affect blood levels of vitamin K–dependent coagulation factors. In this regard, Chiswick and coauthors[124,180] reported that vitamin E (25mg/kg IM daily) reduced the incidence of intraventricular hemorrhage in the newborn, although the overall incidence of subependymal or intraventricular hemorrhage was similar (42.9 versus 43.5%). Hittner and Kretzer[184] also reported a reduced incidence of severe intraventricular hemorrhage with vitamin E treatment. Further studies are needed to examine these preliminary observations.

Therapeutic Indications. Vitamin E has been administered in pharmacologic doses to neonates for treatment or prevention of red blood cell hemolysis, retrolental fibroplasia (RLF), bronchopulmonary dysplasia (BPD), and intraventricular hemorrhage. The rationale for these and other uses of vitamin E in neonates ranges from simple curiosity to elaborate well-conceived theories. For the most part, the therapeutic experience with vitamin E in pediatrics has been on a sound and scholarly basis, but controversy continues regarding its actual clinical value. Part of the difficulty in examining the published results with vitamin E resides in the significant differences in the therapeutic programs utilized: 25 mg/kg to as high as 200 mg/kg of alpha-tocopherol or alpha-tocopheryl acetate given IM, PO, or IV at intervals of every 6 hours, daily, or less often (Tables 9–10, 9–11). The need for multiple large doses (100 to 200 mg/kg/day) of vitamin E to achieve whatever maximum benefits there may be remains to be validated.

The use of vitamin E for the prevention of *hemolytic anemia* has been reviewed by Bell and Filer,[116] Ehrenkranz,[127] and Bieri and colleagues.[120] Hematologic manifestations (e.g., hemolytic anemia) of vitamin E deficiency in the premature infant are of limited clinical significance. Controlled studies have revealed conflicting or equivocal effects of vitamin E on red cell survival. A difference in mean hemoglobin concentration, small but statistically significant, has been demonstrated only in infants with inadequate dietary E:PUFA ratios who also received supplementary iron therapy. Many risk factors are involved in development of anemia (i.e., red blood cell hemolysis) in premature infants: nutritional intake of vitamin E and PUFAs (E:PUFA ratio) and iron; ability to synthesize red blood cells; and the oxidative challenge to and stability of the red blood cells. The rational use of vitamin E for prevention or treatment of hemolytic anemia requires only adequate nutritional intake of vitamin E, not large pharmacologic doses.

Pharmacologic doses of vitamin E have been recommended for prevention of *retrolental fibroplasia* (RLF). Several reviews have been published regarding the use of vitamin E in RLF.[127,148,188] Controlled studies have demonstrated both a statistically significant decrease in the incidence of severe cicatricial RLF (i.e., blindness) and no effect following prophylactic administration of vitamin E (Table 9–11). As noted by Phelps,[148] the routine use of vitamin E prophylaxis, as indicated by appropriate therapeutic criteria (e.g., birth weight < 1500 g, oxygen therapy), would involve an estimated 21,000 infants in the United States; of these, only about 500 would in fact be at risk for the development of severe RLF (blindness), leaving more than 20,000 infants who would receive vitamin E without any anticipated benefit. Therefore, the importance of demonstrating the safety of vitamin E therapy is paramount, particularly since it has not yet been possible to identify those infants who will benefit from vitamin E therapy. [*Early administration of vitamin E should not be considered a guarantee against RLF in premature infants.*] Although a variety of dosing programs have been employed (Table 9–11), there is no consistent relationship between the dose of vitamin E and the plasma levels of vitamin E on the incidence or severity of retinopathy. Differences in analysis of vitamin E in RLF may be responsible. The risk–benefit ratio and appropriate dose, route of administration, and dosage form (alpha-tocopherol versus alpha-tocopheryl acetate) remain to be firmly established.

In the clinical studies of vitamin E in infants with *acute and chronic lung disease* (i.e., RDS and BPD, respectively), very little support for efficacy of vitamin E exists. Ehrenkranz and colleagues[128] found no significant effect of vitamin E on the clinical course in infants with RDS, although preliminary studies by these investigators suggested a shorter requirement for supplemental oxygen therapy, positive pressure ventilation, and endotracheal continuous-distending airway pressure. McClung,[143] Abbasi,[109] and Saldanha[155] and their colleagues were unable to identify a protective effect of vitamin E against the development of BPD in infants with respiratory distress. Experimental studies, on the other hand, have demonstrated protective effects of vitamin E against certain aspects of oxygen-induced lung injury in newborn animals, especially if deprived of normal nutritional sources of vitamin E.[153] The value of vitamin E in pharmacologic doses for prevention of oxidative lung injury in neonates remains to be demonstrated.

Although preliminary reports of protective effects of vitamin E against *intraventricular hemorrhage* in premature newborns are encouraging,[180,184] further studies will be required before vitamin E can be recommended for this purpose.

In summary, the routine employment of pharmacologic doses of vitamin E in all preterm newborns cannot be justified by the available information. The question of efficacy of vitamin E in any clinical problem will be difficult to answer without a clear understanding of the relationship between dosage of vitamin E (dose, dosage form, route of administration, duration of therapy), resulting tissue levels, and antioxidant effect. It is particularly important to establish whether or not pharmacologic doses of vitamin E produce additional advantages (tissue levels, pharmacologic antioxidant effects) beyond that provided by nutritional sources of vitamin E. It may be that vitamin E supplementation will be most beneficial if given at birth to neonates at risk for oxidative injury who are not expected to receive nutritional sources of vitamin E.[122,123] The question of safety of pharmacologic doses of vitamin E is of equal significance in these considerations. Therefore, the use of pharmacologic doses of vitamin E in neonates must still be considered experimental. Newborns most likely to benefit from vitamin E therapy include prematures with risk factors for the development of RLF and who are unable to receive adequate nutrition, including vitamin E. An oral dose of 20 to 100 mg/kg of alpha-tocopherol or alpha-tocopheryl acetate given as soon after birth as possible is probably sufficient to produce vitamin E tissue levels exceeding those achieved by normal nutrition. Subsequently, every other day or twice weekly doses (20 to 100 mg/kg PO) should be sufficient to maintain adequate tissue levels of vitamin E. Parenteral (IM, IV) alpha-tocopherol should be employed only if oral dosing is not possible. The parenteral administration (IM or IV) of alpha-tocopheryl acetate may be less efficacious than oral administration because of poor hydrolysis of the ester (acetate).[185] Unfortunately, most commercial preparations of vitamin E for parenteral administration are the acetate ester (Table 9–9).

Clinical Toxicology. The absence of overt manifestations of toxicity following large doses of vitamin E has been emphasized repeatedly by physicians employing this drug in the clinical setting. The issue of the safety of pharmacologic doses of vitamin E is controversial.[148,152] There are reports of local tissue injury and calcification at IM vitamin E injection sites[186] and unpublished reports to the FDA of increased incidence of sepsis and necrotizing enterocolitis in prematures treated with vitamin E.[183,187] The pharmacologic actions of vitamin E, which have been demonstrated on free radical-based reactions, including neutrophil and platelet function and prostaglandin synthesis (see Pharmacology and Clinical Pharmacology sections), are the basis of other theoretical concerns on vitamin E toxicity.

References

Prostaglandins

1. Bennett A, Fleshler B: Prostaglandins and the gastrointestinal tract. Gastroenterology 59:790, 1970.
2. Benson LN, Olley PM, Patel RG, et al: Role of prostaglandin E₁ infusion in the management of transposition of the great arteries. Am J Cardiol 44:691, 1979.
3. Bray MA, Gordon D: Prostaglandin production by macrophages and the effect of anti-inflammatory drugs. Br J Pharmacol 63:635, 1978.
4. Cassin S: Role of prostaglandins and thromboxanes in the control of the pulmonary circulation in the fetus and newborn. Semin Perinatol 4:101, 1980.
5. Cassin S, Tod M, Philips J, et al: Effects of prostaglandin D₂ on perinatal circulation. Am J Physiol 240:H755, 1981.
6. Chang LCT, Splawinski JA, Oates JA, Nies AS: Enhanced renal prostaglandin production in the dog. II. Effects on intrarenal hemodynamics. Circ Res 36:204, 1975.
7. Christensen NC, Fabricus J: Medical manipulation of the ductus arteriosus. Lancet 2:406, 1975.
8. Clyman RI, Heymann MA: Pharmacology of the ductus arteriosus. Pediatr Clin North Am 28:77, 1981.
9. Coceani F, Olley PM: Role of prostaglandins, prostacyclin, and thromboxanes in the control of prenatal patency and postnatal closure of the ductus arteriosus. Semin Perinatol 4:109, 1980.
10. Coceani F, Olley PM, Lock JE: Prostaglandins, ductus arteriosus, pulmonary circulation: Current concepts and clinical potential. Eur J Clin Pharmacol 18:75, 1980.
11. Elliott RB, Starling MB, Neutze JM: Medical manipulation of the ductus arteriosus. Lancet 1:140, 1975.
12. Feigen LP: Actions of prostaglandins in peripheral vascular beds. Fed Proc 40:1987, 1981.
13. Freed MD, Heymann MA, Lewis AB, et al: Prostaglandin E₁ in infants with ductus arteriosus–dependent congenital heart disease. Circulation 64:899, 1981.
14. Friedman WF, Fitzpatrick KM: Effects of prostaglandins, thromboxanes, and inhibitors of their synthesis on renal and gastrointestinal function in the newborn period. Semin Perinatol 4:143, 1980.
15. Friedman Z, Berman W: Hematologic effects of prostaglandins and thromboxanes, and inhibitors of their synthesis in the perinatal period. Semin Perinatol 4:73, 1980.
16. Gerber JG, Branch RA, Nies AS, et al: Prostaglandins and renin release: II. Assessment of renin secretion following infusion of PGI₂, E₂ and D₂ into the renal artery of anesthetized dogs. Prostaglandins 15:81, 1978.
17. Gorman RR, Shebuski RJ, Aiken JW, Bundy GL: Analysis of the biological activity of azoprostanoids in human platelets. Fed Proc 40:1997, 1981.
18. Heymann MA, Rudolph AM: Ductus arteriosus dilatation by prostaglandin E₁ in infants with pulmonary atresia. Pediatrics 59:325, 1977.
19. Heymann MA, Berman W Jr, Rudolph AM, Whitman V: Dilatation of the ductus arteriosus by prostaglandin E₁ in aortic arch abnormalities. Circulation 59:169, 1979.
20. Heymann MA: Pharmacologic use of prostaglandin E₁ in infants with congenital heart disease. Am Heart J 101:837, 1981.
21. Higgs EA, Moncada S: Prostacyclin—physiology and clinical uses. Gen Pharmacol 14:7, 1983.
22. Hyman AL, Mathe AA, Lippton HL, Kadowitz PJ: Prostaglandins and the lung. Med Clin North Am 65:789, 1981.
23. Kadowitz PJ, Joiner PD, Hyman AL: Physiological and pharmacological roles of prostaglandins. Ann Rev Pharmacol 15:285, 1975.
24. Lands WEM: The biosynthesis and metabolism of prostaglandins. Ann Rev Physiol 41:633, 1979.
25. Lang P, Freed MD, Rosenthal A, et al: The use of prostaglandin E₁ in an infant with interruption of the aortic arch. J Pediatr 91:805, 1977.
26. Lang P, Freed MD, Bierman FZ, et al: Use of prostaglandin E₁ in infants with d-transposition of the great arteries and intact ventricular septum. Am J Cardiol 44:76, 1979.
27. Lewis AB, Takahashi M, Lurie PR: Administration of prostaglandin E₁ in neonates with critical congenital cardiac defects. J Pediatr 93:481, 1978.
28. Lewis AB, Freed MD, Heymann MA, et al: Side effects of therapy with prostaglandin E₁ in infants with critical congenital heart disease. Circulation 64:893, 1981.
29. Lock JE, Olley PM, Coceani F, et al: Use of prostacyclin in persistent fetal circulation. Lancet 1:1343, 1979.
30. Lucas A, Mitchell MD: Plasma-prostaglandins in preterm neonates before and after treatment for patent ductus arteriosus. Lancet 2:130, 1978.
31. McGiff JC, Growshaw K, Terragno NA, et al: Prostaglandin-like substances appearing in canine renal venous blood during renal ischemia. Circ Res 27:765, 1970.

32. Moncada S, Flower RJ, Vane JR: Prostaglandins, prostacyclin, and thromboxane A_2. In Gilman AG, Goodman LS, Gilman A (eds): The Pharmacological Basis of Therapeutics, 6th ed. P 668. New York, Macmillan, 1980.

34. Murphy JD, Freed MD, Lang P, et al: Prostaglandin-E_1 infusion in neonatal persistent pulmonary hypertension. Pediatr Res 14:606, 1980.

35. Neutze JM, Starling MB, Elliott RB, Barratt-Boyes BG: Palliation of cyanotic congenital heart disease in infancy with E-type prostaglandins. Circulation 55:238, 1977.

36. Olley PM, Coceani F, Bodach E: E-type prostaglandins: A new emergency therapy for certain cyanotic congenital heart malformations. Circulation 53:728, 1976.

37. Olley PM, Coceani F: The prostaglandins. Am J Dis Child 134:688, 1980.

38. Olley PM, Coceani F: Use of prostaglandins in cardiopulmonary diseases of the newborn. Semin Perinatol 4:135, 1980.

39. Overturf ML, Druilhet RE, Kirkendall WM: Prostaglandins and the renin–angiotensin–aldosterone system. In Greenberg S, Kadowitz PJ, Burks TF (eds): Modern Pharmacology–Toxicology Series: Prostaglandins: Organ- and Tissue-specific Actions. Vol 21, Chap 7. New York, Marcel Dekker, 1982.

40. Ramwell PW, Foegh M, Loeb R, Leovey EMK: Synthesis and metabolism of prostaglandins, prostacyclin, and thromboxanes: The arachidonic acid cascade. Semin Perinatol 4:3, 1980.

41. Robinson BF, Collier JG, Karim SMM, Somers K: Effect of prostaglandins A_1, A_2, B_1, E_2, and $F_{2\alpha}$ on forearm arterial bed and superficial hand veins in man. Clin Sci 44:367, 1973.

42. Rubin LJ, Lazar JD: Influence of prostaglandin synthesis inhibitors on pulmonary vasodilatory effects of hydralazine in dogs with hypoxic pulmonary vasoconstriction. J Clin Invest 67:193, 1981.

43. Rubin LJ, Groves BM, Reeves JT, et al: Prostacyclin-induced acute pulmonary vasodilation in primary pulmonary hypertension. Circulation 66:334, 1982.

44. Samuelsson B, Goldyne M, Granström E, et al: Prostaglandins and thromboxanes. Ann Rev Biochem 47:997, 1978.

44a. Samuelsson B, Hammarström S: Leukotrienes: A novel group of biologically active compounds. In Munson PL, Diczfalusy E, Glover J, Olson RE (eds): Vitamins and Hormones Vol. 39. P 1. New York, Academic Press, 1982.

45. Silove ED, Coe JY, Shiu MF, et al: Oral prostaglandin E_2 in ductus-dependent pulmonary circulation. Circulation 63:682, 1981.

46. Silver MM, Freedom RM, Silver MD, Olley PM: The morphology of the human newborn ductus arteriosus: A reappraisal of its structure and closure with special reference to prostaglandin E_1 therapy. Hum Pathol 12:1123, 1981.

47. Soifer SJ, Morin FC III, Heymann MA: Prostaglandin D_2 reverses induced pulmonary hypertension in the newborn lamb. J Pediatr 100:458, 1982.

48. Sun FF, Taylor BM, McGuire JC, Wong PYK: Metabolism of prostaglandins in the kidney. Kidney Int 19:760, 1981.

49. Szczeklik A, Gryglewski RJ, Nizankowski R, et al: Circulatory and anti-platelet effects of intravenous prostacyclin in healthy men. Pharmacol Res Comm 10:545, 1978.

50. Tannebaum J, Splawinski JA, Oates JA, Nies AS: Enhanced renal prostaglandin production in the dog. I. Effects on renal function. Circ Res 36:204, 1975.

51. Ueda K, Saito A, Nakano H, et al: Cortical hyperostosis following long-term administration of prostaglandin E_1 in infants with cyanotic congenital heart disease. J Pediatr 97:834, 1980.

52. Venuto RC, Ferris TF: Prostaglandins and renal function. In Greenberg S, Kadowitz PJ, Burks TF (eds): Modern Pharmacology–Toxicology Series: Prostaglandins: Organ- and Tissue-specific Actions. Vol 21, Chap 6. New York, Marcel Dekker, 1982.

53. Yam J, Roberts RJ: Modification of alveolar hyperoxia–induced pulmonary vasodilation by indomethacin. Prostaglandins 11:679, 1976.

Indomethacin

54. Alpert BS, Lewins MJ, Rowland DW, et al: Plasma indomethacin levels in preterm newborn infants with symptomatic patent ductus arteriosus—clinical and echocardiographic assessments of response. J Pediatr 95:578, 1979.

55. Bhat R, Vidyasagar D, Vadapalli M, et al: Disposition of indomethacin in preterm infants. J Pediatr 95:313, 1979.

56. Bhat R, Fisher E, Raju TNK, Vidyasagar D: Patent ductus arteriosus: Recent advances in diagnosis and management. Pediatr Clin North Am 29:1117, 1982.

57. Bianchetti G, Monin P, Marchal F, et al: Pharmacokinetics of indomethacin in the premature infant. Dev Pharmacol Ther 1:111, 1980.

58. Brash AR, Hickey DE, Graham TP, et al: Pharmacokinetics of indomethacin in the neonate: Relation of plasma indomethacin levels to response of the ductus arteriosus. N Engl J Med 305:67, 1981.

59. Campbell AN, Beasley JR, Kenna AP: Indomethacin and gastric perforation in a neonate. Lancet 1:1110, 1981.

60. Catterton Z, Sellers B Jr, Gray B: Insulin clearance in the premature infant receiving indomethacin. J Pediatr 96:737, 1980.

61. Cifuentes RF, Olley PM, Balfe JW, et al: Indomethacin and renal function in premature infants with persistent patent ductus arteriosus. J Pediatr 95:583, 1979.

62. Clyman RI: Ontogeny of the ductus arteriosus response to prostaglandins and inhibitors of their synthesis. Semin Perinatol 4:115, 1980.

63. Clyman RI, Heymann MA: Pharmacology of the ductus arteriosus. Pediatr Clin North Am 28:77, 1981.

64. Coceani F, Olley PM: Role of prostaglandins, prostacyclin, and thromboxanes in the control of prenatal patency and postnatal closure of the ductus arteriosus. Semin Perinatol 4:109, 1980.

65. Coceani F, Olley PM, Lock JE: Prostaglandins, ductus arteriosus, pulmonary circulation: Current concepts and clinical potential. Eur J Clin Pharmacol 18:75, 1980.

66. Curry SH, Brown EA, Kuck H, Cassin S: Preparation and stability of indomethacin solutions. Can J Physiol Pharmacol 60:988, 1982.

67. Evans M, Bhat R, Vidyasagar D, et al: A comparison of oral and intravenous indomethacin dispositions in the premature infant with patent ductus arteriosus. Pediatr Pharmacol 1:251, 1981.

68. Friedman AL, Segar WE: Antiduretic hormone excess. J Pediatr 94:521, 1979.
69. Friedman CA, Parks BR, Rawson JE, et al: Indomethacin and the preterm infant with a patent ductus arteriosus: Relationship between plasma concentration and ductus closure. Dev Pharmacol Ther 4:37, 1982.
70. Friedman WF, Hirschklau MJ, Printz MP, et al: Pharmacologic closure of patent ductus arteriosus in the premature infant. N Engl J Med 295:526, 1976.
71. Friedman WF, Fitzpatrick KM: Effects of prostaglandins, thromboxanes, and inhibitors of their synthesis on renal and gastrointestinal function in the newborn period. Semin Perinatol 4:143, 1980.
72. Friedman Z, Whitman V, Maisels MJ, et al: Indomethacin disposition and indomethacin-induced platelet dysfunction in premature infants. J Clin Pharmacol 18:272, 1978.
73. Gaffney GR, Williamson HE: Effect of indomethacin and meclofenamate on canine mesenteric and celiac blood flow. Res Comm Chem Path Pharmacol 25:165, 1979.
74. Gersony WM, Peckham GJ, Ellison RC, et al: Effects of indomethacin in premature infants with patent ductus arteriosus: Results of a national collaborative study. J Pediatr 102:895, 1983.
75. Gray PH, Pemberton PJ: Gastric perforation associated with indomethacin therapy in a pre-term infant. Aust Paediatr J 16:65, 1980.
76. Halliday HL, Hirata T, Brady JP: Indomethacin therapy for large patent ductus arteriosus in the very low birth weight infant: Results and complications. Pediatrics 64:154, 1979.
77. Harris JP, Merritt TA, Alexson CG, et al: Parenteral indomethacin for closure of the patent ductus arteriosus. Am J Dis Child 136:1005, 1982.
78. Helleberg L: Clinical pharmacokinetics of indomethacin. Clin Pharmacokin 6:245, 1981.
79. Heymann MA: Management of PDA with prostaglandin (PG) synthetase inhibitors. Report of the Seventy-Fifth Ross Conference on Pediatric Research. Columbus, Ohio, Ross Laboratories 1978. p 84.
80. Kääpä P, Lanning P, Koivisto M: Early closure of patent ductus arteriosus with indomethacin in preterm infants with idiopathic respiratory distress syndrome. Acta Paediatr Scand 72:179, 1983.
81. Kwan KC, Breault GO, Umbenhauer ER, et al: Kinetics of indomethacin absorption, elimination, and enterohepatic circulation in man. J Pharmacokin Biopharm 4:225, 1976.
82. Lindemann R, Blystad W, Egge K: Retrolental fibroplasia in premature infants with patent ductus arteriosus treated with indomethacin. Eur J Pediatr 138:56, 1982.
83. Mahony L, Carnero V, Brett C, et al: Prophylactic indomethacin therapy for patent ductus arteriosus in very-low-birth-weight infants. N Engl J Med 306:506, 1982.
84. McCarthy JS, Zies LG, Gelband H: Age-dependent closure of the patent ductus arteriosus by indomethacin. Pediatrics 62:706, 1978.
85. Mehta AC, Calvert RT: An improved high-performance liquid chromatographic procedure for monitoring indomethacin in neonates. Ther Drug Monit 5:143, 1983.
86. Merritt TA, DiSessa TG, Feldman BH, et al: Closure of the patent ductus arteriosus with ligation and indomethacin: A consecutive experience. J Pediatr 93:639, 1978.

87. Merritt TA, Harris JP, Roghmann K, et al: Early closure of the patent ductus arteriosus in very low-birth-weight infants: A controlled trial. J Pediatr 99:281, 1981.
88. Morselli PL, Franco-Morselli R, Bossi L: Clinical pharmacokinetics in newborns and infants: Age-related differences and therapeutic implications. Clin Pharmacokin 5:485, 1980.
89. Mrongovius R, Imbeck H, Wille L, et al: Variability of serum indomethacin concentrations after oral and intravenous administration of preterm infants. Eur J Pediatr 138:151, 1982.
90. Mullet MD, Croghan TW, Myerberg DZ, et al: Indomethacin for closure of patent ductus arteriosus in prematures. Clin Pediatr 21:217, 1982.
91. Nagaraj HS, Sandhu AS, Cook LN, et al: Gastrointestinal perforation following indomethacin therapy in very low birth weight infants. J Pediatr Surg 16:1003, 1981.
92. Neal WA, Kyle JM, Mullett MD: Failure of indomethacin therapy to induce closure of patent ductus arteriosus in premature infants with respiratory distress syndrome. J Pediatr 91:621, 1977.
93. Nestrud RM, Hill DE, Arrington RW, et al: Indomethacin treatment in patent ductus arteriosus: A double-blind study utilizing indomethacin plasma levels. Dev Pharmacol Ther 1:125, 1980.
94. Neu J, Ariagno RL, Johnson JD, et al: A double blind study of the effects of oral indomethacin in preterm infants wih patent ductus arteriosus who failed medical management. Pediatr Pharmacol 1:245, 1981.
95. Obeyesekere HI, Pankhurst S, Yu VYH: Pharmacological closure of ductus arteriosus in preterm infants using indomethacin. Arch Dis Child 55:271, 1980.
96. Peterson S, Christensen NC, Jensen KM, Ryssing E: Serum indomethacin concentrations after intravenous administration to preterm infants with patent ductus arteriosus. Acta Paediatr Scand 70:729, 1981.
97. Procianoy RS, Garcia-Prats JA, Hittner HM, et al: Use of indomethacin and its relationship to retinopathy of prematurity in very low birth weight infants. Arch Dis Child 55:362, 1980.
98. Rasmussen LF, Ahlfors CE, Wennberg RP: Displacement of bilirubin from albumin by indomethacin. J Clin Pharmacol 18:477, 1978.
99. Seyberth HW, Muller H, Wille L, et al: Recovery of prostaglandin production associated with reopening of the ductus arteriosus after indomethacin treatment in preterm infants with respiratory distress syndrome. Pediatr Pharmacol 2:127, 1982.
100. Shankaran S, Pantoja A, Poland RL: Indomethacin and bilirubin-albumin binding. Dev Pharmacol Ther 4:124, 1982.
101. Stein G, Kunze M, Zaumseil J, Traeger A: Zue Pharmakokinetik von Indomethazin und Indomethazin-metaboliten bei wiederholter Applikation an nierengesunde und nierengeschadigten Patienten. Int J Clin Pharmacol 15:470, 1977.
102. Thalji AA, Carr I, Yeh TF, et al: Pharmacokinetics of intravenously administered indomethacin in premature infants. J Pediatr 97:995, 1980.
103. Vert P, Bianchetti G, Marchal F, et al: Effectiveness and pharmacokinetics of indomethacin in premature newborns with patent ductus arteriosus. Eur J Clin Pharmacol 18:83, 1980.
104. Yaffe SJ, Friedman WF, Rogers D, et al: The disposi-

tion of indomethacin in preterm babies. J Pediatr 97:1001, 1980.

105. Yanagi RM, Wilson A, Newfeld EA, et al: Indomethacin treatment for symptomatic patent ductus arteriosus: A double-blind control study. Pediatrics 67:647, 1981.
106. Yeh TF, Luken JA, Thalji A, et al: Intravenous indomethacin therapy in premature infants with persistent ductus arteriosus—a double-blind controlled study. J Pediatr 98:137, 1981.
107. Yeh TF, Wilks A, Singl J, et al: Furosemide prevents the renal side effects of indomethacin therapy in premature infants with patent ductus arteriosus. J Pediatr 101:433, 1982.
108. Yeh TF, Goldbarg HR, Henek T, et al: Intravenous indomethacin therapy in premature infants with patent ductus arteriosus. Am J Dis Child 136:803, 1982.

Vitamin E

109. Abbasi S, Johnson LK, Boggs T: Effect of vitamin E by infusion in sick small premature infants at risk for BPD. Pediatr Res 14:638, 1980.
110. Abrams BA, Gutteridge JMC, Stocks J, et al: Vitamin E in neonatal hyperbilirubinaemia. Arch Dis Child 48:721, 1973.
111. Ali M, Gudbranson G, McDonald JWD: Inhibition of human platelet cyclooxygenase by alpha-tocopherol. Prostaglandins Med 4:79, 1980.
112. Baehner RL, Boxer LA, Allen JM, Davis J: Autooxidation as a basis for altered function of polymorphonuclear leukocytes. Blood 50:327, 1977.
113. Baker H, Frank O, DeAngelis B, Feingold S: Plasma tocopherol in man at various times after ingesting free or acetylated tocopherol. Nutr Rep Int 21:531, 1980.
114. Behrens WA, Thompson JN, Madere R: Distribution of alpha-tocopherol in human plasma lipoproteins. Am J Clin Nutr 35:691, 1982.
115. Bell EF, Brown EJ, Milner R, et al: Vitamin E absorption in small premature infants. Pediatrics 63:830, 1979.
116. Bell EF, Filer LJ Jr: The role of vitamin E in the nutrition of premature infants. Am J Clin Nutr 34:414, 1981.
117. Bieri JG, Evarts RP: Vitamin E activity of γ-tocopherol in the rat, chick and hamster. J Nutr 104:850, 1974.
118. Bieri JG, Farrell PM: Vitamin E. Vitam Horm 34:31, 1976.
119. Bieri JG, Tolliver TJ: On the occurrance of alpha-tocopheryl quinone in rat tissue. Lipids 16:777, 1981.
120. Bieri JG, Corash L, Hubbard VS: Medical uses of vitamin E. N Engl J Med 308:1063, 1983.
121. Boxer LA, Harris RE, Baehner RL: Regulation of membrane peroxidation in health and disease. Pediatrics 64(Suppl):713, 1979.
122. Bucher JR, Roberts RJ: α-Tocopherol (vitamin E) content of lung, liver, and blood in the newborn rat and human infant: Influence of hyperoxia. J Pediatr 98:806, 1981.
123. Bucher JR, Roberts RJ: Effects of α-tocopherol treatment on newborn rat lung development and injury in hyperoxia. Pediatr Pharmacol 2:1, 1982.
124. Chiswick ML, Wynn J, Toner N: Vitamin E and intraventricular hemorrhage in the newborn. Ann NY Acad Sci 293:109, 1982.

125. Colburn WA, Ehrenkranz RA: Pharmacokinetics of a single intramuscular injection of vitamin E to premature neonates. Ped Pharmacol 3:7, 1983.
126. Csallany AS, Draper HH, Shah SN: Conversion of d,1-alpha-tocopheryl-C^{14} to tocopheryl-p-quinone in vivo. Arch Biochem Biophys 98:142, 1962.
127. Ehrenkranz RA: Vitamin E and the neonate. Am J Dis Child 134:1157, 1980.
128. Ehrenkranz RA, Ablow RC, Warshaw JB: Effect of vitamin E on the development of oxygen-induced lung injury in neonates. Ann NY Acad Sci 393:452, 1982.
129. Filer LJ Jr, Wright SW, Manning MP, Mason KE: Absorption of α-tocopherol and tocopheryl esters by premature and full-term infants and children in health and disease. Pediatrics 8:328, 1951.
130. Finer NN, Schindler RF, Grant G, Hill GB: Effect of intramuscular vitamin E on frequency and severity of retrolental fibroplasia. Lancet 1:1087, 1982.
131. Gallo-Torres HE, Miller ON: Tissue uptake and metabolism of d,1-3,4-$^3H_2$-a-tocopheryl nicotinate and d,1-a-tocopheryl-1,2-$^3H_2$-acetate following intravenous administration. J Vitam Nutr 41:339, 1971.
132. Gallo-Torres HE: Absorption, transport and metabolism. In Machlin LJ (ed): Vitamin E: A Comprehensive Treatise. Chap 5A and 5B. New York, Marcel Dekker, 1980.
133. Graeber JE, Williams ML, Oski FA: The use of intramuscular vitamin E in the premature infant. J Pediatr 90:282, 1977.
134. Gross S, Melhorn DK: Vitamin E–dependent anemia in the premature infant. III. Comparative hemoglobin, vitamin E, and erythrocyte phospholipid responses following absorption of either water-soluble or fat-soluble d-alpha tocopheryl. J Pediatr 85:753, 1974.
135. Gross SJ: Vitamin E and neonatal bilirubinemia. Pediatrics 64:321, 1979.
136. Hittner HM, Godio LB, Rudolph AJ, et al: Retrolental fibroplasia: Efficacy of vitamin E in a double-blind clinical study of preterm infants. N Engl J Med 305:1365, 1981.
137. Hittner HM, Godio LB, Speer ME, et al: Retrolental fibroplasia: Further clinical evidence and ultrastructural support for efficacy of vitamin E in the preterm infant. Pediatrics 71:423, 1983.
138. Horwitt MK: Vitamin E: A re-examination. Am J Clin Nutr 29:569, 1976.
139. Krishnamurthy S, Bieri JG: The absorption, storage, and metabolism of α-tocopherol-C^{14} in the rat and chicken. J Lipid Res 4:330, 1963.
140. Lake AM, Stuart MJ, Oski FA: Vitamin E deficiency and enhanced platelet function: Reversal following E supplementation. J Pediatr 90:722, 1977.
141. Lucy JA: Part I. Cellular biochemistry of vitamin E: Functional and structural aspects of biolgical membranes: A suggested structural role for vitamin E in the control of membrane permeability and stability. Ann NY Acad Sci 203:4, 1972.
142. Machlin LJ, Gabriel E: Kinetics of tissue α-tocopherol uptake and depletion following administration of high levels of vitamin E. Ann NY Acad Sci 293:48, 1982.
143. McClung HJ, Backes C, Lavin A, Kerzner B: Prospective evaluation of vitamin E therapy in premature infants with hyaline membrane disease (HMD). Pediatr Res 14:604, 1980.
144. Melhorn DK, Gross S: Vitamin E–dependent anemia in the premature infant. II. Relationships between

gestational age and absorption of vitamin E. J Pediatr 79:581, 1971.

145. Milner RA, Watts JL, Paes B, et al: RLF in 1500 gram neonates: Part of a randomized clinical trial of the effectiveness of vitamin E. Retinopathy of Prematurity Conference Syllabus, Washington DC, Dec 4–6, 1981, Vol 2, p 703.

146. Muller DPR, Manning JA, Mathias PM, Harries JT: Studies on the intestinal hydrolysis of tocopheryl esters. Int J Vitam Nutr Res 46:207, 1976.

147. Nakano M, Sugioka K, Nakamura T, Oki T: Interaction between an organic hydroperoxide and an unsaturated phospholipid and alpha-tocopherol in model membranes. Biochim Biophys Acta 619:274, 1980.

148. Phelps DL: Vitamin E and retrolental fibroplasia in 1982. Pediatrics 70:420, 1982.

149. Prasad JS: Effect of vitamin E supplementation on leukocyte function. Am J Clin Nutr 33:606, 1980.

150. Puklin JE, Simon RM, Ehrenkranz RA: Influence on retrolental fibroplasia of intramuscular vitamin E administration during respiratory distress syndrome. Ophthalmology 89:96, 1982.

151. Reddy CC, Scholz RW, Thomas CE, Massaro EJ: Vitamin E–dependent reduced glutathione inhibition of rat liver microsomal lipid peroxidaton. Life Sci 31:571, 1982.

152. Roberts HJ: Perspective on vitamin E as therapy. JAMA 246:129, 1981.

153. Roberts RJ: Vitamin E in respiratory distress. In Filer LJ, Leathem WD (eds): Parenteral Nutrition in the Infant Patient. North Chicago IL, Abbott Laboratories Hospital Products Division, 1983.

154. Rosenfeld W, Evans H, Jhaveri R, et al: Safety and plasma concentrations of bovine superoxide dismutase administered to human premature infants. Dev Pharmacol Ther 5:151, 1982.

155. Saldanha RL, Cepeda EE, Poland RL: The effect of vitamin E prophylaxis on the incidence and severity of bronchopulmonary dysplasia. J Pediatr 101:89, 1982.

156. Steiner M: Effect of alpha-tocopherol administration on platelet function in man. Thromb Haemost 49:1, 1983.

157. Stuart MJ, Oski FA: Vitamin E and platelet function. Am J Pediatr Hematol Oncol 1:77, 1979.

158. Zipursky A, Milner RA, Blanchette VS, Johnston MA: Effect of vitamin E therapy on blood coagulation tests in newborn infants. Pediatrics 66:547, 1980.

Additional References

Prostaglandins

159. Coe JY, Radley-Smith R, Yacoub M: Management of tricuspid atresia with orally administered prostaglandin E_2. J Pediatr 100:496, 1982.

160. Cole RB, Abman S, Aziz KU, et al: Prolonged prostaglandin E_1 infusion: Histologic effects on the patent ductus arteriosus. Pediatrics 67:816, 1981.

161. Heymann MA, Clyman RI: Evaluation of alprostadil (prostaglandin E_1) in the management of congenital heart disease in infancy. Pharmacotherapy 2:148, 1982.

162. Leffler CW, Tyler TL, Cassin S: Effect of indomethacin on pulmonary vascular response to ventilation of fetal goats. Am J Physiol 234:H346, 1978.

163. Pitlick P, French JW, Maze A, et al. Long-term low-dose prostaglandin E_1 administration. J Pediatr 96:318, 1980.

164. Ringel RE, Haney PJ, Brenner JI, et al: Periosteal changes secondary to prostaglandin administration. J Pediatr 103:251, 1983.

165. Soifer SJ, Morin FC III, Kaslow DC, Heymann MA: The developmental effects of prostaglandin D_2 on the pulmonary and systemic circulations in the newborn lamb. J Develop Physiol 5:237, 1983.

166. Stenmark KR, James SL, Voelkel NF, et al: Leukotriene C_4 and D_4 in neonates with hypoxemia and pulmonary hypertension. New Engl J Med 309:77, 1983.

Indomethacin

167. Bedard MP, Kotagal UR, Kleinman LI: Acute cardiovascular effects of indomethacin in anesthetized newborn dogs. Dev Pharmacol Ther 6:179, 1983.

168. Clyman RI, Brett C, Mauray F: Circulating prostaglandin E_2 concentrations and incidence of patent ductus arteriosus in preterm infants with respiratory distress syndrome. Pediatrics 66:725, 1980.

169. Honoré B, Brodersen R, Robertson A: Interaction of indomethacin with adult human albumin and neonatal serum. Dev Pharmacol Ther 6:347, 1983.

170. Lock JE, Olley PM, Soldin S, Coceani F: Indomethacin-induced pulmonary vasoconstriction in the conscious newborn lamb. Am J Physiol 238:H639, 1980.

171. Rudd P, Montanez P, Hallidie-Smith K, Silverman M: Indomethacin treatment for patent ductus arteriosus in very low birthweight infants: double blind trial. Arch Dis Child 58:267, 1983.

172. Schlegel W, Stein W, Toussaint R, et al: Concentrations of prostaglandin E_2 and F_{2a} in the cardiovascular system of infants with persisting patent ductus arteriosus. Horm metabol Res 15:377, 1983.

173. Seyberth HW, Rascher W, Hackenthal R, Willie L: Effect of prolonged indomethacin therapy on renal function and selected vasoactive hormones in very-low-birth-weight infants with symptomatic patent ductus arteriosus. J Pediatr 103:979, 1983.

174. Tyler T, Wallis R, Leffler C, Cassin S: The effects of indomethacin on the pulmonary vascular response to hypoxia in the premature and mature newborn goat. Proc Soc Exp Biol Med 150:695, 1975.

175. Winther J, Printz MP, Mendoza SA, et al: The influence of indomethacin on neonatal renal function. Pediatr Res 11:402, 1977.

176. Yam J, Roberts RJ: Modification of alveolar hyperoxia induced pulmonary vasodilation by indomethacin. Prostaglandins 11:679, 1976.

177. Yeh TF, Raval D, Lilien LD, et al: Decreased plasma glucose following indomethacin therapy in premature infants with patent ductus arteriosus. Pediatr Pharmacol 2:171, 1982.

178. Yeh TF, Luken J, Raval D, et al: Indomethacin treatment in small versus large premature infants with ductus arteriosus: Comparison of plasma indomethacin concentration and clinical response. Br Heart J 50:27, 1983.

Vitamin E

179. Bieri, JG, Evarts RP, Gart JJ: Relative activity of α-tocopherol and γ-tocopherol in preventing oxidative red cell hemolysis. J Nutr 106:124, 1976

180. Chiswick ML, Johnson M, Woodhall C, et al: Protective effect of vitamin E (DL-alpha-tocopherol) against intraventricular haemorrhage in premature babies. Br Med J 287:81, 1983.

182. Finer NN, Schindler RF, Peters KL, Grant GD: Vitamin E and retrolental fibroplasia: Improved visual outcome with early vitamin E. Ophthalmology 90:428, 1983.

183. Hittner HM, Kretzer FL, Rudolph AJ, et al: Vitamin E in retrolental fibroplasia. New Engl J Med 309:669, 1983.

184. Hittner HM, Kretzer FL: Vitamin E and retrolental fibroplasia: Ultrastructural mechanism of clinical efficacy. In Diplock AT, Porter R (eds): Ciba Foundation Symposium on Biology of Vitamin E. London: Pitman Books, 1983, p 165.

185. Newmark HL, Pool W, Bauernfeind JC, DeRitter E: Biopharmaceutical factors in parenteral administration of vitamin E. J Pharmaceut Sci 64:655, 1975.

186. Smith IJ, Buchanan MFG, Goss I, Congdon PJ: Vitamin E in retrolental fibroplasia. New Eng J Med 309:669, 1983.

187. Sobel S, Gueriguian J, Troendle G, Nevius E: Vitamin E in retrolental fibroplasia. New Eng J Med 306:867, 1982.

188. Weiter JJ: Retrolental fibroplasia: An unsolved problem. New Eng J Med 305:1404, 1981.

TEN

Miscellaneous Drugs

AGENTS FOR REDUCING OR ENHANCING SECRETORY ACTIVITY

See also H_2-Receptor Antagonists: Cimetidine later in this chapter.

Atropine

Pharmacology. Atropine, an alkaloid produced by plants of the Solanaceae family (e.g., deadly nightshade), is one of the older drugs still widely used in medicine. Many attempts have been made to selectively alter the structure–activity relationships of the atropine molecule in an effort to elicit only specific anticholinergic actions.

Atropine is completely ionized ($pK_a = 9.8$) in acid environments ($pH < 2.5$) and as a result is absorbed rapidly from the intestinal tract but not the stomach. The pharmacologic activity of IM or IV administered atropine is two- to threefold greater than that of the drug given PO.[20] About 20% of the drug in plasma is bound to protein.[9] The plasma half-life in adults has been determined, by specific assay for atropine, to be 4 hours.[1] The drug is excreted in the urine primarily unchanged (80% of dose excreted in 8 hr).

Atropine is a competitive inhibitor of the actions of acetylcholine on muscarinic receptors, which include exocrine glands, smooth and cardiac muscle, and postganglionic cholinergic nerve terminals. The physiologic effects of atropine are summarized in Table 10–1. Atropine can produce a biphasic response on heart rate by altering the balance between the accelerator effects of the sympathetic system and the more dominant slowing effects of the parasympathetic system. Bradycardia can occur initially, but this effect is generally transient and

mild; suggested mechanisms include centrally mediated vagal stimulation (not likely), inhibition of cholinesterase at the S-A node receptor site, thereby allowing a transient increase in acetylcholine, and a membrane-depolarizing effect.[19] The heart rate then returns to normal or increases, depending upon the dose given and the extent of vagal influence on heart rate at the time. In infants, vagal tone is believed to be significantly less than in young adults. Thus, minimal increases in heart rate may occur in infants. Usually, tachycardia occurs only with rapid IV injection of atropine over less than 1 minute; the increase in heart rate is a direct result of blockade of vagal (slowing) effects on the S-A node by the drug. Atropine can abolish many types of reflex vagal cardiac slowing, particularly stimulation associated with occular and peritoneal surgical manipulations. An acceleration effect on A-V node conduction is uniform at all doses. The P–R interval is shortened linearly according to the dose of atropine administered. Changes in heart rate correlate best with estimates of tissue levels rather than plasma levels of atropine. The time to peak tachycardia is 12 to 16 minutes, and the duration of action is 6 hours.[1] Factors that can influence the chronotropic action of atropine are shown in Table 10–2.

Atropine can cause cardiac arrhythmias, particularly during the first 2 minutes following IV administration. Lower doses are more apt to cause arrhythymias than large doses, particularly in infants.[3] The arrhythmia is usually a simple atrioventricular (A-V) dissociation with nodal rhythm, atrial rhythm, and ventricular ectopic beats. Atropine in therapeutic doses has little effect on blood pressure or perfusion. Of note is the ability of atropine in vitro to block the constricting effect of oxygen on the ductus arteriosus.[16]

Table 10–1. **PHYSIOLOGIC EFFECTS OF ATROPINE**[a]

Body System	Effect of Atropine
Cardiovascular	
heart	
rate	biphasic effect possible: initial decrease followed by return to normal and progressing to tachycardia; with rapid IV administration, tachycardia only
cardiac output	increased with tachycardia; stroke volume unchanged or decreased
vasculature	
peripheral	resistance unchanged or mildly decreased
pulmonary	fall in pressure
ductus arteriosus	blockade of constricting effect of oxygen in vitro
Gastrointestinal	
esophageal sphincter	lowered tone with increased risk for regurgitation
tone and contraction	reduced but not completely inhibited; parasympathomimetic effects of other drugs completely inhibited
secretions	salivary secretions completely inhibited, gastric secretions (volume and acid content) only partially inhibited; no significant effect on pancreatic, biliary, or intrinsic intestinal secretions
Respiratory	
airways	dilation greater in larger than smaller airways (improved airway conductance), with increase in anatomical dead space by as much as 30%
pharyngeal reflex	no direct action to prevent laryngospasm
CNS	mild to profound depression depending on dose; at clinical doses, lethargy with tendency to sleep and reduced ability to concentrate
Ocular	dilation of pupil, loss of accommodation

[a] Data from Shutt LE, Bowes JB: Anaesthesia 34:476, 1979.

Vagal influences on the gastrointestinal tract are only partially inhibited by atropine. Motor activity in the stomach and small and large bowel is reduced by atropine, causing a decrease in tone and in amplitude and frequency of peristaltic contractions. Because of the existence of complex intrinsic motor activity, complete inhibition of gastrointestinal tone and movement is not observed following even large doses of atropine. Esophageal sphincter tone is reduced sufficiently to increase the risk of esophageal reflux. Atropine does effectively inhibit cholin-

Table 10–2. **FACTORS INFLUENCING THE CHRONOTROPIC RESPONSE TO ATROPINE**

Factor	Atropine Response	Suggested Mechanism
age	less change in heart rate in infants and elderly	diminished vagal "tone"
exercise	less absolute heart rate increase at greater workloads	vagal preponderance reduced by exercise
increased environmental temperature	increased heart rate; in hot dry climate, possible circulatory collapse	inhibition of sweating, further vasodilation, temperature elevation
race	Blacks less susceptible than Caucasians	?genetic variation: lower resting pulse rates
Down's syndrome	increased sensitivity to cardioaccelerator effect	pharmacogenetic abnormality affecting autonomic receptors
hyperthyroidism	smaller-than-normal increase in heart rate from a resting tachycardia	direct rate-increasing effect of thyroxine on S-A node and impairment of vagal inhibition of heart rate
diabetes	small response in patients with autonomic neuropathy	neuropathy affecting cardiac efferent nerves
uremia	flat dose-response curve	impaired vagal function or decreased sensitivity of pacemaker cells to acetylcholine
coronary heart disease	smaller increase in heart rate in patients with two- and three-vessel occlusive disease than in normals.	possibly reduced blood supply to S-A node
digitalis	little response in digitalized patients	vagotonic effect superseded by the direct myocardial effect of digitalis at high doses
morphine, fentanyl	less cardioacceleration after low doses	central vagal stimulation by opiates

ergic actions of parasympathomimetic drugs on the gastrointestinal tract. Salivary secretion is effectively inhibited by atropine, but gastric secretion is only minimally reduced in volume and total acid content. There is little effect of atropine on pancreatic, bile, or intrinsic intestinal secretions.

Atropine relaxes the smooth muscles located in the bronchi and bronchioles, thereby reducing airway resistance and increasing dead space by as much as 30%.[7] The larger airways are affected more than the smaller airways. Atropine is a potent inhibitor of bronchoconstriction produced by parasympathomimetic drugs and is moderately active against histamine. Contrary to popular belief, atropine does not have any intrinsic action on the pharyngeal reflex and therefore has *no direct action in prevention of laryngospasm.*[18] Any observed benefit in this regard probably is related to depression of upper airway secretions, which can precipitate reflex laryngospasm.

Although atropine in therapeutic doses has been considered a CNS stimulant, the proposal for such a pharmacologic role probably relates to reported subjective sensations of its peripheral effects, not to direct central effects. Therapeutic doses can cause lethargy, sedation, and decreased ability to concentrate;[3,19] toxic doses are associated with CNS stimulation. This dose-dependent difference in CNS effects probably relates to the penetration of the drug into the CNS.

Other physiologic effects of atropine include dilation of the pupil and loss of visual accommodation by blockade of cholinergic activation of the ciliary muscle in the eye. Patients with Down's syndrome show a marked sensitivity for mydriasis as well as to the cardioacceleratory effects of atropine.[6] These effects can develop with either local or systemic administration. Little effect on intraocular pressure occurs with systemic administration, but local ocular application can produce significant increases. The increased intraocular pressure can persist for up to 6 days and, rarely, can lead to blindness in patients with narrow-angle glaucoma. High systemic doses can also produce difficulty with micturition and a fall in fasting blood glucose levels.

Clinical Pharmacology. One of the earliest studies of atropine in infants attempted to define sensitivity to the drug at various ages (newborn – 12 yr) by examination of suppression of salivation.[20] In 129 children, the minimal effective dose of atropine was found to be smaller in infants from birth to 12 months of age and in

children from 1 to 3 years old (0.16 and 0.14 mg/kg PO, respectively) than in older children (aged 3 – 12 yr, 0.20 – 0.22 mg/kg PO). The ratio between oral and parenteral dose equivalency was about 3 to 1, respectively, in all age groups. The maximum effect on secretions occurred between 1 and 2 hours after PO administration, and the effect lasted for a period of 4 hours. There was no indication of tolerance with repeated dosing.

Dauchot and Gravenstein[3] observed atropine-induced arrhythmias to be particularly frequent in young children compared with adults. The doses of atropine employed in their study ranged from 0.0018 to 0.0143 mg/kg given IV. The smaller doses shortened the P–R interval and either lowered the heart rate or had no effect; the larger doses increased the heart rate and shortened the P–R interval. The percentage of decrease in heart rate was greatest in adults.

Kattwinkel and coworkers[8] studied the use of atropine for treatment of bradycardia in eight pre-term infants. The bradycardia was associated with feedings (in four infants), surgical manipulation of visceral structures (in three), and chronic lung disease (in one). A wide range of doses were employed (0.02 – 0.09 mg/kg PO), with resolution of the bradycardia in seven infants and further deterioration in one.

Adams and colleagues[1] studied the pharmacokinetics of atropine given IV by radioimmunoassay in six normal adults. Plasma disappearance followed a biexponential curve, with an elimination half-life of 4 hours. The maximum clinical response as measured by pulse rate occurred between 12 and 16 minutes after IV administration, consistent with the time of maximal tissue drug levels. The volume of distribution was estimated to be 3 l/kg.

Therapeutic Indications. Atropine has been employed as a therapeutic agent in a wide variety of clinical problems. Despite this experience, the indications for atropine are few. Its routine use as a premedication in anesthesia can no longer be condoned,[4,11,13,19] for the following reasons cited in various studies: inadequate effect on airway secretions, loss of lower-esophageal spincter tone, lack of protective effect against laryngospasm, and increased incidence of arrhythmias and other side-effects during anesthesia. The exception is ocular surgery, where *oculocardiac-induced reflex bradycardia* and even cardiac arrest can be prevented with anticholinergics.[12]

Reversal of bradycardia is a legitimate use of atropine, particularly when the etiology is a predominance of parasympathetic influences on the heart (digoxin, β-blocker drugs, hyperactive carotid sinus reflex). The recommended dose is 0.01 mg/kg given IV over 1 minute. This dose may be repeated every 10 to 15 minutes to achieve the desired effect, with a maximum total dose of 0.04 mg/kg. For cardiovascular resuscitation, atropine may be given intratracheally for immediate effect if an IV route is not available.

The use of belladonna alkaloids including atropine and synthetic substitutes for gastrointestinal "colic" in the infant has been demonstrated not to result in symptomatic relief.[17]

Clinical Toxicology. The signs and symptoms of atropine toxicity are dose-related. Initial or low-dose toxicities include dilated pupils, dry mucous membranes, blurred vision, flushed skin with rash (upper trunk, neck, and face), and fever. Fever can be a particularly serious problem in infants and children.[19] Larger doses can produce tachycardia and abdominal distention with absent bowel activity. Sedation is followed by excitation with increasing doses. Cardiac arrhythmias can also occur (see under Pharmacology). Systemic toxicities have been reported in neonates following topical instillation of atropine-like drugs into the eye.[2]

Glycopyrrolate

Glycopyrrolate, a relatively new anticholinergic drug compared to atropine, possesses a potent antisialogogue action with minimal cardiovascular effects and absence of CNS effects.[10,15] Comparative studies of atropine and glycopyrrolate indicate that glycopyrrolate produces adequate control of secretions, with one report in adults suggesting better drying effects with glycopyrrolate.[14,15] In clinical trials in children, the incidence of dysrhythmias was similar for glycopyrrolate (5%) and for atropine (3.3%).[10] Fontán and colleagues[256] utilized glycopyrrolate in a 3 week old infant with esophageal spasm associated with apnea and bradycardia. Glycopyrrolate (8 μg/kg IV) reduced the amplitude, frequency, and duration of the esophageal spasms; there was also an associated improvement in apnea and bradycardia. The infant was subsequently treated with an oral dose of glycopyrrolate (1000 μg/kg/day, dosing interval not indicated) sufficient to increase heart rate by 10%. After 5 days of oral therapy, fewer than 5 mild episodes of apnea and bradycardia per day were observed compared with 14 episodes during a control (no drug) period. The use of glycopyrrolate in infants should be considered experimental. The recommended dose of glycopyrrolate is 2.5 to 5 μg/kg IV or IM given every 4 to 8 hours. In children and adults, the recommended PO dose is 10 times the parenteral dose (20 to 50 μg/kg) given 2 to 3 times daily; no PO dosing interval information is available for infants.

Bethanechol

Pharmacology. Bethanechol is a parasympathomimetic agent that produces stimulant actions on the gastrointestinal tract and urinary bladder similar to the effects of acetylcholine. Effects on the gastrointestinal tract include an increase in tone, amplitude of contractions and peristaltic activity of the esophagus, stomach, and intestine, and enhanced secretory activity. In the urinary bladder, bethanechol causes a contraction of the muscle. All of these effects can be competitively antagonized by atropine. Bethanechol produces minimal cardiovascular effects but its potency in ocular effects exceeds that of acetylcholine. Effects on the respiratory system include bronchoconstriction and increased tracheobronchial secretions. Bethanechol is virtually resistant to hydrolysis by acetylcholinesterases.

Clinical Pharmacology. Bethanechol has been used for the treatment of gastroesophageal reflux in infants and children.[21,22,268] In a double-blind crossover study involving 30 infants less than 1 year old, Euler[21] observed a significant symptomatic improvement and weight gain during bethanechol treatment, 3 mg/m² of body surface per dose given PO every 8 hours. The number of vomiting episodes also diminished during drug therapy. Lower esophageal sphincter pressure increased from 12.8 ± 4.2 mm Hg to a maximum of 26.8 ± 3.0 mm Hg 30 minutes after dosing. The number of episodes of gastroesophageal reflux as monitored by an esophageal pH probe decreased from 5.8 ± 1.1 to 1.8 ± 1.3 episodes per hour, and the duration of the episodes decreased from 4.3 ± 1.2 to 1.5 ± 1.3 minutes. Gastric emptying was not evaluated. The duration of treatment was 3 to 4 months in most infants. Strickland and Chang,[22] using the same dose of bethanechol (3 mg/m² PO q 8 hr), noted improvement as measured by a gastroesophageal reflux scoring system in 28 of 37 infants (76%). The frequency of reflux or duration did not decrease with bethanechol treatment during the feeding period but did decrease during the fasted period. These data correlated with testimony of parents that symptoms of restlessness, irritability, and vomiting diminished between feedings, with minimal effects on vomiting of formula immediately after feedings. No significant complications, other than dizziness and headache during the first week of therapy in one 5-year-old child, were noted in these studies.

Sondheimer and colleagues[268] studied 11 infants (0.5 to 7.5 months old) with gastroesophageal reflux who also had symptoms of failure to thrive, emesis, and apnea. Bethanechol (0.1 mg/kg PO 4 times daily 15 minutes before feedings and before sleep) decreased the time that pH was <4 in 8 of 11 patients, decreased the time of individual episodes of reflux in 9 of 11 patients, and improved the acid clearance time in 10 of 11 patients. The frequency of reflux episodes improved in only 4 of 11 patients. In a 6 week outpatient trial in these 11 patients, improvement occurred in 8 of 11 patients. These investigators speculate that the therapeutic effect of bethanechol is the result of improved esophageal motor function rather than improved gastric emptying or augmented lower esophageal sphincter pressure.

Therapeutic Indications. The recommended dose of bethanechol for treatment of *gastroesophageal reflux* is 0.1 to 0.2 mg/kg given PO before each meal (maximum 4 times daily). The dose should be given between 30 minutes to 1 hour prior to feeding. Contraindications for treatment with bethanechol include esophageal stricture and presence of pulmonary disease.[21]

AGENTS FOR CORRECTING METABOLIC IMBALANCES

See also Strychnine Therapy for Nonketotic Hyperglycinemia later in this chapter.

Bicarbonate

Pharmacology. Sodium bicarbonate or $NaHCO_3$ is the alkali most frequently employed for correction of metabolic acidosis. It is generally administered IV for acute management of metabolic acidosis but is also well absorbed from the gastrointestinal tract.[30] From 20% to 60% of an orally administered dose can be recovered in the form of expired carbon dioxide.[33,35] The apparent bicarbonate space has been estimated to be 74% of body weight, with a range of 37% to 134%.[43] Most calculations of

bicarbonate dosage are based on a volume of distribution of 0.3 to 0.4 l/kg body weight.[37] An accurate estimate of the volume of distribution for bicarbonate is difficult because of its rapid metabolism, shifts in solute-free water into the interstitial and intravascular compartments, and the existing endogenous production and pools of bicarbonate.

The capacity of a buffer to minimize changes in pH is greatest when the concentration ratio of the anion form (HCO_3^-) to the acid form (H_2CO_3) is 1:1 (pK_a). For carbonic acid (H_2CO_3), this optimal pH (or pK_a) is 3.6, which is comparable to that of pyruvic and lactic acids. However, because of the dissociation of carbonic acid into water and the volatile gas, carbon dioxide, the actual pK_a for the bicarbonate system (represented by the following set of reactions) is 6.1.

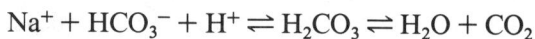

$$Na^+ + HCO_3^- + H^+ \rightleftharpoons H_2CO_3 \rightleftharpoons H_2O + CO_2$$

AT pH 7.4 the ratio of the anion (HCO_3^-) to the acid form (H_2CO_3) is 20:1. This means that the efficiency of the bicarbonate system as a buffer is dependent upon the dissociation of carbonic acid to water and carbon dioxide. Therefore, the regulation of carbon dioxide blood levels (reduction by respiratory excretion) is critical in forcing the bicarbonate system reaction to proceed actively to the right, resulting in maximum buffering activity:

$$pH = 6.1 + \log \frac{[HCO_3] \text{ mEq/l}}{[PaCO_2 \text{ mmHg}] \times (0.03)}$$

where 0.03 is the conversion factor for PCO_2 to millimoles per liter.

From this equation (Henderson-Hasselbalch) it can be appreciated that the pH varies inversely with $PaCO_2$ and is ultimately determined by the ratio of the concentrations of bicarbonate and carbon dioxide. If elevation of $PaCO_2$ occurs with rapid bicarbonate infusion, such as in situations of lung disease or inadequate ventilation where the ability to excrete carbon dioxide is compromised, little or no increase in pH will occur.[35,44] This concern regarding the use of bicarbonate has not been universally accepted.[24,29,37] The renal excretion of bicarbonate is reviewed in Chapter 8.

Clinical Pharmacology. The administration of alkali to neonates for treatment of metabolic acidosis became popular in the late 1950s with the availability of bicarbonate-containing pharmaceutical products. In one of the earliest attempts at a controlled trial, Usher[46] demonstrated that the mortality rate among 35 premature infants with respiratory distress syndrome (RDS) given sodium bicarbonate was 17% compared with 37% in 35 control infants. No significant effect was observed in infants weighing less than 1500 grams at birth. The infants in this study received 1.5–2 mEq/kg of sodium bicarbonate as a constant IV infusion over 24 hours along with 10% glucose. Other studies[32,39,40,43] have examined the question of early correction of acidemia in RDS using infusion and bolus dosing with hyperosmolar bicarbonate solutions. Sinclair and coworkers[43] utilized a slow bicarbonate treatment (dose sufficient to correct pH to >7.3 within 24 hr) and rapid dosing (total correction of pH to >7.3 with bicarbonate, 44.6 mEq/50 ml, given intra-arterially over 5 min) in a randomized study. No significant difference in mortality between the two regimens was observed.

Russell and Cotton[39] employed a bolus dose of bicarbonate calculated from base deficit determinations; they concluded that early correction of acidosis in 19 infants with RDS resulted in improved pulmonary function as a result of decreased pulmonary vascular resistance, reduced right-to-left shunt, and improved pulmonary capillary perfusion. Although the results of these and other studies conflict, the employment of vigorous bicarbonate resuscitation has become widespread.

Ostrea and Odell[35] studied the acid-base properties of blood in vitro and demonstrated that if the carbon dioxide generated from the bicarbonate buffering system cannot escape (closed system), the resulting rise in pH is relatively small. In addition, these studies showed that if hypertonic bicarbonate solutions are employed, more carbon dioxide is produced from bicarbonate owing to increasing acidic properties of hemoglobin. The overall effect of these two factors—retention and increased production of carbon dioxide from bicarbonate—could lead to an actual fall in blood pH with bicarbonate administration rather than the expected rise. Observations from clinical situations analogous to this in vitro study have been conflicting. Evans and colleagues[30] studied the effect of infusions of bicarbonate on asphyxiated newborns who were breathing spontaneously. Bicarbonate given via intragastric tube or IV (2.6–1.3 mEq/kg) failed to correct the low pH and led to elevations of $PaCO_2$.

Baum and Robertson[24] infused 5- or 10-ml volumes of bicarbonate (1 M, equal to 8.4% solution) with an osmolality of 1680 mOsm/kg water into neonates with severe RDS. The overall mean rise in pH over a 10-minute period was 0.1 unit of pH. The $PaCO_2$ rose sharply after bicarbonate infusion and remained elevated throughout the 10-minute observation period. Osmolality of the serum increased also, the greatest rise (25 mOsm/kg H_2O) occurring in neonates receiving a dose of bicarbonate over 30 seconds. No abrupt rise in PaO_2 occurred in any neonate. These authors concluded that severe respiratory distress did not constitute a closed system and that even in the presence of an increased $PaCO_2$, the pH will increase with bicarbonate administration.

Bland and coworkers,[26] in a randomized and a controlled prospective study, evaluated the effectiveness of rapid infusions of sodium bicarbonate given in the first 2 hours of life to premature infants. The dose of bicarbonate was 1.5 or 3.0 ml/kg of a 7.5 gm/100 ml bicarbonate solution. No differences were observed in blood gases or outcome (incidence of respiratory distress, intracranial hemorrhage, mortality) between newborns receiving alkali and those receiving glucose.

Rhodes and colleagues[37] examined the effect of hypertonic sodium bicarbonate on whole blood and red cell pH, body fluid toxicity, and plasma and red cell water and solute. A 1.0 M solution was infused at 0.3 ml/kg per minute to provide a dose of bicarbonate in mEq equal to $(0.4) \times$ (weight in kg) $\times$ (negative base excess). The study involved neonates with acidosis associated with RDS and other forms of neonatal asphyxia. The mean bicarbonate dose was 4.5 ± 1.2 mEq. Significant increases were observed in body fluid tonicity and arterial pH and $PaCO_2$, although the authors noted no clear pattern of change in arterial blood gases. The osmotic load imposed by the hypertonic bicarbonate infusion caused a shift of solute-free water into the interstitial and intravascular fluids. The authors concluded that the results were inconclusive relative to the merits of prompt correction of metabolic acidosis versus the potentially harmful effects of the osmotic load imposed by the infusion of hypertonic bicarbonate.

Corbet and coworkers[27] examined the effects of liberal (average dose of 2.2 mEq/kg at birth plus 3.6 mEq/kg in first 24 hr of life) versus restricted (1.5 mEq/kg at birth only) bicarbonate therapy on mortality and incidence of intraventricular hemorrhage in 62 high-risk neonates. The definition of high-risk included any of the following criteria: birth weight less than 1.5 kg, less than 32 weeks' gestation, Apgar score of less than 3 at 1 minute, diagnosis of hyaline membrane disease, or birth weight less than 2 kg and requiring assisted ventilation. There was no significant difference in the rate at which arterial pH was corrected between the restricted- and liberal-intake groups. No statistically significant differences were observed between treatment groups in intraventricular hemorrhage or mortality. Thus, no supporting evidence was found for continued prophylactic infusion of bicarbonate. The authors noted that with adequate control of blood pressure by means of vascular volume expansion and with blood oxygenation via use of supplemental inspired oxygen and positive airway pressure, the requirement for sodium bicarbonate was not large.

Despite the lack of evidence for its beneficial effects, prophylactic bicarbonate therapy has been employed in increasing numbers of sick infants. The incidence of intracranial hemorrhage has been noted to increase simultaneously, leading to the controversy regarding the relationship between CNS hemorrhage and IV sodium bicarbonate therapy (bolus or infusion of hypertonic solutions).[29,31] Baum and Roberts[24] reported that a single dose of 4 mEq/kg of bicarbonate given over 30 seconds raises the serum osmolality an average of 25 mOsm/kg water. A significant increase in intraventricular hemorrhage was noted in neonates who received a rapid infusion of hyperosmolar (1 to 0.5 M) sodium bicarbonate.[36] CNS hemorrhage secondary to hypertonic sodium bicarbonate infusion appears to be associated with a downward osmolal concentration gradient between plasma and the CNS fluids; this occurs only with rapid infusion of a hypertonic solution, the critical variables being concentration, rate, and total bicarbonate dose. Molar concentrations of sodium bicarbonate are the most dangerous.

Therapeutic Indications. *Persistent and severe metabolic acidosis* (pH < 7.15) despite maximum cardiorespiratory support is an indication for controlled infusion of 0.5 mEq/ml sodium bicarbonate solution. Careful attention to maintenance of thermal neutrality and adequate vascular perfusion by plasma volume expansion or pharmacologic therapy are essential, and ventilatory support with supplemental oxygen therapy if necessary should be in place preferably before, but certainly coincident with, sodium bicarbonate therapy.[24,29]

Dosage recommendations for correction of acidosis are somewhat arbitrary from a therapeutic point of view, since correction of acidosis can be influenced by other supportive procedures. Avoiding toxicity, therefore, becomes a primary objective in dosage considerations. The following dosage calculation is based on minimizing the osmotic challenge yet maximizing the buffering capability:

$$\text{dose (mEq } HCO_3^-) = \text{(weight in kg)} \times (0.4) \times \left(\begin{array}{c} \text{base deficit} \\ \text{in mEq/l} \end{array} \right)$$

The base deficit must be derived from an accurate determination of pH, pCO_2, and pO_2 in an arterial blood sample. Administration of half the calculated dose has been advocated for a variety of reasons including minimizing the dose of sodium and fluid. If the patient is truly a candidate for bicarbonate therapy, this approach seems arbitrary. The recommended rate of infusion is no more rapid than 1 mEq of bicarbonate/kg per minute.[24] The concentration of bicarbonate employed should be no greater than 0.5 mEq/ml (4.2 gm/100 ml).

For emergency *cardiac resuscitation* the recommended procedure is institution of bicarbonate therapy if metabolic acidosis is suspected despite maximal cardiopulmonary resuscitation. Studies by Bishop and Weisfeld[25] demonstrated that metabolic acidosis associated with cardiac arrest can be adequately managed with ventilation and cardiac massage without the use of bicarbonate. The recommended initial dose is 1 mEq/kg by either bolus injection or infusion over 10 minutes.[23] A second dose can be given if effective circulation is not restored, but additional doses should be based on blood gas and pH measurements.

Sodium bicarbonate is effective for correction of bicarbonate deficit due to *renal or gastrointestinal loss*. Infants with low renal bicarbonate threshold (renal tubular acidosis) have been effectively managed with oral bicarbonate therapy.[28,34,38] The recommended dose is 3 to 15 mEq/kg per day given PO with feedings.

The value of bicarbonate therapy in "hypobasemia"[41] or "late metabolic acidosis" in low-birth-weight infants[34] is controversial. In a comparative study of the efficacy of bicarbonate and saline, Schwartz and colleagues[41] found no difference between treatment groups in weight gain by low-birth-weight infants whose condition satisfied the definition of late metabolic acidosis. It would appear that the total serum carbon dioxide content in low-birth-weight infants (mean at birth, 18.6 mEq/l; at 1 mo, 20 mEq/l) is lower than in full-term and older infants and adults.[41,45]

Table 10–3. ADVERSE EFFECTS ASSOCIATED WITH THE USE OF SODIUM BICARBONATE IN NEONATES

local tissue necrosis and thrombosis
excessive increases in vascular volume, serum osmolality, serum sodium
hypercarbia
hypocalcemia
paradoxical acidosis (intracellular, CSF)
intracranial hemorrhage (?)

The side-effects are largely associated with the use of inappropriately excessive doses, infusion rates, or concentrations of sodium bicarbonate. Some of these side-effects, such as intracranial hemorrhage, may not be specific for sodium bicarbonate.
Data from studies by Ostrea and Odell,[35] Simmons et al,[42] Corbet et al,[27] Finberg,[31] and Eidelman and Hobbs.[29]

Clinical Toxicology. The side-effects associated with the administration of sodium bicarbonate are listed in Table 10–3. The most serious of these is intracranial hemorrhage; some evidence points to the use of hypertonic sodium bicarbonate given by rapid infusion as a major contributing factor.[31,36] As a result, a slow infusion of no greater than 0.5 mEq/ml solution of sodium bicarbonate is recommended.

Tromethamine (THAM)

Pharmacology. Tromethamine or THAM (tris-hydroxymethyl-aminomethane) is an organic buffer used for the correction of acidosis. Tromethamine has been purported to be a more effective buffer than bicarbonate for the treatment of metabolic acidosis because it is a stronger base (pK_a 7.84 vs. 6.1) and because it produces more rapid restoration of intracellular acid-base balance.[49] However, metabolic acidosis involves nonvolatile acids with low pK_a values (lactic, pyruvic) that are as effectively buffered by bicarbonate as by tromethamine. The more rapid restoration of intracellular acid-base equilibrium has not been established as a significant factor in clinical efficacy. The molecular reaction involved between tromethamine and carbon dioxide is as follows:

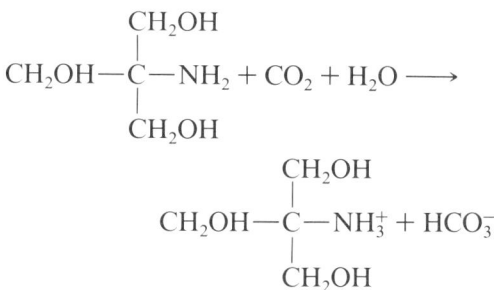

$$CH_2OH-\underset{\underset{CH_2OH}{|}}{\overset{\overset{CH_2OH}{|}}{C}}-NH_2 + CO_2 + H_2O \longrightarrow$$

$$CH_2OH-\underset{\underset{CH_2OH}{|}}{\overset{\overset{CH_2OH}{|}}{C}}-NH_3^+ + HCO_3^-$$

The usefulness of these reactions is extremely limited because 1 mM (millimole) of tromethamine can buffer no more than 1 mM of carbon dioxide. Therefore, an enormous quantity of drug would be necessary to remove a significant quantity of dissolved carbon dioxide.

Tromethamine is ineffective given PO and must be administered by parenteral infusion. It has a large volume of distribution and is rapidly excreted by the kidney. The rate of correction of intracellular pH by tromethamine and bicarbonate is controversial.[52] At physiologic pH, tromethamine is only half as effective a hydrogen ion acceptor as is bicarbonate.[47] It also causes a shift of the oxygen-hemoglobin dissociation curve of whole blood, resulting in an increase in oxygen affinity.

Clinical Pharmacology. The early clinical studies with tromethamine reported increases in PaO_2, with little change in $PaCO_2$.[50,51] In two comparative studies of tromethamine and bicarbonate therapy in neonates with RDS,[48,53] a consistent difference in effect on $PaCO_2$ was noted: Tromethamine treatment caused a decrease or no change, but bicarbonate therapy generally produced an increase. However, clinically important changes were not apparent in either PaO_2 or $PaCO_2$. No differences between these alkalies in efficacy or incidence of toxicity have been clearly established.

Therapeutic Indications. There is no clear advantage of tromethamine over bicarbonate for the treatment of *metabolic acidosis*. The role of alkali infusion in the management of metabolic acidosis in infants remains controversial. The established treatment of choice for respiratory acidosis is assisted ventilation along with correction and support of cardiovascular status. Whether tromethamine or bicarbonate is employed as adjunct therapy for metabolic acidosis, slow infusion must be used to avoid complications of hyperosmolality. The osmolality of 0.3 M tromethamine (3.6%) is about 350 mOsm/kg H_2O; 1 millimole (mM) of tromethamine is equal to 120 mg.

The appropriate dose of tromethamine is arbitrary and based on minimizing the osmotic challenge while maximizing the buffering capacity. One recommended dose is 1 to 2 mM/kg. Other dose recommendations involve consideration of the base deficit:

$$\text{dose (ml of 0.3 M THAM)} = \left(\begin{array}{c}\text{weight} \\ \text{in kg}\end{array}\right) \times (1.1) \times \left(\begin{array}{c}\text{base deficit} \\ \text{in mEq/l}\end{array}\right)$$

The base deficit must be derived from an accurate determination of pH, pCO_2, and pO_2 in an arterial blood sample. As an emergency measure in the absence of information on acid-base status, a dose of 10 ml/kg IV of 0.3 M solution (360 mg/kg) can be utilized. The recommended rate of infusion is no more rapid than 1 mM (120 mg) or 1 ml per minute.[48] Tromethamine is clearly not indicated for the management of metabolic acidosis associated with bicarbonate deficiency (renal tubular acidosis).

Clinical Toxicology. Reported side-effects associated with the use of tromethamine include local tissue reaction and necrosis and respiratory depression. The evidence for hypoglycemia and for hyperkalemia have come only from experimental animal studies. In one group of infants given tromethamine, neither hypoglycemia nor abnormalities in serum potassium were noted.[53] Following slow IV infusion of tromethamine in another patient group, there were no abnormalities in blood glucose or potassium; however, an increased incidence of respiratory depression and apnea was observed.[52]

Bronchodilators

Bronchodilator drugs have limited applicability in infants. Infants with chronic lung disease (e.g., bronchopulmonary dysplasia) have been treated with theophylline (see Chapter 6), pulmonary vasodilators (see Chapter 7), corticosteroids (see section this chapter), and selective beta$_2$-adrenergic agonists.[269]

The *beta$_2$-adrenergic agonists* have become very popular in the treatment of obstructive airway disease (e.g., asthma) in older children because of their excellent bronchodilatory effects and receptor specificity, which minimizes the unpleasant side-effects associated with nonselective adrenergic drug therapy (e.g., epinephrine). Sosulski and colleagues[269] used terbutaline (5 μg/kg subcutaneously) in 7 infants with ventilator-dependent BPD. Lung compliance and inspiratory and expiratory resistance improved significantly. Clinical improvement in pulmonary air exchange and wheezing was noted in 5 of the 7 infants. $PaCO_2$ was decreased in 4 of 6 infants. The work of breathing remained unaffected. Earlier studies with nebulized selective beta agonists in acute wheezing episodes in children indicated that children under 20 months of age fail to respond.[259] The development of tolerance to the bronchodilator effects of terbutaline has been reported, although this phenomenon is controversial.[257] A number of side-effects, many dose-dependent, have been reported with terbutaline, including tachycardia, muscle tremors, myocardial ischemia, pulmonary edema, cerebral hemorrhage, and seizures.[257] Additional studies are needed to examine the long-term value, if any, of bronchodilator therapy in management of BPD.

Calcium

Pharmacology. Calcium, one of the most abundant elements in the body, has many important physiologic roles. Pharmacologic doses of calcium are well absorbed from the intestinal tract. Sutton and coworkers[77] showed that radiolabeled calcium (^{46}Ca) given as a food supplement is almost completely absorbed by 4 hours following PO administration to pre-term infants; in other studies, however, only one third to three fourths of dietary calcium was absorbed from the intestinal tract.[73,76] Vitamin D and parathyroid hormone (PTH) both augment the absorption of dietary calcium, but their effect on pharmacologic doses of calcium is unknown.

Most of the calcium in the body (99%) resides in the skeleton. Calcium is present in plasma in three different fractions: (1) about 40% is bound to plasma proteins (albumin); (2) approximately 10% is complexed with citrate and phosphate, although it is still diffusible; and (3) the remainder is ionized calcium. Ionized calcium is the active fraction that exerts physiologic effects. Only a small percentage (1.5%) of calcium administered in pharmacologic doses is excreted in the urine.[57,58] In the kidney PTH stimulates the reabsorption of calcium by the distal tubule, while the active vitamin D metabolites stimulate proximal tubular reabsorption of calcium. Calcitonin inhibits the proximal renal tubular reabsorption of calcium, thus enhancing its excretion.[79]

The physiologic activity of calcium in the cardiovascular system is reviewed in Chapter 7. Calcium contributes to the maintenance of normal myocardial contractility[60] and the maintenance of normal vascular tone.[61] It has also been implicated as a factor in determining the state of contracture of the ductus arteriosus. Calcium regulates a number of functional and metabolic processes in cells outside those in the cardiovascular system, including the adrenal medulla (release of catecholamines), and the neuromuscular system and

CNS. Hypocalcemia, therefore, can produce a wide range of manifestations in the neonate (see under Therapeutic Indications).

Transition from fetal to neonatal life results in an abrupt termination of an influx of 130 to 150 mg/kg per 24 hours of elemental calcium.[74] This termination of calcium influx is associated with a rapid fall in serum calcium level, especially in premature neonates, in whom manifestations of hypocalcemia may develop (early neonatal hypocalcemia). There is a predisposition for the development of early hypocalcemia in all seriously ill neonates, particularly those with asphyxia or RDS who have received large amounts of citrated blood, those born to mothers with hyperparathyroidism, and those with true hypoparathyroidism or DiGeorge's syndrome. Significant decreases in serum calcium levels may be associated with depressed myocardial function including congestive failure, tachycardia, hypotension, PDA, acidosis, cyanosis, temperature instability, coagulation abnormalities, alteration of consciousness, apnea, and motor nerve excitability.[64,69,78]

Clinical Pharmacology. Early neonatal hypocalcemia has been shown to be prevented by oral and parenteral calcium supplementation. Brown and coworkers[55] administered 75 mg/kg/24 hr of elemental calcium PO (as calcium glubionate) in divided doses every 6 hours. Mean serum calcium levels were higher in the supplemental-therapy group during the treatment period (12–72 hr of age) and up to 36 hours following discontinuation. No differences were observed in serum magnesium, phosphorus, parathyroid hormone, or 25,hydroxy-vitamin D levels. Moya and Domenech[67] gave approximately 100 mg/kg/24 hr of elemental calcium (as calcium lactate) with feedings to eight newborns through the first 5 days of life; in contrast to controls, serum calcium rose on the third day in calcium-supplemented infants. In a study by Sann and colleagues,[72] calcium, 80 mg/kg/24 hr (given as 10% calcium gluconate in water [297 mOsm/kg H_2O]) was added to the milk feedings for the first 5 days of life. A total of 46 pre-term infants (32–37 wk gestation) were randomly assigned to a control or treatment group. Serum calcium concentration remained at the admission baseline level in the treated group, but in controls it fell significantly between 12 to 76 hours and then returned to baseline levels between 92 and 100 hours of life. Of 23 infants in the calcium-supplemented group, 2 became hypercalcemic (>2.8 mmol/l); 4 of 23 in the control group became hypocalcemic (<1.75 mmol/l). The

serum calcitonin levels were significantly increased in the control group at 12 to 16 hours of life but remained unchanged in the treated group. No side-effects were observed. In another study, infusion of calcium (7 mg/kg/hr of elemental calcium) at 2 to 12 hours of life resulted in serum calcium levels in the normal or above-normal range; serum phosphorus and PTH levels were significantly lower than those found in controls.[58]

Continuous infusion of 1 mg/kg/hr of elemental calcium (as gluconate of glucoheptonate) sustained serum calcium levels in the normal range in low-birth-weight neonates with RDS.[68] In a dose-response study in sick premature neonates given calcium gluconate infusions, a dose of 36 or 54 mg/kg/24 hr (elemental calcium) increased serum calcium levels, whereas a dose of 18 mg/kg/24 hr did not.[56]

The maximum increase and rate of decline in serum calcium and ionized calcium concentrations were examined in 24 premature neonates (27–37 wk) given a parenteral infusion of 18 mg/kg of elemental calcium (200 mg/kg of calcium gluconate) over 2 minutes.[57] Serum calcium increased to 7.5 mg/dl at 5 hours. The pre-infusion serum calcium concentration was 6.7 mg/dl. The estimated half-life of the infused calcium was 30 minutes.

Parenteral calcium therapy (18 mg/kg of elemental calcium IV or intra-arterially given at a rate of 9 mg/min) was shown to increase blood pressure and heart rate in 24 moderately ill but normotensive premature infants.[71] Mean and systolic blood pressures increased by 4 and 7 torr, respectively, 20 minutes after completion of dosing. Heart rate increased significantly (8 beats/min over baseline), peaking at 35 minutes. Although direct effects of calcium on the myocardium and vascular smooth muscle cells may account for these effects, a catecholamine-mediated effect could not be ruled out. In a subsequent study, Mirro and Brown[263] infused calcium gluconate (200 mg/kg) over 2 minutes to 16 premature infants (27 to 34 weeks' gestation) with hypocalcemia. All infants had hyaline membrane disease and were less than 48 hours old. The previously reported increase in heart rate and blood pressure were confirmed, and decreased left ventricular systolic time interval ratios (LVSTI) consistent with improved myocardial function were noted in the infants. The improvement in myocardial function was felt to be the result of the positive inotropic effect of calcium. No immediate or delayed complications of calcium therapy were noted in either study.

Therapeutic Indications. *Early neonatal hypocalcemia* can be prevented by supplemental oral or parenteral calcium.[57,67,72] The therapeutic value of such prophylaxis remains controversial. There are several arguments against prophylactic calcium treatment: The infants usually are asymptomatic; the "hypocalcemia" is self-limited; and calcium therapy is potentially dangerous.[71] The recommended doses for supplemental oral calcium therapy are summarized in Table 10–4. For oral calcium supplementation to prevent early decreases of serum calcium levels (not necessarily hypocalcemia) elemental calcium, 80 mg/kg/24 hr (divided equally among feedings), has been employed. Calcium gluconate is believed to be less irritating to the gastrointestinal tract than calcium chloride.

Existing or "late" hypocalcemia can be effectively treated with continuous IV administration of calcium. Although a clear definition of hypocalcemia in neonates remains controversial, most investigators consider values for serum ionized calcium of less than 2.4 mg/dl or for total serum calcium of less than 7.0 mg/dl as consistent with a diagnosis of hypocalcemia.[57,75] The relationship between ionized and total

serum calcium is unpredictable. Bolus doses of calcium shown to be effective in correcting existing hypocalcemia have ranged between 10 and 20 mg/kg of elemental calcium given by slow IV infusion (Table 10–4). The maximum rate of administration is 20 mg/kg/min (1 mEq/kg/min) of elemental calcium. In fact, IV infusion of calcium should be conducted over at least 30 minutes to avoid hypercalcemia and rebound hypocalcemia. Continuous calcium infusion is therapeutically ideal once hypocalcemia has been corrected. The minimal effective parenteral dose of elemental calcium necessary to maintain normocalcemia is about 1 mg/kg per hour (Table 10–4). The serious consequences of extravasation of calcium and the problem of incompatibility of calcium with bicarbonate, parenteral nutrition, and many drugs represent a serious compromise to the use of slow or continuous calcium infusion. The very short 30-minute half-life of calcium given IV over less than 2 minutes is equally undesirable. When feasible, the PO route of administration would appear to be preferable over the IV route for the treatment of hypocalcemia. IV calcium administration is indicated in severe manifestations of hypocalcemia such as sei-

Table 10–4. CALCIUM CONTENT OF SELECTED PHARMACEUTICAL PREPARATIONS AND DOSE RECOMMENDATIONS

Preparations	Description (concentration)	Elemental Calcium (Ca^{2+}) Content	
		mg/ml	*mEq/ml*
calcium chloride	10% injection	27	1.36
calcium gluconate	10% injection	9.3	0.46
calcium glubionate	syrup 6.47% (360 mg/ml)	23	1.16
calcium gluceptate	22% injection	18	0.9
calcium lactate	powder (13%)	130 mg/gm powder	
calcium levulinate	10% injection	13	0.65

Dose Recommendations (given as *elemental calcium* [Ca^{2+}])[a]
PO[b] 80 mg Ca^{2+}/kg q 24 hr (4.0 mEq/kg) divided equally among feedings. Demonstrated effective in preventing early neonatal hypocalcemia. Should not be continued beyond 3 to 5 days of age unless nutritional source of calcium is inadequate or hypocalcemia is demonstrated.
IV *bolus therapy for symptomatic hypocalcemia:* 10–20 mg Ca^{2+}/kg (0.5–1.0 mEq/kg) given by slow infusion over at least 30 minutes. Maximum rate of calcium infusion (bolus) should never exceed 20 mg Ca^{2+}/kg/min (1.0 mEq/kg/min). Monitoring for bradycardia and arrhythmias is essential.
  continuous-infusion maintenance therapy: 1 mg Ca^{2+}/kg/hr (0.05 mEq/kg/hr). Administration of an equivalent dose intermittently can be utilized to avoid incompatibility with other parenteral medications.
  bolus therapy for cardiac resuscitation: 4–8 mg Ca^{2+}/kg/dose (0.2–0.4 mEq/kg/dose) IV or by intracardiac route. Do not exceed 20 mg Ca^{2+}/kg/min.
  exchange transfusion: 9 mg (0.45 mEq) of Ca^{2+} per 100 ml of citrated blood exchanged.

[a] To avoid the serious confusion created by different concentrations of calcium in the various preparations, the doses of calcium are given *as elemental calcium* in both mg/kg and mEq/kg. One mEq of elemental calcium is equivalent to 20 mg of elemental calcium.
[b] Expectant nonintervention versus preventive administration of calcium is controversial in early-onset neonatal hypocalcemia.[56]

zures and cardiovascular decompensation. Repeated measurement of serum calcium should be employed to establish the adequacy of the calcium therapy and the need for its continuation.

The use of calcium in *cardiac resuscitation* is justified by its known role in the maintenance of normal myocardial contractility and of normal vascular tone,[71] as well as its potential value in improving the function of a failing heart.[59,62,78,263] Calcium may be beneficial in restoring an electrical cardiac rhythm in instances of asystole and may enhance the efficacy of cardiac electrical defibrillation.[54] Rapid IV administration of calcium can lead to cardiac arrest, particularly in patients who are fully digitalized. The recommended dose of elemental calcium for cardiac resuscitation is 4 to 8 mg/kg given IV or by intracardiac infusion (Table 10–4); this dose can be repeated at 10-minute intervals, to a maximum of 20 mg/kg of elemental calcium. Bolus IV calcium administration has been shown to effectively reverse hemodynamic and electrophysiologic complications associated with verapamil therapy[66] (see Verapamil in Chap. 7).

Because of substantial differences in calcium content of the available pharmaceutical preparations, great care must be exercised in calculating the appropriate volumes to provide the recommended dose of elemental calcium. Table 10–4 lists the actual calcium content of several commercial preparations as well as dosing recommendations.

Calcium chloride has been recommended over other calcium preparations for parenteral administration because the calcium in calcium chloride is in the ionized form and requires no metabolism of the anion substrate.[69] No clinical studies have critically compared the efficacy or toxicity in neonates of the various calcium-containing preparations. For reasons of safety, a minimum number of calcium-containing preparations should be available in any infant care unit, and the actual elemental calcium concentration should be clearly indicated on each container (Table 10–4).

Clinical Toxicology. Complications following PO administration of calcium are minimal, being restricted essentially to local gastric irritation and diarrhea.[55] IV calcium therapy can produce local calcium deposition and tissue necrosis including nerve damage,[65,70] serious dysrhythmias (especially bradycardia), and deterioration of cardiovascular function.[71] Peripheral arterial administration of calcium should be avoided because of the danger of

tissue necrosis. Prolonged parenteral calcium therapy has been associated with hypercalcemia.[63]

H$_2$-RECEPTOR ANTAGONISTS: CIMETIDINE

Pharmacology. Cimetidine is a reversible, competitive antagonist of the actions of histamine on the H$_2$-receptor but has no effects against the H$_1$-receptor actions. Thus, cimetidine inhibits histamine-dependent gastric acid secretion. It also inhibits secretion induced by gastrin or pentagastrin and partially inhibits the stimulatory actions of acetylcholine and related drugs such as bethanecol or even caffeine. Both the volume and hydrogen ion concentration of gastric secretions are reduced by cimetidine. Cimetidine reportedly does not consistently affect the rate of gastric emptying, lower-esophageal sphincter pressure, or pancreatic secretion.[85] Only a few other physiologic effects of cimetidine have been reported, including interference with the peripheral conversion of T$_4$ to T$_3$ in adults.[87]

Cimetidine is approximately 60% bioavailable from the gastrointestinal tract; peak serum levels are reached within 2 hours of dosing in the adult.[80] The drug is approximately 13% to 25% plasma protein–bound and distributes widely in the body, with the exception of adipose tissue. About 30% of an administered dose is metabolized in the liver, primarily to the sulfoxide, with smaller amounts of hydroxymethyl and amide derivatives also identified. Approximately 70% of the dose is excreted unchanged in the urine; a small percentage is excreted in the bile. In patients with less than 10% to 20% normal renal function, the dosing interval should be doubled.[88] No adjustment in dosage is required with hepatic cirrhosis.[90] Close scrutiny of the clinical responses to cimetidine (gastric pH, CNS toxicity) will aid in establishing the optimal dosage for patients with significant renal or hepatic failure.

Clinical Pharmacology. In adults the reported values for cimetidine elimination half-life range from 1.8 to 6.7 hours.[80] The volume of distribution ranges from 1.4 to 4.3 l/kg. Pharmacokinetic studies following cimetidine administration (4 mg/kg IV) to a one month old premature infant (BW 660 g) revealed a $T\frac{1}{2}$ of 2.6 hr, a clearance rate of 261 mg/kg/hr, and an apparent Vd of 0.95 l/kg.[245] The peak serum cimetidine level was approximately 5 μg/ml. The gastric pH increased by one hour after administration, with a sustained pH above 6 for at least 8 hours. Studies in children (1 to 12 years old) revealed a $T\frac{1}{2}$ of 1.4 ± 0.4 hr (range 0.8 to 2.1 hr) and a Vd of 2.1 l/kg.[252] Mean plasma drug concentrations of 0.78, 2.15, and 6.70 μg/ml have been reported to produce 50%, 80%, and 95% inhibition of pentagastrin-stimulated gastric acid secretion.[86] The sited target plasma level concentration for 50% inhibition of gastric acid secretion is 0.5 to 1.0 μg/ml. Serum cimetidine concentrations of 1.0 μg/ml were found to maintain gastric pH around 4.[252] Mental confusion has been reported to occur with plasma levels of greater than 1.25 μg/ml or sulfoxide metabolite levels greater than 5 μg/ml.

In studies by Chhattriawalla and by Aranda and their colleagues[83,245] cimetidine was administered to premature neonates with evidence of reflux esophagitis or gastrointestinal bleeding suspected to be caused by stress or corticosteroid treatment. The doses employed ranged from 4 mg/kg IV q 12 hours or longer[245] to 10 to 20 mg/kg per day (interval not specified).[83] Gastric pH was maintained between 5 and 6 with these doses, without evidence of drug-induced side-effects. Bar-Maor and coworkers[82] employed cimetidine in the management of neonates diagnosed as having esophageal atresia with lower tracheoesophageal fistula. The purpose of the drug therapy was to reduce the gastric acidity and volume, which are believed to be the major injurious factors in gastric regurgitation–related pulmonary injury. The gastric pH in the four neonates managed with cimetidine was greater than 6. Goudsouzian and colleagues[85] employed cimetidine in 97 infants and children (aged 4 mo–14 yr) as a preanesthetic medication to study its effect on gastric pH and volume. A dose-response relationship was identified: A dose of 2.5 mg/kg PO resulted in a mean gastric pH of 3.9 ± 0.6; a maximum dose of 10 mg/kg PO produced a gastric pH of 6.4 ± 0.3. The volume of gastric aspirate decreased exponentially as the dose of cimetidine was increased. These effects on gastric pH and volume were maximal between 1 and 4 hours after oral dosing.

Therapeutic Indications. Cimetidine has been approved for prophylaxis and treatment of duodenal ulcers and treatment of hypersecretory status in adults. Controversy surrounds the use of cimetidine for prophylaxis against acute upper gastrointestinal hemorrhage secondary to stress or steroid use in critically ill patients.[252] It has been used experimentally in neonates to treat gastric ulcers, gastroesophageal reflux, and upper gastrointestinal bleeding, and to prevent the complications of gastric aspiration.[81,83,85] Studies in infants clearly show a reduction in gastric acidity and volume without obvious complications. However, the use of cimetidine in infants must be considered experimental.

The recommended dosage of cimetidine for preanesthetic prophylaxis against gastroesophageal reflux (pulmonary aspiration) is 7.5 mg/kg PO or IM as a single dose. The daily dosage for infants has not been established. In a case report, Aranda and coauthors[245] employed a dose of cimetidine in a one month old premature infant of 4 mg/kg IV, given every 12 hours or longer based on gastric pH measurements. The recommended dose for children over 1 year old is 24 mg/kg IV daily; because of the rapid elimination of the drug in this age group, divided doses given every 4 or 6 hours or a continuous infusion (1 mg/kg/hr) may be required.[252] The adult dose is 4.3 mg/kg given every 6 hours; this is similar to the reported dose used in infants (2.5–5 mg/kg PO, IM or IV). Toxicity in infants and children has been reported by several investigators with doses of cimetidine of 15 to 40 mg/kg per day. Measurements of gastric pH and volume, monitoring for clinical signs of toxicity (CNS), and measurements of cimetidine plasma levels will be necessary to establish the appropriate dosage in neonates.

Clinical Toxicology. Cimetidine has been reported to be well tolerated in experimental studies in infants. Signs of toxicity include alterations for consciousness, visual hallucinations, myoclonus, carphologia, dysarthria, divergent gaze, and diplopia;[81] these appear to be associated with excessive doses (>15–40 mg/kg q 24 hr) and plasma levels (>1.25 μg/ml) of the drug. Cholestatic jaundice, modification of the peripheral metabolism of thyroid hormones, and a number of interactions with other drugs metabolized by hepatic enzymes have also been reported.[80,87,89] Goldenring has cautioned against the combined use of cimetidine and tolazoline owing to the interference with the H_1 and H_2 receptor–dependent pulmonary vasodilating properties of tolazoline. This is a theoretical consideration, the clinical significance of which remains unestablished.

CORTICOSTEROIDS

Therapeutic Indications. There are only a few well-defined indications for the use of corticosteroid therapy in the infant.[109] The various corticosteroids employed therapeutically have three basic pharmacologic effects: glucocorticoid, mineralocorticoid, and anti-inflammatory action. Table 10–5 summarizes the pharmacologic properties of commonly employed corticosteroids, which have been the subject of several excellent reviews.[91,92,98,110] This discussion is limited to a consideration of the use of the corticosteroids in replacement therapy for endocrine disorders and miscellaneous systemic illnesses where pharmacologic doses of steroids may be of benefit. Antenatal corticosteroid use is discussed in Chapter 11.

Congenital adrenal hyperplasia: The adrenogenital syndromes are hereditary deficiencies of one or more enzymes necessary for cortisol synthesis by the adrenal gland. The anatomy, embryology and clinical presentation of adrenal insufficiency have been reviewed by Gutai and Migeon.[100] Treatment of the acute phases of adrenal insufficiency (electrolyte abnormalities only) can be accomplished with the use of deoxycorticosterone acetate (DOCA) in a dose of 1 mg IM every 12 hours while diagnostic tests are performed. DOCA therapy will not interfere with the measurement of urinary 17-ketosteroids, 17-hydroxycorticosteroids, or pregnanetriol but will provide mineralocorticoid effects.

The most common form of adrenogenital syndrome, 21-hydroxylase deficiency, is easily diagnosed by a single blood sample for 17-OH progesterone. Early diagnosis permits prompt institution of appropriate therapy, which should include mineralocorticoids (see below) along with treatment of shock and repletion of body sodium and water. If the patient demonstrates evidence of continued deterioration, hydrocortisone (Solu-Cortef) should be given IV (2 mg/kg), followed by continuous infusion of hydrocortisone (2 mg/kg over 8 hr) until improvement occurs.

The accepted regimen for maintenance therapy is administration of oral hydrocortisone, 20 mg/m² per 24 hours, or cortisone acetate, 25 mg/m² per 24 hours. It may be preferable to give one half of the daily dose in the morning, followed by one fourth the daily dose 8 and 16 hours later, so that resulting levels of serum cortisol more closely reflect normal diurnal variation.[105] Hydrocortisone acetate has also been used for replacement therapy, given as a single injection IM every third day at a dose equal to 3 times the daily requirement. The proper dose of hydrocortisone must necessarily be adjusted for the individual infant;[103] growth rate, virilization, serum 17-hydroxyprogesterone, and plasma renin values have been used to determine the adequacy of glucocorticoid replacement.[122] If plasma renin activity is normal, the early-morning 17-OH progesterone value should be maintained below 200 mg/dl.

It is now recognized that most patients with congenital adrenal hyperplasia have sufficient impairment of mineralocorticoid function so that body sodium content is decreased and plasma renin activity (PRA) is increased.[115] If ignored, the reduced total body sodium content and increased PRA will stimulate release of ACTH, which in turn will increase the apparent glucocorticoid dosage requirement. Any patient with congenital adrenal hyperplasia determined to have an increased PRA should receive mineralocorticoid in sufficient doses to normalize PRA.[122] This approach will minimize the glu-

Table 10–5. PHARMACOLOGY OF THE CORTICOSTEROIDS

| Corticosteroids | Glucocorticoid Equivalent Dose (mg/m²/day) | Relative Activity or Potency | | | T½ (hr) | |
		Gluco-corticoid	Mineralo-corticoid	Anti-inflammatory	Plasma	Biologic
Short-acting						
cortisol (hydrocortisone)	20	1	1	1	1.5	8–12
cortisone	25	0.8	0.8	0.8	0.5	8–12
prednisone	5	4	<1	4	3	12–36
prednisolone	5	4	<1	4	2	12–36
Intermediate-acting						
triamcinolone	4	5	0	5	5	
Long-acting						
betamethasone	0.6	25	0	25		
dexamethasone	0.75	30	0	25	3–4	36–54
9-alpha-fluorocortisol	0	0	20	10		
deoxycorticosterone acetate (DOCA)	0	0	20	0		

cocorticoid dosage requirements and avoid the consequences of corticoid excess, including growth failure.[97] Either a long-acting DOCA preparation can be employed parenterally (approximately 25 mg administered IM every 3–4 wk), or a synthetic compound may be used orally (9-alpha-fluorocortisol, 0.05–0.20 mg once daily). It is imperative that salt replacement therapy be used in conjunction with the mineralocorticoid treatment. The dose of fluorocortisol should be reduced if elevation of blood pressure occurs or if PRA is below normal for age. Additional doses of hydrocortisone must be administered during periods of stress. Moderate illness requires a doubling of the maintenance dose, whereas major illnesses or surgery require tripling of the maintenance dose.

Infants born with hypoplasia of the adrenal glands present with severe hyponatremia, hyperkalemia, vomiting, and dehydration.[114] Both hydrocortisone and mineralocorticoid therapy should be instituted as discussed for treatment of congenital hyperplasia. Signs of bilateral adrenal hemorrhage may present in such infants within the first few days of life, although the signs of adrenal insufficiency can be subtle and delayed. Management of hypoglycemia is a more frequent requirement than correction of electrolyte disturbances. A state of relative adrenal insufficiency may also occur in infants with neonatal hyperthyroidism.[105] Hydrocortisone acetate in a dose of 15 mg IM every 12 hours has been recommended as replacement therapy for infants when indicated.

Neonatal hypoglycemia: A number of illnesses are associated with or can lead to the development of hypoglycemia in the infant.[101] In most circumstances, an infusion of glucose at a rate of 2 to 14 mg/kg/min will provide adequate glucose blood levels in the infant. In infants who continue to manifest hypoglycemia despite aggressive glucose infusion (> 14 mg/kg/min) and in whom associated fluid overload becomes a problem, the administration of hydrocortisone may be indicated while appropriate diagnostic tests are being conducted.[111] The dose of hydrocortisone employed in these situations is 1 to 2 mg/kg given IV every 8 hours. Occasionally, infants require up to twice this dose of hydrocortisone for control of the hypoglycemia.

Septic gram-negative shock: The indications for the use of high-dose steroid therapy for sepsis or meningitis in neonatal infants is speculative. In cases of gram-negative infection associated with signs and symptoms of cardio-

vascular shock, pharmacologic doses of glucocorticoids may be useful, as suggested by related experience in adults.[116] The recommended dose of hydrocortisone is 30 to 50 mg/kg administered IV over a 10-minute period; this may be repeated as clinically indicated for a total of 4 doses given over a 4-hour period. This treatment has not been evaluated in neonates and should be considered investigational, particularly in other infectious conditions such as sepsis caused by Group B streptococci. In a study of methylprednisolone therapy for bacterial meningitis in infants and children, no statistically significant difference in survival or long-term sequelae was identified between the control and steroid therapy groups.[95]

Dermatologic conditons: A variety of skin conditions in infants, the most common being atopic eczema, are responsive to topical application of corticosteroids. However, significant absorption sufficient to produce systemic toxicity can result.[99]

Laryngotracheobronchitis (croup): Considerable controversy surrounds the use of steroids in the treatment of croup.[120] Major inadequacies in the reported clinical studies have hampered interpretation of the data. At best, steroids appear to shorten by a matter of hours the hospital stay and recovery from symptoms.[106] The dose recommended for therapy is 0.3 mg/kg of dexamethasone given IM on admission and again 2 hours later. Future studies may establish criteria for identifying those infants with croup most likely to benefit from steroid therapy.

Other disorders: Glucocorticoid therapy has been employed in infants for the treatment of a variety of other conditions, including RDS,[102,117,118] hemangiomatosis,[94,108,253,271] dehydration,[104] acute wheezing,[119] and BPD.[107] In most cases, no clear benefit of such therapy has been identified. The exceptions include hemangiomatosis and BPD. Diffuse life-threatening hemangiomatosis has responded to glucocorticoids with stabilization and shrinkage in size of the lesions. The therapeutic effect may be delayed in onset (weeks) and may not be sufficient to avoid the need for additional supportive procedures. High dose prednisone therapy (1 mg/kg given every 12 hr PO) or its equivalent has been recommended.[271] The anticipated duration of therapy in infants with therapeutic response is 1 to 3 months. In a recent study,[107] dexamethasone therapy in infants with BPD resulted in a significant reduction in required respiratory support and in oxygen diffusion gradients. The dose of dexamethasone employed in these studies was 0.25 mg/kg given IV every 12 hours for 3 days. A lower dose (0.10 mg/kg) appeared to be less effective. However, the value of this therapy in altering the outcome of BPD remains unclear, particularly from the standpoint of complications such as infection, cessation of growth and osteoporosis; this use is, therefore, considered experimental. In another report, infants with malignant infantile osteopetrosis, a rare autosomal recessive disorder characterized by decreased hematopoiesis, responded positively to prednisone therapy.[112]

Clinical Toxicology. A number of significant side-effects occur with the administration of pharmacologic doses of corticosteroids (Table 10–6).[93,113,248] Normal adrenal function is significantly suppressed. Acute adrenal insufficiency results from too-rapid withdrawal of corticosteroids after prolonged therapy.[96,251] Any infant receiving steroid therapy (which elevates plasma glucocorticoid levels throughout the day) for more than 7 to 10 days is likely to manifest evidence of pituitary-adrenal suppression. Pituitary-adrenal integrity can best be examined by checking morning plasma cortisol levels before and 2 hours after ACTH adminis-

Table 10–6. COMPLICATIONS OF STEROID THERAPY

ophthalmologic
   posterior subcapsular cataracts
   glaucoma
   reactivation of herpes keratitis
CNS
   pseudotumor cerebri
   psychiatric disturbances and dependency
hematopoietic system
   leukocytosis, neutrophilia, monocytopenia,
      lymphopenia, eosinopenia
   purpura
gastrointestinal system
   pancreatis
   peptic ulcer (?)
   fatty infiltration of the liver
renal system
   nephrocalcinosis
   nephrolithiasis
   uricosuria
musculoskeletal system
   myopathy
   osteoporosis and fractures
   aseptic necrosis of bone
endocrine and metabolic
   diabetes
   adrenal insufficiency
   growth failure
   hyperlipidemia
   lipomatosis
   hypocalcemia
   hypokalemic alkalosis
   sodium retention and hypertension

From Rimza ME: Am J Dis Child 132:806, 1978.

tration (0.25 mg IV).[251] Baseline plasma cortisol levels should be at least 10 μg/dl and greater than 30 μg/dl 2 hours after ACTH. Chamberlin and Meyer[251] have suggested several plans for steroid withdrawal for different clinical situations. Other direct toxicities include severe growth retardation, fluid and electrolyte disturbances, hyperglycemia, increased susceptibility to infections, cataracts, myopathy, and osteoporosis with bone fractures. The inhibition or arrest of growth can result following relatively small doses of glucocorticoids in children. The literature regarding the effects of glucocorticoids on neurologic development and associated concerns has been reviewed by Weichsel.[121]

ANTICOAGULANTS: HEPARIN

Pharmacology. Commercial heparin preparations are prepared from beef lung or porcine intestinal mucosa. The major constituents of commercial heparin contain three molecules of 2,6-disulfo-glucosamine alternating with uronic acids. Heparin is effective when administered by continuous or intermittent IV infusion, by SQ or intraperitoneal injection, or endotracheally as an aerosol.[125,126] Irrespective of the mode of administration, the total amount of heparin required to maintain approximately the same degree of hypocoagulation for the same total time period is equivalent. Differences in individual response to heparin have been proposed to relate to differences in heparin distribution between plasma and cellular compartments and to differences in concentration of the heparin cofactor, Antithrombin-III (AT-III).[127] Intrapulmonary administration of heparin achieves a maximum loading of the cellular compartment and maintains moderate plasma concentrations of heparin for several weeks in humans. In contrast, continuous IV infusion maintains plasma concentrations with minimal cellular distribution and consequently, produces a short duration of action with maximal anticoagulant effect. PO administration of heparin does not produce an alteration of coagulation, although there is some evidence for absorption from the gastrointestinal tract. Following administration, heparin is rapidly taken up by endothelial cells, with the remainder bound to plasma proteins; further redistribution through the reticuloendothelial system then occurs, and antithrombin-inactive chains of the heparin molecules return to the circulation as antithrombin-active chains.[125,128] The locus of the anticoagulation action is the endothelium, not the bloodstream as was originally believed. The major portion of administered heparin is metabolized by N-desulfation. Only small quantities of unchanged heparin and the partially O-desulfated metabolite, uroheparin, have been identified in urine.[125,127]

The ability of heparin to complex with and change the properties of proteins accounts for its ability to modify the activity of many enzymes in a variety of ways. Its marked potency in inhibiting blood coagulation is due to its activation of an inhibitor in plasma, Antithrombin-III. This protein progressively inactivates both thrombin and Factor Xa, key proteolytic enzymes in the clotting of fibrinogen and activation of prothrombin.[127] The variability in anticoagulant activity of different preparations of heparin is due to variations in carbohydrate structure and chain length; standardization by in vitro coagulation testing minimizes but does not eliminate this variability.

Heparin also possesses anticomplementary activity, inhibiting both the classic and the alternative pathways.[254] Several sites have been proposed for the inhibition by heparin of the classic complement pathway, including direct inhibition of C1q binding to immune complexes, inhibition of the interaction of C1s with C_4 and C_2, and potentiation of the effect of C1 inhibitor function by interaction with C1-INH.[250] Heparin inhibition of the alternate pathway occurs by augmentation of the regulatory action of the control proteins, β1H and C3b inactivator. The result is prevention of the formation and function of the amplification convertase C3b,Bb.[258] As a consequence of the anticomplementary activity of heparin, inhibition of both opsonization and neutrophil-mediated phagocytosis of bacterial pathogens is possible. Studies by Edwards and coworkers[254] indicate that the serum heparin levels associated with therapeutic anticoagulant doses of heparin (0.3 to 0.5 U/ml) are not sufficient to inhibit complement-dependent bactericidal activity in neonatal sera. Very high serum heparin concentrations (25 and 250 U/ml) caused 32% and 100% inhibition of bactericidal activity, respectively.

Clinical Pharmacology. The in vitro effect of heparin on the prothrombin time (PT) and partial thromboplastin time (PTT) of plasma from newborns and adults has been studied by Barnard and Hathaway.[124] PT is significantly prolonged in the newborn plasma by 0.5 U/ml compared with 1.0 U/ml in adults. PTT is prolonged by 0.05 U heparin/ml in the newborn plasma and by 0.1 U/ml in adults. In clinical studies, infants have demonstrated an increased or decreased sensitivity to heparin depending upon the assay technique and clinical status. These observations illustrate some of the difficulties involved in heparin therapy.

McDonald and colleagues[129] examined the plasma half-life of heparin in 25 pre-term newborns and 8 normal adults given a single IV bolus dose (100 U/kg in newborns and 75 U/kg in adults). In newborn infants, mean plasma heparin half-life ($T\frac{1}{2}$ = 35.5 min at 29–36 wk gestation; 41.6 min at 25–28 wk gestation) was significantly shorter than that in adults ($T\frac{1}{2}$ = 63.3 min). The volume of distribution of heparin in newborns varied inversely with gestational age (58–81 ml/kg). Heparin clearance was significantly greater in all newborn infants than in adults (newborn, 1.4–1.5 ml/kg/min; adult mean, 0.43 ml/kg/min). Earlier studies in premature and full-term infants demonstrated a half-life of approximately 3 hours.[124]

McDonald and Hathaway[130] administered heparin by continuous IV infusion to newborns and older infants at a rate sufficient to achieve a heparin plasma concentration of 0.3 to 0.5 U/ml. The dose required was 16 to 35 U/kg per hour with a mean of 27 U/kg per hour in newborn infants (25–40 wk gestation) and infants 6 weeks to 28 months of age. A striking increase in heparin clearance rate was noted in infants with thrombosis. The individual clearance values for heparin ranged from 0.4 to 11 ml/kg per minute. Neonates exposed to parenteral fluids containing heparin to maintain patency of venous catheters (1 U/ml of fluid) had heparin levels averaging less than 0.05 U/ml serum (range 0.0 to 0.14 U/ml).[254] The heparin dose received by these neonates averaged between 2.4 and 4.1 U/kg/hr.

Therapeutic Indications. Heparin is an effective antithrombotic agent used for prophylaxis of large-vessel *thromboembolic disease.* Review of its use for clot lysis in adults indicates less than a 20% success rate.[123] In neonates heparin has been largely employed within intensive-care therapy, such as that required for catheter-related thrombosis, and to maintain patency of peripheral and central catheters.[124,131] The value of such uses, although still widely accepted, is questionable. Rasoulpour and McLean[132] emphasize maintenance of fluid and electrolyte balance and general supportive care rather than heparin therapy in the management of renal vein thrombosis in neonates. Heparin

(1–2 U/ml or 1–10 U via flush) does not appear to alter the number of thrombotic complications related to umbilical catheters.[124]

The following recommendations for the use of heparin in newborns were presented by McDonald and Hathaway:[129]

1. Obtain baseline values of coagulation studies including activated PTT, PT, platelet count, fibrinogen, and Laidlaw clotting time (or other whole-blood activated clotting time).
2. Begin with a bolus heparin dose of 50 U/kg, followed by a continuous infusion of 20 to 25 U/kg per hour.
3. Increase or decrease the dose by 5 U/kg per hour depending upon the results of clotting studies (activated whole-blood clotting time, Laidlaw clotting time, or activated PTT). One and one-half to two times baseline Laidlaw clotting time is considered ideal. (The activated PTT in neonates is often prolonged, thus reducing its usefulness as a guide for heparinizaton.[124])
4. Continue heparin therapy 48 hours beyond the point of thrombus resolution.

Heparinization is contraindicated in infants with evidence of intracranial or gastrointestinal bleeding or thrombocytopenia (< 50,000/mm³). IM injections should also be discontinued during heparin therapy. Continuous therapy is safer than and just as effective as intermittent injection.[133] The therapeutic range for serum heparin to produce anticoagulant activity in infants is 0.3 to 0.5 U/ml serum.[254] No control studies have been done to demonstrate the efficacy of heparinization in neonates with thromboembolic disease.

A recent study[134] showed that continuous administration of low-dose heparin (1 U/ml of IV fluid administered) helped to reduce serum triglyceride concentration during infusion of fat emulsion to low-birth-weight infants. Serum-free fatty acids increased significantly as expected. The value of heparin lipolytic activity in improving the utilization of lipid emulsion therapy in low-birth-weight infants remains to be established.

Clinical Toxicology. Very few allergic manifestations have been reported with the use of heparin.[125] The main untoward effect is unpredictable spontaneous hemorrhage. Heparin can also cause transient mild thrombocytopenia, osteoporosis (rarely), hypoaldosteronism, and T-lymphocyte suppression.[126]

Protamine sulfate, a protein of low molecular weight, combines ionically with heparin to form a stable complex devoid of anticoagulant activity; therefore, it is useful in situations of heparin overdose. The dose of protamine sulfate is 1 mg, administered IV by slow infusion, for every 100 U of heparin estimated to remain in the patient. Excessive doses of protamine sulfate can cause serious bleeding problems as a result of binding to platelets and various proteins such as fibrinogen.

NARCOTIC ANALGESICS; SEDATIVES AND HYPNOTICS; LOCAL ANESTHETICS

The value of pain control and mood alteration in sick infants has received little attention, and there is a corresponding lack of data on the use of drugs for this purpose in the literature. The absence of communication between patient and physician unquestionably explains this void, in contrast to the wealth of information available regarding older children and adults. Except for operative procedures conducted under general anesthesia and cardiac catherization, the use of drugs with analgesic or CNS-depressant effects in neonates has been infrequent, particularly when compared with their use in adult patients in analogous intensive-care settings. Newborns do respond to pain stimuli as measured by adrenal cortical response, immediate postoperative behavior, heart rate, and respiratory rate, and by changes in transcutaneous oxygen levels.[189] The following sections are brief summaries of the pharmacology and clinical experience with analgesics, sedatives, and local anesthetics that have been or could be employed in neonates and infants.

Narcotic Analgesics

Morphine and meperidine are two popular narcotic analgesics that have been used in infants. Fentanyl is a potent synthetic narcotic agent used IV in neonates as an anesthetic. The development of tolerance to and physical dependence on morphine, meperidine, and other narcotics has prompted a continuing search for equally effective analgesic agents with fewer serious side-effects. Morphine, however, remains the drug of choice for most situations requiring pain relief. Pharmacologic differences between morphine and the semisynthetic and synthetic agents such as meperidine and fentanyl have largely been overestimated; with equivalent analgesic doses, the incidence or degree of unwanted side-effects, including respiratory depression, is the same.[154,156] However, individual patients may manifest differing responses, including side-effects, to the various narcotic agents. It is, therefore, important to have several narcotic analgesics available for use.

Morphine and Meperidine

Pharmacology. All opioids are well absorbed from the gastrointestinal tract, but high hepatic first-pass clearance significantly reduces the amount reaching therapeutic sites of action (e.g., CNS). Thus, in most cases the parenteral route of administration is preferred. For meperidine, about 50% of the absorbed dose is cleared by first-pass hepatic metabolism in the adult.[168] The onset of action is generally more rapid with parenteral than with oral administration. The protein-bound fraction is about 30% for morphine and 50% to 60% for meperidine.[173]

The major pathway for metabolism of morphine is conjugation with glucuronic acid. Only minor amounts of morphine undergo N-demethylation. Meperidine is hydrolyzed to meperidinic acid, which can then undergo conjugation or N-demethylation to normeperidine, followed by hydrolysis and subsequent conjugation.[145] In adults, only a small percentage of a dose of morphine or meperidine is excreted unchanged in the urine; in newborn infants, significant amounts of unchanged drug can be found in the urine along with metabolites.[157,161,169] Normeperidine can produce excitation, which would oppose the depressant action of meperidine. In the newborn, the rate of formation of normeperidine is relatively slow, so that accumulation to toxic levels occurs only with renal failure or with toxic oral doses of meperidine. The rate of oral absorption of toxic doses of meperidine is slow enough that the hepatic conversion of meperidine to normeperidine can theoretically result in mixed stupor (from meperidine) and excitation (from normeperidine), depending on which compound predominates.

Morphine and related narcotics produce their major pharmacologic effects by stimulating so-called opioid receptors in the CNS that mimic the actions of the endogenous ligands, enkephalins, and β-endorphins.[136] The analgesic effect of morphine can occur without a significant alteration in consciousness. Increasing the dose produces increasing drowsiness and sleep; the incidence of nausea and vomiting is also increased. High doses of opioids can produce muscular rigidity.

The opioids produce respiratory depression primarily by a direct effect on the brain-stem respiratory centers. This respiratory-depressant effect is proportional to the drug dose; the mechanism involved is a reduction in responsiveness of the respiratory center to carbon dioxide tension. Way and colleagues[188] compared the effect of morphine and meperidine on CO_2 response curves in newborn male infants undergoing circumcision. Both drugs depressed or completely suppressed the regular "sigh" in the infant's breathing pattern. Morphine (0.05 mg/kg IM) decreased the resting ventilation rate by 22% and shifted the CO_2 response curve to the right and downward. Meperidine (0.5 mg/kg IM) did not change the resting ventilation rate from control levels and did not appear to produce as great a shift in the CO_2 response curve. At equal end-tidal pCO_2 (35 mm Hg), morphine produced a 57% decrease in minute volume, and meperidine, a 23% depression; whether equal analgesic effects were present was not determined. In general, infants appear to be more sensitive than adults to the respiratory-depressant effects of morphine. Meperidine produces similar effects on respiration in infants and adults. The duration of morphine- and meperidine-induced respiratory depression can be expected to extend several hours beyond the plasma half-life.[156] The time for recovery from the sedative-hypnotic effects is generally much shorter than that from analgesic effects. Romagnoli and coworkers[178] found the mean recovery time for sleep in children given a single dose of meperidine (0.5 mg/kg) plus scopolamine to be about 10 minutes.

In analgesic doses morphine and meperidine have no major effect on the cardiovascular system. Blood pressure will decrease with increasing doses unless hypoxemia is prevented by mechanical ventilation (and oxygen if necessary). Resistance and capacitance vessels are dilated by the opioids; this effect can manifest as orthostatic hypotension. The release of histamine and central suppression of adrenergic tone are primarily responsible for the vasodilating effects of morphine. Myocardial function and cerebral circulation, however, are not ordinarily affected by morphine.[159]

The opioids have significant effects on gastrointestinal secretions, motility, and tone: Secretions and motility are decreased in the stomach, while tone is increased. Gastric emptying can be delayed by up to as long as 12 hours. Resting tone is increased and propulsive contractions are decreased in the small intestine.[159] The tone of the ileocecal valve is enhanced. Propulsive motility in the large intestine is diminished or abolished by opioids, while tone increases (i.e., spasm occurs). Although these gastrointestinal effects are generally considered adverse side-effects, they can be used to advantage in certain patients.

Smooth muscle of the biliary and urinary tract can be stimulated to contract by opioids, resulting in increases in biliary tract pressure and urinary retention.

Clinical Pharmacology. For *morphine,* the minimum concentration in plasma associated with suppression of clinical signs of pain during surgery in infants and children ranges between 46 and 83 ng/ml.[143] The terminal phase of the plasma half-life for infants over 1 month old and children is similar to that for adults ($T\frac{1}{2} = 2-3$ hr). The mean plasma drug clearance is about 6 ml/min/kg; the volume of distribution is 1.1 to 1.4 l/kg. There is no available information on morphine kinetics in newborns.

For *meperidine,* the reported plasma half-life in newborns ranges from 6.5 to 39 hours.[172] Most of this information was obtained from infants exposed to meperidine in utero. One study in 9 infants (3 to 18 months old) given IV doses of meperidine ranging from 0.65 to 1.1 mg/kg revealed a $T\frac{1}{2}$ (beta phase) of 2.3 ± 0.4 hr and a Vd of 5 l/kg.[246] Drug disposition kinetics in adults are largely perfusion-dependent.[167] The terminal phase of the half-life is about 3 to 8 hours.[145] Analgesic effects occur with plasma concentrations between 200 to 700 ng/ml. Marked respiratory depression occurs at plasma drug concentrations of greater than 500 ng/ml.[169] A lower dose given at a more frequent interval would be least likely to produce respiratory depression while maximizing analgesic effects.

Therapeutic Indications. Morphine and meperidine should be reserved for the treatment of *severe pain.* The analgesic effect can be achieved with or without sedation. Different sensitivity among patients to the analgesic effects of morphine has not been observed.[143]

The recommended analgesic/sedative dose for morphine is 0.1 mg/kg repeated every 4 hours IV or IM as needed (Table 10–7). The IV route is recommended to avoid problems with absorption from IM or SQ sites. Continuous infusion of morphine is preferred in some situations because it provides a more uniform relief of pain in children than that achieved with intermittent administration, and because the total dosage required is less.[170,183,264] The recommended dose for continuous infusion of morphine in children is 0.04 to 0.07 mg/kg per hour; the dose required for complete pain control may range from 0.02 to 2.6 mg/kg per hour.[170] The recommended analgesic dose for meperidine in infants and children is 0.5 mg/kg IV repeated as required (Table 10–7).

Clinical Toxicology. Opioids can produce a wide variety of unwanted side-effects including nausea, vomiting, and constipation. Increased sensitivity to pain can also occur after the analgesic effect of the opioid has worn off. Allergic reactions have been reported, but only rarely. Hypotension can develop in patients with inadequate or borderline blood volume. Respiratory depression along with histamine release is an expected effect that may pose a serious risk to infants with respiratory illness, particularly if adequate respiratory support is not provided. Addiction to opioids is discussed in Chapter 11.

The major effects of the opioids, including respiratory depression, can be reversed by *naloxone,* 0.01 to 0.1 mg/kg IV or IM (see Chapter 11).[155]

Fentanyl

Fentanyl has become a popular agent, particularly in cardiovascular surgery (e.g., ligation of PDA), because of its purported lack of cardiovascular effects.[137,177] The dose for induction

Table 10–7. **DOSAGE RECOMMENDATIONS FOR NARCOTIC AGENTS IN INFANTS**

Drug	Indication	Dose[a]
morphine	analgesia ± sedation	bolus: 0.1 mg/kg IV repeated as required (usually q 4 hr) continuous infusion: 0.04–0.07 mg/kg/hr IV; maximum pain relief: 0.02–2.6 mg/kg/hr IV
meperidine (Demerol)	analgesia ± sedation	0.5 mg/kg IV repeated as required (usually q 4 hr); maximum dose: 2.0 mg/kg IV
fentanyl (Sublimaze)	anesthetic major surgery minor surgery analgesia	 30–50 µg/kg IV 2–10 µg/kg IV 2–µg/kg IV

[a] The narcotics can produce respiratory depression severe enough to require mechanical respiratory support, particularly with the larger recommended doses. Specific antidote for narcotic overdose: naloxone, 0.01–0.1 mg/kg IV. (IM administration will delay onset of antidote action 15 minutes or more).

and maintenance of analgesia and anesthesia is 30 to 50 μg/kg administered IV as a single bolus dose or infused over 1 minute.[177] A dose of 100 μg of fentanyl is equivalent to 10 mg of morphine or 75 mg of meperidine. Reported effective doses of fentanyl for a variety of clinical situations range from 2 to 50 μg/kg.[156,177] In adults the half-life of the terminal elimination phase of fentanyl is approximately 4 hours. The half-life is markedly prolonged in elderly patients. Robinson and Gregory[177] reported that prematures anesthetized with fentanyl were awake within 1 hour following completion of surgery. Fentanyl is extensively bound to albumin and undergoes hepatic metabolism. Changes in the CO_2 response curve lasting for up to 3 or 4 hours have been noted to occur with doses of fentanyl of 2 to 9 μg/kg.[156]

As with all narcotics, fentanyl produces nausea and vomiting in over 50% of patients given doses of more than 3.0 μg/kg. High doses of fentanyl can produce severe muscular rigidity requiring reversal with a neuromuscular blocker.[177] Other side-effects are listed above under Clinical Toxicology.

Sedatives and Hypnotics

Experience with sedation in infants and children has largely evolved from cardiac catheterization, angiography, and surgical or other procedures in an attempt to ensure comfort and to allow measurements and procedures to be done with stable hemodynamics. The anecdotal experience with sedatives in infants and children does not provide the opportunity for critical evaluation of the optimal drugs or doses, particularly with regard to the value of single-drug versus multiple-drug regimens. Although the majority of clinical studies focus on drug combinations, the use of more than one drug does not necessarily correlate with maximum therapeutic benefit. The most important element of successful employment of the sedative drugs is sufficient clinical experience with a particular drug or drugs. Little is to be gained by frequent or random changes from one medication or combination to another.

Specific drugs that have been used for sedation or hypnosis in infants and children include the shorter-acting barbiturates (pentobarbital, secobarbital), and nonbarbiturate sedative – hypnotics (chloral hydrate, chlorpromazine, diazepam, hydroxyzine, ketamine, promethazine).

Barbiturates

The barbiturates are capable of producing sedation or hypnosis with either oral or parenteral administration. Because they often produce hyperalgesia and increased reaction to painful stimuli, these agents are contraindicated in patients with pain requiring sedation. Tolerance to barbiturate-induced sedation and hypnosis develops according to the therapeutic regimen employed. Once-a-day sedation with secobarbital or pentobarbital causes negligible tolerance, whereas chronic continuous dosing can increase the dose requirements up to sixfold.[160] The primary use of barbiturates in infants and children has been for preanesthetic sedation and for certain other procedures such as electroencephalography.[146,180] These short-acting barbiturates have a major disadvantage: Too low a dose results in an excited, hyperagitated patient; larger doses may produce the desired sedation but with respiratory depression, prolong narcosis or postanesthetic recovery time.[166,171] The recommended dose for secobarbital and pentobarbital is 2 to 6 mg/kg PO, rectally, IM, or IV (Table 10 – 8); this can be repeated as required for maintenance of sedation.

Chloral Hydrate

Pharmacology. Chloral hydrate has been used extensively as a sedative in pediatric patients for many years. It is well absorbed from

Table 10 – 8. DOSAGE RECOMMENDATIONS FOR SEDATIVES AND HYPNOTICS IN INFANTS[a]

Drug	Recommended Dose[b]
Barbiturates	
pentobarbital	2 – 6 mg/kg PO, rectally, or IM
secobarbital	2 – 6 mg/kg PO, rectally, or IM
Sedative – Hypnotics	
chloral hydrate	25 – 50 mg/kg PO or rectally
chlorpromazine	0.2 – 0.5 mg/kg IV
diazepam	sedation: 0.1 – 0.25 mg/kg IV infused slowly over 3 min; may be repeated after 30 min × 3 as needed for desired sedation effect anesthesia: 0.25 – 1.5 mg/kg IV
ketamine	anesthesia: 1 – 4.5 mg/kg IV infused over 1 min or 6.5 – 13 mg/kg IM

[a] Larger doses may result in respiratory depression sufficient to require mechanical ventilation.

[b] These doses can be repeated as required for maintenance of desired sedative or hypnotic state. Repetitive dosing, however, can lead to drug accumulation and associated respiratory depression.

the gastrointestinal tract and distributes widely in the body. The volume of distribution is approximately 1 to 2 l/kg.[270] The drug is metabolized to the active hypnotic metabolite, trichloroethanol, in the liver by alcohol dehydrogenase.[139] A fraction of both chloral hydrate and trichloroethanol is oxidized to trichloroacetic acid. *In vitro* protein binding studies with adult human plasma found 35 to 41% of trichloroethanol bound to protein and 71 to 88% of trichloroacetic acid protein-bound.[261] Trichloroethanol is conjugated and excreted in the urine as a glucuronide. The major route of excretion is via the urine, although small amounts of metabolites have been identified in the bile. Chloral hydrate should be used with caution in patients with hepatic or renal disease.

Clinical Pharmacology. Reported peak plasma levels of trichloroethanol following chloral hydrate administration to neonates (36–53 mg/kg) range from 10 to 55 μg/ml.[151] The average therapeutic plasma level of trichloroethanol is reported to be 12 μg/ml.[270] The plasma half-life for trichloroethanol in neonates ranges from 8.5 to 64 hours (mean 37 hr); values in adults range from 4 to 14 hours.[139,229] The average plasma trichloroethanol level in adults following a dose of 15 mg/kg of chloral hydrate is 8 μg/ml; this increases to over 80 μg/ml after 7 days of continuous therapy.[184]

When chloral hydrate was employed in children as a preanesthetic sedative with scopolamine, a dose of 30 to 50 mg/kg PO produced sedation by 15 minutes and sleep by 40 minutes in 60% of patients;[185] unfortunately, no controls for chloral hydrate or scopolamine alone were included in this study. Cerebral irritation in the newborn has been reported to be responsive to treatment with chloral hydrate (25 mg/kg PO q 6 hrs).[162] Satisfactory sedation lasting approximately 1 hour, sufficient for electroencephalography, ophthalmologic examination, pulmonary function and CO_2 ventilatory response studies, and CT scans, has been accomplished in neonates with the use of chloral hydrate (30–75 mg/kg PO).[140,141,158,164,186] In various studies, deep sleep ensued within 30 to 45 minutes, and most infants were fully awake 2 hours later. In doses of 50 mg/kg given PO, chloral hydrate significantly increases tidal volume and oxygen consumption (4.9 vs. 6.0 ml/kg and 6.4 vs. 8.2 ml/min/kg, respectively) but has no effect on CO_2 chemoreceptor response in infants.[164]

Therapeutic Indications. The recommended dose of chloral hydrate for *sedation* in infants is 25 to 50 mg/kg given PO (Table 10–8). Like the barbiturates, chloral hydrate has no analgesic properties; therefore, excitement rather than sedation may result from its use in patients with pain. The prophylactic use of a narcotic drug at the end of a painful surgical procedure has been recommended to prevent the excitatory period that occurs during recovery in about 10% to 15% of children given only chloral hydrate.[179]

One of the major disadvantages of chloral hydrate is its irritant properties, which account for its unpleasant taste and the gastrointestinal discomfort, nausea, and vomiting it produces in some patients. These effects can be reduced by giving a small amount of fluid (juice or milk) with the oral dose.

Clinical Toxicology. Chloral hydrate is a relatively safe sedative and hypnotic drug. The lethal–therapeutic dose ratio is lower than for diazepam. Gastric irritation, paradoxical excitement, vasodilation, hypotension, respiratory depression, cardiac arrhythmias, and myocardial depression have been reported as side-effects.[174]

Chlorpromazine

Pharmacology. Phenothiazines (including chlorpromazine and promethazine) have been used as adjuncts in preoperative medication, as agents in combination sedation-anesthesia, and in attempts to reduce peripheral and pulmonary vascular resistance. Among the useful pharmacologic properties of these drugs are tranquilization, potentiation of narcotic analgesic effects, general anesthetic and hypnotic effects, antiemetic and antinausea activity, antihistamine effects, and α-adrenergic blockade.[152]

The absorption of phenothiazines from the gastrointestinal tract is believed to be erratic and unpredictable. Parenteral administration is associated with 4 to 10 times the bioavailability of oral dosing.[181] The drugs are highly lipophilic and distribute widely in the body tissues. Phenothiazines are metabolized in the liver to as many as 12 metabolites and are largely conjugated with glucuronic acid before elimination by renal (major) and hepatic (minor) processes.

In contrast to sedative-hypnotics and opioids, the phenothiazines suppress spontaneous movement and complex behavior while allowing the patient to remain responsive to the environment with intellectual functions intact. The proposed mechanism for this so-called neuroleptic action is antagonism of dopamine-mediated synaptic neurotransmission.[135] The antagonistic action is believed to explain not only the neurologic and antipsychotic effects but also the increase in prolactin secretion as well as the suppression of the activity of the chemoreceptor trigger zone in the medulla (antiemetic effects). Central respiratory function is generally not affected, but vasomotor reflexes mediated by the hypothalamus or brain stem are depressed by relatively low doses. Chlorpromazine also has significant anti−α-adrenergic and anticholinergic actions. As a result of the central and peripheral actions, the drug is capable of producing systemic and pulmonary vasodilation.[138,163] Tolerance to its hypotensive effects can develop. A weak diuretic effect of the drug is believed related to a decrease in ADH or a direct inhibiting action on renal tubular (reabsorption) function. Renal blood flow tends to increase with chlorpromazine therapy.

Clinical Pharmacology. For the phenothiazines, disposition follows multi-compartment pharmacokinetics. The elimination of chlorpromazine from plasma has shown marked variability, with an average half-life of about 30 hours in the adult. Phenothiazine pharmacokinetics have not been reported for infants. The elimination $T\frac{1}{2}$ in a newborn exposed to chlorpromazine *in utero* was 3.2 days.[265] Attempts to correlate plasma levels of chlorpromazine with pharmacologic effects have not been successful. Minimal effective plasma levels have been estimated to be less than 30 ng/ml; toxicity occurs at levels greater than 750 ng/ml.

The major clinical experience with phenothiazines in infants and children has been in their use as preanesthetics and as anesthetics in combination with other agents (see under Drug Combinations). Chlorpromazine has also been used in newborn infants with severe hypoxemia.[163,176] Larsson and coworkers[163] gave chlorpromazine to newborn infants with a variety of illness including RDS, persistent fetal circulation, pneumonia, and diaphragmatic hernia. The dosage used was 0.13 to 0.88 mg/kg over 1 hour; in responders, this was followed by a maintenance dose of 0.03 to 0.21 mg/kg per hour for up to 47 hours. Oxygenation, calculated right-to-left shunt, $PaCO_2$, pH, and PaO_2 showed evidence of improvement in 14 of 18 patients. Mortality, however, was similar in responders and nonresponders. Sedation was apparent only during the first 24 hours. The mechanism for the clinical improvement was hypothesized to be due to reduced pulmonary vascular resistance and increased pulmonary and systemic perfusion. Earlier studies in adult patients showed improvement with chlorpromazine therapy (0.25 mg/kg IV) following cardiopulmonary bypass surgery;[138] a consistent decrease in pulmonary vascular resistance was observed.

Therapeutic Indications. Chlorpromazine appears to be an effective component of drug combinations used for sedation and anesthesia (see under Drug Combinations). The use of chlorpromazine rather than more specific-acting drugs (see Chap. 7) to reduce pulmonary vascular resistance requires further study. The use of chlorpromazine for treatment of drug withdrawal in the neonate is reviewed in Chapter 11.

Clinical Toxicology. A variety of toxic effects have been reported in adult patients given phenothiazines preoperatively, although these agents enjoy a remarkably high therapeutic index.[144] Hypotension, tachycardia, local irritation at the injection site, dizziness, nausea and vomiting, and restlessness are among frequently occurring acute undesirable effects. Hypotension, extrapyramidal reactions (Parkinsonian syndrome, akathisia, acute dystonic reactions, tardive dyskinesia), jaundice, blood dyscrasias (leukocytosis, leukopenia, eosinophilia), skin reactions, and abnormal pigmentation are among the more common reported side-effects with chronic use.[135]

Diazepam

Diazepam has been employed for preanesthetic sedation and as an anesthetic. Doses that provide mild to moderate sedation result in amnesia in up to 60% of adult patients.[149] The effects of diazepam are most predictable with slow IV or PO administration; IM administration is associated with unpredictable absorption and should therefore be avoided. Infusion of the sedative dose (0.1−0.25 mg/kg) should be accomplished over a 3-minute period (Table 10−8). Because of the variability in dose requirements and the delay of 1 to 2 minutes for maximal effect after completion of infusion, the need for repeated doses for sedation should be carefully assessed. The dose required for anesthesia is variable, ranging from 0.25 to 1.5 mg/kg IV (Table 10−8).

Minor or no cardiovascular effects should be expected with diazepam therapy. Tidal volume decreases and respiratory rate will increase, but ventilation is generally unaltered. The average duration of the preoperative sedative effect of diazepam (1 mg/kg) in children averaging 5 years of age has been found to be between 5 and 20 minutes.[178]

The pharmacology of diazepam is reviewed in Chapter 5.

Hydroxyzine

Hydroxyzine is an antihistamine that produces a variable degree of sedation. Because it is an unsatisfactory sedative when used alone, it is always combined with other drugs when employed as a preanesthetic.[171] The most effective combination is hydroxyzine (1.1 mg/kg) and secobarbital (2.2 mg/kg) given IM. Its use alone as a general sedative cannot be recommended.

Ketamine

Pharmacology. Ketamine is a nonbarbiturate anesthetic that is effective when administered IV or IM. The drug is metabolized in the liver by demethylation and hydroxylation followed by conjugation with glucuronic acid and dehydration. Some of the metabolites are active as CNS depressants. Diazepam is known to inhibit the metabolism of ketamine.[190]

The sedation achieved with ketamine is characterized as an amnesic state in which the patient may appear to be awake but is immobile and unresponsive to pain. The anesthesia state is dose-dependent and is reached rapidly even with IM injection. The duration of action ranges from 1 to 10 minutes with doses of 0.5 to 2.0 mg/kg; recovery from the postanesthetic psychic effects is more prolonged.

Cerebral blood flow and CSF and intracranial pressure are markedly increased by ketamine.[190] The cardiovascular effects include an increase in systemic and diastolic blood pressure and pulmonary artery pressure, and an increase in heart rate.[150] All of these effects are associated with an increase in plasma norepinephrine levels. CNS stimulation is believed responsible for these cardiovascular effects. Ketamine also has a direct myocardial-depressant effect that is generally not appreciated because of the sympathomimetic stimulation. Because respiratory rate and tidal volume are decreased by ketamine, oxygen and mechanical ventilatory support may be required. Muscle tone is increased; in some patients this effect may be so great as to resemble seizure activity. Pretreatment with diazepam has been recommended to control the serious circulatory, neuromuscular, and psychic side-effects of ketamine.[190]

Clinical Pharmacology. The disappearance of ketamine from plasma follows a two-compartment open model. The disappearance phase of the $T\frac{1}{2}$ in adults is about 2 hours. The ketamine dose requirements to prevent gross movements are reported to be four times greater in infants under 6 months of age than in 6-year-olds.[165] Studies following a single dose show little metabolism of ketamine by the newborn.[142]

Therapeutic Indications. Ketamine is useful for repeated *anesthesia* in burn patients, for diagnostic studies such as eye examination or CT scans, for *sedating uncontrollable patients* (e.g., mentally impaired), and for *minor surgical procedures.* The analgesic properties of ketamine may contribute significantly to its usefulness. It is also of value when there is a need for sedation without cardiovascular depression (as can be anticipated with the barbiturates).

The recommended dose of ketamine is 1 to 4.5 mg/kg IV given over 1 minute, or 6.5 to 13 mg/kg IM. Induction anesthesia lasting 5 to 10 minutes can be achieved with 2 mg/kg IV. For maintenance of anesthesia, one half of the full induction dose should be given as often as required. Premedication with *diazepam* (0.1–0.2 mg/kg IV) has been shown to be useful in reducing the side-effects of ketamine.[190]

Clinical Toxicology. Muscular rigidity, athetoid motions of the mouth and tongue, swallowing, blinking and nystagmus, random movements of the extremeties, laryngeal spasm, fasciculations, tremors, and generalized extensor spasm have been noted following ketamine administration. Frank convulsions are very rare. Generalized extensor spasm with opisthotonos has been reported in infants.[175] Heart rate and blood pressure may increase by as much as 25%. Acute rises in pulmonary artery pressure have been seen in infants with congenital heart disease when ketamine has been used as the anesthetic for cardiac catheterization.[150] Transient respiratory depression and apnea may occur in neonates immediately following IV administration.[147] Intracranial pressure may rise in infants with hydrocephalus.[165]

Drug Combinations

Combination drug regimens of demonstrated effectiveness include diazepam-morphine, meperidine-promethazine-chlorpromazine, fentanyl-droperidol, and ketamine-pentobarbital-chlorpromazine.[148,153,182,267] Altered oxygen consumption and respiratory depression, inadequate sedation, altered cardiovascular status, and a variety of other problems have been associated with all these combinations. In a double-blind controlled study, Ruckman and coauthors[182] concluded that combinations of meperidine-promethazine-chlorpromazine and fentanyl-droperidol were equally effective for patient management during cardiac catheterization. Of the patients receiving these drug combinations, supplemental sedation was required in less than 20%. Side-effects included respiratory depression, shivering, nausea, hypotension or hypertension, and extrapyramidal reactions. (Reasonable starting doses for each drug combination for sedation during cardiac catheterization are shown in Table 10–9.)

Local Anesthetics

Local anesthetics have been employed in infants for pain control of minor surgical procedures such as insertion of catheters or chest tubes, lumbar puncture, and circumcision.[187,189] The use of lidocaine by direct application to the surface of mucous membranes produces local anesthesia within 2 to 5 minutes, which lasts for 30 to 45 minutes. Systemic absorption through mucous membranes can occur rapidly, resulting in toxic reactions. Infiltration anesthesia by local injection of lidocaine or procaine will provide pain control to deeper structures. The addition of epinephrine (5 mg/ml) will double the duration of infiltration anesthesia. Epinephrine-containing solutions, however, should not be injected into tissues supplied by "end" arteries (i.e., fingers, toes, ears, nose, and penis). Lidocaine solutions, 0.5% to 1.0%, are most frequently employed for infiltration anesthesia. To avoid systemic toxicity, the volume of the infiltrate should be less than 0.5 ml/kg of a 1% lidocaine solution (5 mg/kg). Procaine solutions, 0.5% to 1.0%, may also be effectively employed.

Table 10–9. DRUG COMBINATIONS FOR SEDATION IN CARDIAC CATHETERIZATION

Combination	Dose (IV)
1. meperidine	1.0 mg/kg
promethazine	0.5 mg/kg
chlorpromazine	0.5 mg/kg
2. morphine	0.1 mg/kg
pentobarbital	2.0 mg/kg
chlorpromazine	0.5 mg/kg
3. droperidol	62.5 mg/kg
fentanyl	1.25 μg/kg

Data from studies by Fixler et al[148] Graham et al,[153] and Ruckman et al.[182]

MUSCLE RELAXANTS: NEUROMUSCULAR BLOCKERS

Pharmacology. Several drugs including succinylcholine, pancuronium, d-tubocurarine, and metocurine are capable of interrupting the neuromuscular junction, thereby producing muscle relaxation or paralysis. These drugs are all poorly absorbed from the gastrointestinal tract and must be administered IM or IV to obtain neuromuscular blockade.

Succinylcholine has the most rapid onset and shortest duration of action (4–6 min after IV administration) of all the neuromuscular blockers. Continuous administration over a prolonged period may result in irreversible blockade (Phase I to Phase II block). Succinylcholine is rapidly hydrolyzed by pseudocholinesterase in the liver and plasma.

The onset and duration of action of the competitive antagonists (d-tubocurarine, pancuronium, metocurine) are essentially identical (Table 10–10). Some controversy exists with respect to the extent of protein binding of the neuromuscular blocking drugs; for metocurine, the reported protein-bound fraction ranges from 30% or 40% to as much as 70%.[208]

d-Tubocurarine is metabolized to a small extent, with the majority of the dose excreted unchanged in the urine (50–95%). Pancuronium is partially hydroxylated in the liver, with approximately 40% of the dose excreted in the urine and 10% in bile.[205] Approximately 45% to 60% of the dose of metocurine is excreted unchanged in the urine.[204]

d-Tubocurarine, pancuronium, and metocurine are nondepolarizing agents that interfere with the sequence of transmitting events at the neuromuscular junction. This is the result of competitive inhibition of acetylcholine for receptor sites on the postjunctional membrane. Reversal of muscular paralysis produced by nondepolarizing agents requires the use of an anticholinesterase such as neostigmine, which slows hydrolysis of acetylcholine, allowing accumulation of sufficient quantities of this neurotransmitter to compete more favorably with the nondepolarizing blocker for postsynaptic membrane receptor sites. In contrast, depolarizing muscle relaxants (succinylcholine) cause a depolarization of the postjunctional membrane resembling that of acetylcholine, except that depolarization persists. A transient muscle fasciculation occurs, with subsequent muscle paralysis due to the sustained depolarization. There are no known antagonists for reversal of

Table 10–10. PHARMACOLOGIC PROPERTIES AND DOSE RECOMMENDATIONS OF NEUROMUSCULAR BLOCKING DRUGS

Drug	Metabolism	Protein Binding (%)	Major Route of Excretion	Onset of Action (min)	Duration of Action (min)	Cardiovascular Effects	Histamine Release	Dose Recommendations
succinylcholine (Sux-cert)	rapid, complete		urine (10% unchanged)	<1	4–6 (single dose)	moderate to severe bradycardia ↑ or ↓ BP	weak	1–1.5 mg/kg IV or IM
d-tubocurarine	<25%	30–50	urine (40–90%)	1–2	30–50 ($T1/2 = 174 \pm 60$)	mild to moderate bradycardia	moderate (↓ BP)	0–1 wk: 0.25 mg/kg IV 1–2 wk: 0.4 mg/kg IV 2–4 wk: 0.5 mg/kg IV (infuse slowly >1 min)
pancuronium (Pavulon)	<50%	20–70 (?)	urine (40–50%); bile (10%)	1–2	20–50	none to mild ↑ heart rate ↑ BP	none to weak	0–1 wk: 0.03 mg/kg IV 1–2 wk: 0.06 mg/kg IV 2–4 wk: 0.09 mg/kg IV (infuse slowly >1 min)
metocurine (Metubine)	<50%	30–40	urine (45–60%)	1–2	25	none to mild	none to weak	0–1 wk: 0.25–0.5 mg/kg IV (increase dose if duration of paralysis <2–3 hr; decrease dose if >4–6 hr)

Pharmacology data from studies by Cook et al;[196] Roizen et al;[209] Nugent et al;[205] Ramzan et al;[208] and Fisher et al.[200] Data on dose recommendations for succinylcholine, from Cook et al;[196] for d-tubocurarine and pancuronium, from Bennett et al;[193] and for metocurine, from Nussmeier et al.[206]

the depolarizing block produced by succinylcholine. The actual termination of this blocking effect results from a redistribution of succinylcholine away from the neuromuscular junction. Succinylcholine is then rapidly hydrolyzed by pseudocholinesterase in the plasma.[196]

A variety of factors have been shown to influence the potency and duration of neuromuscular blockade produced by the nondepolarizing drugs. These are summarized in Table 10–11.

Clinical Pharmacology. Comparison of succinylcholine effects in infants and adults indicates that the recovery in infants is faster than that in adults; on a weight basis, however, the infant requires about twice as much succinylcholine to produce 50% neuromuscular blockade.[197] Early clinical studies of the effects of succinylcholine in infants and children reported sinus bradycardia, acquired tolerance, altered response to repeated administration, uneven muscle relaxation, and Phase II block. This experience prompted the use of nonpolarizing agents.

In an unselected series of 215 infants undergoing surgery, d-tubocurarine was administered in doses sufficient to permit adequate control of ventilation and to produce ideal operative conditions.[195] Dose requirements ranged from 0.32 to 0.53 mg/kg, with newborns requiring the lowest dose and older infants the highest. Similar findings have been reported by other investigators.[194] In pharmacokinetic studies of d-tubocurarine, the volume of distribution was 0.74 ± 0.33 l/kg in neonates; this is significantly larger than the values of 0.52 ± 0.22 to 0.30 ± 0.10 l/kg observed in older infants and adults, respectively.[200] The elimination half-life is 174 ± 60 minutes in neonates, compared with 90 minutes in children and adults.

The effect of pancuronium was evaluated in 100 pediatric patients of varying age.[191] In this series, the mean time of onset of paralysis was reached in about 30 seconds, with a mean increase in pulse rate of 28 per minute and in blood pressure of 19 mm Hg. The mean duration of action varied with dose: 0.1 mg/kg, 30 minutes; 0.15 mg/kg, 57 minutes. A double-blind study in children (aged 2 mo–10 yr) comparing pancuronium and d-tubocurarine revealed that their onset of action and heart rate and blood pressure effects were similar, but that pancuronium had a significantly shorter duration of action (30 vs. 42 min.).[192] The average dose of pancuronium was 0.094 mg/kg, and of d-tubocurarine, 0.45 mg/kg. A study of dose requirements of pancuronium in neonates revealed that the newborn is more sensitive to the drug, and that this sensitivity diminishes with age.[193] Infants less than 1 week of age required one third of the dose for those 2 to 4 weeks of age (30 μg/kg vs. 90 μg/kg). The dose required was reduced further by prematurity, acidosis, or hypothermia. Dose requirements and recovery from pancuronium was evaluated in 30 infants ranging in age from 2 to 16 days and 27 to 42 weeks' gestation;[202] the average dose of pancuronium during the 3 to 4 days of study ranged from 0.3 mg/kg per day in 30-week gestation infants (6 days old) to 0.4 to 0.5 mg/kg per day in 35- to 40-week gestation infants (6–17 days of age). The dose required for neuromuscular blockade (95% depression of twitch height) was extremely variable (3.5-fold differences). The daily dose of pancuronium required in individual infants ranged between 0.1 and 1.1 mg/kg per day. The dose of drug and the number of days of treatment did not have a predictable influence on reversibility of the neuromuscular blockade, but immaturity appeared to be an influential factor. Infants appeared to recover fully from the effect of pancuronium after 20 hours. One infant with renal failure showed evidence of neuromuscular blockade 48 hours after the last dose; reversal was accomplished with atropine (0.02 mg/kg) and neostigmine (0.06 mg/kg).

The effect of muscle paralysis on gas exchange and incidence of pneumothorax was examined in 35 infants with a requirement for mechanical ventilation (RDS, pneumonia, persistent fetal circulation, hydrops).[210] Pancuronium was administered IV in a dose of 0.1 mg/kg, repeated as necessary to produce a loss of spon-

Table 10–11. FACTORS AFFECTING NEUROMUSCULAR BLOCKING ACTION OF NONDEPOLARIZING DRUGS

Potentiation (Prolongation)	Antagonism (Shortening)
acidosis	alkalosis
hypothermia	epinephrine, norepinephrine
age	age
neuromuscular disease	increased K^+
tetanus	
hepatic disease	
cardiovascular disease	
other neuromuscular blockers	
antibiotics (aminoglycosides, tetracyclines, lincomycin, colistin)	
decreased K^+ (diuretics)	
$MgSO_4$	
lithium	

taneous respirations; a variety of other supportive measures were provided. In approximately half the patients, arterial oxygenation improved within 6 hours following induction of paralysis with pancuronium.

A study in 20 consecutive admissions of premature infants with severe hyaline membrane disease given pancuronium (0.05 mg/kg initially with the equivalent of 0.03 mg/kg/hr maintenance) showed a significant improvement in oxygenation and reduction of CO_2 retention.[198] The proposed mechanism of action was improvement in distribution of airway ventilation, with better matching of ventilation and perfusion. In 10 pre-term infants, the effect of pancuronium on occurrence and duration of hypoxia and hyperoxia and on intracranial pressure was examined during two 12-hour periods separated by 12-hour rest periods.[199] Pancuronium given IV at an initial dose of 0.1 mg/kg, with subsequent doses of 0.07 mg/kg every 60 to 90 minutes, reduced the amount of time associated with nonoptimal oxygenation and episodes of elevated intracranial pressure, but it produced no significant improvement in blood gas values, fractional inspiratory oxygen, or ventilator settings during muscle relaxation. In a controlled trial of muscle relaxation in infants with hyaline membrane disease, requirement for added oxygen therapy was significantly less in infants receiving pancuronium than in the control infants.[207] The dose of pancuronium was 0.03 mg/kg IV. No differences between treatment groups were observed in ventilator requirements, necessary duration of mechanical ventilation, or incidence of pneumothorax or interstitial emphysema.

The effects of metocurine were examined in 30 infants and children undergoing a variety of surgical procedures. Metocurine in doses of 0.05 to 0.5 mg/kg caused no significant change in blood pressure or pulse rate; no cardiac arrhythmias were noted. The rate of recovery was the same as that of *d*-tubocurarine.[201] The effect of metocurine was evaluated in 25 newborn infants (35-wk gestation or older) who required respiratory support with 100% oxygen and mechanical ventilation.[203] The mean dose of metocurine was 3.5 mg/kg per day (range 1.45–6.79). An increase in the dose requirement was observed in some patients who required paralysis for 1 week or longer. PaO_2 values measured 1 hour following induction of paralysis were significantly higher than pre-paralysis values. Transient decreases in blood pressure were occasionally observed with rapid IV administration of metocurine. With chronic use of metocurine, a dramatic increase in daily dose requirements occurred during the first week of therapy in infants of greater than 38 weeks' gestation.[206] Infants with a gestational age of less than 33 weeks did not demonstrate a statistically significant increase in daily dose requirements; the initial daily dose was approximately 2.5 mg/kg per 24 hours, increasing to 10 mg/kg per 24 hours.

Therapeutic Indications. The use of neuromuscular blockers for routine care of infants requiring mechanical ventilation is not indicated. In those infants who continue to manifest evidence of inadequate oxygenation despite optimal supportive care, a trial of muscle relaxation or paralysis is indicated. Infants who appear to benefit most from neuromuscular blockade therapy are those who are gestationally mature with persistence of right-to-left vascular shunt (persistent fetal circulation). Significant changes in mechanical ventilator settings are sometimes required to prevent serious complications such as a pneumothorax or pulmonary interstitial air in infants responding to such therapy. Other indications for induction of neuromuscular paralysis include severe, unresponsive seizure activity (status epilepticus), including neonatal tetanus. The recommended doses of the neuromuscular blocking drugs are listed in Table 10–10. The IV infusion should be conducted slowly over a 1-minute period to minimize the potential for adverse cardiovascular complications. The administration of the drug at intervals of 2 hours or less should prompt an increase in dose. Paralysis lasting beyond 4 to 6 hours is suggestive of excessive dosing.[206]

Clinical Toxicology. The greatest danger associated with neuromuscular blockade is hypoxemia resulting from inadequate mechanical ventilation. Other complications include cardiovascular disturbances such as bradycardia, tachycardia, hypo- or hypertension and arrhythmias, and malignant hyperthermia.[211]

The neuromuscular blockage induced by neuromuscular blocking drugs can be reversed by *neostigmine,* which inhibits acetylcholinesterase at the neuromuscular junction. The inhibition of acetylcholinesterase allows the accumulation of acetylcholine, which can successfully compete with the neuromuscular blocker at the neuromuscular junction, thus restoring activity.[262] *Atropine* is given in combination with neostigmine to avert the non-neuromuscular effects of neostigmine, including increased tracheobronchial and salivary secretions, bronchoconstriction, and bradycardia.

Dose response and pharmacokinetic studies in infants indicate that the dose requirements for neostigmine in infants are less than those for adults.[255] The lower dose requirement in infants is contrary to impressions held previously. The dose of neostigmine required to produce 70% antagonism of d-tubocurarine-induced neuromuscular depression is about 25 μg/kg IV. The previously recommended dose of neostigmine (70 μg/kg IV) is approximately twice the recommended adult dose. Atropine (0.02 mg/kg IV) is given in combination with neostigmine (25 mg/kg IV). The peak effect after IV bolus doses of neostigmine and atropine occurs within 5 to 10 minutes.[255]

STRYCHNINE THERAPY FOR NONKETOTIC HYPERGLYCINEMIA

Nonketotic hyperglycinemia or glycine encephalopathy in neonates is an inherited metabolic disease; manifestations develop shortly after birth and typically include intractable respiratory failure, muscular hypotonia, myoclonic seizures, spasticity, severe mental dysfunction, and early death.[215] The primary defect is in the glycine cleavage enzyme system, which results in elevated concentrations of glycine in plasma, CSF, urine, and brain. Therapy has been directed toward reducing the high glycine concentrations in these tissues because of the evidence that excess glycine is responsible for the manifestations of the disease.

Early treatments with leucovorin unsuccessfully attempted to enchance the normal folate-dependent cleavage reactions that result in conversion of glycine to serine.[217] Sodium benzoate therapy was subsequently tried because it was known to lower glycine levels in blood by conjugation reactions, resulting in excretion of glycine as hippurate.[214] Despite a significant reduction in serum glycine levels, no change in CSF glycine levels occurred, although some patients showed transient clinical improvement.

Recognition that glycine is not only the precursor of other amino acids in the CNS but the putative transmitter of certain small inhibitory neurons in the CNS prompted experimental trials with strychnine.[212,213,216] Strychnine and benzodiazepines are inhibitors of the glycine receptors and thus can potentially offset some of the effects of excessive glycine in the CNS.[218] Most of the therapeutic trials with strychnine therapy also employed sodium benzoate and usually a benzodiazepine such as clonazepam. The doses of sodium benzoate employed in these studies ranged from 25 mg/kg to 250 mg/kg given PO or IV every 4 to 6 hours. Transient improvement in muscle tone usually occurred with sodium benzoate alone. Strychnine doses employed in neonates range from 25 to 100 μg/kg given PO or IV every 6 to 8 hours. In one patient, the dose used was up to 900 μg/kg per day.[213,272] Strychnine therapy has been associated with variable effects, ranging from complete failure to improved motor and social behavior. Benzodiazepines enhance the hypotonia of the disease but suppress the seizure activity. Attempts to improve the clinical status of patients on these regimens by various manipulations of sodium benzoate, strychnine and benzodiazepine dosages have resulted in some transient success. A truly successful therapy for glycine encephalopathy in neonates has obviously not yet been realized.

THYROID AND ANTITHYROID DRUGS

The dynamic physiology of the thyroid hormones in the newborn is associated with a high incidence of both permanent and transient disorders of thyroid function. Details of the development of normal thyroid function can be found in any of several review articles.[220,222,224,229,232,240,243]

Replacement Therapy for Hypothyroidism

As shown in Table 10–12, neonatal hypothyroidism has multiple causes. Permanent abnormalities leading to hypothyroidism occur once in every 4000 live births.[224] These disorders can generally be identified by measurement of serum thyroxine (T_4), T_3, and thyroid-stimulating hormone (TSH) levels. Normal values for newborns (premature and full-term) and neonates have been published.[224] Transient disorders of thyroid function are thought to evolve largely from immaturity of the hypothalamic-pituitary axis. A particularly high frequency of low serum T_4 values with normal serum TSH levels has been identified in low-birth-weight infants, particularly those with RDS.[243] Repeated determinations of serum T_4 and TSH are required in order to make a decision regarding normality versus the need for treatment for hypothyroidism.[243]

Treatment of hypothyroidism should be accomplished with *levothyroxine*. Although a

Table 10-12. CAUSES OF NEONATAL HYPOTHYROIDISM

Increased TSH
primary hypothyroidism
  aplasia
  hypoplasia
  ectopic gland
  dyshormonogenesis
transient
  fetal exposure (antithyroid drugs, iodide)
  idiopathic
  "sick" premature infant
Normal TSH
hypothalamic–pituitary hypothyroidism
  idiopathic
  aplasia (pituitary)
  dysplasia
low TBG or binding
  hereditary
  generalized
  hypoproteinemia
  drugs
transient
  premature
  SGA
  nonthyroid illness

variety of thyroid hormone preparations are commercially available, this synthetic T_4 preparation has been determined to be the agent of choice.[219,235] The two commercial preparations judged to be of suitable and consistent potency are Synthroid and Levothroid. The recommended doses of levothyroxine are based on age: 0 to 6 months, 8 to 10 μg/kg per day; 6 to 12 months, 6 to 8 μg/kg per day (Table 10-13). The dose is administered PO once daily. Lower doses may be desirable in the presence of severe systemic illness or preexisting cardiac disease, particularly if the infant is susceptible to decompensation from congestive heart failure.

The determination of adequacy of therapy is based on clinical and laboratory information. The half-life of levothyroxine (T_4) is longer than 1 week, necessitating a period of 4 to 6 weeks of therapy before steady state is reached (see Section I). As a consequence, serum T_4 levels, if determined prior to attainment of steady state (1–2 wk), would be expected to be subnormal. Thyrotoxicosis is not an unexpected occurrence with thyroid replacement therapy. Some infants develop clinical and chemical evidence of thyrotoxicosis after periods of apparent stability. Determination of serum T_3 levels can serve to identify hyperthyroidism, particularly if serum T_4 levels have been found to be normal.

Serum T_3 levels are not very useful for moni-

toring for hypothyroidism. Infants with primary congenital hypothyroidism may have elevated levels of TSH for several years following replacement therapy. Lowering of TSH values, therefore, may not occur and should not be interpreted as a reflection of adequacy of replacement therapy. Subnormal serum T_4 values should prompt an immediate increase in levothyroxine dosage (with the exception of pre-steady state conditions). The usual increment of dose increase is 12.5 μg (half of a 25-μg tablet); smaller incremental changes can be accomplished by dosing on alternate days with the additional dose. Dosage adjustment should be monitored at 3- and 6-week periods by both clinical and laboratory assessment. The target T_4 value is 8 to 11 μg/dl;[235] however, because normal values vary from one laboratory to another, an acceptable T_4 value is the upper limit of normal for the laboratory being utilized. The outcome in neonates whose treatment begins before 1 month of age is excellent.[244]

Table 10-13. TREATMENT OF THYROID DYSFUNCTION

Drug	Therapeutic Regimen
Hypothyroidism	
levothyroxine (Synthroid, Levothroid)	
age 0–6 mo:	8–10 μg/kg PO q 24 hr
6–12 mo:	6–8 μg/kg PO q 24 hr
monitoring	Steady-state serum levels of T_4 (levothyroxine) attained approximately 6 wk after initiating or changing dose of levothyroxine. Clinical evaluation (growth and symptoms) and laboratory studies (for T_4) are of equal importance. Serum T_3 levels may be of value in evaluating for thyrotoxicosis. Serum TSH values are unreliable for monitoring therapy.
dose adjustment	increase or decrease by 12.5-μg increments (equal to ½ tablet)
Hyperthyroidism[a]	
iodine solution (Lugol's)	1 drop PO, 1–3 times q 24 hr
propylthiouracil	2–4 mg/kg PO q 8 hr, increasing daily to maximum of 10 mg/kg/dose as required *Note:* Onset of action with initial dosing may take several days.
propranolol	0.25 mg/kg PO q 6 hr, increasing to maximum of 1 mg/kg/dose (see text)

[a] See text for caution on the development of iatrogenic hypothyroidism produced by overly aggressive drug therapy.

Thyroid Inhibitor Therapy for Hyperthyroidism

Most of the reported cases of neonatal hyperthyroidism are associated with a maternal history of hyperthyroidism either during or prior to pregnancy. The exact etiology is unknown but is generally accepted to involve transplacental passage of human thyroid-stimulating immunoglobulin (HTSI).[221] However, a few cases of neonatal hyperthyroidism have been reported in offspring of mothers with no history of thyroid disease.[227] In affected infants, clinical evidence of neonatal hyperthyroidism most often is present at birth or appears within the first 24 hours of life. Signs and symptoms include goiter, tachycardia, hyperkinesis, tachypnea, diarrhea, weight loss or poor weight gain despite good caloric intake, flushing, periorbital edema, and bilateral exophthalmos.[241]

The treatment of neonatal thyrotoxicosis remains controversial. A number of drugs are capable of interfering directly or indirectly with the synthesis of thyroid hormones. The major inhibitors have been classified into three categories: antithyroid drugs, which interfere directly with the synthesis of thyroid hormones; ionic inhibitors, which block the iodide transport mechanism; and iodide itself, which in high concentrations suppresses thyroid gland function. *Propylthiouracil* is the antithyroid drug of choice in the treatment of neonatal thyrotoxicosis.[223] Both propylthiouracil and *methimazole,* another less-used antithyroid drug, inhibit the formation of thyroid hormones by interfering with the incorporation of iodine into thyroglobulin.[231] They also inhibit the formation of iodothyronines by interfering with the coupling of the iodotyrosyl residues. As a result of inhibition of hormone synthesis, depletion of stores of iodinated thyroglobulin occurs over a period of time. As a consequence, circulating thyroid hormone levels begin to decline and clinical manifestations subside. In addition to blocking hormone synthesis, propylthiouracil inhibits the peripheral deiodination of thyroxine to triiodothyronine.[226,238] Methimazole does not have this effect.

The absorption of propylthiouracil and methimazole occurs rapidly following PO administration. In adults the half-life of propylthiouracil in plasma is about 2 hours, compared with 6 to 13 hours for methimazole.[231] The duration of effective inhibition of thyroid hormone synthesis is comparatively brief: For propylthiouracil, this effect lasts for 2 to 3 hours, or at most 6 to 8 hours, in adults; for methimazole,

inhibition is 6 to 8 hours for low doses and as long as 24 hours for a single large dose. Unchanged drug (< 10%) and metabolites are excreted largely in the urine.[228]

Iodide is one of the oldest drugs employed for the treatment of thyroid disorders. The onset of action of iodide in the treatment of hyperthyroidism is often rapid and striking, typically occurring within 24 hours. The mechanism for this effect is interference with release of thyroid hormone into the circulation. Acute inhibition of synthesis of iodotyrosine and iodothyronine also follows iodide administration; the mechanism is not known.[220] The maximum effect is reached by about 2 weeks of continuous therapy. Iodide therapy alone generally does not completely control the manifestations of hyperthyroidism. In addition, hyperthyroidism may return to the original intensity or may become even more severe with continued administration of iodide beyond 2 weeks. The mechanism for this resistant or rebound state is unknown.

Other drugs that have been employed in the treatment of hyperthyroidism include *propranolol.*[233,234,242] The doses of propranolol employed in infants ranged from 0.5 mg 3 to 4 times daily PO increasing over several weeks to a maximum of 7 to 8 mg given 4 times daily. Propranolol and its use in hyperthyroidism is reviewed in Chapter 7.

Pharmacologic management of hyperthyroidism in neonates and older infants is appropriate only when clinical status is judged to be significantly compromised by the disorder. In the vast amount of anecdotal experiences in the literature, quantitative measure of the extent of improvement with a variety of drug therapies is seldom reported. Included among the drugs that have been administered to neonates and infants with hyperthyroidism are digitalis, phenobarbital, diazepam, steroids, thiazides, furosemide, hydralazine, propranolol, reserpine, potassium iodide, propylthiouracil, and methimazole.[230,236,239,266]

A rational approach to management of neonatal thyrotoxicosis is the administration of a saturated solution of potassium iodide (Lugol's solution) in a dose of 1 to 3 drops PO per day. This regimen should result in a clinical response within 24 hours. Propylthiouracil therapy can be instituted simultaneously or after evaluation of the response to the Lugol's solution (Table 10–13). The dose of propylthiouracil is 2 to 4 mg/kg administered PO every 8 hours (10 mg/kg q 24 hr). The latent period for maximum effect of this drug may be a few days to 2 or more weeks. Propranolol clearly should not be employed as the sole therapeutic agent[225] because it fails to inhibit the function of the thyroid; however it may provide suppression of the signs and symptoms of thyrotoxicosis. The initial recommended dose is 0.25 mg/kg given PO every 6 hours, increasing daily to a maximum of 1 mg/kg per dose (see Propranolol in Chap. 7).

It is important to remember that the vast majority of cases of neonatal hyperthyroidism are transient. The half-life of HTSI is 30 to 35 days; therefore, failure to reduce and subsequently to discontinue the antithyroid medication appropriately will result in hypothyroidism. Because normal neurologic development is dependent on normal thyroid hormone concentrations, *this iatrogenic hypothyroidism can result in mental retardation.*

Clinical Toxicology. The incidence of side-effects of the thyroid inhibitors (e.g. propylthiouracil) is relatively low (3%). The most serious side-effect is agranulocytosis.[237] The most common reaction is a purpuric or papular rash. See the preceding paragraph regarding iatrogenic hypothyroidism.

References
Atropine and Glycopyrrolate

1. Adams RG, Verma P, Jackson AJ, Miller RL: Plasma pharmacokinetics of intravenously administered atropine in normal human subjects. J Clin Pharmacol 22:477, 1982.
2. Bauer CR, Trottier MCT, Stern L: Systemic cyclopentolate (Cyclogyl) toxicity in the newborn infant. J Pediatr 82:501, 1973.
3. Dauchot P, Gravenstein JS: Effects of atropine on the electrocardiogram in different age groups. Clin Pharmacol Ther 12:274, 1971.
4. Fassoulaki A, Kaniaris P: Does atropine premedication affect the cardiovascular response to laryngoscopy and intubation? Br J Anaesth 54:1065, 1982.
5. Greenberg MI, Mayeda DV, Chrzanowski R, et al: Endotracheal administration of atropine sulfate. Ann Emerg Med 11:546, 1982.
6. Harris WS, Goodman RM: Hyper-reactivity to atropine in Down's syndrome. N Engl J Med 279:407, 1968.
7. Ingram RHJ, Wellman JJ, McFadden ER, Mead J: Relative contribution of large and small airways to flow limitation in normal subjects before and after atropine and isoproterenol. J Clin Invest 59:696, 1977.
8. Kattwinkel J, Fanaroff AA, Klaus MH: Bradycardia in preterm infants: Indications and hazards of atropine therapy. Pediatrics 58:494, 1976.
9. Kurz H, Mauser-Granshorn A, Stickel HH: Differences in the binding of drugs to plasma proteins from newborn and adult man. I. Eur J Clin Pharmacol 11:463, 1977.
10. Lavis DM, Lunn JN, Rosen M: Glycopyrrolate in children: A comparison between the effects of glycopyrrolate and atropine administered before induction of anaesthesia. Anaesthesia 35:1068, 1980.

11. Leighton KM, Sanders HD: Anticholinergic premedication. Can Anaesth Soc J 23:563, 1976.
12. Meyers EF, Tomeldan SA: Glycopyrrolate compared with atropine in prevention of the oculocardiac reflex during eye-muscle surgery. Anesthesiology 51:350, 1979.
13. Mirakhur RK, Clarke RSJ, Elliott J, Dundee JW: Atropine and glycopyrronium premedication. Anaesthesia 33:906, 1978.
14. Mirakhur RK, Dundee JW, Connolly JDR: Studies of drugs given before anaesthesia. XVII. Anticholinergic premedicants. Br J Anaesth 51:339, 1979.
15. Mirakhur RK, Briggs LP, Clarke RSJ, et al: Comparison of atropine and glycopyrrolate in a mixture with pyridostigmine for the antagonism of neuromuscular block. Br J Anaesth 53:1315, 1981.
16. Oberhansli-Weiss I, Heymann MA, Rudolph AM, Melmon KL: The pattern and mechanism of response to oxygen by the ductus arteriosus and umbilical artery. Pediatr Res 6:693, 1972.
17. O'Donovan JC, Bradstock AS Jr: The failure of conventional drug therapy in the management of infantile colic. Am J Dis Child 133:999, 1979.
18. Rosen M: Atropine in the treatment of laryngeal spasm. Br J Anaesth 32:190, 1960.
19. Shutt LE, Bowes JB: Atropine and hyoscine. Anaesthesia 34:476, 1979.
20. Unna KR, Glaser K, Lipton E, Patterson PR: Dosage of drugs in infants and children: I. Atropine. Pediatrics 6:197, 1950.

Bethanechol

21. Euler AR: Use of bethanechol for the treatment of gastroesophageal reflux. J Pediatr 96:321, 1980.
22. Strickland AD, Chang JHT: Results of treatment of gastroesophageal reflux with bethanechol. J Pediatr 103:311, 1983.

Bicarbonate

23. Anonymous: Advanced life support. JAMA 227:857, 1974.
24. Baum JD, Robertson NRC: Immediate effects of alkaline infusion in infants with respiratory distress syndrome. J Pediatr 87:255, 1975.
25. Bishop RL, Weisfeldt ML: Sodium bicarbonate administration during cardiac arrest. Effect on arterial pH, Pco_2, and osmolality. J Am Med Assoc 235:506, 1976.
26. Bland RD, Clarke TL, Harden LB: Rapid infusion of sodium bicarbonate and albumin into high-risk premature infants soon after birth: A controlled, prospective trial. Am J Obstet Gynecol 124:263, 1976.
27. Corbet AJ, Adams JM, Kenny JD, et al: Controlled trial of bicarbonate therapy in high-risk premature newborn infants. J Pediatr 91:771, 1977.
28. Donckerwolcke RA: Diagnosis and treatment of renal tubular disorders in children. Pediatr Clin North Am 29:895, 1982.
29. Eidelman AI, Hobbs JF: Bicarbonate therapy revisited. A study in therapeutic revisionism. Arch Dis Child 132:847, 1978.
30. Evans RS, Olver RE, Appleyard WJ, Newman CGH: Effects of intragastric and intravenous sodium bicarbonate on rate of recovery from post-asphyxial acidosis in the neonate. Arch Dis Child 45:321, 1970.

31. Finberg L: The relationship of intravenous infusions and intracranial hemorrhage—a commentary. J Pediatr 91:777, 1977.
32. Hobel CJ, Oh W, Hyvarinen MA, et al: Early versus late treatment of neonatal acidosis in low-birth-weight infants: Relation to respiratory distress syndrome. J Pediatr 81:1178, 1972.
33. Irving CS, Lifshitz CH, Wong WW, et al: Bicarbonate/CO_2 pool sizes and flux in infants measured by $NaH^{13}CO_3$ breath tests. Pediatr Res 17:291A, 1983.
34. Nash MA, Torrado AD, Greifer I, et al: Renal tubular acidosis in infants and children. J Pediatr 80:738, 1972.
35. Ostrea EM, Odell GB: The influence of bicarbonate administration on blood pH in a "closed system": Clinical implications. J Pediatr 80:671, 1972.
36. Papile L, Burstein J, Burstein R, et al: Relationship of intravenous sodium bicarbonate infusions and cerebral intraventricular hemorrhage. J Pediatr 93:834, 1978.
37. Rhodes PG, Hall RT, Hellerstein S: The effects of single infusions of hypertonic sodium bicarbonate on body composition in neonates with acidosis. J Pediatr 90:789, 1976.
38. Rodriguez-Soriano J, Vallo A, Castillo G, Oliveros R: Natural history of primary distal renal tubular acidosis treated since infancy. J Pediatr 101:669, 1982.
39. Russell G, Cotton EK: Effects of sodium bicarbonate by rapid injection and of oxygen in high concentration in respiratory distress syndrome of the newborn. Pediatrics 41:1063, 1968.
40. Savignoni PG, Bucci G, Ceccamea A, et al: Intravenous infusion of glucose and sodium bicarbonate in hyaline membrane disease. Acta Paediatr Scand 58:1, 1969.
41. Schwartz GJ, Haycock GB, Edelmann CM Jr, Spitzer A: Late metabolic acidosis: A reassessment of the definition. J Pediatr 95:102, 1979.
42. Simmons MA, Adcock EW, Bard H, Battaglia FC: Hypernatremia and intracranial hemorrhage in neonates. N Engl J Med 291:6, 1974.
43. Sinclair JC, Engel K, Silverman WA: Early correction of hypoxemia and acidemia in infants of low birth weight: A controlled trial of oxygen breathing, rapid alkali infusion, and assisted ventilation. Pediatrics 42:565, 1968.
44. Steichen JJ, Kleinman LI: Studies in acid-base balance. I. Effect of alkali therapy in newborn dogs with mechanically fixed ventilation. J Pediatr 91:287, 1977.
45. Svenningsen NW: Renal acid-base titration studies in infants with and without metabolic acidosis in the postneonatal period. Pediatr Res 8:659, 1974.
46. Usher R: Reduction of mortality from respiratory distress syndrome of prematurity with early administration of intravenous glucose and sodium bicarbonate. Pediatrics 32:966, 1963.

THAM

47. Battaglia FC, Makowski EL, Meschia G, Niernberg MM: Effect of THAM and sodium bicarbonate on the oxygen dissociation curve and pH difference across the red cell. Pediatr Res 2:193, 1968.
48. Baum JD, Roberton NRC: Immediate effects of alkaline infusion in infants with respiratory distress syndrome. J Pediatr 87:255, 1975.
49. Bleich HL, Schwartz WB: TRIS buffer (THAM): An appraisal of its physiologic effects and clinical usefulness. N Engl J Med 274:782, 1966.
50. Gupta JM, Malaya MB: The effect of THAM on the oxygen tension of arterial blood in neonatal respiratory-distress syndrome. Lancet 1:734, 1965.
51. Gupta JM, Dahlenburg GW, Davis JA: Changes in blood gas tensions following administration of amine buffer THAM to infants with respiratory distress syndrome. Arch Dis Child 42:416, 1967.
52. Roberton NRC: Apnoea after THAM administration in the newborn. Arch Dis Child 45:206, 1970.
53. vanVliet PKJ, Gupta JM: THAM versus sodium bicarbonate in idiopathic respiratory distress syndrome. Arch Dis Child 48:249, 1973.

Calcium

54. Anonymous. Advanced life support. JAMA 227:857, 1974.
55. Brown DR, Tsang RC, Chen IW: Oral calcium supplementation in premature and asphyxiated neonates. J Pediatr 89:973, 1976.
56. Brown DR, Steranka BH, Taylor FH: Treatment of early-onset neonatal hypocalcemia. Am J Dis Child 135:24, 1981.
57. Brown DR, Salsburey DJ: Short-term biochemical effects of parenteral calcium treatment of early-onset neonatal hypocalcemia. J Pediatr 100:777, 1982.
58. David L, Salle BL, Putet G, Grafmeyer DC: Serum immunoreactive calcitonin in low birth weight infants. Pediatr Res 15:803, 1981.
59. Drop LJ, Laver MB: Low plasma ionized calcium and response to calcium therapy in critically ill man. Anesthesiology 43:300, 1975.
60. Feinberg H, Boyd E, Katz LN: Calcium effect on performance of the heart. Am J Physiol 202:643, 1962.
61. Frohlick ED, Scott JB, Haddy FJ: Effect of cations on resistance and responsiveness of renal and forelimb vascular beds. Am J Physiol 203:583, 1962.
62. Ginsburg R, Esserman LJ, Bristow MR: Myocardial performance and extracellular ionized calcium in a severely failing human heart. Ann Intern Med 98:603, 1983.
63. Goldsmith MA, Bhatia SS, Kanto WP, Kutner MH, Rudman D: Gluconate calcium therapy and neonatal hypercalciuria. Am J Dis Child 135:538, 1981.
64. Hammerman C, Eidelman AI, Gartner LM: Hypocalcemia and the patent ductus arteriosus. J Pediatr 94:961, 1979.
65. Heckler FR, McGraw JB: Calcium-related cutaneous necrosis. Surgical Forum 27:553, 1976.
66. Morris DL, Goldschlager N: Calcium infusion for reversal of adverse effects of intravenous verapamil. JAMA 249:3212, 1983.
67. Moya M, Domenech E: Calcium intake in the first five days of life in the low birthweight infant. Arch Dis Child 53:784, 1978.
68. Nervez CT, Shott RJ, Bergstrom WH, Williams ML: Prophylaxis against hypocalcemia in low-birth-weight infants requiring bicarbonate infusion. J Pediatr 87:439, 1975.
69. Perkin RM, Levin DL: Shock in the pediatric patient. Part II. Therapy. J Pediatr 101:319, 1982.
70. Ramamurthy RS, Harris V, Pildes RS: Subcutaneous calcium deposition in the neonate associated with intravenous administration of calcium gluconate. Pediatrics 55:802, 1975.
71. Salsburey DJ, Brown DR: Effect of parenteral calcium

treatment on blood pressure and heart rate in neonatal hypocalcemia. Pediatrics 69:605, 1982.

72. Sann L, David L, Chayvialle JA, et al: Effect of early oral calcium supplementation on serum calcium and immunoreactive calcitonin concentration in preterm infants. Arch Dis Child 55:611, 1980.

73. Senterre J, Salle B: Calcium and phosphorus economy of the preterm infant and its interaction with vitamin E and its metabolites. Acta Paediatr Scand 296 (Suppl):85, 1982.

74. Shaw JCL: Parenteral nutrition in the management of sick low birthweight infants. Pediatr Clin North Am 20:333, 1973.

75. Sorell M, Rosen JF: Ionized calcium: Serum levels during symptomatic hypocalcemia. J Pediatr 87:67, 1975.

76. Steichen JJ, Gratton TL, Tsang RC: Osteopenia of prematurity: The cause and the possible treatment. J Pediatr 96:528, 1980.

77. Sutton A, Mole RH, Barltrop D: Urinary and faecal excretion of marker calcium (^{46}Ca) by low birthweight infants. Arch Dis Child 52:50, 1977.

78. Troughton O, Singh SP: Heart failure and neonatal hypocalcaemia. Br Med J 4:76, 1972.

79. Tsang RC, Donovan EF, Steichen JJ: Calcium physiology and pathology in the neonate. Pediatr Clin North Am 23:611, 1976.

Cimetidine

80. Abate MA, Hyneck ML, Cohen IA, Berardi RR: Cimetidine pharmacokinetics. Clin Pharmacol 1:225, 1982

81. Bale JF Jr, Roberts C, Book LS: Cimetidine-induced cerebral toxicity in children. Lancet 1:725, 1979.

82. Bar-Maor JA, Shoshany G, Monies-Chass I: Use of cimetidine in esophageal atresia with lower tracheoesophageal fistula. J Pediatr Surg 16:8, 1981.

83. Chhattriawalla Y, Colon AR, Scanlon JW: The use of cimetidine in the newborn. Pediatrics 65:301, 1980.

84. Goldenring J: Cimetidine and pulmonary hypertension. Pediatrics 66:1029, 1980.

85. Goudsouzian N, Cote CJ, Liu LMP, Dedrick DF: The dose-response effects of oral cimetidine on gastric pH and volume in children. Anesthesiology 55:533, 1981.

86. Gugler R, Fuchs G, Dieckmann M, Somogyi AA: Cimetidine plasma concentration-response relationships. Clin Pharmacol Ther 29:744, 1981.

87. Hugues JN, Perret G, Sebaoun J, Modigliani E: Effects of cimetidine on thyroid hormones. Clin Endocrinol 17:297, 1982.

88. Larsson R, Norlander B, Bodemar G, Walan A: Steady-state kinetics and dosage requirements of cimetidine in renal failure. Clin Pharmacokinet 6:316, 1981.

89. Lilly JR, Hitch DC, Javitt NB: Cimetidine cholestatic jaundice in children. J Surg Res 24:384, 1978.

90. Okolicsanyi L, Venuti M, Orlando R, et al: Oral and intravenous pharmacokinetics of cimetidine in liver cirrhosis. Int J Clin Pharmacol Ther Toxicol 20:482, 1982.

Corticosteroids

91. Axelrod L: Glucocorticoid therapy. Medicine 55:39, 1976.

92. Baxter JD: Glucocorticoid hormone action. Pharmacol Ther (Part B) 2:605, 1976.

93. Bond WS: Toxic reactions and side effects of glucocorticoids in man. Am J Hosp Pharm 34:479, 1977.

94. Cohen SR, Wang CI: Steroid treatment of hemangioma of the head and neck in children. Ann Otol 81:584, 1972.

95. deLemos RA, Haggerty RJ: Corticosteroids as an adjunct to treatment in bacterial meningitis: A controlled clinical trial. Pediatrics 44:30, 1969.

96. Dixon RB, Christy NP: On the various forms of corticosteroid withdrawal syndrome. Am J Med 68:224, 1980.

97. Duck SC: Acceptable linear growth in congenital adrenal hyperplasia. J Pediatr 97:93, 1980.

98. Fauci AS, Dale DC, Balow JE: Glucocorticosteroid therapy: Mechanisms of action and clinical considerations. Ann Intern Med 84:304, 1976.

99. Feinblatt BI, Aceto T Jr, Beckhorn G, Bruck E: Percutaneous absorption of hydrocortisone in children. Am J Dis Child 112:218, 1966.

100. Gutai JP, Migeon CJ: Adrenal insufficiency during the neonatal period. Clin Perinatol 2:163, 1975.

101. Gutberlet RL, Cornblath M: Neonatal hypoglycemia revisited, 1975. Pediatrics 58:10, 1976.

102. Haddad HM, Hsia DYY, Gellis SS: Studies on respiratory rate in the newborn: Its use in the evaluation of respiratory distress in infants of diabetic mothers. Pediatrics 17:204, 1956.

103. Hansen JW, Loriaux DL: Variable efficacy of glucocorticoids in congenital adrenal hyperplasia. Pediatrics 57:942, 1976.

104. Haque KN: Dexamethasone in the treatment of hypernatraemic dehydration. Arch Dis Child 56:223, 1981.

105. Klevit HD: Corticosteroid therapy in the neonatal period. Pediatr Clin North Am 17:1003, 1970.

106. Leipzig B, Oski FA, Cummings CW, et al: A prospective randomized study to determine the efficacy of steroids in treatment of croup. J Pediatr 94:194, 1979.

107. Mammel MC, Green TP, Johnson DE, Thompson TR: Controlled trial of dexamethasone therapy in infants with bronchopulmonary dysplasia. Lancet 1:1356, 1983.

108. Overcash KE, Putney FJ: Subglottic hemangioma of the larynx treated with steroid therapy. Laryngoscope 83:679, 1973.

109. Pearn JH: Use of corticosteroids in childhood disease. Drugs 10:426, 1975.

110. Pickup ME: Clinical pharmacokinetics of prednisone and prednisolone. Clin Pharmacokinet 4:111, 1979.

111. Raivio KO: Neonatal hyperglycemia. II. A clinical study of 44 idiopathic cases with special reference to corticosteroid treatment. Acta Paediatr Scand 57:540, 1968.

112. Reeves JD, Huffer WE, August CS, et al: The hematopoietic effects of prednisone therapy in four infants with osteopetrosis. J Pediatr 94:210, 1979.

113. Rimsza ME: Complications of corticosteroid therapy. Am J Dis Child 132:806, 1978

114. Roselli A, Barbosa LT: Congenital hypoplasia of the adrenal glands. Pediatrics 35:70, 1965.

115. Rosler A, Levine LS, Schneider B, et al: The interrelationship of sodium balance, plasma renin activity, and ACTH in congenital adrenal hyperplasia. J Clin Endocrinol Metab 45:500, 1977.

116. Schumer W: Steroids in the treatment of clinical septic shock. Ann Surg 184:333, 1976.

117. Taeusch HW Jr, Wang NS, Baden M, et al: A controlled trial of hydrocortisone therapy in infants

with respiratory distress syndrome: II. Pathology. Pediatrics 52:850, 1973.

118. Taeusch HW Jr: Glucocorticoid prophylaxis for respiratory distress syndrome: A review of potential toxicity. J Pediatr 87:617, 1975.

119. Tal A, Bavilski C, Yohai D, et al: Dexamethasone and salbutamol in the treatment of acute wheezing in infants. Pediatrics 71:13, 1983.

120. Tunnessen WW Jr, Feinstein AR: The steroid-croup controversy: An analytic review of methodologic problems. J Pediatr 96:751, 1980.

121. Weichsel ME Jr: The therapeutic use of glucocorticoid hormones in the perinatal period: Potential neurological hazards. Ann Neurol 2:364, 1977.

122. Winter JSD: Marginal comment: Current approaches to the treatment of congenital adrenal hyperplasia. J Pediatr 97:81, 1980.

Heparin

123. Arnesen H, Heilo A, Jakobsen E, et al: A prospective study of streptokinase and heparin in the treatment of deep vein thrombosis. Acta Med Scand 203:457, 1978.

124. Barnard DR, Hathaway WE: Neonatal thrombosis. Am J Pediatr Hematol Oncol 1:235, 1979.

125. Coon WW: Some recent developments in the pharmacology of heparin. J Clin Pharmacol 19:337, 1979.

126. Estes JW: Clinical pharmacokinetics of heparin. Clin Pharmacokinet 5:204, 1980.

127. Jacques LB: Heparins—anionic polyelectrolyte drugs. Pharmacol Rev 31:99, 1980.

128. Levy SW, Jacques LB: Appearance of heparin antithrombin-active chains *in vitro* after injection of commercial heparin and in anaphylaxis. Thromb Res 13:429, 1978.

129. McDonald MM, Jacobson LJ, Hay WW Jr, Hathaway WE: Heparin clearance in the newborn. Pediatr Res 15:1015, 1981.

130. McDonald MM, Hathaway WE: Anticoagulant therapy by continuous heparinization in newborn and older infants. J Pediatr 101:451, 1982.

131. Merenstein GB: Heparinized catheters and coagulation studies. J Pediatr 79:117, 1971.

132. Rasoulpour M, McLean RH: Renal venous thrombosis in neonates. Initial and follow-up abnormalities. Am J Dis Child 134:276, 1980.

133. Salzman EW, Deykin D, Shapiro RM, Rosenberg R: Management of heparin therapy: Controlled prospective trial. N Engl J Med 292:1046, 1975.

134. Zaidan H, Dhanireddy R, Hamosh M, et al: Effect of continuous heparin administration on intralipid clearing in very low birth weight infants. J Pediatr 101:559, 1982.

Narcotic Analgesics, Sedatives and Hypnotics, Local Anesthetics

135. Baldessarini RJ: Schizophrenia. N Engl J Med 297:988, 1977.

136. Beaumont A, Hughes J: Biology of opioid peptides. Ann Rev Pharmacol Toxicol 19:245, 1979.

137. Bentley JB, Borel JD, Nenad RE Jr, Gillespie TJ: Age and fentanyl pharmacokinetics. Anesth Analg 61:968, 1982.

138. Borman JB, Merin G, Majblum S, et al: The beneficial effects of chlorpromazine on pulmonary hemodynamics after cardiopulmonary bypass. Ann Thorac Surg 11:570, 1971.

139. Breimer DD: Clinical pharmacokinetics of hypnotics. Clin Pharmacokinet 2:93, 1977.

140. Bryan MH, Hardie MJ, Reilly BJ, Swyer PR: Pulmonary function studies during the first year of life in infants recovering from the respiratory distress syndrome. Pediatrics 52:169, 1973.

141. Carabelle RW: Chloral hydrate: A useful pediatric sedative. Am J Ophthalmol 51:834, 1961.

142. Cook DR: Paediatric anaesthesia: Pharmacological considerations. Drugs 12:212, 1976.

143. Dahlstrom B, Bolme P, Feychting H, et al: Morphine kinetics in children. Clin Pharmacol Ther 26:354, 1979.

144. Dundee JW, Moore J, Love WJ, et al: Studies of drugs given before anaesthesia: VI. The phenothiazine derivatives. Br J Anaesth 37:332, 1965.

145. Edwards DJ, Svensson CK, Visco JP, Lalka D: Clinical pharmacokinetics of pethidine: 1982. Clin Pharmacokinet 7:421, 1982.

146. Ellingson RJ, Houfek EE: Seconal and chloral hydrate as sedatives in clinical electroencephalography. Clin Neurophysiol 1:93, 1952.

147. Eng M, Bonica JJ, Akamatsu TJ, et al: Respiratory depression in newborn monkeys at caesarean section following ketamine administration. Br J Anaesth 47:917, 1975.

148. Fixler DE, Carrell T, Browne R, et al: Oxygen consumption in infants and children during cardiac catheterization under different sedation regimens. Circulation 50:788, 1974.

149. Frumin MJ, Herekar VR, Jarvik ME: Amnesic actions of diazepam and scopolamine in man. Anesthesiology 45:406, 1976.

150. Gassner S, Cohen M, Aygen M, et al: The effect of ketamine on pulmonary artery pressure. Anaesthesia 29:141, 1974.

151. Gershanik JJ, Boecler B, Lertora JJL, et al: Monitoring levels of trichloroethanol (TCE) during chloral hydrate (CH) administration to sick neonates. Clin Res 29:895A, 1981.

152. Gordon M: Psychopharmacological Agents. Vol II. New York, Academic Press, 1974.

153. Graham TP Jr, Atwood GF, Werner B: Use of droperidol-fentanyl sedation for cardiac catheterization in children. Am Heart J 87:287, 1974.

154. Halpern LM: Analgesic drugs in the management of pain. Arch Surg 112:861, 1977.

155. Handal KA, Schauben JL, Salamone RF: Naloxone. Ann Emerg Med 12:438, 1983.

156. Harper MH, Hickey RF, Cromwell TH, Linwood S: The magnitude and duration of respiratory depression produced by fentanyl and fentanyl plus droperidol in man. J Pharmacol Exp Ther 199:464, 1976.

157. Hogg MIJ, Wiener PC, Rosen M, Mapleson WW: Urinary excretion and metabolism of pethidine and norpethidine in the newborn. Br J Anaesth 49:891, 1977.

158. Houser OW, Smith JB, Gomez MR, Baker HL: Evaluation of intracranial disorders in children by computerized transaxial tomography: A preliminary report. Neurology 25:607, 1975.

159. Jaffe JH, Martin WR: Opioid analgesics and antagonists. In Gilman AG, Goodman LS, Gilman A (eds): The Pharmacological Basis of Therapeutics, 6th ed. Chap 22. New York, Macmillan, 1980.

160. Kales A, Hauri P, Bixler EO, Silberfarb P: Effectiveness of intermediate term use of secobarbital. Clin Pharmacol Ther 20:541, 1976.

161. Kuhnert BR, Kuhnert PM, Prochaska AL, Sokol RJ:

Meperidine disposition in mother, neonate, and nonpregnant females. Clin Pharmacol Ther 27:486, 1980.

162. Kuzemko JA, Hartley S: Treatment of cerebral irritation in the newborn: Double-blind trial with chloral hydrate and diazepam. Dev Med Child Neurol 14:740, 1972.

163. Larsson LE, Ekstrom-Jodal B, Hjalmarson O: The effect of chlorpromazine in severe hypoxia in newborn infants. Acta Paediatr Scand 71:399, 1982.

164. Lees MH, Olsen GD, McGilliard KL, et al: Chloral hydrate and the carbon dioxide chemoreceptor response: A study of puppies and infants. Pediatrics 70:447, 1982.

165. Lockhart CH, Jenkins JJ: Ketamine-induced apnea in patients with increased intracranial pressure. Anesthesiology 37:92, 1972.

166. Maguire HT, Aldrete JA: Postanesthetic recovery in infants and children. Anesth Rev 2:9, 1975.

167. Mather LE, Tucker GT, Pflug AE, et al: Meperidine kinetics in man: Intravenous injection in surgical patients and volunteers. Clin Pharmacol Ther 17:21, 1975.

168. Mather LE, Tucker GT: Systemic availability of orally administered meperidine. Clin Pharmacol Ther 20:535, 1976.

169. Mather LE, Meffin PJ: Clinical pharmacokinetics of pethidine. Clin Pharmacokinet 3:352, 1978.

170. Miser AW, Miser JS, Clark BS: Continuous intravenous infusion of morphine sulfate for control of severe pain in children with terminal malignancy. J Pediatr 96:930, 1980.

171. Mojdehi E, Mauro AL, Labartino L, Reynolds B: Clinical evaluation of hydroxyzine hydrochloride in pediatric anesthesia and its effect on arousal time. Anesth Analg 47:685, 1968.

172. Morselli PL, Rovei V: Placental transfer of pethidine and norpethidine and their pharmacokinetics in the newborn. Eur J Clin Pharmacol 18:25, 1980.

173. Nation RL: Meperidine binding in maternal and fetal plasma. Clin Pharmacol Ther 29:472, 1981.

174. Nordenberg A, Delisle G, Izukawa T: Cardiac arrhythmia in a child due to chloral hydrate ingestion. Pediatrics 47:134, 1971.

175. Radnay PA, Badola RP: Generalized extensor spasm in infants following ketamine anesthesia. Anesthesiology 39:459, 1973.

176. Riemenschneider TA, Nielson HC, Ruttenberg HD, Jaffe RB: Disturbances of the transitional circulation: Spectrum of pulmonary hypertension and myocardial dysfunction. J Pediatr 89:622, 1976.

177. Robinson S, Gregory GA: Fentanyl-air-oxygen anesthesia for ligation of patent ductus arteriosus in preterm infants. Anesth Analg 60:331, 1981.

178. Romagnoli A, Cuison S, Cohen M: The use of diazepam in paediatric premedication. Can Anaesth Soc J 15:603, 1968.

179. Root B: Oral premedication of children with chloral hydrate and scopolamine. Anesth Analg 41:194, 1962.

180. Root B: Oral premedication for children: Experience with glutethimide, ethchlorvynol, and secobarbital. Anesth Analg 46:481, 1967.

181. Root B, Loveland JP: Premedication of children with promethazine, propiomazine, and mepazine: Comparison of oral and intramuscular routes. J Clin Pharmacol 10:182, 1970.

182. Ruckman RN, Keane JF, Freed MD, et al: Sedation for cardiac catheterization: A controlled study. Pediatr Cardiol 1:263, 1980.

183. Rutter PC, Murphy F, Dudley HAF: Morphine: A controlled trial of different methods of administration for postoperative pain relief. Br Med J 280:12, 1980.

184. Sellers EM, Lang ML, Cooper SD, Koch-Weser J: Chloral hydrate and triclofos metabolism. Clin Pharmacol Ther 14:147, 1973.

185. Stetson JB, Jessup GVS: Use of oral chloral hydrate mixtures for pediatric premedication. Anesth Analg 41:203, 1962.

186. Stocks J, Godfrey S: The role of artificial ventilation, oxygen, and CPAP in the pathogenesis of lung damage in neonates: Assessment by serial measurements of lung function. Pediatrics 57:352, 1976.

187. Ward RJ, Crawford EW, Stevenson JD: Anesthetic experiences for infants under 2500 grams weight. Anesth Analg 49:767, 1970.

188. Way WL, Costley EC, Way EL: Respiratory sensitivity of the newborn infant to meperidine and morphine. Clin Pharmacol Ther 6:454, 1965.

189. Wiliamson PS, Williamson ML: Physiologic stress reduction by a local anesthetic during newborn circumcision. Pediatrics 71:36, 1983.

190. Zsigmond EK, Domino EF: Ketamine: Clinical pharmacology, pharmacokinetics, and current clinical uses. Anesth Rev 7:13, 1980.

Neuromuscular Blockers

191. Bennett EJ, Daugherty MJ, Bowyer DE, Stephen CR: Pancuronium bromide: Experiences in 100 pediatric patients. Anesth Analg 50:798, 1971.

192. Bennett EJ, Bowyer DE, Giesecke AH, Stephen CR: Pancuronium bromide: A double-blind study in children. Anesth Analg 52:12, 1973.

193. Bennett EJ, Ramamurthy S, Dalal FY, Salem MR: Pancuronium and the neonate. Br J Anaesth 47:75, 1975.

194. Bennett EJ, Ignacio A, Patel K, et al: Tubocurarine and the neonate. Br J Anaesth 48:687, 1976.

195. Bush GH, Stead AL: The use of d-tubocurarine in neonatal anaesthesia. Br J Anaesth 34:721, 1962.

196. Cook DR, Wingard LB Jr, Taylor FH: Pharmacokinetics of succinylcholine in infants, children, and adults. Clin Pharmacol Ther 20:493, 1976.

197. Cook DR: Muscle relaxants in infants and children. Anesth Analg 60:335, 1981.

198. Crone RK, Favorito J: The effects of pancuronium bromide on infants with hyaline membrane disease. J Pediatr 97:991, 1980.

199. Finer NN, Tomney PM: Controlled evaluation of muscle relaxation in the ventilated neonate. Pediatrics 67:641, 1981.

200. Fisher DM, O'Keeffe C, Stanski DR, et al: Pharmacokinetics and pharmacodynamics of d-tubocurarine in infants, children, and adults. Anesthesiology 57:203, 1982.

201. Goudsouzian NG, Liu LMP, Savarese JJ: Metocurine in infants and children: Neuromuscular and clinical effects. Anesthesiology 49:266, 1978.

202. Goudsouzian NG, Crone RK, Todres ID: Recovery from pancuronium blockade in the neonatal intensive care unit. Br J Anaesth 53:1303, 1981.

203. Henry GW, Stevens DC, Schreiner RL, et al: Respiratory paralysis to improve oxygenation and mortality in large newborn infants with respiratory distress. J Pediatr Surg 14:761, 1979.

204. Meijer DKF, Weitering JG, Vermeer GA, Scaf AHJ: Comparative pharmacokinetics of d-tubocurarine

and metocurine in man. Anesthesiology 51:402, 1979.

205. Nugent SK, Laravuso R, Rogers MC: Pharmacology and use of muscle relaxants in infants and children. J Pediatr 94:481, 1979.

206. Nussmeier N, Henry GW, Stevens DC, et al: Dose requirement of *d*-tubocurarine and metocurine used for chronic respiratory paralysis in neonates. J Pediatr Surg 16:700, 1981.

207. Pollitzer MJ, Reynolds EOR, Shaw DG, Thomas RM: Pancuronium during mechanical ventilation speeds recovery of lungs of infants with hyaline membrane disease. Lancet 1:346, 1981.

208. Ramzan MI, Somogyi AA, Walker JS, et al: Clinical pharmacokinetics of the non-depolarising muscle relaxants. Clin Pharmacokinet 6:25, 1981.

209. Roizen MF, Feeley TW: Pancuronium bromide. Ann Intern Med 88:64, 1978.

210. Stark AR, Bascom R, Frantz ID III: Muscle relaxation in mechanically ventilated infants. J Pediatr 94:439, 1979.

211. Taylor P: Neuromuscular blocking agents. In Gilman AG, Goodman LS, Gilman A (eds): The Pharmacological Basis of Therapeutics, 6th ed. Chap. 11. New York, Macmillan, 1980.

Strychnine, Sodium, Benzoate, and Benzodiazepine Therapy

212. Arneson D, Ch'ien LT, Chance P, Wilroy RS: Strychnine therapy in nonketotic hyperglycinemia. Pediatrics 63:369, 1979.

213. Gitzelmann R, Steinmann B, Otten A, et al: Nonketotic hyperglycinemia treated with strychnine, a glycine receptor antagonist. Helv Paediatr Acta 32:517, 1977.

214. Krieger I, Winbaum ES, Eisenbrey AB: Cerebrospinal fluid glycine in nonketotic hyperglycinemia. Effect of treatment with sodium benzoate and a ventricular shunt. Metabolism 26:517, 1977.

215. Perry TL, Urquhart N, MacLean J, et al: Nonketotic hyperglycinemia: Glycine accumulation due to absence of glycine cleavage in brain. N Engl J Med 292:1269, 1975.

216. Sankaran K, Casey RE, Zaleski A, Mendelson IM: Glycine encephalopathy in a neonate. Clin Pediatr 21:636, 1982.

217. Spielberg SP, Lucky AW, Schulman JD, et al: Failure of leucovorin therapy in nonketotic hyperglycinemia. J Pediatr 89:681, 1976.

218. Young AB, Zukin SR, Snyder SH: Interaction of benzodiazepines with central nervous glycine receptors: Possible mechanism of action. Proc Natl Acad Sci USA 71:2246, 1974.

Thyroid and Antithyroid Drugs

219. Committee on Drugs: Treatment of congenital hypothyroidism. Pediatrics 62:413, 1978.

220. Degroot LJ, Niepomniszcze H: Biosynthesis of thyroid hormone: Basic and clinical aspects. Metabolism 26:665, 1977.

221. Dirmikis SM, Munro DS: Placental transmission of thyroid-stimulating immunoglobins. Br Med J 2:665, 1975

222. Erenberg A: Thyroid function in the preterm infant. Pediatr Clin North Am 29:1205, 1982.

223. Fisher DA: Pathogenesis and therapy of neonatal Graves disease. Arch Dis Child 130:133, 1976.

224. Fisher DA, Klein AH: Thyroid development and disorders of thyroid function in the newborn. N Engl J Med 304:702, 1981.

225. Gardner LI: Is propranolol alone really beneficial in neonatal thyrotoxicosis? Am J Dis Child 134:819, 1980.

226. Geffner DL, Azukizawa M, Hershman JM: Propylthiouracil blocks extrathyroidal conversion of thyroxine to triiodothyronine and augments thyrotropin secretion in man. J Clin Invest 55:224, 1975.

227. Hollingsworth DR, Mabry CC: Congenital Graves' disease: Four familial cases with long-term follow-up and perspective. Am J Dis Child 130:148, 1976.

228. Kampmann JP, Hansen JM: Clinical pharmacokinetics of antithyroid drugs. Clin Pharmacokinet 6:401, 1981.

229. MacGillivray MH: Thyroid dysfunction in the neonatal period. Clin Perinatol 2:15, 1975.

230. Mahoney CP, Pyne GE, Stamm SJ, Bakke JL: Neonatal Graves' disease. Am J Dis Child 107:516, 1964.

231. Marchant B, Lees JFH, Alexander WD: Antithyroid drugs. Pharmacol Ther [B] 3:305, 1978.

232. Novogroder M: Neonatal screening for congenital hypothyroidism. Pediatr Clin North Am 27:881, 1980.

233. Pearl KN, Chambers TL: Propranolol treatment of thyrotoxicosis in a premature infant. Br Med J 2:739, 1977.

234. Pemberton PJ, McConnell B, Shanks RG: Neonatal thyrotoxicosis treated wih propranolol. Arch Dis Child 49:813, 1974.

235. Redmond GP: Therapy of congenital hypothyroidism in the era of mass screening. Semin Perinatol 6:181, 1982.

236. Rosenberg D, Grand MJH, Silbert D: Neonatal hyperthyroidism. N Engl J Med 268:292, 1963.

237. Rosove MH: Agranulocytosis and antithyroid drugs. West J Med 126:339, 1977.

238. Saberi M, Sterling FH, Utiger RD: Reduction in extrathyroidal triiodothyronine production by propylthiouracil in man. J Clin Invest 55:218, 1975.

239. Samuel S, Pildes RS, Lewison M, Rosenthal IM: Neonatal hyperthyroidism in an infant born of an euthyroid mother. Am J Dis Child 121:440, 1971.

240. Schonberger W, Grimm W, Gempp W, Dinkel E: Transient hypothyroidism associated with prematurity, sepsis, and respiratory distress. Eur J Pediatr 132:85, 1979.

241. Singer J: Neonatal thyrotoxicosis. J Pediatr 91:749, 1977.

242. Smith CS, Howard NJ: Propranolol in treatment of neonatal thyrotoxicosis. J Pediatr 83:1046, 1973.

243. Uhrmann S, Marks KH, Maisels MJ, et al: Frequency of transient hypothyroxinaemia in low birthweight infant. Arch Dis Child 56:214,1981.

244. Virtanen M, Maenpaa J, Santavuori P, et al: Congenital hypothyroidism: Age at start of treatment versus outcome. Acta Paediatr Scand 72:197, 1983.

Additional References

245. Aranda JV, Outerbridge EW, Schentag JJ: Pharmacodynamics and kinetics of cimetidine in a premature newborn. Am J Dis Child 137:1207, 1983.

246. Atwood GF, Evans MA, Harbison RD: Pharmacokinetics of meperidine in infants. Pediatr Res 10:328, 1976.

247. Baldessarini RJ: The "neuroleptic" antiphychotic drugs. 2. Neurologic side effects. Postgrad Med 65:123, 1979.

248. Baylink DJ: Glucocorticoid-induced osteoporosis. New Engl J Med 309:306, 1983.

249. Berry DJ: Determination of trichlorethanol at therapeutic and overdose levels in blood and urine by electron capture gas chromatography. J Chromatography 107:107, 1975.

250. Caughman GB, Boackle RJ, Vesley J: A postulated mechanism for heparin's potentiation of C1 inhibitor function. Molec Immunol 19:287, 1982.

251. Chamberlin P, Meyer WJ III: Management of pituitary-adrenal suppression secondary to corticosteroid therapy. Pediatrics 67:245, 1981.

252. Chin TWF, MacLeod SM, Fenje P, et al: Pharmacokinetics of cimetidine in critically ill children. Pediatr Pharmacol 2:285, 1982.

253. Edgerton MT: The treatment of hemangiomas: With special reference to the role of steroid therapy. Ann Surg 183:517, 1976.

254. Edwards MS, Buffone GJ, Rench MA, et al: Effect of continuous heparin infusion on bactericidal activity for group B streptococci in neonatal sera. J Pediatr 103:787, 1983.

255. Fisher DM, Cronnelly R, Miller RD, Sharma M: The neuromuscular pharmacology of neostigmine in infants and children. Anesthesiology 59:220, 1983.

256. Fontán JP, Heldt GP, Heyman MB, et al: Esophageal spasm associated with apnea and bradycardia in an infant. Pediatrics 73:52, 1984.

257. Friedman R, Zitelli B, Jardine D, Fireman P: Seizures in a patient receiving terbutaline. Am J Dis Child 136:1091, 1982.

258. Kazatchkine MD, Fearon DT, Silbert JE, Austen KF: Surface-associated heparin inhibits zymosan-induced activation of the human alteration complement pathway by augmenting the regulatory action of the control proteins on particle-bound C3b. J Exp Med 150:1202, 1979.

259. Lenney W, Milner AD: At what age do bronchodilator drugs work? Arch Dis Child 53:532, 1978.

260. Lockhart CH, Nelson WL: The relationship of ketamine requirement to age in pediatric patients. Anesthesiology 40:507, 1974.

261. Marshall EK Jr, Owens AH Jr: Absorption, excretion and metabolic fate of chloral hydrate and trichloroethanol. Bull Johns Hopkins Hosp 95:1, 1954.

262. Miller RD: Antagonism of neuromuscular blockade. Anesthesiology 44:318, 1976.

263. Mirro R, Brown DR: Parenteral calcium treatment shortens the left ventricular systolic time intervals of hypocalcemic neonates. Pediatr Res 18:71, 1984.

264. Miser AW, Davis DM, Hughes CS, et al: Continuous subcutaneous infusion of morphine in children with cancer. Am J Dis Child 137:383, 1983.

265. Nielsen HC, Wiriyathian S, Rosenfeld CR, et al: Chlorpromazine excretion by the neonate following chronic in utero exposure. Pediatr Pharmacol 3:1, 1983.

266. Schonwetter BS, Libber SM, Jones MD Jr, et al: Hypertension in neonatal thyroidism. Am J Dis Child 137:954, 1983.

267. Sigurdsson G, Lindahl S, Norden N: Influence of premedication on plasma ACTA and cortisol concentrations in children during adenoidectomy. Br J Anaesth 54:1075, 1982.

268. Sondheimer JM, Mintz HL, Michaels M: Bethanecol treatment of gastroesophageal reflux in infants. Effect on continuous esophageal pH records. J Pediatr 104:128, 1984.

269. Sosulski R, Abbasi S, Fox WW: Therapeutic value of terbutaline in bronchopulmonary dysplasia. Pediatr Res 16:309A, 1982.

270. Stalker NE, Gambertoglio JG, Fukumitsu CJ, et al: Acute massive chloral hydrate intoxication treated with hemodialysis: A clinical pharmacokinetic analysis. J Clin Pharmacol 18:136, 1978.

271. Stillman AE, Hansen RC, Hallinan V, Strobel C: Diffuse neonatal hemangiomatosis with severe gastrointestinal involvement. Clin Pediatr 22:589, 1983.

272. von Wendt L, Simila S, Saukkonen AL, Koivisto M: Failure of strychnine treatment during the neonatal period in three Finnish children with nonketotic hyperglycinemia. Pediatrics 65:1166, 1980.

ELEVEN

Fetal and Infant Intoxication

Drug- or chemical-induced intoxication of the fetus or infant can be the consequence of inadvertent or intentional exposure of the fetus to certain drugs or chemicals prior to or during birth, or may be the result of intentional drug therapy in the sick infant. The character of the intoxication can include any of a wide variety of reversible or irreversible abnormal states such as dysmorphology, and cellular or organ injury and dysfunction. The consequence may be incompatible with life or may be a benign unobtrusive abnormality. Intoxication in the neonate can have an additional important dimension not found in adults: Development or maturational processes can be perturbed, with potentially serious consequences.[178] This unique potential toxicity and the fact that other adverse effects may not be revealed by experience in adults or animals are serious concerns. The toxicities associated with thalidomide, DES, and the preservative benzyl alcohol are a few poignant examples of the reality of this concern.[101,160]

Not only are certain toxic reactions life-threatening, but the frequency of any form of intoxication of the fetus or infant is alarmingly high. The high frequency is related in part to the current extent of drug and chemical exposure of the fetus and infant. Despite the wide publicity surrounding abnormalities resulting from drug contamination of the fetal environment, drug consumption during pregnancy continues at a distressing frequency.[22,44,399] Surveys of pregnant American females have shown that an average of 7 or more different drug products containing up to 4 or 5 ingredients are taken during pregnancy.[44] Studies of drug utilization in newborn infants admitted to a neonatal intensive-care unit demonstrated that 76% of neonates received from 1 to 26 different drugs for diagnostic or therapeutic purposes; the average neonate was given 6 different drugs during hospitalization.[3] In a related study,[4] adverse drug reactions occurred in 30% of neonates admitted to an intensive-care unit. Of those neonates, 15% incurred life-threatening reactions, and the hospital stay was prolonged because of the adverse reaction in 25%. These figures are not that dissimilar to those from surveys of children and adult populations, where up to 20% of all admissions have been reported to be caused by drug-related illness.[124] Examination of normalized data from hospitalized children and adults (number of adverse drug reactions per drug administered) has revealed that 5.8% of the physician-ordered drugs administered to children were associated with an adverse reaction, in comparison with 4.8% of such drugs administered to adults.[13]

A most difficult problem is the issue of environmental pollution and effects on the fetus and infant.[100,108,425] Proof of cause-and-effect relationships subsequent to known exposure to a drug has often been a major obstacle to gaining satisfactory remedies in order to reduce the incidence of episodes of toxicity in the fetus or infant. In the case of environmental chemicals, the cause-and-effect issue is substantially more ambiguous. Investigations on the subject of the toxic hazards of environmental pollution for infants have not yet materialized much beyond the level of concern, despite its obvious importance. The inability to predict toxicity in infants from adult experience is just as much a problem with environmental chemicals as with drugs. This chapter examines the most commonly encountered situations of intoxication of the fetus and infant.

DRUGS, CHEMICALS, AND PREGNANCY

Table 11-1 outlines potential outcomes of exposure of the fetus to toxic drugs or environ-

Table 11–1. POTENTIAL HAZARDS OF FETAL
EXPOSURE TO DRUGS AND ENVIRONMENTAL
CHEMICALS

altered fertility
spontaneous abortion
chromosomal abnormalities
dysmorphology (major, minor)
altered sex ratio
late fetal or neonatal death
prenatal or postnatal growth retardation
developmental or behavioral disorders
childhood malignancies
childhood death

mental pollutants. Drugs and chemical substances reported to be toxic to the fetus are listed in Table 11–2; injurious physical factors, in Table 11–3. Textbooks and review articles are available that are devoted to the subject of fetal toxicity of drugs and chemicals.[21,71,73,81,82,140,148,399,429,438,456,481]

As mentioned earlier, assessment of the risks to the fetus of exposure to any drug or chemical is fraught with difficulties. Case reports and epidemiologic studies usually suffer from one or more major deficiencies, so that extrapolation to similar situations of other patient populations carries a high degree of risk for error. Therefore, caution must be exercised in interpretation of the information presented in Tables 11–2 and 11–3. A large number of variables undoubtedly influence the toxicity of any drug or chemical on the fetus. Dose and duration of exposure, gestational age of the fetus, genetic predisposition, and other coexisting factors may alter the characteristics and extent of the toxicity.[73,81]

Analgesics and Antipyretics

Currently recognized problems associated with maternal *aspirin* ingestion within 5 days of delivery include prolonged gestation and labor, excessive blood loss at delivery, and impairment of hemostasis (platelet adhesiveness and aggregation) in newborns.[34,162] Whether this salicylate-induced bleeding tendency in the newborn leads to complications is unknown. The incidence of intracranial hemorrhage has been shown to be greater in prematures born to mothers who ingested aspirin within 1 week of delivery;[138] no statistical correlation has been found with *acetaminophen* ingestion. Neonates exposed to aspirin in utero within 5 days of birth should be carefully evaluated for evidence of bleeding. Confusion re-

garding aspirin-induced dysmorphology is the result of the high incidence of aspirin use in pregnancy, with consequent biasing of epidemiologic studies.[34,145,153,418] A number of authors have strongly incriminated salicylate as a cause of congenital anomalies in human infants. McNiel[453] reported that eight infants exposed in utero to aspirin or other salicylate-containing medications during the first trimester had significant congenital anomalies, including one with anencephaly. Nelson and Forfar[458] reported an increased incidence of significant malformations in infants of mothers who ingested aspirin during the first month of pregnancy. Benawra and colleagues[402] reported on one infant with cyclopia and other major anomalies whose mother had taken aspirin daily throughout the first trimester of pregnancy. On the basis of information gathered in a large collaborative study, Slone and colleagues[153] concluded that aspirin ingestion during pregnancy is not associated with congenital anomalies. They did, however, consider the possibility of excessive exposure to aspirin as being teratogenic. Corby,[418] after a review of the literature, concluded that "indiscriminate use of aspirin during pregnancy is contraindicated" despite the lack of direct conclusive evidence of adverse effects.

Indomethacin and *naproxen* are known to result in closure of the ductus arteriosus in utero; indomethacin has been reported to cause morphologic changes in the pulmonary vasculature in human infants exposed in utero.[38,92,172] These observations have prompted experimental animal studies of the possible relationship between in utero ductal closure induced by aspirin, indomethacin, and naproxen and persistent fetal circulation in the newborn.[68,93,137] Further examination of this relationship is warranted.

The time of administration of *meperidine* relative to delivery of the infant and the dose and the rate of maternal meperidine metabolism are very important determinants of CNS and respiratory depression in the newborn.[113] If meperidine is given between 1 and 3 hours of delivery or in large doses, a significant increase in the incidence of such depression is observed in the newborn; if the drug is given IV in small repeated doses within 1 hour of birth, however, little or no compromise of respiratory effort may occur.[53] Differences in maternal and neonatal metabolism of meperidine, and in the rates of placental transfer of the drug and its major metabolite, normeperidine, are responsible for the dosage-related effects. The ratio be-

Table 11-2. EFFECTS OF DRUGS ON THE FETUS OR NEWBORN REPORTED IN CLINICAL STUDIES

Drug	Effect[a]	Author(s) of Published Study[b]
Analgesic, Antipyretic, Anti-inflammatory Agents		
non-addicting	dysmorphogenic effects (?): large number of associations but no absolute proof	Slone et al,[153] Collins[34]
aspirin	aspirin: platelet dysfunction (? intracranial bleeding)	Rumack et al,[138] Stuart et al[162]
phenacetin		
salicylamide		
acetaminophen		
indomethacin	in utero ductus arteriosus closure (? pulmonary vascular anomalies, increased morbidity)	Levin et al,[92] Howard and Hill,[77] Rudolph[137]
addicting		
narcotics	acute: respiratory and CNS depression in newborn	
	chronic: see abused drugs under CNS Drugs and Table 11-7	
codeine	respiratory malformations (?)	Heinonen et al[73]
Anticoagulants		
dicumarol	embryotoxic or CNS abnormality (17%), fetal mortality and premature birth (17%)	Shaul and Hall,[146] Hall et al[63]
warfarin		
heparin	fetal mortality and premature birth (33%)	
Anticonvulsants		
phenytoin	coagulation defects	Hawkins[70]
	fetal hydantoin syndrome: craniofacial anomalies, hypoplasia of nails and digits, growth deficiency, mental deficiency	Hanson and Smith,[65] Smith,[154] Committee on Drugs,[35] Albengres and Tillement[395]
trimethadione	syndrome: craniofacial abnormalities, cardiac anomalies, mental deficiency	Feldman et al[49]
phenobarbital	acute: CNS depression	Blumenthal and Lindsay,[15] Smith[154]
	chronic: teratogenicity (? low incidence); newborn withdrawal (see tranquilizers and sedatives under CNS Drugs)	
valproic acid	spina bifida (?)	Robert,[131] Bjerkedal[11]
Antihypertensives		
beta-blockers (propranolol)	controversial: IUGR, hypoglycemia, bradycardia, polycythemia, hypocalcemia, apnea	Rubin,[136] Witter[175]
diazoxide	hypoglycemia, alopecia (?)	
reserpine	nasal obstruction, lethargy hypothermia, bradycardia	
Antimalarials		
quinine	abortion (?), thrombocytopenia	Howard and Hill,[77] Ledward[91]
chloroquine	damage to retina (?), cranial nerve VIII (?)	
Antimicrobials		
aminoglycosides	ototoxicity (?) (streptomycin only)	
chloramphenicol	aplastic anemia (?)	
novobiocin	interference with bilirubin conjugation	Sutherland and Keller[163]
sulfonamides	methemoglobinemia (G6PD deficiency), predisposing to kernicterus (?)	
tetracyclines	dental discoloration, enamel hypoplasia (?) retardation of bone growth (?), cataracts (?)	Cohlan et al,[33] Kline et al,[84] Genot et al,[56] Ravid and Toaff[129]
Antithyroid Drugs		
iodine	goiter, thyroid ablation	Carswell et al,[24] l'Allemand et al[88]
carbamazole	goiter, hypothyroidism, IUGR with poor maternal thyroid control	Chahal et al[25]
methimazole		
propylthiouracil		
Beta-Agonists (Tocolytics)		
fenterol	hypoglycemia, hypotension (?), hypocalcemia (?), ileus (?), neonatal death (?), decreased incidence of RDS (?)	Brazy and Pupkin,[19] Epstein et al,[46] Olver[119]
isoxsuprine		
ritodrine		
terbutaline		
Antineoplastics		
alkylating agents	IUGR (?) abortion (?), various fetal abnormalities (?), bone marrow suppression	Sweet and Kinzie,[164] Barber,[7] Hawkins[70]
busulfan		
chlorambucil		

Table 11-2. EFFECTS OF DRUGS ON THE FETUS OR NEWBORN REPORTED IN CLINICAL STUDIES
(Continued)

Drug	Effect[a]	Author(s) of Published Study[b]
nitrogen mustard		
cyclophosphamide		
antimetabolites		
methotrexate	Abortion (1st trimester), craniofacial	Barber,[7] Hanson[67]
aminopterin	abnormalities	
6-MP		
5-FU		
CNS Drugs		
abused drugs	IUGR, increased fetal mortality (?)	
LSD	limb defects (?)	Long[98]
opiates	withdrawal syndrome, various malformations (?)	Ostrea and Chaves[120]
phencyclidine	various malformations (?), neurobehavioral abnormalities	Golden et al,[58] Chasnoff et al[413]
lithium	cardiac anomalies (Ebstein's, coarctation, tricuspid valve), cyanosis and hypotonia, diabetes insipidus; persistent pulmonary hypertension (?), atrial flutter (?)	Schou et al,[142,143] Schardein,[140] Mizrahi et al,[110] Arnon et al,[5] Filtenborg,[51] Wilson et al[173]
stimulants		
amphetamines	prematurity, IUGR, increased fetal mortality (?), various malformations (?)	Schardein,[140] Bolton,[16] Naeye[116]
tranquilizers and sedatives		
diazepam	cleft lip and palate (?), newborn withdrawal	Safra and Oakley,[139] Rosenberg et al[470]
meprobamate	cardiac (?)	Hartz et al[69]
phenobarbital	various malformations (?), newborn withdrawal	Palmer[121]
phenothiazines	various malformations (?), extrapyramidal dysfunction, functional GI obstruction	Schardein,[140] Tamer et al,[475] Falterman and Richardson,[424] Slone et al[477]
haloperidol	various malformations (?)	
thalidomide	limb and other anomalies	Stern[160]
tricyclic antidepressants	limb anomalies (?)	Schardein[140]
Diuretics	respiratory tract malformations (?)	Witter et al[175]
acetazolamide	various malformations (?)	Schardein[140]
thiazides	thrombocytopenia, hypoglycemia, hyperbilirubinemia (rare)	Rodriguez et al,[132] Witter et al[175]
General Anesthetics	acute: CNS depression; occupational hazard: abortions, various malformations (?)	Vessey and Nunn[169]
Local Anesthetics	bradycardia, apnea, hypotonia, mydriasis, early-onset seizures, neurobehavioral disturbances, metabolic acidosis	Dodson,[43] Ralston and Shnider,[123] Merkow et al[105]
Steroids		
clomiphene	neural tube defect (?), Down's syndrome (?), multiple births	Oakley,[118] Schardein[141]
corticosteroids:	increased incidence of IUGR, stillbirths	Taeusch,[165]
betamethasone	cleft palate (?), increased lung maturity and	Taeusch et al,[166] Clyman et al,[31] Sidhu,[149]
dexamethasone	risk of infection, decreased incidence PDA, increased theophylline metabolism	Jager-Roman et al[79]
diethylstilbestrol (DES)	vaginal adenosis and adenocarcinoma, cervical and uterine abnormalities, genitourinary abnormalities in males	Henderson et al,[74] Herbst[75]
estrogens	feminization of male fetus	Bongiovanni and McPadden[17]
oral contraceptives	congenital heart disease (?), limb abnormalities (?), CNS abnormalities (?)	Ferencz et al,[50] Kalter and Warkany[82]
progestins, androgens	masculinization of female fetus	Schardein[141]
Miscellaneous Drugs		
aminopterin	multiple defects, abnormal osseous development (skull deformity characteristic), early death, normal mental development	Shaw[147]
atropine	tachycardia, dilated nonreactive pupils	Mendez-Bauer and Poseiro[104]

Table continued on following page

Table 11-2. EFFECTS OF DRUGS ON THE FETUS OR NEWBORN REPORTED IN CLINICAL STUDIES
(Continued)

Drug	Effect[a]	Author(s) of Published Study[b]
cholinesterase inhibitors	myasthenia-like symptoms (muscle weakness)	Blackhall et al[12]
cimetidine	gonadal and sexual dysfunction (animal studies only)	Anand and Thiel[2]
ephedrine	fetal tachycardia	Wright et al[177]
ergot, ergotamine	spontaneous abortion, CNS symptoms, Poland syndrome, jejunal atresia (?)	Graham et al[431]
isotretinoin (vitamin A isomer)	spontaneous abortion, hydrocephalus, microtia, cardiac abnormalities	Rosa[133]
magnesium sulfate	hypotonia, hyporeflexia, CNS and respiratory depression, neurobehavioral impairment	Lipsitz and English,[96] Lipsitz,[97] Rasch et al[128]
penicillamine	abnormal connective tissue (Ehlers-Danlos syndrome ?)	Solomon et al[157]
oxytocin	increased bilirubin levels	Davies et al,[41] Lamont[89]
scopolamine	lethargy, tachycardia, fever	Evens and Leopold[423]
theophylline	tachycardia, vomiting, jitteriness (?)	Arwood et al[6]

[a] (?) indicates unsubstantiated or questionable cause-and-effect relationship. Additional discussion of most of the known or suspected adverse drug effects on the fetus can be found in the text.
[b] See References at end of chapter.

tween cord-blood meperidine concentration and maternal venous concentration increases with time. Ratios of 1 or greater are usually observed 1 to 5 hours after administration.[114,126] The ratio is higher after IV than after IM administration. The half-life for meperidine in the newborn has been reported to range from 6.5 to 39 hours,[23,114,115] which is significantly longer than that reported for adults (2.5–3 hr).[86] The concentration of normeperidine in the maternal circulation increases during the first 4 hours

after administration of meperidine.[8] But because placental transfer of normeperidine is slower than that of meperidine, cord-blood concentrations of the metabolite are usually less than meperidine concentrations.[8,446] Normeperidine elimination rate in the newborn infant is slower than that for meperidine ($T\frac{1}{2} = 20-36$ hr).[114] Thus, meperidine and normeperidine acquired during the time of labor may be present in the neonate for up to 3 days because of the slow elimination rate.[446] The combina-

Table 11-3. PHYSICAL AND CHEMICAL (ENVIRONMENTAL) AGENTS AND INJURY TO THE FETUS REPORTED IN CLINICAL STUDIES

Agent	Effects[a]	Author(s) of Published Study[b]
Physical		
radiation	IUGR, CNS damage, ocular defects (exposure at < 1 mo gestation), mutation (?), carcinogenic (?)	Hutchison,[440] Longo,[100] Hanson,[67] Kalter and Warkany[81]
heat	neurotube defects (?)	Miller et al,[107] Layde et al[90]
mechanical	deformations	Jones[441]
Chemical (Environmental)		
alcohol (ethanol)	fetal alcohol syndrome (IUGR, dysmorphic facial features, neurologic defects, various anomalies)	Smith,[155] Bolton,[16] Shaywitz et al[471]
smoking	spontaneous abortion, preterm delivery, IUGR, increased perinatal mortality, decreased mental function (?)	Miller et al,[106] Rantakallio,[127] Witter and King,[175] Longo,[100] Merritt[454]
heavy metals		
mercury (organic)	major motor and mental dysfunction	Snyder,[156] Amin-Zaki et al[1]

[a] (?) indicates unsubstantiated or questionable cause-and-effect relationship.
[b] See References at end of chapter.

tion of low concentration and low pharmacologic activity of normeperidine compared with meperidine argues against a major role for normeperidine in respiratory depression in the newborn associated with maternal meperidine use. In addition, normeperidine has more excitatory and fewer depressant effects than meperidine.[8] However, placental transfer, plus slow elimination and increasing capacity for formation of normeperidine by the neonate after birth, can result in the development of substantial blood levels of the metabolite by 1 to 2 days of age. It has been proposed that normeperidine may cause some of the nonrespiratory adverse effects seen in the neonate exposed to meperidine during labor and delivery.[113]

Treatment of Narcotic-induced Depression: Naloxone

Pharmacology. Treatment of narcotic-induced depression in the newborn infant can be accomplished with the administration of naloxone. Naloxone, a pure narcotic antagonist that lacks intrinsic agonist properties, is virtually free of toxic side-effects;[64] it has also been reported to be of value in selected cases of nonnarcotic overdose. Onset of action occurs within 1 to 2 minutes of IV administration and within 15 to 40 minutes of IM or SQ administration. An even greater delay in onset of action may occur in patients with shock or hypotension when the drug is given by the IM or SQ route. Despite naloxone's greater affinity for the opiate receptor (12 times that of morphine) and approximately equivalent half-lives, duration of action is significantly shorter for naloxone than for morphine; effects of naloxone in adults usually last 45 to 90 minutes, although there are reports in neonates of antagonist effects for many hours.[20,47] PO administration of naloxone in the adult is associated with a high first-pass hepatic extraction, so that only a small percentage of the administered dose reaches the systemic circulation unchanged.[54] Naloxone is metabolized to glucuronide conjugates in the liver, with subsequent excretion of the metabolites in the urine.

Clinical Pharmacology. In neonates, reported peak plasma levels of naloxone in a dose of 0.01 to 0.02 mg/kg given IV range from 4 to 20 ng/ml (mean 11 ng/ml) within 40 minutes of administration.[20] Plasma concentrations at the end of 4 hours range from 1.4 to 6.6 ng/ml (mean 4.2 ng/ml). The elimination half-life is 185 ± 108 minutes ($\pm$ SD); the volume of distribution, 2 ± 0.3 l/kg; and the plasma clear-

ance rate 0.6 ± 0.1 l/kg per hour. In adults the reported elimination half-life ranges from 30 to 100 minutes.[117]

Several controlled trials have demonstrated significant differences between narcotic-exposed infants given naloxone (0.04 mg IV) and controls in alveolar PCO_2 and tidal volume[48,171] and in ventilation response to breathing CO_2-enriched air.[57] Rapid improvement in ventilatory activity, sucking behavior, and response to auditory stimuli resulted from IV administration of 0.2 mg of naloxone, but the duration of effect was less than 1 hour.[171] Intramuscular doses of 0.2 mg produced effects that lasted for 48 hours. Studies of the effects of naloxone (0.02 mg/kg IM) in newborn infants whose mothers received routine narcotic analgesia within 6 hours of delivery revealed a higher alertness score and general behavior assessment score with naloxone treatment than did placebo controls;[118] no differences in Apgar scores or capillary blood gas determinations were found. None of the infants in these controlled studies were significantly depressed at birth.

Brice and coworkers[20] examined the effect of naloxone doses of 0.01 and 0.02 mg/kg IV in a randomly designed study in neonates born to mothers receiving meperidine during labor. No significant effect was observed on respiratory function or neurobehavioral states with the 0.01-mg/kg dose until 90 minutes after dosing; an improved and more rapid effect was seen with the 0.02-mg/kg dose. These authors recommended use of an IV dose of 0.02 mg/kg or more of naloxone in newborn infants with narcotic-induced depression.

In two uncontrolled studies, the IV dose of naloxone required to reverse narcotic-induced depression in newborns ranged from 0.005 to 0.026 mg/kg.[30,52] In another study, improvement was noted in 8 of 11 depressed newborns given 0.01 to 0.015 mg of naloxone intralingually.[36] No adverse effects of naloxone were observed in any of these studies.

Therapeutic Indications. Naloxone is indicated as an agent in adjunctive therapy to the customary resuscitation efforts immediately initiated for signs of inadequate oxygenation due to *narcotic-induced respiratory (CNS) depression* in newborn. There is no clearcut evidence to support the routine administration of naloxone to newborn infants who have been exposed to narcotic analgesia during labor but who show no overt clinical signs of CNS or respiratory depression.[36] The recommended dose is 0.02 mg/kg given IV as a bolus injection. The pediatric naloxone preparation, 0.02 mg/ml, should be employed. The initial dose may be repeated without risk to the newborn infant in 3 to 5 minutes if there is no response. Because of the relatively short duration of action of naloxone, subsequent doses may be necessary and should be based on repeated clinical assessments. With IM or SQ administration of naloxone, a 15-minute or more delay in onset of action is likely.[64]

Administration of naloxone to the mother just prior to delivery to reverse the effects of administered narcotic analgesics on the fetus or newborn infant is not recommended. Naloxone should also not be given routinely to narcotic-exposed but normal newborn infants, or to symptomatic infants born to narcotic-dependent mothers, in whom it may precipitate withdrawal symptoms.

The use of naloxone for neonatal depression caused by asphyxia during labor and delivery has been examined in experimental animals.[29,59,72] These and other studies suggest that certain manifestations or antepartum asphyxia (depressed cardiorespiratory function) may be a reflection of increased effects of endogenous opioids on central vascular and ventilatory control.[28,87] The use of naloxone in the asphyxiated human newborn has not been examined.

Naloxone has also been shown to reverse hypotension associated with hemorrhagic and septic shock.[64] The proposed mechanism for this effect is antagonism of the hypotensive action of endorphins that are released in shock. There has not been any published experience regarding this effect of naloxone in infants.

Clinical Toxicology. Naloxone has a history of being remarkably free of side-effects, with the exception of precipitating manifestations of withdrawal in physically dependent adults and newborns. In addition, there have been a few case reports in adults of hypertension, sudden cardiac arrest, and cardiac arrhythmias associated with the administration of naloxone. These phenomena have been proposed to involve the sudden release of catecholamines.[64] There are no similar reports in infants. The long-term effects of naloxone in infants are unknown, but studies in experimental animals have raised a concern regarding interference with opiate receptors and endogenous opioid substances.[36]

Anticoagulants

Published reports estimate that 25% to 50% of fetuses exposed to coumarin derivatives such as *dicumarol* or *warfarin* in the first trimester will have the following congenital anomalies ("warfarin embryopathy"): hypoplastic (saddle) nose, stippling of various epiphyses (chondrodysplasia punctata), broad short hands, short distal phalanges, eye abnormalities (optic atrophy, cataracts, microophthalmia, hypertelorism), and mental retardation.[63,146,161] Exposure during the second or third trimester appears to predispose to the development of a spectrum of CNS abnormalities.[63] Besides the increased risk of abnormal live-born infants, about one sixth of the pregnancies in which coumarin derivatives are used will result in abortion or stillbirth; the remaining pregnancies will be apparently normal.

Heparin is considered preferable to oral anticoagulant therapy in pregnancy primarily because it does not cross the placenta. Heparin therapy, when well controlled (preferably by use of continuous infusion), has not been associated with an identifiable syndrome as have the oral anticoagulants; however, a marked rate of maternal complications, including hemorrhage (10%) and death (2%), has been observed.[63] Excluding the maternal complications, pregnancy outcome with heparin therapy is not much different from that with coumarin-derivative therapy. Whether to use heparin or coumarin derivatives in those cases where pregnancy is to be continued is not nearly as important as careful monitoring of maternal coagulation status. Approximately 10% to 15% of the fetuses from women receiving heparin are stillborn, and 20% are born premature. This adverse fetal outcome appears to be due to the underlying maternal coagulation disorder, not to the heparin therapy.[63]

The recommendation to use heparin therapy during pregnancy cannot be based on the likelihood of a better outcome than with the coumarin derivatives. Hall and coworkers[63] suggest the risks to mother and fetus warrant preconceptual counseling and pregnancy prevention or therapeutic abortion.

Anticonvulsants

Considerable controversy has surrounded the teratogenic potential of anticonvulsants.[144] Babies of mothers with seizure disorders treated with phenytoin, barbiturates, or trimethadione are believed to have an increased incidence of congenital anomalies, particularly facial clefts and congenital heart disease.[154] The underlying seizure disorder and genetic and environmental factors are believed to contribute to the teratogenicity.[35,71,159]

Phenytoin therapy in the pregnant woman carries a 10% risk for a serious defect in the infant (mild to moderate mental deficiency, clefts of lip and/or palate, congenital heart disease, renal defects).[434] There is a 30% risk for one or more of the following features associated with the *fetal hydantoin syndrome:* craniofacial abnormalities including broad, low nasal bridge, epicanthic folds, short upturned nose, hypertelorism, ptosis or strabismus, ear abnormalities, and variations in head size and shape with wide fontanels; limb defects including finger-like thumbs and hypoplasia of distal phalanges and nails; and growth deficiency of prenatal onset, with postnatal linear growth 75% of normal.[65,154] There is substantial evidence for genetic variation in fetal susceptibility to the teratogenic effects of phenytoin.[464] Some investigators, however, have concluded that parental epilepsy (mother or father) itself rather than its treatment is responsible for the teratogenicity.[73] An increased incidence of neoplasms (neuroblastoma, Wilms' tumor, mesenchymoma) has been reported in cases of fetal hydantoin syndrome, suggesting that exposure of the fetus to phenytoin carries a risk of carcinogenic effects.[395,396] There have been no reports of neural crest tumors in normal offspring of mothers taking phenytoin during pregnancy.

Trimethadione, like phenytoin, has been reported to cause a specific syndrome of anomalies that includes craniofacial abnormalities (ear anomalies, cleft lip and/or palate), cardiac anomalies, and mental deficiency.[49] Because of the high incidence of fetal loss and abnormalities (over 80%), its use in the pregnant woman should be avoided.

The data on malformations with *phenobarbital* are less conclusive than those on trimethadione and phenytoin.[154] *Carbamazepine* has not been found to cause an increase in fetal malformations in limited clinical experience.

Valproic acid given during the first trimester has been associated with an increased incidence of spina bifida.[11,131] One case of a dysmorphic infant born to a mother who had received valproic acid has been reported.[39]

Although interference with folic acid has been offered as a biochemical explanation for the teratogenicity of the various anticonvulsants, there is little direct evidence to support this hypothesis. Anticonvulsant therapy during pregnancy has been reported to produce coagulation defects in the newborn that are responsive to vitamin K therapy and a withdrawal syndrome characterized by hypotonia, hypothermia, and apnea in the first 2 days of life.[14,70,167] The risk of having a malformed infant for a mother with a seizure disorder who is treated with anticonvulsants has been estimated to be about 1 in 10.[154]

Antihypertensives

Treatment of essential hypertension in pregnancy is important for both mother and fetus. *Methyldopa* is the only antihypertensive that has clearly been shown to improve fetal prognosis.[94] A number of case reports have cautioned that chronic therapy with *beta-blockers* (propranolol) may cause intrauterine growth retardation (IUGR), bradycardia, polycythemia, hypocalcemia, hyperbilirubinemia, and apnea at birth.[136] Controversy, however, has arisen regarding the cause-and-effect relationship between these observations in the newborn and propranolol and the underlying maternal hypertension. Pruyn and colleagues[122] concluded that hypoglycemia, hyperbilirubinemia, polycythemia, neonatal apnea, and bradycardia did not correlate statistically with chronic propranolol therapy, whereas there was a causal relationship with IUGR. Upon review of existing literature, Rubin[136] concluded that there are no clear adverse effects in the fetus resulting from intrauterine exposure to propranolol, with the exception of transient bradycardia and hypoglycemia in the newborn. Evidently, the use of beta-blockers in moderate doses for control of mild to moderate hypertension, arrhythmias, or other disorders will be well tolerated by the fetus. This is in contrast to large dose propranol therapy for the treatment of severe hypertension, where fetal prognosis is poor at the onset. With severe hypertension it is difficult to differentiate the consequences of drug therapy from those of hypertensive disease. The more cardioselective β-adrenoceptive blocking agents currently under development may be of less risk to the infant.[476]

Hydralazine has been primarily used during the third trimester of pregnancy as a second drug to control hypertension. It has the advantage of not affecting uterine blood flow in the hypertensive pregnant patient.[175] No clear adverse effects on the fetus have been reported with hydralazine.

Reserpine therapy during pregnancy has been associated with nasal discharge and stuffiness, lethargy, and hypothermia in newborns. This condition lasts 1 to 5 days and occurs in 10% of neonates exposed in utero, if the exposure includes the last 2 days before birth.[175] Because of the multiple adverse effects reported, reserpine should not be used in pregnancy. Administration of *diazoxide* during pregnancy has been associated with alopecia and impaired glucose tolerance in the neonate.[70,109]

Antimalarials

Quinine in high doses is believed to be toxic to the fetus by a direct action of drug on the myometrium or on the fetus, resulting in abortion[70] and congenital malformations.[140] It has also been reported to cause thrombocytopenia.[102] *Chloroquine* has been reported to be associated with fetal retinal damage as a result of high drug concentrations in the fetal eye and retina. Damage to cranial nerve VIII has been produced experimentally in animal studies and has also been reported in humans.[77] Effective treatment of malaria, however, is a more important consideration relative to the fetus than the potential or real teratogenic hazard.

Antimicrobials

Reports of toxic effects of antimicrobial drugs on the fetus are few despite their frequent use in the care of pregnant females. Teratogenic effects through direct actions on the developing fetus might be expected because many antimicrobial agents pass freely into the fetal environment. Because of their known ototoxicity, there is concern that *aminoglycosides* could produce damage to cranial nerve VIII in the fetus. However, no such findings have been reported in newborns exposed in utero. The *sulfonamides* undergo rapid placental transfer and may displace bilirubin from albumin binding sites in the fetus and newborn. Although it is conceivable that the result of this effect could be a predisposition to kernicterus, no actual reports confirming this possibility have appeared in the literature. Patients predisposed to methemoglobinemia as a consequence of glucose 6-phosphate dehydrogenase (G6PD) deficiency should not be given sulfonamides. The association of *chloramphenicol* with aplastic anemia, though rare, is a significant consideration with respect to the fetus. *Novobiocin* has been associated with interference with bilirubin conjugation and should therefore be avoided in late pregnancy.[163]

Tetracyclines can cause brownish, grayish, or yellow staining of the child's teeth if administered to the mother after the fourth month of pregnancy. Usually only deciduous teeth are involved, but crowns of permanent teeth may also be stained.[84,148,170] Enamel hypoplasia and mottling of the enamel have been commonly associated with the dental discoloration, but the causal relationship of these abnormalities to tetracyclines has been challenged.[56] In contrast to other teratogenic agents, the dental staining effect of tetracyclines occurs only after week 25 of gestation and is least pronounced when the exposure occurs during the first trimester of human pregnancy.[129] The fluorescence in bone and inhibition of linear bone growth associated with deposition of tetracyclines appears to be reversible. At present no definitive evidence exists for the production of any permanent skeletal defects in humans by tetracycline antibiotics.[33,56]

Penicillins, cephalosporins, and *erythromycin* have all been employed in pregnancy without reported significant adverse effects in the fetus.

Auditory defects and ocular nerve damage have been observed in infants exposed to *streptomycin* in utero.[479] Severe encephalopathies have been reported in children whose mothers had been treated with *isoniazid* during pregnancy.[479] Minimal dose therapy and supplemental vitamin B_6 should be employed when these tuberculostatic drugs are required for treatment of pregnant women with tuberculosis.

Antithyroid Drugs

Iodine and drugs containing this element are contraindicated in pregnancy. Iodide is concentrated in the thyroid gland of the fetus as well as of the mother and may produce fetal goiter and hypothyroidism.[24] The fetal thyroid remains suppressed secondary to iodide uptake, while the adult thyroid gland appears to be able to avoid the inhibitory effects. Therapy with thyroxin is recommended for transient neonatal hypothyroidism associated with fetal iodine exposure if it persists beyond a 2-week period.[88] The incidence or degree of adverse effects on the fetus associated with the treatment of maternal hyperthyroidism by *carbamizole, methimazole,* or *propylthiouracil* (PTU) is small as long as minimal effective therapy is utilized.[25] Sitar and coworkers[152] found no abnormalities in serum TSH or thyroxine levels and no clinical abnormalities in three neonates exposed in utero to PTU. Goiter and hypothyroidism may occur in the neonate if the maternal therapy is not carefully monitored and regulated. With proper management of maternal hyperthyroidism, these problems affect only about 3% of newborns.[70] Growth and development of children exposed in utero to carbamizole was found to be normal when they were examined at 3 to 13 years of age.[103]

Beta-Agonists (Tocolytics)

Beta-sympathomimetic drugs, including *fenterol, isoxsuprine, ritodrine,* and *terbutaline,* are clinically useful for inhibition of premature labor. A variety of conditions in newborns have been associated with the use of tocolytics. A lower incidence of respiratory distress syndrome has been observed in preterm infants exposed to terbutaline or ritodrine in utero.[403,409] Such an effect is consistent with animal studies in preterm fetuses and newborns showing an increase in airway surfactant after in utero exposure to beta-agonists.[404,405,442] Up to two thirds of exposed newborns may develop hypoglycemia within 90 minutes of delivery.[46] Adequate parenteral glucose administration immediately after delivery and for at least 12 hours can prevent the development of neonatal hypoglycemia.[467] Elevation of cord serum insulin concentration has been observed in both short-term and long-term tocolytic therapy.[467] Hansen and coworkers[433] observed lower insulin clearances and higher plasma renin activity and urinary arginine vasopression excretion in neonates born to mothers treated with ritodrine. No significant physiologic change in cardiovascular or renal performance was associated with these changes resulting from ritodrine therapy. Other more questionable effects in the newborn attributed to in utero exposure to beta-agonists include hypotension, hypocalcemia, ileus, and neonatal death.[19,119] A retrospective review of two consecutive cohorts of newborn infants did not reveal any statistical differences between a study group exposed to ritodrine in utero and a control group in umbilical venous pH, Apgar scores, and neurologic assessment.[439]

Antineoplastics

Increasing experience with chemotherapy in successful pregnancies has resulted in some insight into the relative risks. Administration of antineoplastic agents during the first trimester of pregnancy carries a significant risk for the fetus. Reviews of cytotoxic drugs given in the second and third trimesters indicate no fetal abnormalities, although low birth weight was

observed in 40% of infants in one study.[7,164] Suppression of bone marrow in the newborn can be expected with chemotherapy near the time of delivery. Questionable fetal abnormalities have been recorded with several of the alkylating agents, including *busulfan, chlorambucil, cyclophosphamide,* and *nitrogen mustard.* Antimetabolite-type drugs appear to be the most dangerous to the fetus. Abortions have been reported in patients receiving *aminopterin* or *methotrexate* during the first trimester. As many as 50% of the surviving infants exposed in utero to antimetabolites are reported to be abnormal;[71] the abnormalities include hydrocephalus, cleft palate and lip, and meningomyelocele. The use of methotrexate for treatment of psoriasis, although approved by the FDA, must be carefully evaluated since psoriasis is a problem not uncommon in young women of childbearing age.

Little information is available on other antineoplastic (chemotherapeutic) agents. Most are teratogenic in animals, but the implications with respect to human pregnancies are unknown. Although it has been proposed that combination cancer chemotherapy is more hazardous than single-drug therapy, supporting evidence is not available. One case report involving the use of MOPP therapy (nitrogen mustard, vincristine, procarbazine, prednisone) beginning at 26 weeks' gestation resulted in an uneventful outcome of the pregnancy.[80]

Cardiac Glycosides

Digitalis preparations have not been associated with teratogenic effects in humans. They do cross the placenta and may produce cardiac effects in the fetus, although such effects are beneficial in the fetus with paroxysmal atrial tachycardia. No adverse effects of maternal digoxin therapy have been seen in the fetus or neonate.[175]

CNS Drugs

Exposure of the fetus to *drugs of abuse* including opioids (discussed in detail later in this chapter) is generally associated with coexisting factors that complicate attempts to isolate the causative agent responsible for fetal or infant abnormalities (nutrition, infectious diseases, multiple drug exposure). A review of the literature has shown an incidence of congenital anomalies among offspring of drug addicts (the majority on heroin) of between 2.7% and 3.2%, which is in the high-normal range.[71] Drug addicts who are not under medical supervision have an increased incidence of low-birth-weight babies.

Although there is no strong evidence that *LSD* is teratogenic in humans, limb defects in babies born to mothers who have used this drug indicate the need for continued surveillance.[98] Cohen and colleagues[32] noted chromosomal aberrations in children exposed to LSD in utero, but all appeared healthy and had no obvious birth defects. There is no evidence that *marijuana* causes congenital abnormalities in humans, although several reports have raised this concern and others, including low birth weight and Apgar scores and increased incidence of fetal alcohol syndrome.[437,447] In a series of 35 pregnancies a significant increase in abnormal labor (prolonged, protracted, arrested, precipitate) and in meconium staining in infants born to known marijuana users has been reported.[62] Fried[55] found no relationship between marijuana use during pregnancy and maternal weight gain, length of gestation, duration of labor, or birth weight but did note certain neurologic differences between the newborn infants of users and those of nonusers; since most marijuana users are also taking other drugs and using alcohol and regular cigarettes, a cause-and-effect relationship with the use of marijuana cannot be determined with any confidence.

Opiate abuse has been associated with IUGR and perinatal mortality. Socioeconomic factors appear to be more involved in causation than the drugs themselves. Abruptio placentae has been associated with *cocaine* use.[394] Cocaine-induced transient hypertension was proposed as the causative mechanism. There is little evidence to link the opiates with fetal malformations. Ostrea and Chavez[120] reported 20 major abnormalities in babies born to 803 patients with a history of exposure to narcotics during pregnancy. Abuse of other drugs and low incidence of abnormalites in the control population complicate the interpretation of the observations.

Phencyclidine ("angel dust" or PCP) has been reported to produce miscellaneous abnormalities, including gross malformations, abnormal behavior and spastic quadriparesis.[58,413,474] Neurobehavioral effects are consistent with studies in experimental animals, but the association between PCP and gross malformations remains to be verified.

Considerable controversy exists in the literature regarding the teratogenicity of antidepressant drugs, especially the *tricyclic compounds*.[140] Review of the literature involving the tricyclic antidepressants has failed to reveal adequate evidence of a causal relationship to fetal abnormalities in humans.[71]

Of the numerous *tranquilizers and sedatives* employed in pregnancy, only thalidomide has produced unequivocal evidence of teratogenicity. *Diazepam* has been associated with a possible increase in the risk for clefts of the lip and palate. In a retrospective study a history of ingestion of diazepam was found to be four times more frequent in mothers of infants with cleft lip than in mothers of infants with other defects;[139] in most of the cases with abnormalities, however, other potentially teratogenic factors could be identified. Rosenberg and colleagues[470] found no increased risk of cleft lip or palate with first-trimester exposure to diazepam. Cardiac malformations, along with other abnormalites, have been reported to be increased in frequency in association with *meprobamate* ingestion during pregnancy. However, one of the largest epidemiologic series reported no increase in any particular catagory of anomaly among children exposed prenatally to meprobamate or to *chlordiazepoxide*.[69] Thus, substantial doubt remains regarding the teratogenicity of these drugs.

Prospective surveys of pregnancies have revealed an increased incidence of malformations in babies exposed to *barbiturates* in early gestation.[121] No consistent relationship, however, was identified among the drug used, time of administration, and the abnormality observed. Although the risk is two to four times the background risk, controversy continues over what proportion is related to barbiturate use versus maternal or constitutional factors (see additional discussion in Anticonvulsant section of this chapter). Barbiturate withdrawal syndrome is reviewed in a later section of this chapter.

Prospective studies of large numbers of pregnancies suggest but do not prove that under certain circumstances some *phenothiazines* may present teratogenic hazard to the human fetus.[140,472] There have been several isolated reports of defects, particularly of the limbs, associated with maternal ingestion of phenothiazines in early pregnancy.[121] Extrapyramidal dysfunction and decreased intestinal motility have been observed in newborns exposed in utero to many psychotropic drugs that have potent anticholinergic activity.[424,435,475]

The risk of malformation following *thalidomide* ingestion during pregnancy has been estimated to range from 2% to 25%.[160] The pattern of malformation involves upper extremity (especially absence of radius) in about 65% to 75% of cases; both upper and lower extremities are affected in 10% to 25%, and in 2% to 5% only the legs are affected. In addition to those of the limbs (phocomelia), various other anomalies have been described, including hydrocephaly, eye and ear defects, cardiovascular anomalies, intestinal and urogenital malformations, and capillary hemangiomata.

Several reports have suggested an increased incidence of congenital abnormalities in babies born to mothers who have taken *amphetamines* during pregnancy.[16] Although these reports deserve serious consideration, an unequivocal teratogenic effect of amphetamines remains to be established. A history of maternal amphetamine use during pregnancy has been associated with prematurity and an increase in incidence of IUGR.[116] These effects are undoubtedly related to socioeconomic circumstances generally surrounding maternal amphetamine abuse.

Fetal exposure to *lithium* during the first trimester has been associated with an increased proportion of congenital cardiovascular abnormalities.[5,125] The cardiac malformations associated with fetal exposure includes Ebstein's anomaly, coarctation of the aorta, VSD, mitral and tricuspid atresia, tricuspid regurgitation, and dextrocardia. The cardiac defects appear to involve primarily the right side. Congenital abnormalities associated with lithium appeared in 9 of 18 infants in a registry for newborns exposed to lithium in the first trimester.[142,143] One case report has attributed the occurrence of persistent pulmonary hypertension to lithium intoxication of the fetus.[51] In addition, lithium exposure late in pregnancy has resulted in cardiac, renal, and neuromuscular dysfunction in the newborn. Serum lithium levels in excess of 1 mEq/l in the newborn are associated with hypotonia, poor Moro and suck reflexes, respiratory distress, decreased cardiac contractility, atrial flutter, cyanosis, euthyroid goiter, and nephrogenic diabetes insipidus.[5,110,111,173,176] The multi-organ system effects of lithium may relate to an incomplete ion substitution for other extracellular and intracellular cations (K^+, Na^+), and interference with cyclic AMP–mediated processes that are regulated by polypeptide hormones. The mechanisms of lithium action have been comprehensively reviewed by Singer and Rotenberg.[151]

Diuretics

In general, there is no evidence of a relationship between diuretic use during pregnancy and congenital malformations, although concern has been raised by retrospective case studies of an association between diuretic use and respiratory tract malformations.[175] Several cases of neonatal thrombocytopenia, hypoglycemia, and hyperbilirubinemia have been reported with the use of *thiazide* diuretics.[133,175] No toxic or teratogenic effects have been noted with maternal *furosemide* therapy. Retrospective surveys of the use of carbonic anhydrase inhibitors such as *acetazolamide* diuretics in pregnancy have not demonstrated any increased fetal risk.[21]

General Anesthetics

Inconsistent observations have been reported regarding occupational exposure to anesthetic agents and the outcome of pregnancy in operating room personnel.[169] Although the information appears to support the contention that operating room personnel have an increased risk of abortion, there is no clear evidence that congenital abnormalities result from the occupational exposure.

Local Anesthetics

Administration of certain local anesthetics during labor has resulted in apnea, hypotonia, bradycardia (common), tachycardia (rare), vomiting, hypotension, convulsions, CNS depression, fixed and dilated pupils, loss of oculocephalic reflexes (doll's eyes), and death in newborns.[43,83,123,134,150,436] Early onset of mydriasis, loss of eye movements on the "doll's head" maneuver, and loss of pupillary light reflexes at birth, persisting after a period of resuscitation and stabilization of the infant, are strongly suggestive of local anesthetic intoxication.[43] Seizures due to local anesthetic toxicity typically develop within the first 6 hours of life, which is earlier than for seizures associated with hypoxemic insults. Neurobehavioral disturbances have been observed as a consequence of penetration of local anesthetics into the fetal environment prior to birth.[105] Most of the reported intoxications have been associated with *mepivacaine,* although a few cases have been reported for *lidocaine.* The initial reports of newborn intoxication due to local anesthetics were attributed primarily to inadvertent administration of drug directly into the unborn baby during caudal, paracervical, and pudendal anesthesia; however, the local anesthetic drugs can cross the placenta and thereby produce more mild degrees of intoxication.[478] The threshold serum level for toxicity with lidocaine and mepivacaine is believed to be 3 μg/ml or greater.[478] Blood levels of mepivacaine or lidocaine in intoxicated newborns have generally been between 10 and 30 μg/ml;[27,83,123,436] one report describes an infant who survived with a level of 75 μg/ml.[150] Deaths caused by local anesthetics have been reported in association with serum levels as low as 10 μg/ml.[42]

Treatment of intoxicated newborns includes appropriate supportive care and promotion of elimination of the local anesthetic, by forced diuresis and repeated or continuous gastric aspiration.[436] Enhancement of elimination is particularly important for the amide-type local anesthetics such as mepivacaine, lidocaine, and bupivacaine, since they are not hydrolyzed by cholinesterase and are slowly metabolized or not metabolized at all by the liver.[115] The basicity of the local anesthetics favors their concentration by ion trapping mechanisms in acidic fluids such as acidic urine and the gastric secretions.[27,452] Ion trapping phenomena also favor greater accumulation of a local anesthetic in an asphyxiated acidotic fetus.[123,410] Exchange transfusion is of questionable value in the treatment of local anesthetic intoxication in the newborn.[42] Seizures induced by local anesthetics are particularly responsive to diazepam therapy.[457]

Steroids

Corticosteroid administered to the mother appears in the fetal blood within 1 hour of administration and remains for as long as 2 weeks after the last dose.[398,401] Generally, no measurable quantities of glucocorticoid can be found in fetal or cord blood by 72 hours after maternal administration. Numerous retrospective examinations of clinical experience involving maternal *corticosteroid* therapy have suggested a small risk of fetal malformation (cleft palate) and IUGR. Whether the corticosteroid therapy produces improvement in the mother's status sufficient to enhance the overall well-being of the fetus, or whether the therapeutic benefit outweighs potentially harmful effects of the corticosteroid on placental function, remains questionable.[149] Despite concern regarding the long-term effects of corticosteroids given to the mother antenatally to reduce the risks of RDS in the neonate, no significant complications have been demonstrated in the offspring to date.[10,449] There is no question regarding the

ability of corticosteroids to reduce the incidence of RDS in infants born between 28 and 34 weeks' gestation.[10,416,445] The potential toxicity of glucocorticoid prophylaxis has been reviewed.[165]

Studies of pituitary-adrenal and testicular function in preterm infants exposed in utero to dexamethasone have revealed no differences from controls.[78] Antenatal betamethasone therapy has been associated with a reduced incidence of PDA in premature infants.[31] Concern has been raised regarding a possible increased risk of infection in the newborn as well as the mother subsequent to corticosteroid prophylaxis against RDS.[166] Maternal administration of dexamethasone can induce a leukocytosis in the newborn female infant which must be distinguished from that caused by an infectious process.[397,462] The rise in neutrophil count, which tends to peak by the second or third day of life and persist for up to 1 week, is caused by accelerated release of neutrophils from the mature neutrophil pool in the bone marrow and by reduced egress from the circulation.[407] Infants prenatally exposed to betamethasone show evidence of activation of the hepatic mono-oxygenase enzyme system as determined by studies of theophylline metabolism.[79]

Diethylstilbestrol (DES) has been clearly established as a cause of vaginal and cervical clear cell adenocarcinoma in female fetuses exposed early in pregnancy.[75,76] An increased risk for cervical abnormality and uterine malformations predisposing to reproductive wastage, ectopic pregnancy, and premature birth during later reproductive life has also been reported.[67] An increased incidence of genital tract abnormalities including epididymal cysts and hypoplasia of the testes has been reported in exposed male fetuses.[74,130]

Other *estrogens* have been reported to produce feminization of male fetuses; *progestin* exposure during pregnancy has been associated with masculinization of external genitalia in female fetuses.[17,149]

Controversial reports regarding the effects of *oral contraceptives* can be found in the literature. The more carefully done epidemiologic studies do not suggest an increased risk for significant cardiac, limb, or CNS defects in fetuses exposed to low-dose oral contraceptives.[50,141] The risks of congenital abnormalities in association with oral contraceptives appear to be extremely low and could be spurious associations arising from the high frequency of use of contraceptive drugs.

Clomiphene has been associated with an increased risk of Down's syndrome and neural tube defects.[141] The underlying maternal disorder requiring treatment with such fertility agents confounds the interpretation of a cause-and-effect relationship. Multiple births associated with the use of clomiphene may predispose to an increased risk of mechanical deformities.

Other Drugs

A variety of drugs have been reported to be associated with adverse reactions affecting the fetus; these are outlined in Table 11–2. Although some of the adverse reactions are clearly drug-related, a number represent single instances not verified by other evidence.[158]

Magnesium sulfate is generally regarded as having minimal or no effects on the fetus and newborn except in situations of hypermagnesemia.[60] Reports of neonatal depression, flaccidity, hyporeflexia, and neurobehavioral impairments have been associated with newborn magnesium serum levels greater than 4 mg/dl.[96,97,128] Serum magnesium levels in full-term non-asphyxiated newborns less than 3.6 ± 0.5 mg/dl have not been associated with any abnormal neurologic findings.[60] Ulnar nerve stimulation studies to evaluate muscle activity have shown the presence of muscle fatigue. Sustained muscle activity is impaired longer than single or intermittent muscle activity.[128] These results with nerve stimulation are consistent with neurobehavioral observations. The inconsistencies between serum magnesium levels and signs of magnesium toxicity may be explained by the sophistication of the clinical assessment, the contribution of coexisting asphyxial insults or prematurity, or the fact that serum magnesium concentrations do not reflect intracellular and total body burden of magnesium.[45,60,128]

The manifestations of magnesium intoxication reflect its ability to decrease CNS excitability by suppressing neuronal firing and inhibiting the release of acetylcholine in the peripheral neuromuscular junction.[128] The half-life of the elevated serum magnesium levels in newborns whose mothers received magnesium therapy prior to delivery is greater than 40 hours, which is similar to the time required for recovery from the clinical manifestations of hypermagnesemia.[41,45] Although maternal calcium levels consistently decrease with magnesium sulfate therapy, neonatal calcium levels generally remain stable.[37] There are, however, reports of elevated serum calcium levels and reduced serum parathyroid hormone levels in newborns with hypermagnesemia.[45]

The high probability of fetal exposure to *caffeine* heightens the concern regarding its potential adverse effects. This issue has been reviewed by Morris and Weinstein.[112] Two epidemiologic retrospective studies, however, have failed to implicate caffeine as a major teratogen, nor was caffeine shown to significantly alter the outcome of pregnancy.[95,135] *Antihistamines* are another group of drugs that are widely employed during pregnancy and for which considerable concern regarding potential fetal toxicity has been expressed; despite the vast clinical experience, no evidence of a significant risk to the developing human fetus exists.[61,140]

The retinoid derivative *isotretinoin* (Accutane, used in the treatment of acne) has been associated with major fetal anomalies and spontaneous abortion.[133] Reported fetal abnormalities include hydrocephalus, cardiac defects, and microtia. The drug should not be used by any female of childbearing age without adequate warning and contraceptive precautions.

Atropine and *scopolamine* have produced symptoms of cholinergic inhibition in newborns following maternal administration.[104,423] Symptoms include tachycardia, lethargy, ileus, and fever. Experimentally, atropine increased the heart rate in an already severely hypoxemic fetus, but cardiac output was not improved.[415] The evidence for the safety and value of scopolamine for sedation in labor and delivery is insufficient to warrant its use.

The influence of drug exposure during pregnancy on incidence of neonatal jaundice has been reviewed by Lamont.[89] Drug influences on neonatal jaundice include in utero exposure to agents known to induce hepatic conjugation of bilirubin and thereby to reduce serum bilirubin levels *(phenobarbital)* or to increase red cell hemolysis (G6PD deficiency) and thereby increase neonatal jaundice. Other drugs can increase the risks of kernicterus as a consequence of displacement of bilirubin from albumin binding sites *(sulfonamides)*; inhibition or competition with bilirubin conjugation in the liver *(novobiocin, chloramphenicol)*; and other unknown mechanisms *(oxytocin)*. Although controversy exists with respect to the increased incidence of neonatal jaundice with maternal *diazepam* or *oxytocin* administration,[26,41,422] the effect is minimal, particularly if the possible serious consequences of withholding oxytocin when indicated are considered.

FETAL INJURY BY PHYSICAL FACTORS AND CHEMICAL (ENVIRONMENTAL) AGENTS

A great deal has been written about the effects of environmental factors on the fetus, and a number of experimental studies have been conducted to determine such effects. Despite the increasing amount of attention, it has been difficult for new knowledge to keep pace with the proliferation of both physical and chemical sources of pollution of the fetal environment. Relatively little is known with absolute certainty about the potential of physical and chemical factors to injure the fetus.

Physical Factors

Injury to the fetus by radiation, heat, and mechanical insults has been reported.[67,81,441] *Radiation* in sufficient doses is known to affect fertility, embryogenesis, and fetal development.[100] An absorbed dose of 10 rads by the fetus at any time during gestation is considered a practical threshold for the induction of congenital defects. The maximum allowable occupational exposure to radiation for the pregnant woman is 0.5 rem (= rad × relative biological effectiveness). Exposure to high-energy radiation from diagnostic x-ray examination or other similar low-dose exposures (<5 rad) are thought to be of low risk to the fetus, although there are reports of increased incidence of malignancy in childhood following in utero exposure to a few rads.[81,440] A prospective study of 972 children identified a significantly greater number of trisomal defects following maternal abdominal radiation exposure.[168] Very high doses of high-energy radiation (e.g., nuclear explosions) with radiation doses of 10 to 50 rads produce IUGR, CNS damage including microcephaly, and ocular defects; the sensitive period

for these effects is considered to be from the 2nd to the 18th week after conception.[455]

A number of anecdotal reports of neural tube closure defects and errors in neuromigration have been reported in offspring of women encountering significant *hyperthermia* in early pregnancy.[90,107] Many structural defects (deformations) in the fetus are now recognized as resulting from mechanical insults occurring in utero.[67,441] Normal structural development requires an adequate amount of space for and a normal ability of the fetus to move. The type of deformation produced by compromise of space or fetal movement is dependent upon the time of occurrence in gestation.

Chemical (Environmental) Agents

Ethanol has been clearly shown to produce damage to the fetus when taken in excess during pregnancy.[155] Four main categories of abnormality are associated with excessive ethanol intake: a characteristic facial appearance (broad flat midface, a broad low nasal bridge, epicanthic folds, short upturned nose, short philtrum, narrow palpebral fissures, and frequently facial hirsutism); neurologic defects (abnormal behavior, mental deficiency); IUGR; and other major anomalies (ear anomalies, large hemangiomata, small nails, altered palmar crease patterns, limited joint movements). For a diagnosis of *fetal alcohol syndrome* at least two of these major features should be present, especially short palpebral fissures or multiple dysmorphic facial features. The effects appear to be dose-dependent, with about a 20% risk for occurrence of the fetal alcohol syndrome if maternal intake is in excess of 60 ml of absolute ethanol per day.[66] Pregnancies are considered to be at risk if the average daily intake exceeds 30 ml of absolute ethanol (Table 11-4). An alcohol intake of

Table 11-4. MATERNAL ETHANOL INTAKE[a] AND ABNORMALITIES IN THE NEWBORN

Newborn Clinical Status	Daily Ethanol Intake before Pregnancy (ml)		Daily Ethanol Intake during 0-5 Months of Pregnancy (ml)	
	Mean	*Range*	*Mean*	*Range*
abnormal with features of fetal alcohol syndrome	129	0-774	36	0-250
minor anomalies	42	0-207	27	0-150
normal	24	0-258	18	0-78

[a] Values shown are for absolute ethanol.
Modified from Hanson JW et al: J Pediatr 92:457, 1978.

two or more drinks per day increases the risk of abruptio placentae and stillbirth.[451] The risk of a serious problem in the offspring of chronically alcoholic women is thought to be in the range of 30% to 50%.[155] Also at risk are pregnancies associated with "binge" drinking — that is, the intake of 5 or more drinks per occasion resulting in intoxication. Although the majority of infants born to women who drink heavily appear to be normal morphologically,[451] serious behavioral and learning difficulties have been identified in children with normal intelligence born to alcoholic mothers.[471] Decreased birth weight has also been observed in infants of alcoholic mothers who abstained during pregnancy.[448] Two case reports have raised the concern of a possible relation between maternal gestational alcohol abuse and neoplasia in the offspring.[444] The fetal alcohol syndrome appears to be related to ethanol intake and is not secondary to malnutrition in the mother. Whether the toxicity is due to ethanol or to its breakdown product, acetaldehyde, is not yet clear. The influence of ethanol on the fetus has been reviewed in detail by Smith[155] and Bolton.[16]

Smoking presents real risks to the fetus, including spontaneous abortion, preterm delivery, IUGR, low Apgar scores, and death (Table 11–3).[454] No increase in fetal malformations have been noted, but delayed developmental skills and hyperkinetic syndrome have been linked to smoking during pregnancy.[174,441,420] Chronic intrauterine stress associated with maternal smoking has been linked to a lower incidence of respiratory distress syndrome in newborns.[419] In one study, mortality and morbidity were increased up to the age of 5 years in offspring of smokers.[127] Sudden infant death syndrome (SIDS) has also been linked to smoking during pregnancy.[9] Although tobacco smoke is a mixture of a very large number of toxic substances, including carbon monoxide, nicotine, and cyanide, substantial weight has been given to the contribution of carbon monoxide to the detrimental effects of smoking on the fetus.[99] *Carbon monoxide* intoxication during pregnancy has resulted in fetal death and brain injury.[430] Neurologic abnormalities in newborns surviving fetal carbon monoxide intoxication include seizures and mental and motor dysfunction (rigidity, athetosis, clonus).

Disastrous consequences from epidemic poisoning with *heavy metals* have occurred throughout the world. Organic mercury compounds have been the most notorious in producing fetal toxicity, although all forms of mercury are considered toxic.[85] One of the more alarming features of fetal toxicity due to mercury is the fact that the mothers may show little evidence of toxicity, while the offspring are markedly affected.[1] In fact, levels of mercury in the blood of newborns are often higher than maternal levels. Gross impairment of motor and mental development with evidence of cerebral palsy, chorea, ataxia, tremors, seizures, mental retardation, deafness, and blindness can be found. The lowest measured blood level of mercury in infants associated with signs of poisoning is 564 parts per billion.[1] The usual source of fetal exposure to mercury is the consumption of contaminated food, including seed grain treated with mercury fungicides.

Available information on prenatal exposure to other environmental chemicals of concern (lead, cadmium, and other heavy metals; polychlorinated biphenyls (PCBs) and polybrominated biphenyls (PBBs); various herbicides and industrial solvents) is inadequate to establish clearly the risks to the infant.[100]

NEONATAL DRUG WITHDRAWAL (NEONATAL WITHDRAWAL SYNDROME)

Maternal dependence on various drugs will result in the *neonatal withdrawal syndrome;* these agents are listed in Table 11–5. The prevalence of multiple drug abuse and smoking and alcohol use during pregnancy complicates attempts to analyze any single agent's contribution to the manifestations of withdrawal in the neonate. Many other drugs that are abused during pregnancy have not been associated with physical dependency and neonatal withdrawal (LSD, cocaine, amphetamines). Several reviews on drug dependency in pregnancy and neonatal withdrawal have appeared in the literature.[185,197,199,206,214,417]

The pregnant drug-dependent female as well as the product of her pregnancy has a high likelihood of encountering a number of difficulties. The perinatal problems associated with maternal drug dependency are summarized in Table 11–6. Although the majority of clinical experience has been with the opiate-addicted pregnancy, similar complications have been observed with non-opiate drug abuse. With the exception of jaundice, which has been reported to be diminished in frequency in infants of addicted mothers,[185] these problems can result in serious consequences for both mother and infant. Conflicting information exists regarding the incidence of RDS in infants of drug-depen-

Table 11-5. DRUGS CAUSING NEONATAL WITHDRAWAL SYNDROMES IN CLINICAL STUDIES

Drug	Author(s) of Published Study[a]
Opiates (all have potential for causing addiction)	
codeine	Kahn et al,[192] Zelson,[214] Rothstein and Gould,[206] Neumann
heroin	and Cohen,[197] Fricker and Segal,[185] Mangurten and Ben-
morphine	awra[450]
meperidine	
methadone	
pentazocin	Goetz and Bain,[187] Preis et al[202]
pentazocin + tripelennamine (T's and Blues)	Chasnoff et al[183]
Barbiturates	
phenobarbital	Desmond et al,[184]
	Blumenthal and Lindsay[181]
amobarbital (?)	
secobarbital	Bleyer and Marshall[408]
Miscellaneous	
alcohol	Pierog et al[466]
chlordiazepoxide (Librium)	Athinarayanan et al[179]
chlorpromazine (Thorazine)	Hill et al,[435] Tamer et al,[475] O'Connor et al[459]
desmethylimipramine	Webster[211]
diazepam (Valium)	Rementeria and Bhatt[205]
diphenhydramine (Benadryl)	Parkin[200]
ethchlorvynol (Placidyl)	Rumack and Walravens[207]
glutethimide (Doriden)	Reveri et al[469]
hydroxyzine (Atarax)	Prenner[203]
phencyclidine (PCP)	Strauss et al,[474] Chasnoff et al[413]
propoxyphene (Darvon)	Tyson[209]

[a] See References at end of chapter.

dent mothers.[186,199] The influence of the drug(s) on birth weight (small for gestational age — SGA) may influence the incidence of RDS by affecting the selection of the control population as well as accelerating pulmonary matura-

Table 11-6. PERINATAL PROBLEMS ASSOCIATED WITH MATERNAL DRUG ADDICTION

Antenatal/Birth
fetal asphyxia (meconium-stained amniotic fluid, low
  Apgar scores, cesarean section for fetal distress)
anemia (mother and fetus)
premature rupture of membranes
hemorrhage (abruptio placentae, placenta previa)
infertility
maternal infections (hepatitis, pulmonary and skin
  infections, gonorrhea, syphilis)
prematurity
low birth weight (SGA, IUGR)
stillbirths
Postnatal
RDS (conflicting information: increased or decreased
aspiration pneumonia (meconium)
thrombocytosis
congenital malformations (? drug-related)
neonatal withdrawal syndrome (Table 11-7)
delayed motor development
disturbances of growth
disturbances of behavior
SIDS (increased incidence)

tion.[208] Thrombocytosis has been observed in infants born to mothers dependent on multiple drugs;[182] this effect, along with increased circulating platelet aggregates, may explain in part the pathogenesis of focal infarcts and subarachnoid and germinal plate hemorrhages observed in addicted infants at autopsy. Sudden infant death syndrome (SIDS) is another major medical complication of prenatal drug addiction.[414,468] The incidence rate for SIDS is over five times greater in addicted infants than in the normal population. Decreased sensitivity to carbon dioxide may contribute to the increased incidence of SIDS among infants exposed to methadone in utero.[460]

Incidence and Manifestations

The available information on incidence of neonatal withdrawal and its manifestations reflects the wide variation in the patient populations examined. In addition, the accuracy of the information provided by the drug-dependent mother may be questionable; multiple drug use is commonly involved (often including alcohol and cigarettes); the type and amount of drug(s) consumed are often unknown; and investigators differ on the definition of withdrawal (i.e., signs and symptoms).

Values in the literature for incidence of withdrawal in infants born to opiate-dependent mothers range from 55% to 94%. A higher incidence of withdrawal is reported with methadone than with heroin.[180,185,204,214] The onset of withdrawal manifestations is usually apparent within 1 to 4 days of birth with all drugs except phenobarbital.[184] Late presentations occurring between 2 and 4 weeks of age have been reported for about 10% of methadone-addicted neonates.[193,206] A more prolonged withdrawal period has also been reported for methadone compared with heroin.[204] The duration of the more acute withdrawal signs may be a few days to several weeks.[197]

Table 11–7 summarizes the more acute manifestations of neonatal withdrawal from opiate dependency. The cardinal signs of neonatal withdrawal syndrome are coarse tremors (jitteriness), hyperactivity, and irritability. The sleep cycle is episodic, with varying periods of restless sleep (usually less than 1 hr) interrupted by periods of crying and constant movement (resulting in skin abrasions). There is a marked increase in muscle tone, so that the infant is "stiff." The sucking activity is increased, but the swallowing reflex mechanism is uncoordinated

Table 11–7. MANIFESTATIONS OF NEONATAL WITHDRAWAL[a]

Major Manifestations
(observed in 20–90% of infants during withdrawal)

coarse tremors
diarrhea
excessive diaphoresis
hyperactivity (including increased Moro response)
hypertonicity
irritability (including high-pitched cry)
poor feeding (despite vigorous sucking activity)
skin abrasions (secondary to hyperactivity)
sleeplessness
sneezing

Other Manifestations
(observed in <20% of infants during withdrawal)

fever
hiccups
nasal stuffiness
salivation
seizures (myoclonic jerks)
tachypnea (with respiratory alkalosis)
vomiting
yawning

[a] These major and minor manifestations represent a summary of the reported experience in opiate-addicted infants. Similar manifestations have been reported for non-opiate drugs.

and ineffectual, resulting in decreased nutritional intake. (Kron and coworkers[195] found that pharmacotherapy significantly influenced the abnormal sucking behavior, although differences existed among the various drugs. Paregoric resulted in the greatest improvement followed by phenobarbital. Diazepam appeared to eliminate all spontaneous nutritive sucking behavior.) The combination of marked irritability, tremors, high-pitched cry, and hypertonicity makes seizure activity difficult to identify. Myoclonic jerks have been considered evidence of seizure activity, although this is not universally accepted.[189] Seizures have been reported to occur in 2% to 11% of addicted neonates.[189] A higher incidence of seizures is reported for methadone-addicted than for heroin-addicted neonates. Perinatal mortality figures for drug-dependent pregnancies are two- to threefold higher than for the control populations.[185,199]

Withdrawal manifestations in infants born to non-opiate-addicted mothers (Table 11–5) are similar to those of opiate withdrawal. Barbiturate withdrawal tends to resemble heroin withdrawal, but the signs begin at a later age.[184] IUGR is not a feature of barbiturate addiction in the neonate.[181]

The use of diazepam prior to and during labor can result in hypothermia, poor suck, hypotonia, respiratory depression, and asphyxia in the newborn.[205] Prolonged exposure to diazepam during pregnancy can result in neonatal withdrawal signs indistinguishable from those associated with the opiates: tremors, irritability, hyperactivity, hypertonicity, tachypnea, vigorous sucking activity, loose stools, vomiting, and poor weight gain. Initial signs occur early (2–6 hr) compared with onset of signs of opiate withdrawal. IUGR has not been a notable feature in the few cases reported.

Long-term neurobehavioral effects associated with drug-dependency during pregnancy have been reported. Behavioral disturbances (irritability, hyperactivity, feeding difficulties) and growth impairment are likely to persist for 6 months to several years.[191,212,213] Although mean developmental scores were no different in methadone and control groups, a higher incidence of low scores was found in methadone-addicted infants.[191]

Treatment

The withdrawal syndrome in the addicted neonate can be a self-limited condition, subsiding in a few days without the need for definitive therapy. Therefore, treatment of the neonate should be primarily supportive.[417] Criteria for determining the need for pharmacologic intervention have been the subject of debate, and have varied considerably as has the drug of choice. Imperative is differentiation of the drug withdrawal syndrome from other causes that could produce a similar clinical condition. Prophylactic therapy in infants born to drug-dependent mothers cannot be justified. Infants with progressive irritability, feeding difficulty, and weight loss in excess of 10% of birth weight are most likely to benefit from drug therapy. Opiates, phenobarbital, chlorpromazine, and diazepam have all been successfully employed in suppressing neonatal drug withdrawal.[194,197,206,215] More recently, clonidine has been shown to control the signs of withdrawal in infants of methadone-addicted mothers.[190] Clonidine is used in adults to control signs of acute opiate withdrawal.[188,210]

There have been few efforts to critically examine and compare the effectiveness of the various pharmacologic therapies. Comparison of existing data is hampered by the different criteria used to judge the severity of the signs of neonatal withdrawal. Some investigators feel that tapering doses of opiate (diluted opium solution, not camphorated opium tincture) is the preferred treatment, rather than a nonspecific sedative. Kandall and colleagues[194] found that phenobarbital treatment was superior to paregoric in suppressing gross signs of neonatal drug abstinence; however, abstinence-associated seizures occurred in greater numbers in the phenobarbital-treated group. Another study found no major differences in the efficacy of phenobarbital and paregoric in the treatment of methadone withdrawal in neonates.[412] Nevertheless, because of the difficulties of obtaining a reliable drug history, caution must be exercised to prevent the use of opiates in situations of dependency on non-opiate drugs.

The necessary *duration of therapy* varies widely, depending on the extent of the addiction and other factors poorly understood. Usually, 50% of neonates will require 10 to 20 days of therapy, 25% less, and 25% more.[215]

Chlorpromazine

Despite being relatively ineffective in management of adult narcotic withdrawal, chlorpromazine has enjoyed considerable success in symptomatic neonates.[192,197] Its use has been discouraged because of its diffuse pharmacologic activity including effects on the cardiovascular, endocrine, and central and autonomic nervous systems. Despite this broad pharmacologic activity, no significant side-effects or problems have been encountered with its use.[206,215] The dosage recommendations are shown in Table 11–8.

Clonidine

Clonidine has been shown to markedly reduce signs of withdrawal in opiate-addicted adults.[188,210] Experimental trials with clonidine (approximately 1 μg/kg PO q 6 hr) in two infants born to methadone-addicted mothers resulted in rapid amelioration of the major signs of withdrawal.[190] Careful monitoring of the infants revealed no adverse effects or complications associated with clonidine therapy. This treatment must be considered experimental, however.

Diazepam

Diazepam has been shown to control effectively the signs and symptoms of neonatal withdrawal syndrome.[196] It apparently has no advantages over the other drugs, and because there is some evidence that it diminishes or eliminates nutritive sucking behavior,[195] its use should probably be restricted to cases refractory to the other agents. The dose recommendations are shown in Table 11–8. See Chapter 5 for a full discussion of the pharmacology of this drug.

Table 11–8. **DRUGS USED FOR TREATMENT OF NEONATAL WITHDRAWAL SYNDROME**

Drug	Dosage[a]
chlorpromazine	0.5–0.7 mg/kg PO, IM, or slow IV infusion, q 6 hr as required
clonidine	experimental; see text
diazepam	0.2–1 mg/kg PO or slow IV infusion, q 6–8 hr as required
opium solution[b] (0.4%)	initial dose: 0.2 ml PO q 3 hr; increase by 0.05-ml increments to 1 ml as required
phenobarbital	loading dose: 10–20 mg/kg PO, IM, or slow IV infusion maintenance dose: 2.5–5 mg/kg q 6–8 hr as required

[a] Tapering of dose: For all these drugs, the effective dosage should be maintained for a period of 3 to 5 days before reducing the dose. Dosage reduction should be attempted every 1 to 2 days as long as the infant sleeps well, eats effectively, and gains weight. Irritability and tremors should not be used as sole criteria for regulating dose.

[b] A 25-fold dilution of tincture of opium; contains an amount of narcotic equal to paregoric (see text).

Opiate Therapy

Signs of narcotic withdrawal are specifically suppressed by a narcotic, not by non-narcotics. Methadone and morphine have been tried in a few infants, but the majority of experience is with opium preparations. Some investigators consider opium preparations the treatment of choice only when diarrhea is a part of the withdrawal syndrome.[215] Paregoric (0.4 mg/ml morphine equivalent) has been found to be superior to diazepam and phenobarbital in the prevention and treatment of abstinence-related seizures.[189,194] Kron and coworkers[195] have observed a more rapid normalization of sucking in infants treated with paregoric compared to those treated with diazepam or phenobarbital. The doses of paregoric employed have ranged from 0.2 to 0.8 ml (0.08 to 0.32 mg morphine equivalent) given PO every 3 hours (Table 11–8). Carin and colleagues[412] found little difference between phenobarbital (5 to 16 mg/kg/day PO in 3 divided doses) and paregoric (0.42 to 2.1 ml/kg/day PO) therapy in 31 infants with withdrawal symptoms resulting from in utero exposure to methadone. Paregoric-treated infants required a significantly longer period of treatment than phenobarbital-treated infants (22 versus 17 days). Neumann and Cohen[197] have pointed out that the composition of paregoric includes several undesirable constituents (anise oil, benzoic acid, camphor) along with opium tincture. They advise diluting opium tincture 25-fold to yield the same concentration of opium as that in paregoric (0.4% opium = 0.4 mg/ml morphine equivalent), thus avoiding the undesirable substances. Complications of opium preparations include constipation and CNS depression.

Phenobarbital

Phenobarbital has been shown to control effectively signs of neonatal withdrawal associated with opiates and barbiturates.[192,194] However, refractory cases have been reported despite very high phenobarbital serum levels.[201] Although phenobarbital has been considered to be particularly valuable in neonates with abstinence-related seizures, in a recent study a greater number of seizures occurred in infants receiving phenobarbital compared to those receiving paregoric.[194] It has also been used in combination with opium preparations in particularly severe withdrawal cases.[189] Because phenobarbital dosage requirements can vary considerably among neonates, close clinical observations and determination of serum phenobarbital levels are advisable. Serum phenobarbital levels associated with control of signs of withdrawal are between 20 and 30 μg/ml.[427] Dosage recommendations are given in Table 11–8. The major side-effect of phenobarbital therapy is CNS depression. See Chapter 5 for a full discussion of the pharmacology of phenobarbital.

Other Measures

Modification of the infant's environment (light and noise control), swaddling, and frequent feedings have been utilized with mixed success in neonates with signs of withdrawal. Ostrea and colleagues[198] could not diminish the severity of neonatal narcotic withdrawal by alterations in the environment to reduce external stimuli. Other important aspects of care have been previously reviewed.[206,417]

CLINICAL TOXICOLOGY IN THE NEONATE

Extrauterine exposure of the neonate to a number of drugs and chemicals has resulted in the development of toxic reactions. The clinical toxicology experience with drugs intentionally administered to the neonate for therapeutic reasons is reviewed under the specific agents in earlier chapters. The following discussion relates to inadvertent or accidental exposure of neonates to toxic amounts of various other drugs or chemicals (Table 11–9).

Alcohols

Intoxication of the neonate by alcohols has been confined to unusual situations of exposure. Case reports of *methanol* intoxication occurring subsequent to percutaneous absorption or accidental use in formula preparation have resulted in the classic manifestations of methanol poisoning including metabolic acidosis.[245,269] Methanol poisoning in infants could obviously be confused with other disorders involving severe metabolic acidosis, including diabetes mellitus, acute renal failure, inborn errors of metabolism, and other toxicities (e.g., with salicylates, phenols, or glycols). Diagnosis is based on the identification of methanol in blood level.

Intoxications with other alcohols have arisen through employment of *ethanol* as an IV nu-

Table 11–9. CHEMICAL-INDUCED TOXICITY IN NEONATES REPORTED IN CLINICAL STUDIES

Agent	Manifestations[a]	Author(s) of Published Study[b]
alcohols		
methanol	vomiting, lethargy, metabolic acidosis, blindness, organ necrosis; topical-skin necrosis	Wenzl et al,[269] Kahn and Blum,[245] Harpin and Rutter[241]
ethanol	CNS depression, hypoglycemia	Peden et al[261]
isopropanol	CNS depression, hypoglycemia	Moss[256]
benzyl alcohol	Progressive CNS dysfunction and metabolic acidosis, seizures, apnea, coma, intracranial hemorrhage, death ("gasping syndrome")	Gershanik et al,[235] Brown et al[222]
baby powder	pulmonary complications following inhalation (cough, dyspnea, sneezing, cyanosis)	Brouillette and Weber,[221] Motomatsu et al,[257] Mofenson et al[255]
boric acid (borate)	skin: erythematous desquamation CNS: irritability, restlessness, seizures gastrointestinal: loss of appetite, vomiting, diarrhea (bloody) renal: oliguria, anuria, cardiovascular collapse	Goldbloom and Goldbloom,[238] Rubenstein and Musher,[263] Gordon et al,[240] O'Sullivan and Taylor[461]
hexachlorophene	muscle twitching, nystagmus, irritability, decreased alertness, seizures, vacuolation of CNS tissue	Lockhart,[252] Mullick,[259] Gluck,[237] Shuman et al[264]
iodine	skin necrosis, transient hypothyroidism, goiter	Chabrolle and Rossier,[223] Wilkinson et al,[270] l'Allemand et al[249]
mercury		
inorganic	acute exposure: severe pulmonary injury following inhalation of metallic vapor	Moutinho et al[258]
	chronic exposure: acrodynia (extreme irritability and restlessness, apathy, insomnia, anorexia, profuse perspiration, thirst, pink color of palms, rosy cheeks, skin rash with desquamation, photophobia, pruritus)	Warkany and Hubbard,[268] Blattner[219]
organic	primarily associated with CNS and peripheral neurologic manifestations	Zepp et al,[272] Chisolm[225]
nitrates and nitrites, aniline dyes, benzocaine, resorcin	methemoglobin formation (nitrites) with cyanosis, respiratory distress	Cornblath and Hartman,[229] Committee on Nutrition,[227] Etteldorf,[234] Johnson et al,[244] Wolff,[271] Cunningham[230]
phenolic disinfectants (pentachlorophenol)	diaphoresis, fever, tachycardia, tachypnea, metabolic acidosis, hepatomegaly	Robson et al,[262] Armstrong,[218] Doan et al[232]
hyperosmolar solutions (bicarbonate, contrast media, formulas, glucose, various medications, propylene glycol, salt)	hepatic necrosis, necrotizing enterocolitis, intracranial hemorrhage	Simmons et al,[265] Book et al,[220] Cooke et al,[228] Devlieger et al,[231] Ernst et al,[233] Glasgow et al[236]

[a] See text for additional details.
[b] See References at end of chapter.

trient,[261] following "alcohol sponging" with ethanol or *isopropanol* to reduce body temperature,[256] and with the use of *methanol spirits* (ethanol, methanol) for antiseptic preparation of the skin prior to an invasive procedure.[241]

The toxicity of *benzyl alcohol,* employed as a preservative in parenteral medications and fluids, was first recognized in 1982.[235] The reported manifestations associated with intoxication with benzyl alcohol in premature infants

included progressive CNS depression and hypoactivity, increasing respiratory distress, severe metabolic acidosis, "gasping" respiration, thrombocytopenia, hepatic and renal failure, hypotension, and cardiovascular collapse followed by death. Infants with manifestations of toxicity received average daily quantities of benzyl alcohol of 99 to 234 mg/kg compared with 27 to 99 mg/kg in a matched control group with no evidence of toxicity. Subsequent reports of benzyl alcohol poisoning in neonatal intensive-care units have appeared.[222] Brown and colleagues[222] estimated the minimal intake of benzyl alcohol resulting in toxicity to be 130 mg/kg per day. In their patients the onset of symptoms appeared to occur sometime after the second to fourth day of exposure at these doses. Seizures commonly occurred in the early phases of intoxication, followed by progressive CNS depression. The clinical picture is that of an infant with severe metabolic acidosis and progressive encephalopathy unresponsive to treatment. The prevalence of benzyl alcohol as a preservative in IV medications and fluids (typical concentrations range from 0.9 to 1.5 mg/ml) has resulted in some difficulty in completely eliminating the exposure of neonates to this substance.

Benzyl alcohol, an aromatic alcohol, is oxidized to benzoic acid and subsequently conjugated in the liver with glycine, resulting in the production of hippuric acid. This product is excreted largely in the urine along with the oxidized product benzoic acid. Serum benzoic acid values in intoxicated neonates have ranged from 8.4 to 28.7 mmol/l.[222] In a recent study,[235] levels of benzyl alcohol in serum showed a mean concentration of 1 mmol/l; urine levels of benzoic acid and hippuric acid were also elevated in intoxicated infants. The levels of benzoic acid in the urine were 0.38 mmol/l versus normal of 0.03 mmol/l, and of hippuric acid, 1.5 mmol/l versus normal of 0.8 mmol/l. Several reports have shown that the oxidative processes and conjugation reactions involved in the metabolism of benzyl alcohol are reduced in infants. The combination of prematurity coupled with very large doses of benzyl alcohol in IV solutions and drugs could result in the accumulation of benzyl alcohol and its metabolites in the blood.[226] At risk would be infants receiving the equivalent of 100 mg/kg or more of benzyl alcohol daily. The exact etiology for the toxic manifestations subsequent to benzyl alcohol administration remains to be elucidated.[253] It is interesting that the toxicity of benzyl alcohol was examined in 1971 by Kimura[246] in experimental animals from the standpoint of its potential toxicity as a component of IV therapy.

Baby Powders

Inhalation of toxic quantities of baby powder by infants has been the subject of several recent articles.[221,255,257] The true incidence of baby powder inhalation toxicity is thought to be grossly underestimated. The manifestations of such toxicity include cough, dyspnea, sneezing, vomiting, and cyanosis. The estimated mortality has been as high as 20%.[221] There is no adequate treatment for the pulmonary complications resulting in morbidity and mortality with baby powder inhalation.

Boric Acid

Boric acid is a colorless, odorless, compound that has been widely used in medicine for centuries. Cases of boric acid poisoning have been reported following injection, ingestion, enemas, lavage of serous cavities, application of powders and ointments to burned or abraded skin including diaper dermititis and when used as a "soother for tender gums."[238,461] Boric acid is rapidly absorbed from the gastrointestinal tract and mucosal surfaces, and extensive absorption has been documented through burned or abraded areas of skin. The most frequent cause of intoxication in infants involves chronic topical application of boric acid with subsequent absorption through the skin. Cutaneous manifestations (generalized erythematous desquamation) resembling toxic epidermal necrolysis develop regardless of the route of poisoning.[263] Other prominent manifestations of toxicity are CNS effects, including irritability and seizures, and gastrointestinal effects, including nausea, vomiting, and diarrhea. In severe poisoning, vomitus and stools may be bloody. Oliguria or anuria from renal tubular necrosis is present in moderate to severe poisonings. Death, which occurs several days following the onset of major manifestations, is usually the result of circulatory collapse and shock. Reported lethal blood level concentrations of boron range from 200 to 1,000 μg/ml, although symptoms have occurred with blood boron concentrations of 80 μg/ml.[428] O'Sullivan and Taylor[461] reported blood boron levels of 2.6 to 8.5 μg/ml in intoxicated infants. Blood boron levels in human infants exposed only to nutritional sources of borates range between 0.0 and 1.3 μg/ml.[428,461] The total fatal dose from acute boric acid ingestion in infants ranges from 4.5 to 15 grams. Severe chronic intoxication has been reported with ingestion of over 2 grams per week.[461]

Treatment involves discontinuation of boric acid exposure and supportive care. Adequate urine output is important for the excretion of boric acid and borates in the urine. The estimated mortality in infancy from exposure to boric acid is 55 to 70%. Gordon and coworkers[240] noted striking differences in the presentation of chronic borate intoxication, ranging from the classic presentation as described here to recurrent convulsions with minimal other manifestations.

Hexachlorophene

Hexachlorophene (HCP), an effective bacteriostatic agent, came under regulatory restrictions as an aftermath of concerns regarding its toxicity.[252] Prior to that time, products containing hexachlorophene were among the most commonly used topical antiseptics. Although toxicities (muscle twitching and coma) were noted in burn patients bathed with hexachlorophene products, it was the results of animal studies demonstrating topical absorption and cerebral edema and "spongy-appearing" microscopic lesions in the brain and spinal cord that heightened the level of concern regarding its use in infants. Prophylactic skin care with hexachlorophene was summarily discontinued following a warning statement by the FDA that was endorsed by the American Academy of Pediatrics.[243] Absorption of hexachlorophene was demonstrated to occur in burn patients who developed CNS symptoms during the course of topical washings with 3% hexachlorophene.[250] Gluck,[237] on reviewing the literature existing at that time, concluded that no evidence existed for untoward effects of hexachlorophene in full-term newborns; however, light microscopy studies of brains of premature infants weighing less than 1.4 kg revealed lesions similar to those seen in experimental animals treated with hexachlorophene. Evidence that hexachlorophene caused the microscopic changes in brain tissue following topical application in infants appears convincing.[259,264] Whether the CNS lesions explain the manifestations of intoxication in premature infants (focal and generalized seizures, decreased alertness) is less clear. Manifestations of hexachlorophene intoxication in neonates following poisoning by mouth closely resemble the signs and symptoms associated with topical intoxication.[242]

Heavy Metals

Metallic *mercury* not only is a prevalent contaminant in the environment but is ubiquitous in clinical medicine as a component of devices such as thermometers, sphygmomanometers, and the Miller-Abbott tube. Among the earliest reports of inorganic mercury poisoning in infants was the description of *acrodynia*.[219] This syndrome has a distinctive clinical presentation and course. Manifestations include extreme irritability and restlessness alternating with periods of apathy, insomnia, anorexia, profuse perspiration and thirst, variable skin rashes with desquamation, rosy cheeks, and a characteristic pink flush of the palms. Extreme pruritus is characteristic, as well as photophobia, which is often pronounced. Pain of the extremities may be severe. Loss of hair and nails may occur. Warkany and Hubbard[268] determined that the cause of acrodynia was mercury, which was a component of lotions, diaper rinses, and teething powders. Acute exposure to metallic mercury vapors can produce severe pulmonary injury and death.[258] Contamination of infant incubators has been reported as a consequence of damage to mercury expansion switches and mercury thermometer breakage.[254,266] Although no obvious adverse effects were identified from these exposures, the possibility of serious consequences clearly exists. A new standard for threshold limit value (TLV) for mercury in infant environments is needed.[432]

Organomercurials including *methyl mercury* have been associated with epidemic catastrophes in thousands of individuals in Minamata Bay, Iraq, and New Mexico.[216,217,225,248,272] These poisonings occurred as a result of contamination of the food chain with industrial waste and the tragic use of seed grain treated with methyl mercury, a fungicide. In contrast to inorganic mercury poisoning, the symptoms of organomercurial poisoning may take weeks or months to develop. Manifestations include paresthesias (tingling sensations of extremities, lips and mouth); visual disturbances, including blindness; deafness; signs of cerebral palsy; emotional instability; chorea and athetoid movements and ataxia; and stupor, coma, or death.

Cases of *lead* intoxication before the age of 6 months are rare, probably because the ingestion of significant quantities of lead-contaminated substances such as paint is unlikely in very young infants.

Iodine

The use of iodine-containing topical disinfectants (povidone-iodine) has been associated with necrosis of the skin in infants, particularly premature newborns.[270] The tissue injury is most likely to develop when excess amounts of the disinfectant are inadvertently left in contact with the skin for prolonged periods. Recent studies found that exposure to providone-iodine solutions during delivery resulted in increased iodine levels in serum and urine in newborn infants.[249,400] TSH levels were elevated and T_4 levels were reduced within the first week of life but returned to control levels by 2 weeks of age. None of the infants developed goiter or exhibited typical clinical signs of hypothyroidism. However, repeated applications of an alcohol-iodine (1%) solution has been shown to induce goiter and hypothyroidism in neonates.[223]

Nitrates and Nitrites, Aniline Dyes, Benzocaine

Over a century ago the first reports of cyanosis in infants exposed to agents capable of inducing methemoglobin formation appeared. The earliest reports have been repeated with astonishing similarity through modern times (Table 11-9). Methemoglobinemia has been reported in infants after consumption of well-water nitrates, the use of aniline dyes for marking diapers, and use of "sweet spirits of nitre" and benzocaine.[224,267,271]

The potential hazard of nitrate is derived through its conversion to *nitrite* either prior to or after ingestion. The nitrite ion oxidizes ferrous iron in hemoglobin to the ferric state (methemoglobin), which is incapable of carrying oxygen. As a consequence, hypoxemia and cyanosis develop. Infants are particularly vulnerable to oxidant agents because of the incomplete maturation of the methemoglobin reductase system and increased susceptibility of fetal hemoglobin to oxidation.[224] Nitrate poisoning in infants appears to be associated only with ingestion of nitrate in water rather than naturally occurring nitrate in foods.[227,229,267] Pursuit of an explanation for the variability in the relationship between content of nitrate in drinking water and formation of methemoglobin in infancy resulted in the conclusion that contamination of water or food with organisms capable of converting the nitrate to nitrite was a critical ingredient.[247] The influence of intestinal pH relates to the proliferation and growth of organisms capable of converting nitrate to nitrites. Current drinking water standards for nitrate levels deemed to be safe for infants are less than 45 ppm (45 μg/l). Nonprotein nitrogen should be less than 10 ppm (10 μg/l).

Methemoglobin formation has also followed exposure to aniline dyes and nitrate- or nitrite-containing medicines.[224,239,244,271] Fatal results in various reports were associated with methemoglobin levels in excess of 80%.

Treatment of methemoglobinemia involves the regeneration of hemoglobin from methemoglobin by the administration of *methylene blue* and oxygen. The dose of methylene blue is 1.5 mg/kg IV.[234]

Phenolic Disinfectants (Pentachlorophenol)

Compounds chemically related to hexachlorophene that are also used as disinfectants have been associated with serious adverse effects in neonates. The use of pentachlorophenol in the laundry of infant diapers resulted in intoxications characterized by perfuse generalized diaphoresis, fever, tachycardia, tachypnea, metabolic acidosis, and hepatomegaly.[218,262] High concentrations of pentachlorophenol were found in the nursery linens and in the serum and autopsy tissues of the infants involved. Phenolic disinfectant detergents have also been reported to increase neonatal jaundice.[232]

Hyperosmolar Solutions

Administration of hyperosmolar preparations to infants has been associated with a number of adverse effects including hepatic necrosis,[231] intracranial hemorrhage,[260,265] and necrotizing enterocolitis.[220,228] The preparations involved include hyperosmolar solutions of bicarbonate and THAM, infant nutritional formulas, glucose, radiographic contrast material, and various drug formulations. The osmolality of these preparations have been found to be as high as 36,800 mOsm/kg H_2O. The majority of drug solutions intended for parenteral administration have an osmolality in the range of 100 to 1,000 mOsm/kg H_2O.[233,251] The major contributor to the osmolality is the drug concentration itself. However, propylene glycol, used as a vehicle in many pharmaceutical preparations, can produce hyperosmolality in infants when given in substantial quantities.[236] No adverse effects have been observed following such treatment. DiSessa and associates[421] examined the effects of two contrast materials, diatrizoate and metrizamide, on various cardiovascular parameters and serum osmolality in neonates. Diatrizoate increased serum osmolality, but neither contrast material changed serum sodium, potassium, or creatinine levels. No serious side-effects were observed with either agent.

BREAST-FEEDING AND DRUGS

The question is not whether a medicated mother should be allowed to nurse, but whether a nursing mother really needs to be medicated.

Sumner J. Yaffe

The need for accurate assessment of the effects of drugs in human milk on the infant has arisen from concern about and analytic confirmation of the presence of drugs in human milk. Unfortunately, the improving sophistication in measurement of drugs in human milk has far exceeded the determination of the clinical relevance of their presence. The increased acceptance of breast-feeding in our highly drug-oriented society further emphasizes the importance of gathering information on drug consumption by nursing mothers and the resulting impact on the well-being of the breast-fed infant.

The older literature reviewing the subject reflects an attitude of conservatism; the mere presence of a drug in breast milk, especially if it had been shown to have toxic effects in adults or children, often prompted a recommendation that it be used with caution or avoided entirely, particularly in the absence of direct information on effects in breast-fed infants. Such recommendations have been found in many cases to be inconsistent with the best interests of both mother and baby. For example, when actual studies were finally conducted to examine the pharmacodynamic effects of oral anticoagulants (dicumarol, warfarin) in infants breast-fed by mothers taking these drugs, no effects on coagulation in the infants could be identified.[293,302,338] The importance of considering the overall value of breast-feeding versus the unknown effects of the drugs incurred by breast-feeding has been emphasized in more recent reviews that champion breast-feeding even though a drug may reach human milk.[385] Which philosophy (conservative vs. liberal) should prevail in decisions regarding individual drugs must be based on a number of issues other than what is known or not known about the adverse consequences associated with the use of the drug by nursing mothers.

Excellent reviews have been written regarding the factors involved in how drugs reach breast milk.[296,333,382,390,391] These factors are summarized in Table 11–10. The most important factors determining drug excretion into

Table 11–10. FACTORS AFFECTING THE AMOUNT OF DRUG REACHING THE BREAST MILK AND THE BREAST-FED INFANT

Maternal Therapeutic Regimen and Drug Disposition
drug dose, frequency and route of administration
rate and route of drug clearance
extent of protein binding of drug
metabolism of drug: consideration of active metabolites
Breast Milk Production
blood flow
milk and plasma pH
milk composition (fat, protein, carbohydrate)
rate of milk production versus plasma drug concentration at that time
ion and other transport mechanisms
drug metabolism and reabsorption from milk
Infant Feeding Schedule
amount and frequency of feeding relative to the amount of drug present in mother's plasma and milk at time of feeding
Drug Characteristics
physico-chemical properties
    pK_a (ionization) versus pH of milk and plasma
    solubility: lipid versus water
protein-binding characteristics
molecular weight

milk are the physicochemical characteristics of the drug (degree of ionization, pK_a and lipid solubility) and the molecular weight; the drug must cross several membrane structures before reaching the milk, including the capillary endothelium, alveolar cell wall, and plasma membrane, and may subsequently pass into the milk by simple diffusion or carrier-mediated or facilitated diffusion, or by active transport. The pH of the plasma, intracellular environment, and milk will affect the movement of drug based on its pK_a and inherent lipid solubility. If the pH differences in these environments favor the drug's becoming less and less ionized, the drug will tend to diffuse more readily from plasma to milk. Normally, breast milk is more acidic (pH 6.8–7.3, average 7.0) than plasma (pH 7.4).[382] Therefore, drugs that are weak bases tend to concentrate more in breast milk relative to plasma than do drugs that are weak acids (Table 11–11). This is the so-called "ion trapping" phenomenon. Protein binding of drugs, which can be altered by pH, either can hinder the movement of drugs into milk by "trapping," and thereby prevent diffusion from plasma into milk, or can facilitate diffusion into milk by acting as a carrier or by capturing the drug in the milk compartment. Protein binding probably does not play a major role in determining the amount of drug reaching the breast milk. Ma-

Table 11-11. DRUG CONCENTRATIONS IN BREAST MILK COMPARED WITH THERAPEUTIC SERUM DRUG LEVELS[a]

Drug	Reported Concentrations in Breast Milk	Therapeutic Serum or Plasma Levels
acetaminophen	10–15 μg/ml	10–20 μg/ml
aminoglycosides	40–70% of maternal serum	
amitriptyline	30–150 ng/ml	160–240 ng/ml
ampicillin	0.01–1 μg/ml	1–25 μg/ml
aspirin	40–80% of maternal serum	10–30 μg/ml
atropine	<0.1 mg/dl	1–20 μg/dl
caffeine	50% of maternal serum	1–20 μg/dl
captopril	0.005 μg/ml	0.7 $\pm$ 0.1 μg/ml
carbamazepine	0.5–2 μg/ml	5–10 μg/ml
cephalosporins	<2.5 μg/ml (maximum reported value)	3–90 μg/ml
chloral hydrate	<10 μg/ml	10–55 μg/ml
chloramphenicol	50% of maternal serum	10–20 μg/ml
chlorothiazide	<0.1 μg/ml	2.3 μg/ml
chlorpromazine	7–98 ng/ml	40–350 ng/ml
cimetidine	5–6 mcg/ml	0.5–1 μg/ml
clindamycin	1–4 mcg/ml	2–10 μg/ml
clonidine	1.5 ng/ml	1 ng/ml
codeine	2 times maternal serum	30–110 ng/ml
corticosteroids	<1% of maternal serum	
diazepam	0.2–1 μg/ml	>600 ng/ml
digoxin	60–70% of maternal serum	1–2 ng/ml
ethanol	equal to maternal serum	
erythromycin	0.4–3.2 μg/ml	1–20 μg/ml
ethosuximide	80–100% of maternal serum	40–100 μg/ml
gentamicin	40–70% of maternal serum	1–10 μg/ml
haloperidol	2–24 ng/ml	10–100 ng/ml
heparin	not present	
hydralazine	760–1270 nmol/l	580–6000 nmol/l
hydrochlorothiazide	50–120 ng/ml	100–600 ng/ml
ibuprofen	<0.5 μg/ml	30–70 μg/ml
imipramine	4–30 ng/ml	>200 ng/ml
insulin	not present	
isoniazid	1–3 times maternal serum	3–5 μg/ml
lincomycin	equal to maternal serum	10–100 μg/ml
lithium	30–50% of maternal serum	>0.7 mEq/l
lorazepam	12 ng/ml	20–80 ng/ml
marijuana (THC)	60–105 ng/ml	5–180 ng/ml
meperidine	<200 ng/ml	200–500 ng/ml
meprobamate	2–4 times maternal serum	10–30 μg/ml
methadone	1–1.5 times maternal serum	70–500 ng/ml
methimazole	equal to maternal serum	50–100 ng/ml
metronidazole	equal to maternal serum	2–10 μg/ml
methotrexate	6×10^{-9} M	10^{-8} to 5×10^{-6} M
morphine	1–1.5 times maternal serum	65 $\pm$ 80 ng/ml
naproxen	0.7–1.3 μg/ml	30–90 μg/ml
nitrofurantoin	<0.5 μg/ml	1 μg/ml
nortriptyline	0.06 μg/ml	0.05–0.15 μg/ml
oral contraceptives	<0.5–12% of maternal serum	
penicillins	<1 IU/ml	2–40 IU/ml
phenytoin	25–45% of maternal serum	10–20 μg/ml
prednisolone	0.007 μg/ml	
prednisone	0.03 μg/ml	
primidone	70–85% of maternal serum	5–10 μg/ml
propranolol	3–150 ng/ml	50–1000 ng/ml
propylthiouracil	<0.7 μg/ml	6–8 μg/ml
quinidine	6–8 μg/ml	2–7 μg/ml
quinine	0.4–1.6 μg/ml	7 μg/ml
rifampin	1–3 μg/ml	1–20 μg/ml
sulfonamides	5–130 μg/ml	40–60 μg/ml
theophylline	60–70% of maternal serum	5–20 μg/ml
tobramycin	0–0.5 μg/ml	1–10 μg/ml
valproic acid	1–2% of maternal serum	50–100 μg/ml
warfarin	<0.024 μg/ml	2 μg/ml

[a] Values for breast milk represent ranges or peak levels. These data were collected under a variety of conditions and therefore should be considered very general approximations of the levels obtainable in the milk. Approximate therapeutic plasma or serum drug levels are provided for comparison.

ternal blood flow to the breast and concentration of drug in the plasma at the time of milk formation (nursing) have obvious influences on the amount of drug reaching the gastrointestinal tract of the nursing infant. Metabolites of the administered drug must also be considered in evaluating extent of infant exposure.

General Recommendations

The critical ingredient required for the recommendation to discontinue breast-feeding during maternal drug therapy is the documentation of a real and substantial risk to the infant. It is no longer acceptable for the physician to intervene arbitrarily with the mother's wish to breast-feed her infant merely because maternal drug therapy is clearly indicated. Nor does it seem reasonable to discontinue breast-feeding solely because the drug in question has been implicated in one or two case reports of toxic side-effects in primary recipients. There are few drugs that have been well documented to cause significant toxicity in infants as a result of breast-feeding.[294] Anecdotal single case reports of reversible side-effects such as sedation with phenobarbital hardly seem to justify denying the mother with a phenobarbital-controlled seizure disorder the opportunity to nurse her infant. Drugs without any known history of causing adverse effects in nursing infants should not be arbitrarily labeled "dangerous until proven safe." On the other hand, total disregard for a potential drug toxicity could lead to disasters in breast-feeding infants. A systematic approach to decisions regarding breast-feeding and maternal drug therapy is outlined in Table 11–12.

Specific Agents

The following sections and Table 11–13 summarize the available information on the advisability of breast-feeding by mothers receiving drug therapy.[294] A historical examination of published reviews and recommendations on individual drugs is also provided in Table 11–13.

Anticoagulants

Conflicting information exists with respect to the effect of maternal oral anticoagulant therapy on breast-feeding infants. Earlier literature recommended avoiding the use of oral antico-

Table 11–12. PROCEDURE FOR ASSESSING ACCEPTABILITY OF BREAST-FEEDING DURING MATERNAL DRUG THERAPY

1. Determine if the drug(s) is *required* for the benefit of the mother, by consultation with informed physician(s).
2. Carefully examine the literature regarding the drug.
   a. If drug is nontoxic (not present in milk) or known to be safe in previous clinical use, (see Table 11–13), breast-feeding is appropriate.
   b. If toxic potential exists, is there an alternative drug with less or no toxicity?
   c. If potential for toxicity exists or is unknown, proceed to step 3.
3. Can toxicity of drug be detected by signs or symptoms or by monitoring infant drug blood levels? Are toxic effects reversible? Is there a history of allergic or idiosyncratic-type drug reactions?
4. Advise the parents of possible problems and of availability of monitoring for adverse effects in the infant. Consider the advantages of breast-feeding to the infant and mother versus the known or possible toxicity associated with the drug.

Additional Considerations

5. It may be possible to minimize infant drug exposure by instructing the mother to take the medication immediately *after* completing breast feeding or by collecting breast milk for subsequent feeding just prior to taking medication.
6. If drug therapy in the mother is to be of short duration, interruption rather than complete termination of breast-feeding should be advised.

agulants because of the possibility of bleeding disorders in the breast-fed infant. However, studies in nursing mothers and their infants has revealed that *warfarin* is not present in significant quantities in breast milk. This is consistent with the observation that prothrombin time (PT) is normal in infants nursed by mothers receiving warfarin.[302,330,338] *Dicumarol* administration to nursing mothers does not affect PT in breast-fed infants, nor have hemorrhages been observed.[293] *Heparin* does not pass into maternal milk.[273]

Anticonvulsants

Every effort possible should be made to allow the mother with a seizure disorder who wishes to breast-feed her infant to do so. Exposure of the infant to anticonvulsants may be minimized by breast-feeding just prior to the next dose whenever possible.[315] The quantities of *phenobarbital* and *phenytoin* present in milk are insufficient under ordinary circumstances to produce symptomatology in the infant who is breast-feeding.[344] The amount of phenobarbital likely to be administered to the nursing infant via the breast milk is less than 5 mg/kg per

Text continued on page 366

Table 11–13. DRUGS AND BREAST-FEEDING: HISTORICAL REVIEW OF RECOMMENDATIONS AND EFFECTS ON INFANT REPORTED IN CLINICAL STUDIES

Drug	Author(s) of Review Article[a]							Recommendations[b]
	Knowles[324,325]	O'Brien[348]	Vorherr[382]	Anderson[276]	White and White[385]	Wilson[390]	Committee on Drugs[301]	
acetaminophen (e.g., Tylenol)			nontoxic levels in milk		no harmful effects known		no effect	no anticipated adverse effects with intermittent use; minimize exposure by nursing prior to dose[287]
acetazolamide (Diamox)		close observation	nontoxic levels in milk		no harmful effects known			no anticipated adverse effects; minimize exposure by nursing prior to dose
alcohol (ethanol)	no problems expected except in large doses	little to no effect with moderate amounts	potential vomiting, drowsiness	low to moderate intake: no toxicity prolonged to large intake: may be detrimental	moderation: no harmful effects	occasional use of moderate dose: no harm; breast-feeding by intoxicated mother CONTRAINDICATED	CNS effects noted with large doses	avoid breast-feeding during and for several hours after drinking alcoholic beverages
amantadine			CONTRAINDICATED		CONTRAINDICATED		usually compatible with nursing	insufficient information available; present in milk (manufacturer)
amikacin	*see gentamicin*							
aminophylline	*see theophylline*							
amitriptyline (Elavil)				undetectable amounts in milk	no harmful effects known	not detected in milk	no effect	present in milk, no anticipated adverse effects; monitor serum drug level in infant[295]
amphetamines	no effect	not present in milk	potential: tremor, insomnia		no evidence of harmful effects; caution if abused	no adverse effects observed	usually compatible with breast-feeding	avoid breast-feeding or drug

Table continued on following page

Table 11–13. DRUGS AND BREAST-FEEDING: HISTORICAL REVIEW OF RECOMMENDATIONS AND EFFECTS ON INFANT REPORTED IN CLINICAL STUDIES *(Continued)*

Drug	Knowles[324,325]	O'Brien[348]	Vorherr[382]	Anderson[276]	White and White[385]	Wilson[390]	Committee on Drugs[301]	Recommendations[b]
				Author(s) of Review Article[a]				
ampicillin	temporarily discontinue breast-feeding (sensitization)	no anticipated effects	nontoxic levels in milk	present in milk (1–30% of maternal serum level)	no known harmful effects			no anticipated adverse effects, but sensitization may justify temporary discontinuation[276]
antacids					no known harmful effects	avoid bicarbonate-containing preparations		no anticipated adverse effects
antihistamines		no anticipated effects	nontoxic levels in milk		no known harmful effects	no severe adverse reactions reported	usually compatible with breast-feeding	no anticipated adverse effects; minimize exposure by nursing prior to dose
aspirin	caution with large doses	could cause bleeding tendency	nontoxic levels in milk	peak levels in milk at 9 hr; milk conc. < plasma; no expected toxicity	no harmful effects reported; caution: high doses, check infant PT	caution with chronic use	usually compatible with breast-feeding	occasional dose: no problems expected chronic use: monitor salicylate levels in infants[284]
atropine	decreased bowel activity	CONTRA-INDICATED	potential: decrease in milk supply; in infant, pupil dilation, tachycardia, constipation, urinary retention	poor documentation of effects on infants	no known harmful effects	avoid use	no effect	monitor for signs and symptoms of anticholinergic effects; dose after nursing
barbiturates	*see* phenobarbital							
belladonna	*see* atropine CONTRA-INDICATED							
busulfan (Myleran)	CONTRA-INDICATED		potential: bone marrow depression		no known harmful effects			insufficient information available

Drug							
caffeine	no anticipated effects		nontoxic levels in milk	no effect on infant	harmless to infant	present in milk	usually compatible with breast-feeding
captopril						low milk/plasma ratio	no effect
carbamazepine (Tegretol)				present in milk (60% of plasma)		no adverse effects noted	no effect
carbenicillin	no anticipated effects				no known harmful effects		
cephalosporins	not excreted in milk				no known harmful effects	low amounts in milk	no effect
chloral hydrate	no anticipated effects		present in milk; can produce sedation in infant	no known harmful effects			usually compatible with breast-feeding
chloramphenicol	temporarily discontinue	caution	potential: jaundice	CONTRA-INDICATED: bone marrow effects possible, (?) symptoms in infant	consider alternative drug	CONTRA-INDICATED	no effect

Drug	Comments
caffeine	no anticipated adverse effect with moderate use[288,379]
captopril	no anticipated adverse effects[303]
carbamazepine (Tegretol)	no adverse effects expected; minimize exposure by nursing prior to dose[357]
carbenicillin	no anticipated adverse effects; minimize exposure by nursing prior to dose
cephalosporins	no anticipated adverse effects; minimize exposure by nursing prior to dose
chloral hydrate	no anticipated serious adverse effects with intermittent use; minimize exposure by nursing prior to dose[329]
chloramphenicol	seek alternative drug; presence in breast milk may indicate risk of bone marrow suppression (?);[312] if used, monitor serum levels in infant

Table continued on following page

Table 11–13. DRUGS AND BREAST-FEEDING: HISTORICAL REVIEW OF RECOMMENDATIONS AND EFFECTS ON INFANT REPORTED IN CLINICAL STUDIES (Continued)

Drug	Author(s) of Review Article[a]							Recommendations[b]
	Knowles[324,325]	O'Brien[348]	Vorherr[382]	Anderson[276]	White and White[385]	Wilson[390]	Committee on Drugs[301]	
chlordiazepoxide (Librium)		no anticipated effects			no known harmful effects	inadequate information	usually compatible with breast-feeding	serious adverse effects unlikely with intermittent use; minimize exposure by nursing prior to dose
chloroquine (Aralen)		no anticipated effects		some data on milk conc. probably faulty			no effect	insufficient information available
chlorothiazide (Diuril)		CONTRA-INDICATED (mfr.'s recommendation)	potential: thrombocytopenia	low amounts in milk; consider possible idiosyncratic reactions	no known harmful effects	safe	avoid use in first month of lactation	no anticipated adverse effects[342,383]
chlorpheniramine	see antihistamines							
chlorpromazine (CPZ)	small amount in milk	may cause galactorrhea		no expected toxicity	no ill effects (1 case: drowsiness)		usually compatible with breast-feeding	no anticipated adverse effects; rare cause of mild CNS depression[327,389]
cimetidine (Tagamet)					no known harmful effects but consider alternative drug	CONTRA-INDICATED	CONTRA-INDICATED	maximum dose possible 1.5 mg/kg/day; avoid use if possible[368]
clindamycin	temporarily discontinue			present in milk	no known harmful effects	low conc. in milk; no effect on infant	no effect	avoid drug if possible until more information available[367] (? gastrointestinal toxicity[337])
clonidine (Catapres)								insufficient information available
cocaine			nontoxic levels in milk		unknown; consider alternative drug CONTRA-INDICATED	present in milk		avoid drug or breastfeeding

codeine	not present in milk	no significant effects	no or trace amounts in milk	levels too low in milk to cause toxicity		no effect	no anticipated adverse effects with single clinical doses; minimize exposure by nursing prior to dose[309,313]
corticosteroids	CONTRA-INDICATED			insufficient information available; most advise against breast-feeding	small amounts in milk not harmful		use with caution: very low amounts in milk, but insufficient information on possible long-term effects with chronic exposure[321,339]
coumarin	*see dicumarol and warfarin*						
cromolyn					no known harmful effects		Insufficient information available
cyclophosphamide		CONTRA-INDICATED	potential: bone marrow suppression	CONTRA-INDICATED	excreted in milk, effects unknown; consider alternative drugs	CONTRA-INDICATED	avoid drug or nurse 24 hr after therapy to minimize exposure[388]
dexamethasone	*see corticosteroids*						
diazepam (Valium)		CONTRA-INDICATED (sedation, hyperbilirubinemia)	not present in milk	can cause symptoms of sedation in infant	present in milk; sedation possible	usually compatible with breast-feeding	continuous use by mother could result in CNS depression in infant[299]
diazoxide					safe		insufficient information available
dicumarol	CONTRA-INDICATED	infant should be monitored with mother	potential: bleeding	use with caution	caution with high doses or if infant to have surgery	no effect	no anticipated adverse effects;[293] dose after nursing; monitoring of infant PT usually not necessary

Table continued on following page

Table 11–13. DRUGS AND BREAST-FEEDING: HISTORICAL REVIEW OF RECOMMENDATIONS AND EFFECTS ON INFANT REPORTED IN CLINICAL STUDIES (Continued)

Drug	Author(s) of Review Article[a]							Recommendations[b]
	Knowles[324,325]	O'Brien[348]	Vorherr[382]	Anderson[276]	White and White[385]	Wilson[390]	Committee on Drugs[301]	
diethylstilbestrol (DES)					CONTRA-INDICATED			no data available; see corticosteroids
digitalis preparations					no known harmful effects	no potential for therapeutic levels to be reached; effects unknown	no effect	no anticipated adverse effects[297,310,358]
diphenhydramine (Benadryl)	see antihistamines							
diphenoxylate (Lomotil)					consider alternative drug			avoid drug or breast-feeding
doxepin					use with caution or select alternative drug			insufficient information available
ephedrine					no known harmful effects			insufficient information available
epinephrine			safe		no known harmful effects	destroyed in gastrointestinal tract		no anticipated adverse effects
ergotamine	symptoms of ergotism in 90% of infants	avoid if possible	potential: nausea, vomiting, diarrhea, weakness	signs of toxicity in 90% of nursing infants	ergotism; consider alternative drug		CONTRA-INDICATED	avoid breast-feeding during course of therapy
erythromycin	temporarily discontinue	high concentrations in milk		levels in milk equal 50% of plasma	not harmful	low levels in milk; not harmful		no adverse effects anticipated; minimize exposure by nursing prior to dose
estrogens	see oral contraceptives							
ethacrynic acid								no adverse effects anticipated

354

Drug							
ethchlorvynol (Placidyl)					present in milk (milk/plasma ratio 0.8)	no effect	insufficient information available[318]
ethosuximide			present in milk	less toxic than trimethadione			insufficient information available
	see chlordiazepoxide						
fenoprofen				no known harmful effects			no adverse effects anticipated; minimize exposure by nursing prior to dose
furosemide (Lasix)		not present in milk	decreased milk production; no adverse effects likely	not found in milk			no adverse effects anticipated
gentamicin	temporarily discontinue	monitor for ototoxicity		no known harmful effects	safe		no anticipated adverse effects; nurse prior to dose
griseofulvin				not found in milk			no anticipated effects; nurse prior to dose
haloperidol				no reported adverse effects	present in milk in concentrations less than mother's plasma	no effect	no adverse effects reported[373,384]
heparin				not found in milk	not present in milk		no adverse effects anticipated
heroin	will not prevent withdrawal in nursing infant	potential: addiction, prevention of withdrawal	present in milk; causes addiction; lessens withdrawal	CONTRA-INDICATED		no effect	detoxification of mother before allowing breastfeeding
hydralazine				probably safe; consider alternative drug		no effect	no adverse effects anticipated[334]
hydrochlorothiazide (HydroDiuril)	CONTRA-INDICATED (mfr.'s recommendation)						*see* chlorothiazide
hyoscyamine				no known harmful effects			*see* atropine

Table continued on following page

Table 11–13. DRUGS AND BREAST-FEEDING: HISTORICAL REVIEW OF RECOMMENDATIONS AND EFFECTS ON INFANT REPORTED IN CLINICAL STUDIES (Continued)

Drug	Author(s) of Review Article[a]							Recommendations[b]
	Knowles[324,325]	O'Brien[348]	Vorher[382]	Anderson[276]	White and White[385]	Wilson[390]	Committee on Drugs[301]	
ibuprofen (Motrin)					not found in milk (?)		no effect	no anticipated adverse effects[377]
imipramine		not present in milk			no known harmful effects			no anticipated adverse effects[306]
indomethacin		no anticipated effects			caution		no effect	insufficient information available
insulin			no problem with good control					no anticipated adverse effects; destroyed in infants gastrointestinal tract
iodine		CONTRA-INDICATED	nontoxic with therapeutic doses to mother; potential hypothyroidism, goiter	CONTRA-INDICATED	no harmful effects	CONTRA-INDICATED	affects thyroid activity	avoid use of iodine; see text
isoniazid (INH)		monitor for toxicity		levels in milk equal to plasma	no reports of harmful effects		no effect	avoid breast-feeding unless infant also treated with INH[287]
isoproterenol					insignificant amount in milk	insignificant amount in milk		no anticipated adverse effects
kanamycin	see gentamicin							
laxatives		potential: loose stools	nontoxic levels in milk	no problems with nonabsorbable; avoid cascara, danthron, and high doses of aloe and senna	no known harmful effects		usually compatible with breast-feeding	no anticipated adverse effects if used in moderation intermittently

Drug								
lincomycin	temporarily discontinue nursing	no anticipated effects			no known harmful effects			use with caution; no adverse effects reported[340]
lithium		monitor for toxicity	no harmful effects reported	present in milk (50–225% of serum); no reported adverse effects	CONTRA-INDICATED	low concentration in milk; no effect	usually compatible with breast-feeding	consider individual risk vs. benefit factors (see text); monitor serum levels[374]
lorazepam					no known harmful effects			no adverse effects reported[386]
LSD					CONTRA-INDICATED			avoid drug or breast-feeding
marijuana					CONTRA-INDICATED		unknown	avoid exposure (milk or air)
meclizine	see antihistamines							
meperidine		no anticipated effects			no known harmful effects		no effect	see morphine
meprobamate		monitor for toxicity	potential: jaundice	present in milk			usually compatible with breast-feeding	insufficient information available
metaproterenol					no known harmful effects	may be available for excretion in milk		insufficient information available
methadone				breast-feeding permissible; conc. in milk: 83% of plasma	breast-feeding permitted		no effect if maternal dose <20 mg/24 hr	nurse with caution; monitor infant
methicillin	see penicillins							
methimazole				CONTRA-INDICATED	caution: monitor infant thyroid function; consider alternative drugs (PTU)		CONTRA-INDICATED	avoid; consider PTU[375]

Table continued on following page

Table 11–13. DRUGS AND BREAST-FEEDING: HISTORICAL REVIEW OF RECOMMENDATIONS AND EFFECTS ON INFANT REPORTED IN CLINICAL STUDIES (Continued)

Drug	Author(s) of Review Article[a]						Committee on Drugs[301]	Recommendations[b]
	Knowles[324,325]	O'Brien[348]	Vorherr[382]	Anderson[276]	White and White[385]	Wilson[390]		
methotrexate	CONTRA-INDICATED		potential: bone marrow depression	CONTRA-INDICATED	not contraindicated	present in milk		avoid if possible; nurse during periods of low or absent serum conc.[317]
methyldopa		no information available			not excreted in milk (trace)		no effect	insufficient information available
metrizamide							no effect	no adverse effects anticipated
metronidazole	CONTRA-INDICATED	caution: high concentrations in milk	potential: anorexia, vomiting, blood dyscrasias	avoid drug owing to possible carcinogenicity	caution; but probably no effect on infant	CONTRA-INDICATED	interrupt feedings for 12–24 hr	no serious side-effects; discontinue breast-feeding for 12 hr following single-dose therapy[307]
morphine		no anticipated effects	no trace amounts in milk; potential: jaundice	insignificant amounts in milk with clinical use, ? with abuse	no known harmful effects	present in milk; inadequate information available on effects	no effect	adverse effects unlikely with single clinical doses; minimize exposure if possible by nursing prior to dose[309]
nafcillin	see penicillins							
naproxen					no information available		no effect	no reported adverse effects[316]

Drug							
nitrofurantoin	not present in milk	no anticipated effects		caution in G6PD deficiency	no known harmful effects	usually compatible with breast-feeding	no anticipated adverse effect; avoid in G6PD deficiency[381] insufficient information available
nortriptyline					not found in milk		use with caution; insufficient information available
novobiocin	temporarily discontinue breast-feeding	no anticipated effects		present in milk (3–7 µg/ml)	no known harmful effects		
opium	*see* paregoric						
oral contraceptives	may decrease milk production	caution: risks *vs.* maternal benefits	potential: jaundice, vaginal epithelium proliferation, gynecomastia, decreased milk supply	controversial literature reviewed	CONTRA-INDICATED	usually compatible with breast-feeding	very low levels (<1% of maternal dose) of estrogens and progestins found in breast milk;[331] no clinically significant effect on composition and quantity of breast milk in well-nourished mothers; long-term effects unknown; seek alternative means of birth control (see text)
oxacillin					no known harmful effects, caution in first 2 wk of life	present in milk	*see* penicillins
oxazepam	temporarily discontinue					usually compatible with breast-feeding	*see* diazepam
paregoric					not found in milk	CONTRA-INDICATED	avoid drug or breast-feeding

Table continued on following page

Table 11-13. DRUGS AND BREAST-FEEDING: HISTORICAL REVIEW OF RECOMMENDATIONS AND EFFECTS ON INFANT REPORTED IN CLINICAL STUDIES (Continued)

Drug	Author(s) of Review Article[a]							Recommendations[b]
	Knowles[324,325]	O'Brien[348]	Vorherr[382]	Anderson[276]	White and White[385]	Wilson[390]	Committee on Drugs[301]	
penicillins	temporarily discontinue breast-feeding	possible sensitization		present in milk (<1 IU/ml); possible allergic sensitization: temporarily discontinue breast-feeding	no effect on infant	low amounts in milk		no anticipated effects, but possible sensitization may justify temporary discontinuation[276]
pentazocine (Talwin)				not found in milk				insufficient information available[276]
pentobarbital perphenazine	see phenobarbital							insufficient information available
phencyclidine					no known harmful effects	high concentrations reached in milk		avoid drug or breast-feeding[345]
phenobarbital	caution	best to avoid nursing (induces metabolizing enzymes)	potential: sedation, decreased sucking, enzyme stimulation	present in milk; reports of drowsiness in nursing infants	trace amounts in milk; no known harmful effects; caution with large doses	present in milk; symptoms unlikely to develop	no expected effects with usual doses	no anticipated adverse effects; monitor infant including drug blood levels if symptoms of CNS depression develop
phenothiazines	see chlorpromazine							
phenylbutazone (Butazolidin)		monitor for toxicity		present in milk (13% of serum); possible: blood dyscrasias			no effect	avoid if possible; insufficient information available
phenylephrine phenylpropanolamine	see ephedrine				destroyed in infant gastrointestinal tract			insufficient information available

Drug							Comments
phenytoin (Dilantin)	safe in most situations	potential: vomiting, tremors, rash, blood dyscrasias			present in milk; adverse effects in infant possible	usually compatible with breast-feeding	no serious adverse effects anticipated; monitor drug blood levels in infant if signs of drug toxicity develop[315,318]
prazosin				no specific information available			insufficient information available
prednisolone and prednisone					not adequately studied	no effect	see corticosteroids
primidone			low amount in milk found in single dose study		present in milk (milk/plasma = 0.8 ± 0.2)	no effect	monitor drug blood levels in infant if signs of drug toxicity develop; minimize exposure by nursing prior to dose[318]
progesterone	CONTRA-INDICATED	CONTRA-INDICATED		CONTRA-INDICATED			see oral contraceptives
propoxyphene (Darvon)		no anticipated effects		no known harmful effects	present in milk (50% of plasma)	no effect	avoid; minimize exposure by nursing prior to dose
propranolol		not present in milk	no effects in infants	no known harmful effects	present in milk; no side-effects reported	no effect	no adverse effects anticipated; minimize exposure by nursing prior to dose[283,477]
propantheline (Pro-Banthine)		not found in milk			insufficient information		insufficient information available
propylthiouracil (PTU)	CONTRA-INDICATED	potential hypothyroidism, goiter		no contraindication reported	use with caution; monitor infant thyroid status	no effect	very little present in milk; no alteration of infant thyroid function[319,336,375]

Table continued on following page

Table 11–13. DRUGS AND BREAST-FEEDING: HISTORICAL REVIEW OF RECOMMENDATIONS AND EFFECTS ON INFANT REPORTED IN CLINICAL STUDIES *(Continued)*

Drug	Author(s) of Review Article[a]						Committee on Drugs[301]	Recommendations[b]
	Knowles[324,325]	O'Brien[348]	Vorherr[382]	Anderson[276]	White and White[385]	Wilson[390]		
pyribenzamine	*see* antihistamines							
quinacrine					no known harmful effects			insufficient information available
quinidine		no anticipated effects			no known harmful effects		no effect	non-therapeutic dose in milk[314]
quinine				amount in milk probably insignificant	no known harmful effects		no effect	monitor infant; minimize exposure by nursing prior to dose
radiopharmaceuticals Gallium (67Ga)		avoid; temporarily stop breast-feeding		CONTRA-INDICATED	2-wk interruption; consider alternative drug		interrupt breast-feeding for 2 wk	interrupt breast-feeding for 2 wk[376]
125I	temporarily discontinue breast-feeding		interrupt breast-feeding for at least 10 days	avoid breast-feeding for 10 days	see Recommendations	CONTRA-INDICATED		discontinue breast-feeding for up to 4 wk; monitor levels of 125I in milk; give Lugol's solution (1 drop) to infant before reinstating breast-feeding[292,350,365]
131I	27% of dose in milk; temporarily discontinue breast-feeding	CONTRA-INDICATED	interrupt breast-feeding for 10 days	avoid breast-feeding for 1–12 days	test done: discontinue breast-feeding for 24–36 hr treatment dose: discontinue breast-feeding for 1–3 wk			discontinue breast-feeding for 2 wk[392]

Drug								
technetium (⁹⁹mTc)	present at 24 hr but gone by 48 hr			discontinue breast feeding for 24–72 hr	interrupt feeding for 24 hr		interrupt breast-feedings for up to 3 days	interrupt breast-feeding for 2–3 days[354,392]
reserpine	may produce galactorrhea		potential: nasal stuffiness, lethargy, diarrhea	nasal stuffiness, increased secretions		no known harmful effects	usually compatible with breast-feeding	avoid use if possible
rifampin		not present in milk				not found in milk	no effect	no anticipated effects; reduce exposure by nursing prior to dose
scopolamine	no anticipated effects	none or trace amounts in milk		no adverse effects expected		no known harmful effects	no effect	monitor infant (see atropine)
secobarbital (Seconal)			*see* phenobarbital					
spironolactone		not present in milk				not found in milk	no effect	present in milk, monitor serum electrolytes in infant[465]
sulfonamides	temporarily discontinue breast-feeding	CONTRA-INDICATED: sulfapyridine, sulfisoxazole; no anticipated effects: sulfathiazole, sulfanilamide	potential: hemolytic anemia (G6PD deficiency), jaundice, bacterial resistance	not absolutely contraindicated; present in milk; causes anemia (G6PD deficiency) and jaundice	enhanced hyperbilirubinemic encephalopathy; G6PD-deficient hemolysis	no contraindications reported except in G6PD-deficient population; amount in milk small	usually no effect; caution with sulfapyridine and sulfisoxazole in G6PD deficiency	contraindicated in G6PD deficiency; allergic reactions possible but rare; increased susceptability to kernicterus very unlikely except with Rh or ABO incompatability[273,276,322]
terbutaline	no anticipated effects					no known harmful effects	no information available	insufficient information available
tetracyclines	temporarily discontinue breast-feeding	CONTRA-INDICATED		probably not absorbed by infant; caution against use	use alternative therapy if possible	harmless to infant	no effect	adverse effects unlikely[355]
theophylline	no adverse effects			no need to avoid in most patients	present in milk	no known harmful effects	usually compatible with breast-feeding	no adverse effects anticipated; minimize exposure by

Table continued on following page

Table 11–13. DRUGS AND BREAST-FEEDING: HISTORICAL REVIEW OF RECOMMENDATIONS AND EFFECTS ON INFANT REPORTED IN CLINICAL STUDIES (Continued)

Drug	Knowles[324,325]	O'Brien[348]	Vorherr[382]	Anderson[276]	White and White[385]	Wilson[390]	Committee on Drugs[301]	Recommendations[b]
Theophylline (continued)								nursing prior to dose;[288] monitor drug blood levels in infant if signs of drug toxicity appear[293]
thiazides		CONTRA-INDICATED (mfr.'s recommendations)		decreased milk production; idiosyncratic reaction possible; no reports of adverse effects	no known harmful effects		avoid use in first month of lactation	no anticipated adverse effects; minimize exposure by nursing prior to dose[393]
thioridazine (Mellaril)		no anticipated effects					usually compatible with breast-feeding	insufficient information available
thyroxine		no anticipated effects		not detected in milk	no known harmful effects			no anticipated adverse effects if maternal thyroid condition well-controlled
tobramycin	see gentamicin							
tolbutamide	present in milk	no anticipated effects		present in milk (9–40% of serum level)	no known harmful effects		jaundice	insufficient information available[343]
trifluoperazine (Stelazine)		no anticipated effects						insufficient information available
trimeprazine (Temaril)	see antihistamines							
trimethoprim				newborns absorb about 0.75–1 mg/day	insignificant amounts in milk		no effect	use with caution (Bactrim: allergic reactions; avoid)

Drug							
tripelennamine (Pyrabenzamine)	see antihistamines						
valproic acid				appears to be safe		no effects	limited experience; low conc. in breast milk but possible side-effects not excluded;[304] use with caution; monitor drug blood levels in infant if signs of drug toxicity develop
warfarin (Coumadin)	CONTRA-INDICATED	monitor PT in infant and mother	potential: bleeding	no known harmful effects; monitor PT with surgery or high doses	not present in milk or infant serum	no effect	no anticipated adverse effects; monitor infant PT if surgery anticipated or high-dose therapy required[302,330,338]

[a] The information given in the review article cited is generally not the result of individual investigations conducted by the author(s); therefore, the recommendations often are a review of the original report(s) rather than new available information.

[b] These recommendations are presented as a general overview of available information; the key reference(s) cited is the report by author(s) conducting clinical study.

day.[315] Questions regarding the extent of exposure of the infant to the drug can be easily answered by measurement of the amount of drug in the infant's serum. Concern regarding enzyme induction by the drug appears unrealistic; infants are exposed to a host of environmental substances known to alter similarly enzyme activity.

Carbamazepine has been reported to be present in breast milk in concentrations equal to 60% of maternal serum concentration.[357] The calculated intake by a nursing infant has been estimated to be 0.7 mg per day. Concern has been raised over the possibility of drug accumulation in nursing infants; however, no discernible adverse effects have been observed in infants nursed by mothers receiving carbamazepine. Ratios of milk to maternal plasma concentration (m/p) have been reported for *valproic acid* (0.1), *primidone* (0.8 ± 0.2), and *ethosuximide* (0.8 ± 0.3), but little other information is available.[304,318]

Antihistamines

An absence of reports of adverse effects despite their widespread use supports the conclusion that antihistamines are safe for breast-feeding infants. Their presence in milk has been documented in one study, but no significant adverse effects were noted.[348,426]

Antihypertensives

There is not a great deal of information available on the effects on breast-fed infants of antihypertensive agents administered to lactating mothers. Use of *reserpine* has traditionally been contraindicated in nursing mothers because of reports that it causes lethargy, diarrhea, and nasal stuffiness in infants subsequent to intrauterine exposure. Although reserpine is known to be present in breast milk, no adverse effects in neonates have been reported as a consequence of this means of exposure. *Hydralazine* and *propranolol* are also found in breast milk, but the quantities are insufficient to produce drug levels anticipated to produce pharmacologic effects in the nursing infant.[283,334,477] Less than 0.002% of the dose of *captopril* administered to the mother is ingested by the breast-feeding infant;[303] no untoward effects have been found in the nursing infant. Little information is available on other antihypertensives (Table 11–13).

Antimicrobials

The concern regarding breast-feeding by mothers receiving antibiotics relates primarily to the possibility of sensitization of the neonate (penicillins and related drugs) and the reports of ototoxicity, renal toxicity, and hematologic complications noted with the use of certain antimicrobials in adults or children (aminoglycosides, chloramphenicol). A strong family history of drug sensitization should weigh significantly in the decision about the advisability of breast-feeding by mothers receiving penicillins and related drugs. The risk of developing resistant strains of bacteria as a result of small amounts of antibiotic in human milk is a serious issue in need of resolution. In addition, the traditional concern regarding the aggravation of kernicterus by the sulfa drugs has been extended to the breast-fed infant (see Chaps. 1 and 4). There is no direct evidence that the use of sulfa drugs by nursing mothers will result in an increased potential for kernicterus in the breast-fed infant. Concern regarding the tetracyclines has likewise arisen because of the reports of toxicity with the use of this drug in pregnancy and in infants and young children.

Whether the mother receiving *chloramphenicol* should breast-feed her baby is a particularly difficult question. Concentrations equivalent to as much as 50% of maternal serum chloramphenicol levels have been reported in breast milk.[312] Up to 50% of the drug present in milk may be an inactive metabolite without antimicrobial activity, however. Maximum concentrations reached in the milk average 6.1 μg/ml by chemical assay and 3.6 μg/ml by microbiologic assay.[312] There is no information on plasma levels of chloramphenicol in nursing infants. Because of the quantities of drug in breast milk and the potential for accumulation of chloramphenicol levels sufficient to produce dose-dependent or dose-independent toxicity, most authors consider chloramphenicol contraindicated in breast-feeding mothers (Table 11–13). As an alternative, chloramphenicol levels can be easily monitored in both infant and mother, although this will not preclude the development of idiosyncratic reactions.

Metronidazole has long been considered contraindicated in lactating mothers who are breast-feeding. In an early study in 10 women given a dose one tenth of that commonly employed (200 mg),[311] milk and maternal serum drug concentrations were found to be equivalent; the serum levels in the nursing infants ranged from 0 (five infants) to 0.4 μg/ml. No obvious effects of the drug were noted in the infants. Studies by Erickson and coworkers[306] showed a similar relationship between milk and serum concentrations in lactating females given a single 2-gm therapeutic dose of metronidazole. These authors calculated that the average infant would consume approximately 22 mg of drug via the breast milk within the first 24 hours after dosing. Discontinuation of breast feeding for 12 hours following drug administration to the mother would reduce the estimated intake by half (10 mg). The authors indicate that the use of a single 2-gm dose of metronidazole, previously shown to be as effective as 250 mg given 3 times daily for 7 days, would allow continuation of breast-feeding with only a 12-hour period of interruption rather than 1 week. No serious complications have been reported in infants receiving metronidazole at therapeutic doses (see Chap. 4).

The potential harm from *sulfonamide* antimicrobial agents appears to have been overestimated. The quantities in breast milk are sufficiently low that significant disruption of bilirubin binding with aggravation of kernicterus does not seem a realistic possibility. Kauffman and colleagues[322] found less than 1% of the maternal dose of sulfisoxazole in breast milk, which would not be expected to effect adversely an otherwise healthy infant. Measurement of sulfasalazine levels (Azulfidine), used in the treatment of inflammatory bowel disease, has revealed that infants will absorb approximately 2 mg per day, an amount that is very unlikely to be harmful, with the exception of sulfa allergy.[284]

The recommendation that breast-feeding be discontinued with *tetracycline* therapy appears unwarranted. The lack of gastrointestinal absorption of tetracyclines in conjuction with breast-feeding ought to render these agents essentially harmless with a usual 2-week course of therapy. In fact, no significant tetracycline activity has been identified in the serum of infants nursed by mothers taking the drug.[355]

Isoniazid (INH) is found in breast milk at concentrations equal to or greater than maternal plasma levels.[284] In addition, its metabolite, acetylisoniazide, which is thought to mediate the hepatitis-like toxicity of INH, is found in breast milk. Because of the high concentrations in breast milk, including the toxic metabolite, isoniazid should not be employed during the period of breast-feeding unless the infant is also receiving INH.

See Table 11–13 for recommendations for other antimicrobial agents.

Antineoplastics

Drugs used in the treatment of neoplastic disease (alkylating agents, antimetabolites, antibiotics, vinca alkaloids) have generally been considered contraindicated in women breast-feeding their infants. The rationale for the recommendation relates primarily to their potent pharmacologic effects on DNA or RNA metabolism, protein synthesis, and selected cellular functions. However, there are no definitive data to support or discourage breast-feeding.[282] *Cyclophosphamide* and *methotrexate* have been detected in milk obtained from mothers receiving these agents.[317,388] Exposure of the nursing infant to these potent agents can be minimized by breast-feeding during times when maternal drug blood levels are minimal.

Psychotherapeutic Agents

The use of major tranquilizers (phenothiazine, haloperidol), antidepressants (tricyclics), and lithium must be viewed from a different perspective than that for the sedative-hypnotics, as they are generally employed on a continuous basis for treatment of serious mental disorders. Therfore, major therapeutic benefits for the mother can be jeopardized if the drug is discontinued solely to permit the mother to breast-feed her infant. If the medication is aiding in a more substantial relationship between mother and infant, then the benefits of continuing the drug may outweigh any potential adverse effects of the drug on the nursing infant.

Chlorpromazine has been reported to have no effects or to cause mild CNS depression in an occasional nursing infant.[291,389] The level of chlorpromazine in the breast milk consumed by one asymptomatic infant was 7 ng/ml but was 92 ng/ml in milk consumed by a second symptomatic infant. Follow-up studies of infants who were breast-fed by mothers on chlorpromazine therapy reveal them to be normally developed and healthy 16 months to 5 years later.[327] *Haloperidol* has been identified in breast milk in low levels.[373,384] No adverse effects were observed in the breast-feeding infants. Considerable confusion exists regarding data on the concentration of *tricyclic antidepressants* in human milk.[275] It would appear that the concentration of antidepressants present in breast milk is less than or equal to maternal serum concentrations (Table 11–11).[295] Although the dose received by the infant via breast-feeding is likely to be "subtherapeutic," opinions about the advisability of breast-feeding vary.[278,306,369]

Concentrations of *lithium* in the serum of nursing infants have been found to be one half to one third of maternal serum levels.[364,374] In general, breast-feeding has been listed as contraindicated in the literature (Table 11–13), probably because of the reports of side-effects in newborns exposed to lithium in utero, as well as the presence of lithium in breast milk and in the serum of nursing infants.[276,378] Sykes and co-workers[374] advised continuation of breast-feeding in their patient because the therapeutic benefits to the mother in their judgment outweighed the risks to the infant. No adverse effects were noted, including studies of thyroid function and bone chemistry. Obviously, more information is needed to establish the risks of maternal lithium therapy to the nursing infant.

Diuretics

Although diuretics have been reported to decrease milk production,[276] no adverse effects in nursing infants have been reported. The *thiazide* diuretics have been quantitated in breast milk, but the levels appear clinically insignificant.[310] Werthmann and Krees[383] examined breast milk samples from 11 mothers who took a single 500-mg chlorothiazide tablet. The milk samples collected contained insignificant quantities of chlorothiazide. Miller and colleagues[342] found between 50 and 125 ng/ml of hydrochlorothiazide in breast milk of a mother receiving 50-mg doses. No detectable levels of drug were found in her breast-fed infant. The milk to maternal serum concentration ratios for the principal metabolite of *spironolactone* have been reported to range between 0.7 and 0.5.[465] Although the estimated intake for the nursing infant is less than 0.2% of the maternal dose, electrolyte balance in the nursing infant should be monitored periodically.

Narcotic and Nonnarcotic Analgesics

Aspirin is known to be present in breast milk in proportion to the mother's plasma level, which in turn is dependent upon the dose and frequency of administration. In one study, an aspirin dose of 650 mg resulted in measurable breast milk levels, which would theoretically deliver between 9% and 21% of the actual maternal dose to the breast-fed infant. Studies of chronic administration of aspirin to lactating mothers have shown breast milk salicylate levels to range between 0.2 and 1.0 mg/dl.[280] The estimated dose of aspirin to the nursing

infant based on these results was calculated to be 1 mg/kg. The occasional use of aspirin has not been associated with adverse effects in nursing infants. However, since salicylates have the potential to alter platelet function, side-effects could conceivably occur with high-dose chronic aspirin therapy such as for rheumatoid arthritis. Studies of this potential side-effect have not been reported in nursing infants. *Acetaminophen* is excreted into breast milk in concentrations approximately equal to maternal plasma concentrations.[285] Exposure to these nonnarcotic analgesics can be minimized by withholding drug administration until the feeding has been accomplished.

At least one non-salicylate anti-inflammatory drug has been found in breast milk of treated mothers: *Naproxen* levels in breast milk range from 70 to 125 μg/dl; at these levels, the drug is unlikely to cause significant effects in the breast-fed infant exposed either acutely or intermittently.[316] No measurable amounts of *ibuprofen* have been found in breast milk.[377]

Information on opiates is surprisingly meager. Observations in narcotic-addicted mothers breast-feeding their infants have prompted the conclusion that opiates are present in breast milk in low quantities.[313] Single doses of *codeine, meperidine,* and *morphine* all appear to be excreted in quantities insufficient to produce symptoms in the nursing infant. Findlay and coworkers[309] have found concentrations of codeine and morphine in breast milk, following PO administration of codeine, that exceeded maternal plasma drug levels by as much as twofold. The maximum codeine concentration in breast milk was 455 ng/ml versus a peak maternal plasma level of 179 ng/ml. The total dose of codeine recovered in breast milk over a 12-hour period after dosing was estimated to be less than 3% of the maternal dose. Further studies of these agents in the lactating mother are needed. In the interim, it would seem prudent to delay administration of these narcotic analgesics if feasible until breast-feeding has been accomplished or to collect breast milk during periods of low or no opiate in mother's blood and milk for subsequent feeding.

Oral Contraceptives

There is considerable controversy regarding the use of oral contraceptives in lactating women. Studies of the effect of oral contraceptives on the quantity and quality of breast milk have presented conflicting information.[298,326,335] Much of the difficulty in interpretation of the published data resides in the employment of the older, higher-dose preparations and the lack of suitable control groups. Close inspection of these studies reveals that oral contraceptives have clinically insignificant effects on the composition and quantity of breast milk in adequately nourished lactating mothers.[301] The issue regarding long-term effects on the breast-feeding infant of the estrogens and progestins present in oral contraceptives that appear in breast milk remains unresolved. L'E Orme and colleagues[331] have reviewed the literature on the measurements of estrogens and progestins in breast milk. The reported findings indicate that generally less than 0.1% of the dose of estrogen or progestin appears in the breast milk. There is very little information on the resulting blood levels in the breast-feeding infants. An infant consuming 600 ml of breast milk per 24 hours from a mother receiving low-dose oral contraceptives, 50 μg of ethinyl estradiol, will ingest approximately 0.01 μg of ethinyl estradiol; this is equivalent to the amount of natural estradiol a breast-feeding infant would receive from the mother not taking an oral contraceptive.

The progestin component of oral contraceptives has also been found in breast milk.[346,363] An infant consuming 600 ml of breast milk will receive an estimated 0.01 μg per 24 hours for each 10 μg of d-norgestrel contained in the oral contraceptive tablet.

There are no reports of overt adverse manifestations in breast-feeding infants with the currently employed oral contraceptive preparations. If alternative contraception is not possible, the mother who wishes to continue breast-feeding should be encouraged to do so but informed of the lack of sufficient information that would allow absolute assurance of the long-term safety in breast-feeding her infant. The lowest effective dose of oral contraceptive should be employed, and the nutritional adequacy of the mother's diet should be established.

Radiopharmaceuticals

The use of radiopharmaceuticals for diagnostic and therapeutic purposes has become an increasingly important aspect of medical care. The nursing mother should not be denied the use of these medical tools, nor the opportunity to breast-feed her infant indefinitely. Considering the ease of measurement of radiopharmaceuticals in milk, definitive judgments should be possible for establishing the period of interruption in breast-feeding necessary to safeguard against significant contamination in the nursing infant.

Gallium (^{67}Ga) has been found in breast milk for a 2-week period following administration of a 3-mCi (millicurie) dose.[376] With a 2-week delay before resumption of breast-feeding, the estimated dose to the nursing infant would be about 0.04 rad to the whole body and 0.07 rad to the skeleton. The half-life for radioactive decay of ^{67}Ga is 76 hours.

The presence of radiolabeled *iodide* (^{125}I, ^{131}I) in breast milk has been well documented. Radioactive iodine given to a nursing mother in therapeutic doses can reach sufficient concentrations in the breast milk to result in injury to the nursing infant's thyroid gland.[292,365] Radioactivity was observed in breast milk for over 12 days following the administration of ^{125}I to the lactating mother.[350] The half-life for radioactive decay of ^{125}I is 60 days.

The estimated dose of radiation to the adult thyroid from a ^{131}I thyroid scan is approximately 100 rads, compared with 2.8 rads for a ^{125}I scan. Administration of a dose of ^{125}I should prompt discontinuation of breast-feeding for a period no less than 24 hours. Bland and co-workers[292] recommend delaying breast-feeding for a 10-day period; Palmer[350] recommends a delay of 4 weeks before resuming breast-feeding after ^{125}I administration. Before resumption of breast-feeding the milk should be analyzed for ^{125}I content, and a drop of Lugol's solution should be given to the infant to prevent residual ^{125}I from being taken up by the thyroid. The major excretion of ^{131}I in breast milk occurs within 1 to 7 hours, with an exponential decay equivalent to a $T\frac{1}{2}$ of about 24 hours.[320,392] Approximately 3% of the dose of ^{131}I administered to the mother can be found in breast milk within a 48-hour period.[341] The half-life for radioactive decay of ^{131}I is 8 days. Wyburn[392] selected the level for resumption of breast-feeding with ^{131}I to be one tenth of the level accepted for continuous occupational exposure — that is, 2×10^{-6} μCi/ml. Based on observations in nursing mothers given ^{131}I, this level would be reached in 10 to 12 days after dosing. Therefore, the recommendation that breast-feeding be interrupted for a 2-week period following the administration of ^{131}I appears reasonable.

Technetium (^{99m}Tc) content of breast milk has been examined in lactating mothers.[354,380,392] Extrapolation from the data presented in several reports indicates that the majority of radioactivity is absent from breast milk by 48 hours. These and other reports suggest that unbound technetium reaches greater concentrations in breast milk and has a longer period of excretion than that seen with albumin-bound technetium. Interruption of breast feeding for a 2- to 3-day period should be more than adequate, particularly since the radioactive half-life for ^{99m}Tc is 66 hours.[354,380,392]

Sedative-Hypnotics

The vast majority of the sedative-hypnotic agents are employed for more minor anxiety disorders or sleep disturbances. Drugs in this category include chlordiazepoxide, diazepam, lorazepam, meprobamate, barbiturates, and chloral hydrate. Drug accumulation in the infant, particularly with *diazepam* and its metabolite desmethyldiazepam, is a possibility with chronic intake or if excessive doses are used by the breast-feeding mother.[299,351] *Lorazepam* has been found in small amounts in breast milk; the estimated dose received by the infants ranges between 3 and 30 μg/kg per day.[386] A bedtime hypnotic dose of *chloral hydrate* has been associated with drowsiness in a nursing infant.[329] Chloral hydrate and its metabolites can be identified in breast milk for up to 24 hours after dosing.[289] Shorter-acting barbiturates *(secobarbital, pentobarbital)* are present in lower concentrations in breast milk than that of the longer-acting barbiturates such as *phenobarbital.*

Although these drugs appear to pose a low risk to the nursing infant, exposure should be minimized by avoiding their administration for as long as possible (4–24 hr, depending on the pharmacokinetics of the drug) prior to breast-feeding. Monitoring the ability of the mother to function adequately as a care provider is another reason for this interlude period. When questions arise regarding signs of drug intoxication in the nursing infant, drug blood level determinations will aid in establishing the cause-and-effect relationship.

Substances of Abuse

There can be no rational encouragement for the mother who is abusing drugs to breast-feed her infant. Although there is no overt evidence of direct harm to the infant as a result of contamination of the milk by stimulants, sedative-hypnotics, marijuana, LSD, phencyclidine, and so on, the clear choice is to avoid breast-feeding

or to avoid the drugs. Tetrahydrocannabinol (THC), believed to be the active component of *marijuana,* is concentrated and secreted in human milk and is absorbed by the nursing infant.[352] The effects of THC on infants are unknown.

One large study involving more than 100 lactating mothers receiving *amphetamine* failed to detect any behavioral stimulation or alteration in the nursing infants.[277] In a single case report, *caffeine* was reported to achieve levels in breast milk sufficient to produce jitteriness.[280] However, the vast experience with the use of caffeine for apnea in neonates has demonstrated its apparent safety. Moderate consumption of caffeine-containing beverages should not predispose the nursing infant to adverse effects (see later section, Environmental Toxins in Breast Milk).

Examination of the *ethanol* content in milk from mothers given known doses of ethanol (0.6 g ethanol/kg body weight) revealed concentrations of alcohol in the milk similar to those in the mother's plasma.[323] There was some delay in the distribution of alcohol from plasma into breast milk. The major metabolite of ethanol, acetaldehyde, was not found in milk. Information relative to alcohol concentrations in the blood of breast-fed infants is unfortunately lacking. Calculations based on the experimental data on milk alcohol content, however, support the impression of many investigators that only with intoxicating levels of blood alcohol in the mother will the infant be likely to ingest amounts of alcohol sufficient to cause mild sedation.[390] Chronic excessive intake of alcohol, however, may result in other harmful effects. Binkiewicz and colleagues[290] described the development of a pseudo–Cushing's syndrome in a 4-month-old female breast-fed by a mother who chronically consumed large amounts of alcohol (alcohol milk content, 100 mg/dl). The infant gained excessively in weight and appeared markedly obese, with a moon-shaped facial appearance, but virilization was not noted. The signs disappeared rapidly after the mother discontinued ethanol intake. The most reasonable conclusion from available information is that occasional, moderate ingestion of ethanol by the mother is not harmful to the nursing infant. However, intoxicated mothers should not breast-feed, not only for reasons of the physical safety of the infant but because of the anticipated high alcohol content in the milk. Chronic alcoholic mothers should be made aware of the significant risk regarding breast-feeding of their infant.

Thyroid Drugs

Examination of milk samples obtained from two mothers on thiouracil therapy revealed drug levels in milk three times those of maternal blood taken at the same time;[480] these findings formed the basis for the long-held recommendation that antithyroid drugs are contraindicated in breast-feeding. Two recent studies have now clearly documented that the quantity of *propylthiouracil* (PTU) excreted in breast milk is clinically insignificant.[319,336] Less than 0.08% to 0.03% of the administered PTU dose was excreted in breast milk in 24 hours. Thyroid function parameters (serum T_4, T_3, and TSH and T_3-resin-uptake test) were unchanged in one infant monitored over a 5-month period.

Studies with *methimazole* indicate that 7% to 16% of the dose may reach the infant through the breast milk.[375] These studies suggest that methimazole may not be appropriate for use in the breast-feeding mother, and that PTU is the preferred agent. Further studies are needed to verify these observations.

Iodine- or *iodide-containing* products have long been considered contraindicated in breast-feeding mothers because of the possibility of effects on the nursing infant's thyroid function. Postellon and Aronow[356] observed a significant increase in breast milk iodine levels following the use of a povidone-iodine vaginal gel by the mother. The nursing infant's serum and urine iodine levels were grossly elevated, but T_4 and TSH levels were normal. Thus, there appears to be little actual documentation in the literature for the recommendation against breast-feeding.

Other Drugs

Bronchodilator therapy is not uncommon in mothers nursing their infants. Studies of *theophylline* therapy in lactating mothers indicate that about 1% of the maternal dose is excreted in the breast milk. The milk-to-plasma ratio is in the range of 0.6 to 0.7.[370,393] The best time to nurse the infant to minimize drug exposure is the period just prior to the next oral dose.[288] However, the newer sustained-release preparations, which minimize fluctuations in maternal serum levels, will largely eliminate this opportunity. Information on the use of beta-agonists, such as *terbutaline,* in lactating mothers is not available.

The use of *corticosteroids* in lactating mothers who wish to breast-feed is difficult to resolve. Although there are no reports of adverse manifestations in breast-fed infants nursed by mothers receiving corticosteroids over brief periods of time, there is no information on the long-term effects that would be associated with chronic steroid therapy. It is clear that very small amounts of *prednisone* or *prednisolone* are found in breast milk.[287,321,339] Less than 8% of the normal daily adrenal output of the infant has been estimated to be delivered in the milk of a mother taking 120 mg of prednisone in a single morning dose. By delaying nursing for 2 hours after maternal dosing, this amount is cut in half, and after 4 hours virtually no steroid is detectable in the milk.

Several studies have examined *digoxin* concentration in maternal plasma and breast milk.[297,332,358] The concentrations in breast milk ranged from 60% to 75% of maternal plasma. Finley and coworkers[310] identified small nontherapeutic amounts of digoxin in infants breast-fed by mothers receiving digoxin, 0.75 mg daily for 7 days. Various investigators conclude that digoxin does not reach therapeutic plasma concentrations in the nursing infant. According to these studies and the clinical experience with direct administration of digoxin to infants, no significant adverse effects should be expected in infants with digoxin exposure via breast-feeding.

Environmental Toxins in Breast Milk

There have been a number of environmental agents identified in human milk, several of which have been associated with significant symptomatology in nursing infants.[301,360] Serious intoxications have been reported subsequent to consumption of seed grain treated with fungicidal agent *hexachlorobenzene.*[353] Breast-fed infants developed pink-colored sores of the skin and an associated progressive loss of weight; death occurred within 1 year. Cessation of breast-feeding was associated with less rapid deterioration. Examination of the breast milk revealed the presence of hexachlorobenzene. Despite the serious and sometimes lethal effects observed with food contaminated with *methyl mercury,* breast-feeding has not been associated with toxic manifestations, even though blood mercury levels have been largely found to increase in the nursing infants.[274] Table 11–14 is a list of environmental agents found in human breast milk. The relevance of most of these substances to the welfare of the nursing infant remains to be established.

Nicotine levels between 20 to 500 ppb have been found in milk of women who smoke be-

Table 11–14. EFFECTS OF NON-THERAPEUTIC AGENTS IN HUMAN MILK ON BREAST-FED INFANT

Agent	Reported Effect or Recommendation
Food Substances	
aspartame	caution in PKU[372]
caffeine	none[379]
chocolate (theobromine)	none[286,359]
fava beans	hemolysis in infant with G6PD deficiency[305]
fluorides	none[366,473]
monosodium glutamate	none[371,379]
Environmental Chemicals	
herbicides and insecticides	
chlorinated hydrocarbons (DDT and metabolites), Aldrin, Chlordane, Dieldrin, Mirex, Lindane, Parathion, Paroxon, PCBs and PBBs	none[281,328,347,349,361,387,443]
hexachlorobenzene	skin rash, diarrhea, vomiting, neurotoxicity, death[301,353]
lead	no toxicity due to contaminated breast milk[362]
mercurial compounds (methyl mercury)	neurotoxicity[274]
nicotine (source: smoking)	no clear evidence of clinical effects[308]
tetrachlorethylene	cholestatic jaundice (?)[279]

tween 10 and 30 cigarettes per day.[308] No evidence of clinical effects of nicotine was found in the nursing infants. *Caffeine* may achieve levels in breast milk of about half to equal to that of the maternal serum level.[280,309,379,406] Because caffeine clearance in the neonate may be several-fold less than that in the adult, chronic exposure of the nursing infant could conceivably result in cumulative levels of caffeine in the blood.[288,406] Studies have not been done to substantiate this concern. Fortunately, experience in infants receiving caffeine therapy for apnea suggests that caffeine is reasonably safe. However, the long-term effects of chronic exposure are unknown.

References
Drugs, Chemicals, and Pregnancy

1. Amin-Zaki L, Elhassani S, Majeed MA, et al: Intrauterine methylmercury poisoning in Iraq. Pediatrics 54:587, 1974.
2. Anand S, Van Thiel DH: Prenatal and neonatal exposure to cimetidine results in gonadal and sexual dysfunction in adult males. Science 218:493, 1982.
3. Aranda JV, Collinge JM, Clarkson S: Epidemiologic aspects of drug utilization in a newborn intensive care unit. Semin Perinatol 6:148, 1982.
4. Aranda JV, Portuguez-Malavasi A, Collinge JM, et al: Epidemiology of adverse drug reactions in the newborn. Dev Pharmacol Ther 5:173, 1982.
5. Arnon RG, Marin-Garcia J, Peeden JN: Tricuspid valve regurgitation and lithium carbonate toxicity in a newborn infant. Am J Dis Child 135:941, 1981.
6. Arwood LL, Dasta JF, Friedman C: Placental transfer of theophylline: Two case reports. Pediatrics 63:844, 1979.
7. Barber HRK: Fetal and neonatal effects of cytotoxic agents. Obstet Gynecol 58:41S, 1981.
8. Belfrage P, Boreus LO, Hartvig P, et al: Neonatal depression after obstetrical analgesia with pethidine. The role of the injection-delivery time interval and of the plasma concentrations of pethidine and norpethidine. Acta Obstet Gynecol Scand 60:43, 1981.
9. Bergman AB, Wiesner LA: Relationship of passive cigarette-smoking to sudden infant death syndrome. Pediatrics 58:665, 1976.
10. Bishop EH: Acceleration of fetal pulmonary maturity. Obstet Gynecol 58:48S, 1981.
11. Bjerkedal T, Czeizel A, Goujard J, et al: Valproic acid and spina bifida. Lancet 2:1096, 1982.
12. Blackhall MI, Buckley GA, Roberts DV, et al: Drug-induced neonatal myasthenia. J Obstet Gynaecol Brit Cwlth 76:157, 1969.
13. Bleyer WA: Surveillance of pediatric adverse drug reactions: A neglected health care program. Pediatrics 55:308, 1975.
14. Bleyer WA, Skinner AL: Fatal neonatal hemorrhage after maternal anticonvulsant therapy. JAMA 235:626, 1976.
15. Blumenthal I, Lindsay S: Neonatal barbiturate withdrawal. Postgrad Med J 53:157, 1977.
16. Bolton PF: Drugs of abuse. In Hawkins DF (ed): Drugs and Pregnancy. Chap 11, p 128 Churchill Livingstone, New York, 1983.
17. Bongiovanni AM, McPadden AJ: Steroids during pregnancy and possible fetal consequences. Fertil Steril 11:181, 1960.
18. Bonta BW, Gagliardi JV, Williams V, Warshaw JB: Naloxone reversal of mild neurobehavioral depression in normal newborn infants after routine obstetric analgesia. J Pediatr 94:102, 1979.
19. Brazy JE, Pupkin MJ: Effects of maternal isoxsuprine administration on preterm infants. J Pediatr 94:444, 1979.
20. Brice JEH, Moreland TA, Walker CHM: Effects of pethidine and its antagonists on the newborn. Arch Dis Child 54:356, 1979.
21. Briggs GG, Bodendorfer TW, Freeman RK, Yaffe SJ (eds): Drugs in Pregnancy and Lactation. Baltimore, Williams & Wilkins, 1983.

22. Brocklebank JC, Ray WA, Federspiel CF, Schaffner W: Drug prescribing during pregnancy: A controlled study of Tennessee Medicaid recipients. Am J Obstet Gynecol 132:235, 1978.

23. Caldwell J, Wakile LA, Notarianni LJ, et al: Maternal and neonatal disposition of pethidine in childbirth — a study using quantitative gas chromatography – mass spectrometry. Life Sci 22:589, 1978.

24. Carswell F, Kerr MM, Hutchison JH: Congenital goitre and hypothyroidism produced by maternal ingestion of iodides. Lancet 1:1241, 1970.

25. Chahal P, Sidhu R, Joplin GF, Hawkins DF: Treatment of thyrotoxicosis in pregnancy. J Obstet Gynaecol 2:11, 1981.

26. Chalmers I, Campbell H, Turnbull AC: Use of oxytocin and incidence of neonatal jaundice. Br Med J 2:116, 1975.

27. Chase D, Brady JP, Chir B: Ventricular tachycardia in a neonate with mepivacaine toxicity. J Pediatr 90:127, 1977.

28. Chernick V: Endorphins and ventilatory control. N Engl J Med 304:1227, 1981.

29. Chernick V, Craig RJ: Nalosone reverses neonatal depression caused by fetal asphyxia. Science 216:1252, 1982.

30. Clark RB, Beard AG, Barclay DL: Naloxone in the newborn infant. Anesth Rev 2:9, 1975.

31. Clyman RI, Ballard PL, Sniderman S, et al: Prenatal administration of betamethasone for prevention of patent ductus arteriosus. J Pediatr 98:123, 1981.

32. Cohen MM, Hirschhorn K, Verbo S, et al: The effect of LSD-25 on the chromosomes of children exposed in utero. Pediatr Res 2:486, 1968.

33. Cohlan SQ, Bevelander G, Bross S: Effect of tetracycline on bone growth in the premature infant. Antimicrob Agents Chemother, p. 668, 1965.

34. Collins E: Maternal and fetal effects of acetaminophen and salicylates in pregnancy. Obstet Gynecol 58:57S, 1981.

35. Committee on Drugs: Anticonvulsants and pregnancy. Pediatrics 63:331, 1979.

36. Committee on Drugs: Naloxone use in newborns. Pediatrics 65:667, 1980.

37. Cruikshank DP, Pitkin RM, Reynolds WA, et al: Effects of magnesium sulfate treatment of perinatal calcium metabolism. Am J Obstet Gynecol 134:243, 1979.

38. Csaba IF, Sulyok E, Ertl T: Relationship of maternal treatment with indomethacin to persistence of fetal circulation syndrome. J Pediatr 92:484, 1978.

39. Dalens B, Raynaud E, Gaulme J: Teratogenicity of valproic acid. J Pediatr 97:332, 1980.

40. Dangman BC, Rosen TS: Magnesium levels in infants of mothers treated with MgSO$_4$. Pediatr Res 11:415, 1977.

41. Davies DP, Gomersall R, Robertson R, et al: Neonatal jaundice and maternal oxytocin infusion. Br Med J 3:476, 1973.

42. Dodson WE, Hillman RE, Hillman LS: Brain tissue levels in a fatal case of neonatal mepivacaine (Carbocaine) poisoning. J Pediatr 86:624, 1975.

43. Dodson WE: Neonatal drug intoxication: Local anesthetics. Pediatr Clin North Am 23:399, 1976.

44. Doering PL, Stewart RB: The extent and character of drug consumption during pregnancy. JAMA 239:843, 1978.

45. Donovan EF, Tsang RC, Steichen JJ, et al: Neonatal hypermagnesemia: Effect of parathyroid hormone and calcium homeostasis. J Pediatr 96:305, 1980.

46. Epstein MF, Nicholls E, Stubblefield PG: Neonatal hypoglycemia after beta-sympathomimetic tocolytic therapy. J Pediatr 94:449, 1979.

47. Evans JM, Hogg MIJ, Lunn JN, Rosen M: Degree and duration of reversal by naloxone of effects of morphine in conscious subjects. Br Med J 2:589, 1974.

48. Evans JM, Hogg MIJ, Rosen M: Reversal of narcotic depression in the neonate by naloxone. Br Med J 2:1098, 1976.

49. Feldman GL, Weaver DD, Lovrien EW: The fetal trimethadione syndrome. Am J Dis Child 131:1389, 1977.

50. Ferencz C, Matanoski GM, Wilson PD, et al: Maternal hormone therapy and congenital heart disease. Teratology 21:225, 1980.

51. Filtenborg JA: Persistent pulmonary hypertension after lithium intoxication in the newborn. Eur J Pediatr 138:321, 1982.

52. Fischer CG, Cook DR: The respiratory and narcotic antagonistic effects of naloxone in infants. Anesth Analg (Cleve) 53:849, 1974.

53. Fishburne JI: Systemic analgesia during labor. Clin Perinatol 9:29, 1982.

54. Fishman J, Roffwarg H, Hellman L: Disposition of naloxone-7, 8-^{3}H in normal and narcotic-dependent men. J Pharmacol Exp Ther 187:575, 1973.

55. Fried PA: Marijuana use by pregnant women — neurobehavioral effects in neonates. Drug Alcohol Depend 6:415, 1980.

56. Genot MT, Golan HP, Porter PJ, Kass EH: Effect of administration of tetracycline in pregnancy on the primary dentition of the offspring. J Oral Med 25:75, 1970.

57. Gerhardt T, Bancalari E, Cohen H, Rocha LF: Use of naloxone to reverse narcotic respiratory depression in the newborn infant. J Pediatr 90:1009, 1977.

58. Golden NL, Sokol RJ, Rubin IL: Angel dust: Possible effects on the fetus. Pediatrics 65:18, 1980.

59. Goodlin RC: Naloxone administration and newborn rabbit response to asphyxia. Am J Obstet Gynecol 140:340, 1981.

60. Green KW, Key TC, Coen R, Resnik R: The effects of maternally administered magnesium sulfate on the neonate. Am J Obstet Gynecol 146:29, 1983.

61. Greenberger P, Patterson R: Safety of therapy for allergic symptoms during pregnancy. Ann Intern Med 89:234, 1978.

62. Greenland S, Staisch KJ, Brown N, Gross SJ: The effects of marijuana use during pregnancy. I. A preliminary epidemiologic study. Am J Obstet Gynecol 143:408, 1982.

63. Hall JG, Pauli RM, Wilson KM: Maternal and fetal sequelae of anticoagulation during pregnancy. Am J Med 68:122, 1980.

64. Handal KA, Schauben JL, Salamone FR: Naloxone. Ann Emerg Med 12:438, 1983.

65. Hanson JW, Smith DW: The fetal hydantoin syndrome. J Pediatr 87:285, 1975.

66. Hanson JW, Streissguth AP, Smith DW: The effects of moderate alcohol consumption during pregnancy on fetal growth and morphogenesis. J Pediatr 92:457, 1978.

67. Hanson JW: Teratogenic agents. In Emergy AEH, Rimoin DL (eds): Principles and Practice of Medical Genetics. Chap 12. London, Longman Group Ltd, 1983.

68. Harker LC, Kirkpatrick SE, Friedman WF, Bloor CM: Effects of indomethacin on fetal rat lungs: A

possible cause of persistent fetal circulation (PFC). Pediatr Res 15:147, 1981.

69. Hartz SC, Heinonen OP, Shapiro S, et al: Antenatal exposure to meprobamate and chlordiazepoxide in relation to malformations, mental development, and childhood mortality. N Engl J Med 292:726, 1975.

70. Hawkins DF: Drug treatment of medical disorders in pregnancy. In Hawkins DF (ed): Drugs and Pregnancy. Chap 7, p 76. New York, Churchill Livingstone, 1983.

71. Hawkins DF (ed): Drugs and Pregnancy. New York, Churchill Livingstone, 1983.

72. Hazinski TA, Grunstein MM, Schlueter MA, Tooley WH: Effect of naloxone on ventilation in newborn rabbits. J Appl Physiol 50:713, 1981.

73. Heinonen OP, Slone D, Shapiro S: Birth Defects and Drugs in Pregnancy. Littleton, MA, Publishing Sciences Group, 1977.

74. Henderson BE, Benton B, Cosgrove M, et al: Urogenital tract abnormalities in sons of women treated with diethylstilbestrol. Pediatrics 58:505, 1976.

75. Herbst AL, Ulfelder H, Poskanzer DC: Adenocarcinoma of the vagina: Association of maternal stilbestrol therapy with tumor appearance in young women. N Engl J Med 284:878, 1971.

76. Herbst AL: Diethylstilbestrol and other sex hormones during pregnancy. Obstet Gynecol 58:35S, 1981.

77. Howard FM, Hill JM: Drugs in pregnancy. Obstet Gynecol Surv 34:643, 1979.

78. Huhtaniemi I, Koivisto M, Pakarinen A, et al: Pituitary–adrenal and testicular function in preterm infants after prenatal dexamethasone treatment. Acta Paediatr Scand 71:425, 1982.

79. Jager-Roman E, Doyle PE, Thomas D, et al: Increased theophylline metabolism in premature infants after prenatal betamethasone administration. Dev Pharmacol Ther 5:127, 1982.

80. Jones RT, Weinerman BH: MOPP (nitrogen mustard, vincristine, procarbazine, and pregnidone) given during pregnancy. Obstet Gynecol 54:477, 1979.

81. Kalter H, Warkany J: Congenital malformations: Etiologic factors and their role in prevention. N Engl J Med 308:424, 1983.

82. Kalter H, Warkany J: Congenital malformations. N Engl J Med 308:491, 1983.

83. Kim WY, Pomerance JJ, Miller AA: Lidocaine intoxication in a newborn following local anesthesia for episiotomy. Pediatrics 64:643, 1979.

84. Kline AH, Blattner RJ, Lunin M: Transplacental effect of tetracyclines on teeth. JAMA 188:178, 1964.

85. Koos BJ, Longo LD: Mercury toxicity in the pregnant woman, fetus, and newborn infant. Am J Obstet Gynecol 126:390, 1976.

86. Kuhnert BR, Kuhnert PM, Prochaska AL, Sokol RJ: Meperidine disposition in mother, neonate, and nonpregnant females. Clin Pharmacol Ther 27:486, 1980.

87. LaGamma EF, Itskovitz J, Rudolph AM: Effects of naloxone on fetal circulatory responses to hypoxemia. Am J Obstet Gynecol 143:933, 1982.

88. l'Allemand D, Gruters A, Heidemann P, Schurnbrand P: Iodine-induced alterations of thyroid function in newborn infants after prenatal and perinatal exposure to povidone-iodine. J Pediatr 102:935, 1983.

89. Lamont RF: Drugs in pregnancy and neonatal jaundice. In Hawkins DF (ed): Drugs and Pregnancy. Chap 13, p 184. New York, Churchill Livingstone, 1983.

90. Layde PM, Edmonds LD, Erickson JD: Maternal fever and neural tube defects. Teratology 21:105, 1980.

91. Ledward RS: Antimicrobial drugs in pregnancy. In Hawkins DF (ed): Drugs and Pregnancy. Chap 9, p. 102. New York, Churchill Livingstone, 1983.

92. Levin DL, Fixler DE, Morriss FC, Tyson J: Morphologic analysis of the pulmonary vascular bed in infants exposed in utero to prostaglandin synthetase inhibitors. J Pediatr 92:478, 1978.

93. Levin DL, Mills LJ, Weinberg AG: Hemodynamic, pulmonary vascular, and myocardial abnormalities secondary to pharmacologic constriction of the fetal ductus arteriosus: A possible mechanism for persistent pulmonary hypertension and transient tricuspid insufficiency in the newborn infant. Circulation 60:360, 1979.

94. Lewis PJ, Bulpitt CJ, Zuspan FP: A comparison of current British and American practice in the management of hypertension in pregnancy. J Obstet Gynaecol 1:78, 1980.

95. Linn S, Schoenbaum SC, Monson RR, Rosner B, Stubblefield PG, Ryan KJ: No association between coffee consumption and adverse outcomes of pregnancy. N Engl J Med 306:141, 1982.

96. Lipsitz PJ, English IC: Hypermagnesemia in the newborn infant. Pediatrics 40:856, 1967.

97. Lipsitz PJ: The clinical and biochemical effects of excess magnesium in the newborn. Pediatrics 47:501, 1971.

98. Long SY: Does LSD induce chromosomal damage and malformations? A review of the literature. Teratology 6:75, 1972.

99. Longo LD: The biological effects of carbon monoxide on the pregnant woman, fetus, and newborn infant. Am J Obstet Gynecol 129:69, 1977.

100. Longo LD: Environmental pollution and pregnancy: Risks and uncertainties for the fetus and infant. Am J Obstet Gynecol 137:162, 1980.

101. Lovejoy FH: Fatal benzyl alcohol poisoning in neonatal intensive care units. Am J Dis Child 136:974, 1982.

102. Mauer AM, DeVaux W, Lahey ME: Neonatal and maternal thrombocytopenic purpura due to quinine. Pediatrics 19:84, 1956.

103. McCarroll AM, Hutchinson M, McAuley R, Montgomery DAD: Long-term assessment of children exposed in utero to carbimazole. Arch Dis Child 51:532, 1976.

104. Mendez-Bauer C, Poseiro JJ, Arellano-Hernandez G, et al: Effects of atropine on the heart rate of the human fetus during labor. Am J Obstet Gynecol 85:1033, 1963.

105. Merkow AJ, McGuinness GA, Erenberg A, Kennedy RL: The neonatal neurobehavioral effects of bupivacaine, mepivacaine, and 2-chloroprocaine used for pudendal block. Anesthesiology 52:309, 1980.

106. Miller HC, Hassanein K, Hensleigh PA: Fetal growth retardation in relation to maternal smoking and weight gain in pregnancy. Am J Obstet Gynecol 125:55, 1976.

107. Miller P, Smith DW, Shepard TH: Maternal hyperthermia as a possible cause of anencephaly. Lancet 1:519, 1978.

108. Miller RW: The susceptibility of the fetus and child to chemical pollutants. Part II (Supplement). Pediatrics 53:792, 1974.

109. Milner RDG, Chouksey SK: Effects of fetal exposure to diazoxide in man. Arch Dis Child 47:537, 1972.

110. Mizrahi EM, Hobbs JF, Goldsmith DI: Nephrogenic diabetes insipidus in transplacental lithium intoxication. J Pediatr 94:493, 1979.

111. Morrell P, Sutherland GR, Buamah PK, Bain HH: Lithium toxicity in a neonate. Arch Dis Child 58:539, 1983.

112. Morris MB, Weinstein L: Caffeine and the fetus: Is trouble brewing? Am J Obstet Gynecol 140:607, 1981.

113. Morrison JC, Whybrew WD, Rosser SI, et al: Metabolites of meperidine in the fetal and maternal serum. Am J Obstet Gynecol 126:997, 1976.

114. Morselli PL, Rovei V: Placental transfer of pethidine and norpethidine and their pharmacokinetics in the newborn. Eur J Clin Pharmacol 18:25, 1980.

115. Morselli PL, Franco-Morselli R, Bossi L: Clinical pharmacokinetics in newborns and infants: Age-related differences and therapeutic implications. Clin Pharmacokinet 5:485, 1980.

116. Naeye RL: Maternal use of dextroamphetamine and growth of the fetus. Pharmacology 26:117, 1983.

117. Ngai SH, Berkowitz BA, Yang JC, Hempstead J, Spector S: Pharmacokinetics of naloxone in rats and in man: Basis for its potency and short duration of action. Anesthesiology 44:398, 1976.

118. Oakley GP Jr: Drug influences on malformations. Clin Perinatol 6:403, 1979.

119. Olver RE: Beta-adrenergic agonists, labour and adaptation of the lungs at birth. Dev Pharmacol Ther 4 (Suppl 1):144, 1982.

120. Ostrea EM Jr, Chavez CJ: Perinatal problems (excluding neonatal withdrawal) in maternal drug addiction: A study of 830 cases. J Pediatr 94:292, 1979.

121. Palmer PG: Sedatives in Pregnancy. In Hawkins DF (ed): Drugs and Pregnancy. Chap 8, p 93. New York, Churchill Livingstone, 1983.

122. Pruyn, SC, Phelan JP, Buchanan GC: Long-term propranolol therapy in pregnancy: Maternal and fetal outcome. Am J Obstet Gynecol 135:485, 1979.

123. Ralston DH, Shnider SM: The fetal and neonatal effects of regional anesthesia in obstetrics. Anesthesiology 48:34, 1978.

124. Ramsay LE, Freestone S, Silas JH: Drug-related acute medical admissions. Hum Toxicol 1:379, 1982.

125. Rane A, Tomson G, Bjarke B: Effects of maternal lithium therapy in a newborn infant. J Pediatr 93:296, 1978.

126. Rane A, Tomson G: Prenatal and neonatal drug metabolism in man. Eur J Clin Pharmacol 18:9, 1980.

127. Rantakallio P: Relationship of maternal smoking to morbidity and mortality of the child up to the age of five. Acta Paediatr Scand 67:621, 1978.

128. Rasch DK, Huber PA, Richardson CJ, et al: Neurobehavioral effects of neonatal hypermagnesemia. J Pediatr 100:272, 1982.

129. Ravid R, Toaff R: On the possible teratogenicity of antibiotic drugs administered during pregnancy—a prospective study. Adv Exp Med Biol 27:505, 1972.

130. Robboy SJ, Noller KL, Kaufman RH, et al: Prenatal diethylstilbestrol (DES) exposure. Clin Pediatr 22:139, 1983.

131. Robert E: Valproic acid in pregnancy: Association with spina bifida: A preliminary report. Clin Pediatr 22:336, 1982.

132. Rodriguez SU, Leikin SL, Hiller MC: Neonatal thrombocytopenia associated with ante-partum administration of thiazide drugs. N Engl J Med 270:881, 1964.

133. Rosa FW: Teratogenicity of isotretinoin. Lancet 2:513, 1983.

134. Rosefsky JB, Petersiel MF: Perinatal deaths associated with mepivacaine paracervical-block anesthesia in labor. N Engl J Med 278:530, 1968.

135. Rosenberg L, Mitchell AA, Shapiro S, Slone D: Selected birth defects in relation to caffeine-containing beverages. JAMA 247:1429, 1982.

136. Rubin P: Beta-blockers in pregnancy. N Engl J Med 305:1323, 1981.

137. Rudolph AM: The effects of nonsteroidal antiinflammatory compounds on fetal circulation and pulmonary function. Obstet Gynecol 58:63S, 1981.

138. Rumack CM, Guggenhein MA, Rumack BH, et al: Neonatal intracranial hemorrhage and maternal use of aspirin. Obstet Gynecol 58:52S, 1981.

139. Safra MJ, Oakley GP Jr: Association between cleft lip with or without cleft palate and prenatal exposure to diazepam. Lancet 2:478, 1975.

140. Schardein JL: Drugs as Teratogens. Cleveland, OH, CRC Press, 1977.

141. Schardein JL: Congenital abnormalities and hormones during pregnancy: A clinical review. Teratology 22:251, 1980.

142. Schou M, Goldfield MD, Weinstein MR, Villeneuve A: Lithium and pregnancy—I, report from the register of lithium babies. Br Med J 2:135, 1973.

143. Schou M, Amdisen A, Sttenstrup OR: Lithium and pregnancy—II, hazards to women given lithium during pregnancy and delivery. Br Med J 2:137, 1973.

144. Shapiro S, Hartz SC, Siskind V, et al: Anticonvulsants and parental epilepsy in the development of birth defects. Lancet 1:272, 1976.

145. Shapiro S, Monson RR, Kaufman DW, et al: Perinatal mortality and birth-weight in relation to aspirin taken during pregnancy. Lancet 1:1375, 1976.

146. Shaul WL, Hall JG: Multiple congenital anomalies associated with oral anticoagulants. Am J Obstet Gynecol 127:191, 1977.

147. Shaw EB: Fetal damage due to maternal aminopterin ingestion: Follow-up at age 9 years. Am J Dis Child 124:93, 1972.

148. Shepard TH: Catalog of Teratogenic Agents, 3rd ed. Baltimore, Johns Hopkins University Press, 1980.

149. Sidhu RF: Corticosteroids in pregnancy. In Hawkins DF (ed): Drugs and Pregnancy. Chap 10, p 116. New York, Churchill Livingstone, 1983.

150. Sinclair JC, Fox HA, Lentz JF, et al: Intoxication of the fetus by a local anesthetic: A newly recognized complication of maternal caudal anesthesia. N Engl J Med 273:1173, 1965.

151. Singer I, Rotenberg D: Mechanisms of lithium action. N Engl J Med 289:254, 1973.

152. Sitar DS, Abu-Bakare A, Gardiner RJ: Propylthiouracil disposition in pregnant and post-partum women. Pharmacology 25:57, 1982.

153. Slone D, Heinonen OP, Kaufman DW, et al: Aspirin and congenital malformations. Lancet 1:1373, 1976.

154. Smith DW: Teratogenicity of anticonvulsive medications. Am J Dis Child 131:1337, 1977.

155. Smith DW: Alcohol effects on the fetus. In Schwarz RH, Yaffe SJ (eds): Drug and Chemical Risks to the Fetus and Newborn. P 73. New York, Alan R Liss Inc, 1980.

156. Snyder RD: Congenital mercury poisoning. N Engl J Med 284:1014, 1971.

157. Solomon L, Abrams G, Dinner M, Berman L: Neonatal abnormalities associated with D-penicillamine treatment during pregnancy. N Engl J Med 296:54, 1977.

158. Soyka LF: Caffeine ingestion during pregnancy: In utero exposure and possible effects. Semin Perinatol 5:305, 1981.

159. Speidel BD, Meadow SR: Epilepsy, anticonvulsants and congenital malformations. Drugs 8:354, 1974.

160. Stern L: In vivo assessment of the teratogenic potential of drugs in humans. Obstet Gynecol 58:35, 1981.

161. Stevenson RE, Burton OM, Ferlanto GJ, Taylor HA: Hazards of oral anticoagulants during pregnancy. JAMA 243:1549, 1980.

162. Stuart MJ, Gross SJ, Elrad H, Graeber JE: Effects of acetylsalicylic-acid ingestion on maternal and neonatal hemostasis. N Engl J Med 307:909, 1982.

163. Sutherland JM, Keller WH: Novobiocin and neonatal hyperbilirubinemia. Am J Dis Child 101:447, 1961.

164. Sweet DL, Kinzie J: Consequences of radiotherapy and antineoplastic therapy for the fetus. J Reprod Med 17:241, 1976.

165. Taeusch HW Jr: Glucocorticoid prophylaxis for respiratory distress syndrome: A review of potential toxicity. J Pediatr 87:617, 1975.

166. Taeusch HW Jr, Frigoletto F, Kitzmiller J, et al: Risk of respiratory distress syndrome after prenatal dexamethasone treatment. Pediatrics 63:64, 1979.

167. Truog WE, Feusner JH, Baker DL: Association of hemorrhagic disease and the syndrome of persistent fetal circulation with the fetal hydantoin syndrome. J Pediatr 96:112, 1980.

168. Uchida IA, Holunga R, Lawler C: Maternal radiation and chromosomal aberrations. Lancet 2:1045, 1968.

169. Vessey MP, Nunn JF: Occupational hazards of anaesthesia. Br Med J 281:696, 1980.

170. Wallman IS, Hilton HB: Teeth pigmented by tetracycline. Lancet 1:827, 1962.

171. Wiener PC, Hogg MIJ, Rosen M: Effects of naloxone on pethidine-induced neonatal depression. Part I: Intravenous naloxone. Br Med J 2:228, 1977.

172. Wilkinson AR, Aynsley-Green A, Mitchell MD: Persistent pulmonary hypertension and abnormal prostaglandin E levels in preterm infants after maternal treatment with naproxen. Arch Dis Child 54:942, 1979.

173. Wilson N, Forfar JC, Godman MJ: Atrial flutter in the newborn resulting from maternal lithium ingestion. Arch Dis Child 58:538, 1983.

174. Witter F, King TM: Cigarettes and pregnancy. In Schwarz RH, Yaffe SJ (eds): Drug and Chemical Risks to the Fetus and Newborn. P 83. New York, Alan R Liss Inc, 1980.

175. Witter FR, King TM, Blake DA: Adverse effects of cardiovascular drug therapy on the fetus and neonate. Obstet Gynecol 58:100S, 1981.

176. Woody JN, London WL, Wilbanks GD Jr: Lithium toxicity in a newborn. Pediatrics 47:94, 1971.

177. Wright RG, Shnider SM, Levinson G, Rolbin SH, Parer JT: The effect of maternal administration of ephedrine on fetal heart rate and variability. Obstet Gynecol 57:734, 1981.

178. Yaffe SJ: Clinical implications of perinatal pharmacology. Eur J Clin Pharmacol 18:3, 1980.

Neonatal Drug Withdrawal

179. Athinarayanan P, Pierog SH, Nigam SK, Glass L: Chlordiazepoxide withdrawal in the neonate. Am J Obstet Gynecol 124:212, 1976.

180. Blinick G, Wallach RC, Jerez E, Ackerman BD: Drug addiction in pregnancy and the neonate. Am J Obstet Gynecol 125:135, 1976.

181. Blumenthal I, Lindsay S: Neonatal barbiturate withdrawal. Postgrad Med J 53:157, 1977.

182. Burnstein Y, Giardina PJV, Rausen AR, et al: Thrombocytosis and increased circulating platelet aggregates in newborn infants of polydrug users. J Pediatr 94:895, 1979.

183. Chasnoff IJ, Hatcher R, Burns WJ, Schnoll SH: Pentazocine and tripelennamine ('T's and Blues's'): Effects on the fetus and the neonate. Dev Pharmacol Ther 6:162, 1983.

184. Desmond MM, Schwanecke RP, Wilson GS, et al: Maternal barbiturate utilization and neonatal withdrawal symptomatology. J Pediatr 80:190, 1972.

185. Fricker HS, Segal S: Narcotic addiction, pregnancy, and the newborn. Am J Dis Child 132:360, 1978.

186. Glass L, Rajedowda BK, Evans HE: Absence of respiratory distress syndrome in premature infants of heroin-addicted mothers. Lancet 2:685, 1971.

187. Goetz RL, Bain RV: Neonatal withdrawal symptoms associated with maternal use of pentazocine. J Pediatr 86:887, 1974.

188. Gold MS, Redmond DE Jr, Kleber HD: Clonidine blocks acute opiate-withdrawal symptoms. Lancet 2:599, 1978.

189. Herzlinger RA, Kandall SR, Vaughn HG Jr: Neonatal seizures associated with narcotic withdrawal. J Pediatr 91:638, 1977.

190. Hoder EL, Leckman JF, Ehrenkranz R, et al: Clonidine in neonatal narcotic-abstinence syndrome. N Engl J Med 305:1284, 1981.

191. Johnson HL, Rosen TS: Prenatal methadone exposure: Effects on behavior in early infancy. Pediatr Pharmacol 2:113, 1982.

192. Kahn EJ, Neumann LL, Polk GA: The course of the heroin withdrawal syndrome in newborn infants treated with phenobarbital or chlorpromazine. J Pediatr 75:495, 1969.

193. Kandall SR, Gartner LM: Late presentation of drug withdrawal symptoms in newborns. Amer J Dis Child 127:58, 1974.

194. Kandall SR, Doberczak TM, Mauer KR, et al: Opiate versus CNS depressant therapy in neonatal drug abstinence syndrome. Am J Dis Child 137:378, 1983.

195. Kron RE, Litt M, Phoenix MD, Finnegan LP: Neonatal narcotic abstinence: Effects of pharmacotherapeutic agents and maternal drug usage on nutritive sucking behavior. J Pediatr 88:637, 1976.

196. Nathenson G, Golden GS, Litt IF: Diazepam in the management of the neonatal narcotic withdrawal syndrome. Pediatr 48:523, 1971.

197. Neumann LL, Cohen SN: The neonatal narcotic withdrawal syndrome: A therapeutic challenge. Clin Perinatol 2:99, 1975.

198. Ostrea EM Jr, Chavez CJ, Strauss ME: A study of

factors that influence the severity of neonatal narcotic withdrawal. Addict Dis 2:187, 1975.

199. Ostrea EM Jr, Chavez CJ: Perinatal problems (excluding neonatal withdrawal) in maternal drug addiction: A study of 830 cases. J Pediatr 94:292, 1979.

200. Parkin DE: Probable Benadryl withdrawal manifestations in a newborn infant. J Pediatr 85, 580, 1974.

201. Pippinger CE, Rosen TS: Phenobarbital plasma levels in neonates. Clin Perinatol 2:111, 1975.

202. Preis O, Choi SJ, Rudolph N: Pentazocine withdrawal syndrome in the newborn infant. Am J Obstet Gynecol 127:205, 1977.

203. Prenner BM: Neonatal withdrawal syndrome associated with hydroxyzine hydrochloride. Am J Dis Child 131:529, 1977.

204. Rajegowda BK, Glass L, Evans HE, et al: Methadone withdrawal in newborn infants. J Pediatr 81:532, 1972.

205. Rementeria JL, Bhatt K: Withdrawal symptoms in neonates with intrauterine exposure to diazepam. J Pediatr 90:123, 1977.

206. Rothstein P, Gould JB: Born with a habit: Infants of drug-addicted mothers. Pediatr Clin North Am 21:307, 1974.

207. Rumack BH, Walravens PA: Neonatal withdrawal following maternal ingestion of ethchlorvynol (Placidyl). Pediatrics 52:714, 1973.

208. Taeusch HW Jr, Carson SH, Wang NS, Avery ME: Heroin induction of lung maturation and growth retardation in fetal rabbits. J Pediatr 82:869, 1973.

209. Tyson HK: Neonatal withdrawal symptoms associated with maternal use of propoxyphene hydrochloride (Darvon). J Pediatr 85:684, 1974.

210. Washton AM, Resnick RB: Clonidine in opiate withdrawal: Review and appraisal of clinical findings. Pharmacotherapy 1:140, 1981.

211. Webster PAC: Withdrawal symptoms in neonates associated with maternal antidepressant therapy. Lancet 2:318, 1973.

212. Wilson GS, Desmond MM, Verniaud WM: Early development of infants of heroin-addicted mothers. Am J Dis Child 126:457, 1973.

213. Wilson GS, McCreary R, Kean J, Baxter JC: The development of preschool children of heroin-addicted mothers: A controlled study. Pediatrics 63:135, 1979.

214. Zelson C: Infant of the addicted mother. N Engl J Med 288:1393, 1973.

215. Zelson C: Acute management of neonatal addiction. Addict Dis 2:159, 1975.

Clinical Toxicology in the Neonate

216. Amin-Zaki L, Elhassani S, Majeed MA, et al: Studies of infants postnatally exposed to methylmercury. J Pediatr 85:81, 1974.

217. Angle CR, McIntire MS: Lead, mercury, and cadmium toxicity in children. Paediatrician 6:204, 1977.

218. Armstrong RW, Eichner ER, Klein DE, et al: Pentachlorophenol poisoning in a nursery for newborn infants. II. Epidemiologic and toxicologic studies. J Pediatr 75:317, 1969.

219. Blattner RJ: Acrodynia. J Pediatr 64:607, 1964.

220. Book LS, Herbst JJ, Atherton SO, Jung AL: Necrotizing enterocolitis in low-birth-weight infants fed an elemental formula. J Pediatr 87:602, 1975.

221. Brouillette F, Weber ML: Massive aspiration of tal-

cum powder by an infant. Can Med Assoc J 119:354, 1978.

222. Brown WJ, Buist NRM, Gipson HTC, et al: Fatal benzyl alcohol poisoning in a neonatal intensive care unit. Lancet 1:1250, 1982.

223. Chabrolle JP, Rossier A: Goitre and hypothyroidism in the newborn after cutaneous absorption of iodine. Arch Dis Child 53:495, 1978.

224. Chilcote RR, Williams B, Wolff LJ, Baehner RL: Sudden death in an infant from methemoglobinemia after administration of "sweet spirits of nitre." Pediatrics 59:280, 1977.

225. Chisolm JJ Jr: Poisoning from heavy metals (mercury, lead, and cadmium). Pediatr Ann 9:458, 1980.

226. Committee on Fetus and Newborn and Committee on Drugs: Benzyl alcohol: Toxic agent in neonatal units. Pediatrics 72:356, 1983.

227. Committee on Nutrition: Infant methemoglobinemia: The role of dietary nitrate. Pediatrics 46:475, 1970.

228. Cooke RWI, Meradji M, De Villeneuve VH: Necrotising enterocolitis after cardiac catheterisation in infants. Arch Dis Child 55:66, 1980.

229. Cornblath M, Hartmann AF: Methemoglobinemia in young infants. J Pediatr 33:421, 1948.

230. Cunningham AA: Resorcin poisoning. Arch Dis Child 31:173, 1956.

231. Devlieger H, Snoeys R, Wyndaele L, et al: Liver necrosis in the newborn infant: Analysis of some precipitating factors in neonatal care. Eur J Pediatr 138:113, 1982.

232. Doan HM, Keith L, Schennan AT: Phenol and neonatal jaundice. Pediatrics 64:324, 1979.

233. Ernst JA, Williams JM, Glick MR, Lemons JA: Osmolality of substances used in the intensive care nursery. Pediatrics 72:347, 1983.

234. Etteldorf JN: Methylene blue in the treatment of methemoglobinemia in premature infants caused by marking ink. J Pediatr 38:24, 1951.

235. Gershanik J, Boecler B, Ensley H, et al: The gasping syndrome and benzyl alcohol poisoning. N Engl J Med 307:1384, 1982.

236. Glasgow AM, Boeckx RL, Miller MK, et al: Hyperosmolality in small infants due to propylene glycol. Pediatrics 72:353, 1983.

237. Gluck L: A perspective on hexachlorophene. Pediatrics 51:400, 1973.

238. Goldbloom RB, Goldbloom A: Boric acid poisoning: Report of four cases and a review of 109 cases from the world literature. J Pediatr 43:631, 1953.

239. Goluboff N, MacFadyen DJ: Methemoglobinemia in an infant associated with application of a tar-benzocaine ointment. J Pediatr 47:222, 1955.

240. Gordon AS, Prichard JS, Freedman MH: Seizure disorders and anemia associated with chronic borax intoxication. Can Med Assoc J 17:719, 1973.

241. Harpin V, Rutter N: Percutaneous alcohol absorption and skin necrosis in a preterm infant. Arch Dis Child 57:477, 1982.

242. Herskowitz J, Rosman NP: Acute hexachlorophene poisoning by mouth in a neonate. J Pediatr 94:495, 1979.

243. James LS: Hexachlorophene. Pediatrics 49:492, 1972.

244. Johnson RR, Navone R, Larson EL: An unusual epidemic of methemoglobinemia. Pediatrics 31:222, 1963.

245. Kahn A, Blum D: Methyl alcohol poisoning in an

8-month-old boy: An unusual route of intoxication. J Pediatr 94:841, 1979.

246. Kimura ET, Darby TD, Krause RA, Brondyk HD: Parenteral toxicity studies with benzyl alcohol. Toxicol Appl Pharmacol 18:60, 1971.

247. Knotek Z, Schmidt P: Pathogenesis, incidence, and possibilities of preventing alimentary nitrate methemoglobinemia in infants. Pediatrics 34:78, 1964.

248. Kurland LT, Faro SN, Siedler H: Minamata disease. World Neurol 1:370, 1960.

249. l'Allemand D, Gruters A, Heidemann P, Schurnbrand P: Iodine-induced alterations of thyroid function in newborn infants after prenatal and perinatal exposure to povidone iodine. J Pediatr 102:935, 1983.

250. Larson DL: Studies show hexachlorophene causes burn syndrome. Hospitals 42:63, 1968.

251. Leff RD, Roberts RJ: Effects of intravenous fluid and drug solution coadministration of final-infusate osmolality, specific gravity, and pH. Am J Hosp Pharm 39:468, 1982.

252. Lockhart JD: How toxic is hexachlorophene? Pediatrics 50:229, 1972.

253. Lovejoy FH: Fatal benzyl alcohol poisoning in neonatal intensive care units. Am J Dis Child 136:974, 1982.

254. McLaughlin JF, Telzrow RW, Scott CM: Neonatal mercury vapor exposure in an infant incubator. Pediatr 66:988, 1980.

255. Mofenson HC, Greensher J, DiTomasso A, Okun S: Baby powder—a hazard! Pediatrics 68:265, 1981.

256. Moss MH: Alcohol-induced hypoglycemia and coma caused by alcohol sponging. Pediatrics 46:445, 1970.

257. Motomatsu K, Adachi H, Uno T: Two infant deaths after inhaling baby powder. Chest 75:448, 1979.

258. Moutinho ME, Tompkins AL, Rowland TW, et al: Acute mercury vapor poisoning: Fatality in an infant. Am J Dis Child 135:42, 1981.

259. Mullick FG: Hexachlorophene toxicity—human experience at the Armed Forces Institute of Pathology. Pediatrics 51:395, 1973.

260. Papile L, Burstein J, Burstein R, et al: Relationship of intravenous sodium bicarbonate infusions and cerebral intraventricular hemorrhage. J Pediatr 93:834, 1978.

261. Peden VH, Sammon TJ, Downey DA: Intravenously induced infantile intoxication with ethanol. J Pediatr 83:490, 1973.

262. Robson AM, Kissane JM, Elvick NH, Pundavela L: Pentachlorophenicol poisoning in a nursery for newborn infants. I. Clinical features and treatment. J Pediatr 75:309, 1969.

263. Rubenstein AD, Musher DM: Epidemic boric acid poisoning simulating staphylococcal toxic epidermal necrosis of the newborn infant: Ritter's disease. J Pediatr 77:884, 1970.

264. Shuman RM, Leech RW, Alvord EC Jr: Neurotoxicity of hexachlorophene in humans. II. A clinicopathological study of 46 premature infants. Arch Neurol 32:320, 1975.

265. Simmons MA, Adcock EW, Bard H, Battaglia FC: Hypernatremia and intracranial hemorrhage in neonates. N Engl J Med 291:6, 1974.

266. Waffarn F, Hodgman JE: Mercury vapor contamination of infant incubators: A potential hazard. Pediatrics 64:640, 1979.

267. Walton G: Survey of literature relating to infant methemoglobinemia due to nitrate-contaminated water. Am J Public Health 41:986, 1951.

268. Warkany J, Hubbard DM: Acrodynia and mercury. J Pediatr 42:365, 1953.

269. Wenzl JE, Mills SD, McCall JT: Methanol poisoning in an infant: Successful treatment with peritoneal dialysis. Am J Dis Child 116:445, 1968.

270. Wilkinson AR, Baum JD, Keeling JW: Superficial skin necrosis in babies prepared for umbilical arterial catheterisation. Arch Dis Child 56:237, 1981.

271. Wolff JA: Methemoglobinemia due to benzocaine. Pediatrics 20:915, 1957.

272. Zepp EA, Thomas JA, Knotts GR: The toxic effects of mercury. Clin Pediatr 13:783, 1974.

Breast Feeding and Drugs

273. Abramowicz M: Update: Drugs in breast milk. Med Lett 21:21, 1979.

274. Amin-Zaki L, Elhassani S, Majeed MA, et al: Studies of infants postnatally exposed to methylmercury. J Pediatr 85:81, 1974.

275. Ananth J: Side effects in the neonate from psychotropic agents excreted through breast-feeding. Am J Psychiatry 135:801, 1978.

276. Anderson PO: Drugs and breast feeding—a review. Drug Intell Clin Pharm 11:208, 1977.

277. Ayd FJ (ed): Excretion of psychotropic drugs in human breast milk. Int Drug Ther Newslett 8:33, 1973.

278. Bader TF, Newman K: Amitriptyline in human breast milk and the nursing infant's serum. Am J Psychiatry 137:855, 1980.

279. Bagnell PC, Ellenberger HA: Obstructive jaundice due to a chlorinated hydrocarbon in breast milk. Can Med Assoc J 117:1047, 1977.

280. Bailey, DN, Weibert RT, Naylor AJ, Shaw RF: A study of salicylate and caffeine excretion in the breast milk of two nursing mothers. J Anal Toxicol 6:64, 1982.

281. Bakken AF, Seip M: Insecticides in human breast milk. Acta Paediatr Scand 65:535, 1976.

282. Barber HRK: Fetal and neonatal effects of cytotoxic agents. Obstet Gynecol 58:41S, 1981.

283. Bauer JH, Pape B, Zajicek J, Groshong T: Propranolol in human plasma and breast milk. Am J Cardiol 43:860, 1979.

284. Berlin CM: Drugs and chemicals in human milk. In Lawrence RA (ed): Counseling the Mother on Breast-Feeding, Report of the Eleventh Ross Roundtable on Critical Approaches to Common Pediatric Problems. P 59. Columbus, OH, Ross Laboratories, 1980.

285. Berlin CM Jr, Yaffe SJ, Ragni M: Disposition of acetaminophen in milk, saliva, and plasma of lactating women. Pediatr Pharmacol 1:135, 1980.

286. Berlin CM Jr, Pascuzzi BS, Yaffe SJ: Excretion of salicylate in human milk. Clin Pharmacol Ther 27:245, 1980.

287. Berlin CM Jr: Pharmacologic considerations of drug use in the lactating mother. Obstet Gynecol 58:17S, 1981.

288. Berlin CM Jr: Excretion of the methylxanthines in human milk. Semin Perinatol 5:389, 1981.

289. Bernstine JB, Meyer AE, Bernstine RL: Maternal blood and breast milk estimation following the administration of chloral hydrate during the puerperium. J Obstet Gynaecol 63:228, 1956.

290. Binkiewicz A, Robinson, MJ, Senior B: Pseudo-Cushing syndrome caused by alcohol in breast milk. J Pediatr 93:965, 1978.

291. Blacker KH, Weinstein BJ, Ellman GL: Mother's milk and chlorpromazine. Am J Psychiatry 119:178, 1962.

292. Bland EP, Crawford JS, Docker MF, Farr RF: Radioactive iodine uptake by thyroid of breast-fed infants after maternal blood-volume measurements. Lancet 2:1039, 1969.

293. Brambel CE, Hunter RE: Effect of dicumarol on the nursing infant. Am J Obstet Gynecol 59:1157, 1950.

294. Briggs GG, Bodendorfer TW, Freeman RK, Yaffe SJ (eds): Drugs in Pregnancy and Lactation. Baltimore, Williams & Wilkins, 1983.

295. Brixen-Rasmussen L, Halgrener J, Jorgensen A: Amitriptyline and nortriptyline excretion in human breast milk. Psychopharmacology (Berlin) 76:94, 1982.

296. Catz CS, Giacoia GP: Drugs and breast milk. Pediatr Clin North Am 19:151, 1972.

297. Chan V, Tse TF, Wong V: Transfer of digoxin across the placenta and into breast milk. Br J Obstet Gynaecol 85:605, 1978.

298. Chopra JG: Effect of steroid contraceptives on lactation. Am J Clin Nutr 25:1202, 1972.

299. Cole AP, Hailey DM: Diazepam and active metabolite in breast milk and their transfer to the neonate. Arch Dis Child 50:741, 1975.

300. Committee on Drugs: Breast feeding and contraception. Pediatrics 68:138, 1981.

301. Committee on Drugs: The transfer of drugs and other chemicals into human breast milk. Pediatrics 72:357, 1983.

302. De Swiet M, Lewis PJ: Excretion of anticoagulants in human milk. N Engl J Med 297:1471, 1977.

303. Devlin RG, Fleiss PM: Selective resistance to the passage of captopril into human milk. Clin Pharmacol Ther 27:250, 1980.

304. Dickinson RG, Harland RC, Lynn RK, Smith WB, Gerber N: Transmission of valproic acid (Depakene) across the placenta: Half-life of the drug in mother and baby. J Pediatr 94:832, 1979.

305. Emanuel B, Schoenfeld A: Favism in a nursing infant. J Pediatr 58:263, 1961.

306. Erickson SH, Smith GH, Heidrich F: Tricyclics and breast feeding. Am J Psychiatry 136:1483, 1979.

307. Erickson SH, Oppenheim GL, Smith GH: Metronidazole in breast milk. Obstet Gynecol 57:48, 1981.

308. Ferguson BB, Wilson DJ, Schaffner W: Determination of nicotine concentrations in human milk. Am J Dis Child 130:837, 1976.

309. Findlay JWA, DeAngelis RL, Kearney MF, et al: Analgesic drugs in breast milk and plasma. Clin Pharmacol Ther 29:625, 1981.

310. Finley JP, Waxman MB, Wong PY, Lickrish GM: Digoxin excretion in human milk. J Pediatr 94:339, 1979.

311. Gray MS, Kane PO, Squires S: Further observations on metronidazole (Flagyl). Br J Vener Dis 37:278, 1961.

312. Havelka J, Hejzlar M, Popov V, et al: Excretion of chloramphenicol in human milk. Chemotherapy 13:204, 1968.

313. Hervada AR, Feit E, Sagraves R: Drugs in breast milk. Perinat Care 2:19, 1978.

314. Hill LM, Malkasian GD Jr: The use of quinidine sulfate throughout pregnancy. Obstet Gynecol 54:366, 1979.

315. Horning MG, Stillwell WG, Nowlin J, et al: Identification and quantification of drugs and drug metabolites in human breast milk using GC-MS-COM methods. Mod Probl Paediatr 15:73, 1975.

316. Jamali F, Tam YK, Stevens RD: Naproxen excretion in breast milk and its uptake by suckling infant. Drug Intell Clin Pharm 16:475, 1982.

317. Johns DG, Rutherford LD, Leighton PG, Vogel CL: Secretion of methotrexate into human milk. Am J Obstet Gynecol 112:978, 1972.

318. Kaneko S, Sato T, Suzuki K: The levels of anticonvulsants in breast milk. Br J Clin Pharmacol 7:624, 1979.

319. Kampmann JP, Johansen K, Hansen JM, Helweg J: Propylthiouracil in human milk. Lancet 1:736, 1980.

320. Karjalainen P, Penttilä IM, Pystynen P: The amount and form of radioactivity in human milk after lung scanning, renography and placental localization by ^{131}I-labelled tracers. Acta Obstet Gynec Scand 50:357, 1971.

321. Katz RH, Duncan BR: Entry of prednisone into human milk. N Engl J Med 293:1154, 1975.

322. Kauffman RE, O'Brien C, Gilford P: Sulfisoxazole secretion into human milk. J Pediatr 97:839, 1980.

323. Kesaniemi YA: Ethanol and acetaldehyde in the milk and peripheral blood of lactating women after ethanol administration. J Obstet Gynaecol Br Cwlth 81:84, 1974.

324. Knowles JA: Excretion of drugs in milk — a review. J Pediatr 66:1068, 1965.

325. Knowles JA: Effects on the infant of drug therapy in nursing mothers. Drug Ther 3:57, 1973.

326. Koetsawang S, Bhiraleus P, Chiemprajert T: Effect of oral contraceptives on lactation. Fertil Steril 23:24, 1972.

327. Kris EB, Carmichael DM: Chlorpromazine maintenance therapy during pregnancy and confinement. Psychiatr Q 31:690, 1957.

328. Kroger M: Insecticide residues in human milk. J Pediatr 80:401, 1972.

329. Lacey JH: Dichloralphenazone and breast milk. Br Med J 4:684, 1971.

330. L'E Orme M, Lewis PJ, De Swiet M, et al: May mothers given warfarin breast feed their infants? Br Med J 1:1564, 1977.

331. L'E Orme M, Back DJ, Breckenridge AM: Clinical pharmacokinetics of oral contraceptive steroids. Clin Pharmacokinet 8:95, 1983.

332. Levy M, Granit L, Laufer N: Excretion of drugs in human milk. N Engl J Med 297:789, 1977.

333. Lewis PJ, Hurden EL: Drugs and Breast Feeding. In Hawkins DF (ed): Drugs and Pregnancy. Chap 14, p 204. New York, Churchill Livingstone, 1983.

334. Liedholm H, Wahlin-Boll E, Hanson A, et al: Transplacental passage and breast milk concentrations of hydralazine. Eur J Clin Pharmacol 21:417, 1982.

335. Lonnerdal B, Forsum E, Hambraeus L: Effect of oral contraceptives on composition and volume of breast milk. Am J Clin Nutr 33:816, 1980.

336. Low LCK, Lang J, Alexander WD: Excretion of carbimazole and propylthiouracil in breast milk. Lancet 2:1011, 1979.

337. Mann CF: Clindamycin and breast feeding. Pediatrics 66:1030, 1980.

338. McKenna R, Cole ER, Vasan U: Is warfarin sodium contraindicated in the lactating mother? J Pediatr 103:325, 1983.

339. McKenzie SA, Selley JA, Agnew JE: Secretion of prednisolone into breast milk. Arch Dis Child 50:894, 1975.

340. Medina A, Fiske N, Hjelt-Harvey I, et al: Absorption, diffusion, and excretion of a new antibiotic lincomycin. Antimicrob Agent Chemother, P 189, 1963.

341. Miller H, Weetch RS: The excretion of radioactive iodine in human milk. Lancet 269:1013, 1955.

342. Miller ME, Cohn RD, Burghart PH: Hydrochlorothiazide disposition in a mother and her breast fed infant. J Pediatr 101:789, 1982.

343. Moiel RH, Ryan JR: Tolbutamide orinase in human breast milk. Clin Pediatr 6:480, 1967.

344. Nau H, Kuhnz W, Egger HJ, et al: Anticonvulsants during pregnancy and lactation: Transplacental, maternal, and neonatal pharmacokinetics. Clin Pharmacokinet 7:508, 1982.

345. Nicholas JM, Lipshitz J, Schreiber EC: Phencyclidine: Its transfer across the placenta as well as into breast milk. Am J Obstet Gynecol 143:143, 1982.

346. Nilsson S, Nygren KG, Johansson EDB: d-Norgestrel concentrations in maternal plasma, milk, and child plasma during administration of oral contraceptives to nursing women. Am J Obstet Gynecol 129:178, 1977.

347. Noren K: Organochlorine contaminants in Swedish human milk from the Stockholm region. Acta Paediatr Scand 72:259, 1983.

348. O'Brien TE: Excretion of drugs in human milk. Am J Hosp Pharm 31:844, 1974.

349. Olszyna-Marzys AE: Contaminants in human milk. Acta Paediatr Scand 67:571, 1978.

350. Palmer KE: Excretion of ^{125}I in breast milk following administration of labelled fibrinogen. Br J Radiol 52:672, 1979.

351. Patrick MJ, Tilstone WJ, Reavey P: Diazepam and breast feeding. Lancet 1:542, 1972.

352. Perez-Reyes M: Presence of Δ^9-tetrahydrocannabinol in human milk. N Engl J Med 307:819, 1982.

353. Peters HA: Hexachlorobenzene poisoning in Turkey. Fed Proc 35:2400, 1976.

354. Pittard WB III, Merkatz R, Fletcher BD: Radioactive excretion in human milk following administration of technetium Tc 99m macroaggregated albumin. Pediatrics 70:231, 1982.

355. Posner AC, Prigot A, Konicoff NG: Further observations on the use of tetracycline hydrochloride in prophylaxis and treatment of obstetric infections. Antibiotics Annual, P 594. New York, Medical Encyclopedia, 1954–55.

356. Postellon DC, Aronow R: Iodine in mother's milk. JAMA 247:463, 1982.

357. Pynnönen S, Kanto J, Sillanpää M, Erkkola R: Carbamazepine: Placental transport, tissue concentrations in foetus and newborn, and level in milk. Acta Pharmacol Toxicol 41:244, 1977.

358. Reinhardt D, Richter O, Genz T, Potthoff S: Kinetics of the translactal passage of digoxin from breast feeding mothers to their infants. Eur J Pediatr 138:49, 1982.

359. Resman BH, Blumenthal P, Jusko WJ: Breast milk distribution of theobromine from chocolate. J Pediatr 91:477, 1977.

360. Rogan WJ: The sources and routes of childhood chemical exposures. J Pediatr 97:861, 1980.

361. Rogan WJ, Bagniewska A, Damstra T: Pollutants in breast milk. N Engl J Med 302:1450, 1980.

362. Ryu JE, Ziegler EE, Fomon SJ: Maternal lead exposure and blood lead concentration in infancy. J Pediatr 93:476, 1978.

363. Saxena BN, Shrimanker K, Grudzinskas JG: Levels of contraceptive steroids in breast milk and plasma of lactating women. Contraception 16:605, 1977.

364. Schou M, Amdisen A: Lithium and pregnancy—III, lithium ingestion by children breast fed by women on lithium treatment. Br Med J 2:138, 1973.

365. Siegel AJ: Workup of thyroid nodules in nursing mothers. Drug Ther 9:115, 1979.

366. Simpson WJ, Tuba J: An investigation of fluoride concentration in the milk of nursing mothers. J Oral Med 23:104, 1968.

367. Smith JA, Morgan JR, Rachlis AR, Papsin FR: Clindamycin in human breast milk. Can Med Assoc J 112:806, 1975.

368. Somogyi A, Gugler R: Cimetidine excretion into breast milk. Br J Clin Pharmacol 7:627, 1979.

369. Sovner R, Orsulak PJ: Excretion of imipramine and desipramine in human breast milk. Am J Psychiatry 136:451, 1979.

370. Stec GP, Greenberger P, Ruo TI, et al: Kinetics of theophylline transfer to breast milk. Clin Pharmacol Ther 28:404, 1980.

371. Stegink LD, Filer LJ Jr, Baker GL: Monosodium glutamate: Effect on plasma and breast milk amino acid levels in lactating women. Proc Soc Exp Biol Med 140:836, 1972.

372. Stegink LD, Filer LJ Jr, Baker GL: Plasma, erythrocyte and human milk levels of free amino acids in lactating women administered aspartame or lactose. J Nutr 109:2173, 1979.

373. Stewart RB, Karas B, Springer PK: Haloperidol excretion in human milk. Am J Psychiatry 137:849, 1980.

374. Sykes PA, Quarrie J, Alexander FW: Lithium carbonate and breast feeding. Br Med J 2:1299, 1976.

375. Tegler L, Lindstrom B: Antithyroid drugs in milk. Lancet 2:591, 1980.

376. Tobin RE, Schneider PB: Uptake of ^{67}Ga in the lactating breast and its persistence in milk: Case report. J Nucl Med 17:1055, 1976.

377. Townsend RJ, Benedetti T, Erickson S, et al: A study to evaluate the passage of ibuprofen into breast milk. Drug Intell Clin Pharm 16:482, 1982.

378. Tunnessen WW Jr, Hertz CG: Toxic effects of lithium in newborn infants: A commentary. J Pediatr 81:804, 1972.

379. Tyrala EE, Dodson WE: Caffeine secretion into breast milk. Arch Dis Child 54:787, 1979.

380. Vagenakis AG, Abreau CM, Braverman LE: Duration of radioactivity in the milk of a nursing mother following ^{99m}Tc administration. J Nucl Med 12:188, 1971.

381. Varsano I, Fishl J, Shochet SB: The excretion of orally ingested nitrofurantoin in human milk. J Pediatr 82:886, 1973.

382. Vorherr H: Drug excretion in breast milk. Postgrad Med 56:97, 1974.

383. Werthmann MW Jr, Krees SV: Excretion of chlorothiazide in human breast milk. J Pediatr 81:781, 1972.

384. Whalley LJ, Blain PG, Prime JK: Halperidol secreted in breast milk. Br Med J 282:1746, 1981.

385. White GJ, White MK: Breast feeding and drugs in human milk. Vet Hum Toxicol 22:1, 1980.

386. Whitelaw AGL, Cummings AJ, McFadyen IR: Effect of maternal lorazepam on the neonate. Br Med J 282:1106, 1981.

387. Wickizer TM, Brilliant LB, Copeland R, Tilden R: Polychlorinated biphenyl contamination of nursing mothers' milk in Michigan. Am J Public Health 71:132, 1981.

388. Wiernik PH, Duncan JH: Cyclophosphamide in human milk. Lancet 1:912, 1971.

389. Wiles DH, Orr MW, Kolakowska T: Chlorpromazine levels in plasma and milk of nursing mothers. Br J Clin Pharmacol 5:272, 1978.

390. Wilson JT, Brown RD, Cherek DR, et al: Drug excretion in human breast milk: Principles, pharmacokinetics, and projected consequences. Clin Pharmacokinet 5:1, 1980.

391. Wilson JT (ed): Drugs in Breast Milk. Sydney, ADIS Press, 1981.

392. Wyburn JR: Human breast milk excretion of radionuclides following administration of radiopharmaceuticals. J Nucl Med 14:115, 1973.

393. Yurchak AM, Jusko WJ: Theophylline secretion into breast milk. Pediatrics 57:518, 1976.

Additional References

394. Acker D, Sachs BP, Tracey KJ, Wise WE: Abruptio placentae associated with cocaine use. Am J Obstet Gynecol 146:220, 1983.

395. Albengres E, Tillement JP: Phenytoin in pregnancy: A review of the reported risks. Biol Res Preg 4:71, 1983.

396. Allen RW, Ogden B, Bentley FL, Jung AL: Fetal hydantoin syndrome, neuroblastoma, and hemorrhagic disease in a neonate. JAMA 244:1464, 1980.

397. Anday EK, Harris MC: Leukemoid reaction associated with antenatal dexamethasone administration. J Pediatr 101:614, 1982.

398. Anderson ABM, Gennser G, Jeremy JY, et al: Placental transfer and metabolism of betamethasone in human pregnancy. Obstet Gynecol 49:471, 1977.

399. Aranda JV, Stern L: Clinical aspects of developmental pharmacology and toxicology. Pharmacol Ther 20:1, 1983.

400. Bachrach LK, Burrow GN, Gare DJ: Maternal-fetal absorption of povidone-iodine. J Pediatr 104:158, 1984.

401. Ballard PL, Granberg P, Ballard RA: Glucocorticoid levels in maternal and cord serum after prenatal betamethasone therapy to prevent respiratory distress syndrome. J Clin Invest 56:1548, 1975.

402. Benawra R, Mangurten HH, Duffell DR: Cyclopia and other anomalies following maternal ingestion of salicylates. J Pediatr 96:1069, 1980.

403. Bergman B, Hedner T: Antepartum administration of terbutaline and the incidence of hyaline membrane disease in preterm infants. Acta Obstet Gynecol Scand 57:217, 1978.

404. Bergman B, Hedner T, Samsioe G: Terbutaline and pulmonary surfactant release in the rabbit fetus. Gynecol Obstet Invest 13:44, 1982.

405. Bergman B, Freyschuss U, Grossmann G, Hedner T: Effect of terbutaline on lung mechanics and morphology in the preterm rabbit neonate. Clin Physiol 3:111, 1983.

406. Berlin CM Jr, Denson HM, Daniel CH, Ward RM: Disposition of dietary caffeine in milk, saliva, and plasma of lactating women. Pediatrics 73:59, 1984.

407. Bishop CR, Athens JW, Boggs DR, et al: Leukokinetic studies. XIII. A non-steady-state kinetic evaluation of the mechanism of cortisone-induced granulocytosis. J Clin Invest 47:249, 1968.

408. Bleyer WA, Marshall RE: Barbiturate withdrawal syndrome in a passively addicted infant. JAMA 221:185, 1972.

409. Boog G, Brahim MB, Gandar R: Beta-mimetic drugs and possible prevention of respiratory distress syndrome. Br J Obstet Gynaecol 82:285, 1975.

410. Brown WU Jr, Bell GC, Alper MH: Acidosis, local anesthetics and the newborn. Obstet Gynecol 48:27, 1976.

411. Butler NR, Goldstein H: Smoking in pregnancy and subsequent child development. Br Med J 4:573, 1973.

412. Carin I, Glass L, Parean H et al: Neonatal methadone withdrawal. Effect of two treatment regimes. Am J Dis Child 137:1166, 1983.

413. Chasnoff IJ, Burns WJ, Hatcher RP, Burns KA: Phencyclidine: Effects on the fetus and neonate. Dev Pharmacol Ther 6:404, 1983.

414. Chavez CJ, Ostrea EM Jr, Stryker JC, Smialek Z: Sudden infant death syndrome among infants of drug-dependent mothers. J Pediatr 95:407, 1979.

415. Cohn HE, Piasecki GJ, Jackson BT: The effect of fetal heart rate on cardiovascular function during labor. Am J Obstet Gynecol 138:1190, 1980.

416. Collaborative Group on Antenatal Steroid Therapy: Effect of antenatal dexamethasone administration on the prevention of respiratory distress syndrome. Am J Obstet Gynecol 141:276, 1981.

417. Committee on Drugs: Neonatal drug withdrawal. Pediatrics 72:895, 1983.

418. Corby DG: Aspirin in pregnancy: Maternal and fetal effects. Pediatrics 62(Suppl): 930, 1978.

419. Curet LB, Rao AV, Zachman RD, et al: Collaborative Group on Antenatal Steroid Therapy: Maternal smoking and respiratory distress syndrome. Am J Obstet Gynecol 147:446, 1983.

420. Denson R, Nanson JL, McWatters MA: Hyperkinesis and maternal smoking. Can Psychiatr Assoc J 20:183, 1975.

421. DiSessa TG, Zednokova M, Hiraishi S, et al: The cardiovascular effects of metrizamide in infants. Radiology 148:687, 1983.

422. Drew JH, Kitchen WH: The effect of maternally administered drugs on bilirubin concentrations in the newborn infant. J Pediatr 89:657, 1976.

423. Evens RP, Leopold JC: Scopolamine toxicity in a newborn. Pediatrics 66:329, 1980.

424. Falterman CG, Richardson CJ: Small left colon syndrome associated with maternal ingestion of psychotropic drugs. J Pediatr 97:308, 1980.

425. Finberg L (ed): Chemical and Radiation Hazards to Children. Report of the eighty-fourth Ross Conference on Pediatric Research. Columbus, Ohio, Ross Laboratories, 1982.

426. Findlay JWA: The distribution of some commonly used drugs in human breast milk. Drug Metab Rev 14:653, 1983.

427. Finnegan LP, Mitros TF, Hopkins LE: Comparison of two high initial oral doses of phenobarbital (PB) used for control of neonatal abstinence syndrome (NAS). Pediatr Res 13:368, 1979.

428. Fisher RS, Freimuth HC: Blood boron levels in human infants. J Invest Dermatol 30:85, 1958.

429. Forfar JO, Nelson MM: Epidemiology of drugs taken by pregnant women: Drugs that may affect

the fetus adversely. Clin Pharmacol Ther 14:632, 1973.

430. Ginsberg MD, Myers RE: Fetal brain injury after maternal carbon monoxide intoxication: Clinical and neuropathologic aspects. Neurology 26:15, 1976.

431. Graham JM Jr, Marin-Padilla M, Hoefnagel D: Jejunal atresia associated with Cafergot ingestion during pregnancy. Clin Pediatr 22:226, 1983.

432. Greene RJ: Mercury in incubators: Detecting "safe" levels. Pediatrics 67:312, 1981.

433. Hansen NB, Oh W, LaRochelle F, Stonestreet BS: Effects of maternal ritodrine administration on neonatal renal function. J Pediatr 103:774, 1983.

434. Hanson JW, Myrianthopoulos NC, Harvey MAS, Smith DW: Risks to the offspring of women treated with hydantoin anticonvulsants, with emphasis on the fetal hydantoin syndrome. J Pediatr 89:662, 1976.

435. Hill RM, Desmond MM, Kay JL: Extrapyramidal dysfunction in an infant of a schizophrenic mother. J Pediatr 69:589, 1966.

436. Hillman LS, Hillman RE, Dodson WE: Diagnosis, treatment, and follow-up of neonatal mepivacaine intoxication secondary to paracervical and pudendal blocks during labor. J Pediatr 95:472, 1979.

437. Hingson R, Alpert JJ, Day N, et al: Effects of maternal drinking and marijuana use on fetal growth and development. Pediatrics 70:539,1982.

438. Holt GR, Mabry RL: ENT medications in pregnancy: Otolaryngol Head Neck Surg 91:338, 1983.

439. Huisjes HJ, Touwen BCL: Neonatal outcome after treatment with ritodrine: A controlled study. Am J Obstet Gynecol 147:250, 1983.

440. Hutchison GB: Late neoplastic changes following medical irradiation. Cancer 37:1102, 1976.

441. Jones MC: Intrinsic versus extrinsically derived deformational defects: A clinical approach. Sem Perinatol 7:247, 1983.

442. Kanjanapone V, Hartig-Beecken I, Epstein MF: Effect of isoxsuprine on fetal lung surfactant in rabbits. Pediatr Res 14:278, 1980.

443. Kendrick E: Testing for environmental contaminants in human milk. Pediatrics 66:470, 1980.

444. Kinney H, Faix R, Brazy J: The fetal alcohol syndrome and neuroblastoma. Pediatrics 66:130, 1980.

445. Kuhn RJP, Speirs AL, Pepperell RJ, et al: Betamethasone, albuterol, and threatened premature delivery: benefits and risks. Obstet Gynecol 60:403, 1982.

446. Kuhnert BR, Kuhnert PM, Lu AI, Lin DCK: Meperidine and normeperidine levels following meperidine administration during labor. II Fetus and neonate. Am J Obstet Gynecol 133:909, 1979.

447. Linn S, Schoenbaum SC, Monson RR, et al: The association of marijuana use with outcome of pregnancy. Am J Public Health 73:1161, 1983.

448. Little RE, Streissguth AP, Barr HM, Herman CS: Decreased birth weight in infants of alcoholic women who abstained during pregnancy. J Pediatr 96:974, 1980.

449. MacArthur BA, Howie RN, Dezoete JA, Elkins J: School progress and cognitive development of 6-year-old children whose mothers were treated antenatally with betamethasone. Pediatrics 70:99, 1982.

450. Mangurten HH, Benawra R: Neonatal codeine withdrawal in infants of nonaddicted mothers. Pediatrics 65:159, 1980.

451. Marbury MC, Linn S, Monson R, et al: The association of alcohol consumption with outcome of pregnancy. Am J Public Health 73:1165, 1983.

452. Mawji F, Joyce TH III: Are local anesthetics safe for mother, fetus, and neonates? Perinatol Neonatal 7:52, 1983.

453. McNiel JR: The possible teratogenic effect of salicylates on the developing fetus: Brief summaries of eight suggestive cases. Clin Pediatr 12:347, 1973.

454. Merritt TA: Smoking mothers affect little lives. Am J Child 135:501, 1981.

455. Miller RW, Mulvihill JJ: Small head size after atomic irradiation. Teratology 14:355, 1976.

456. Moya F, Thorndike V: The effects of drugs used in labor on the fetus and newborn. Clin Pharmacol Ther 4:628, 1963.

457. Munson ES, Wagman IH: Diazepam treatment of local anesthetic-induced seizures. Anesthesiology 37:523, 1972.

458. Nelson MM, Forfar JO: Associations between drug administered during pregnancy and congenital abnormalities of the fetus. Br Med J 1:523,1971.

459. O'Connor M, Johnson GH, James DI: Intrauterine effect of phenothiazines. Med J Aust 1:416, 1981.

460. Olsen GD, Lees MH: Ventilatory response to carbon dioxide of infants following chronic prenatal methadone exposure. J Pediatr 96:983, 1980.

461. O'Sullivan K, Taylor M: Chronic boric acid poisoning in infants. Arch Dis Child 58:737, 1983.

462. Otero L, Conlon C, Reynolds P, et al: Neonatal leukocytosis associated with prenatal administration of dexamethasone. Pediatrics 68:778, 1981.

463. Parkin DE: Probable benadryl withdrawal manifestations in a newborn infant. J Pediatr 85:580, 1974.

464. Phelan MC, Pellock JM, Nance WE: Discordant expression of fetal hydantoin syndrome in heteropaternal dizygotic twins. New Engl J Med 307:99, 1982.

465. Phelps DL, Karim A: Spironolactone: Relationship between concentrations of dethioacetylated metabolite in human serum and milk. J Pharmaceut Sci 66:1203, 1977.

466. Pierog S, Chandavasu O, Wexler I: Withdrawal symptoms in infants with fetal alcohol syndrome. J Pediatr 90:630, 1977.

467. Procianoy RS, Pinheiro CEA: Neonatal hyperinsulinism after short-term maternal beta-sympathomimetic therapy. J Pediatr 101:612, 1982.

468. Rajegowda BK, Kandall SR, Falciglia H: Sudden unexpected deaths in infants of narcotic-dependent mothers. Early Hum Develop 2:219, 1978.

469. Reveri M, Pyati SP, Pildes RS: Neonatal withdrawal symptoms associated with glutethimide (Doriden) addiction in the mother during pregnancy. Clin Pediatr 16:424, 1977.

470. Rosenberg L, Mitchell AA, Parsells JL, et al: Lack of relation of oral clefts to diazepam use during pregnancy. New Engl J Med 309:1282, 1983.

471. Shaywitz SE, Cohen DJ, Shaywitz BA: Behavioral and learning difficulties in children of normal intelligence born to alcoholic mothers. J Pediatr 96:978, 1980.

472. Slone D, Siskind V, Heinonen OP, et al: Antenatal exposure to the phenothiazines in relation to congenital malformations, perinatal mortality rate, birth weight, and intelligence quotient score. Am J Obstet Gynecol 128:486, 1977.

473. Spak CJ, Hardell LI, De Chateau P: Fluoride in human milk. Acta Pediatr Scand 72:699, 1983.

474. Strauss AA, Modanlou HD, Bosu SK: Neonatal man-

ifestations of maternal phencyclidine (PCP) abuse. Pediatrics 68:550, 1981.

475. Tamer A, McKey R, Arias D, et al: Phenothiazine-induced extrapyramidal dysfunction in the neonate. J Pediatr 75:479, 1969.

476. Tardoux H,Gerard J, Bazquez G, Flouvat B: Which beta-blocker in pregnancy-induced hypertension? Lancet 2:1194, 1983.

477. Thorley KJ, McAinsh J: Levels of the beta-blockers atenolol and propranolol in the breast milk of women treated for hypertension in pregnancy. Biopharm Drug Disposition 4:299, 1983.

478. Walson PD, Ott MA, Carter DE: Lidocaine and mepivacaine in cord blood. Pediatr Pharmacol 2:341, 1982.

479. Warkany J: Antituberculosis drugs. Teratology 20:133, 1979.

480. Williams RH, Kay GA, Jandorf BJ: Thiouracil, its absorption, distribution and excretion. J Clin Invest 23:613, 1944.

481. Witter FR, King TM, Blake DA: The effects of chronic gastrointestinal medication on the fetus and neonate. Obstet Gynecl 58:79S, 1981.

INDEX

Note: Page numbers in *italics* refer to illustrations; those followed by (t) indicate tables, and those in **boldface** refer to drug dosages.

Methicillin *(Continued)*
  antimicrobial spectrum of, 42(t)
  clinical pharmacology of, 51
  clinical toxicology of, 51
  dosage recommendation for, **44(t)**
  plasmid-mediated resistance to, 41(t)
  structural and pharmacologic properties of, 46(t)
  therapeutic indications for, 51
Methimazole, and breast-feeding during maternal drug therapy, 357(t), 371
Methotrexate, and breast-feeding during maternal drug therapy, 358(t), 367
Methyl mercury, as an environmental toxin in breast milk, 371, 372(t)
Methyl mercury poisoning, in neonates, 342(t), 344
Methyl xanthine. See also specific agents.
  use of, in apnea, 120, 121(t)
Methyldopa, clinical toxicology of, 198
  pharmacology of, 198
    clinical, 198
  therapeutic indications for, 180(t), 198
Metocurine, dosage recommendations for, **309(t)**
  pharmacologic properties of, 309(t)
Metolazone, clinical toxicology of, 243
  commercial pharmaceutical preparation for, 229(t), 230(t)
  dosage recommendation for, **229(t)**
  pharmacology of, 242
    clinical, 242–243
  therapeutic indications for, 243
Metoprolol, pharmacologic properties of, 194(t)
Metronidazole, and breast-feeding during maternal drug therapy, 358(t), 366–367
  and dosage adjustment in neonates with kidney or liver dysfunction, 43(t)
  antimicrobial spectrum of, 42(t)
  clinical toxicology of, 77
  dosage recommendation for, **44(t)**
  effect on microbial cells of, 40(t)
  pharmacology of, 76
    clinical, 76
  therapeutic indications for, 76–77
Metubine. See *Metocurine.*
Miconazole, antimicrobial spectrum of, 42(t)
  clinical toxicology of, 84
  pharmacology of, 83
    clinical, 83
  therapeutic indications for, 83–84
Milrinone. See *Bipyridines.*
Minimum bactericidal concentration (MBC), testing of microbial sensitivity for, 41
Minimum inhibitory concentration (MIC), testing of microbial sensitivity for, 41
Minipress. See *Prazosin.*
Minoxidil, clinical toxicology of, 182–183
  pharmacology of, 175(t), *178,* 182
    clinical, 182
  dosage recommendation for, **180(t), 182**
  therapeutic indications for, 180(t), 182
Morphine, and breast-feeding during maternal drug therapy, 358(t), 368
  clinical toxicology of, 303
  "dilution intoxication" and, 28, 30(t)
  dosage recommendation for, **303, 303(t)**
  pharmacology of, 302
    clinical, 303
  therapeutic indications for, 303, 303(t)
Motrin. See *Ibuprofen.*

Moxalactam, and dosage adjustment in neonates with kidney or liver dysfunction, 43(t)
  clinical toxicity of, 59
  dosage recommendation for, **44(t)**
  pharmacology of, 59
    clinical, 59
  therapeutic indications for, 59
Multiple dosing, maximum safe concentration in, 18, *19*
  minimum effective concentration in, 18, *19*
  optimal therapeutic regimen in, 18, *19*
Multi-Vitamin Infusion. See also *Vitamin E.*
  form and concentration of, 272(t)
Muscle relaxants. See *Neuromuscular blockers.*
Mutational resistance, antimicrobial agents and, 40–41, 41(t)
Myocardial contractility, diminished, use of digoxin in, *149,* 152–153
Myocardial dysfunction, drugs of choice for, 173(t)
Myocarditis, digoxin dosage adjustment due to, 154(t)

Nadolol, pharmacologic properties of, 194(t)
Nafcillin, and dosage adjustment in neonates with kidney or liver dysfunction, 43(t)
  antimicrobial spectrum of, 42(t)
  clinical pharmacology of, 51–52
  clinical toxicology of, 52
  dosage recommendation for, **44(t)**
  structural and pharmacologic properties of, 46(t)
  therapeutic indications for, 52
Naloxone, clinical toxicology of, 328
  pharmacology of, 327
    clinical, 327
  therapeutic indications for, 327–328
  use of, to reverse the effects of opioids, 303
Naproxen, and breast-feeding during maternal drug therapy, 358(t), 368
  maternal ingestion of, and associated problems in newborn, 323
Narcotic analgesics. See *Analgesics.*
Narcotic withdrawal, neonatal, use of clonidine in, 197–198
Neostigmine, use of, to reverse drug-induced neuromuscular blockage, 311–312
Nephron, functional anatomy of, 226, *227*
Netilmicin, as an antibacterial agent, 69–70
  dosage recommendation for, **44(t)**
Neuromuscular blockers.
  clinical toxicology of, 311–312
  dosage recommendation for, **309(t), 311**
  pharmacologic properties of, 309(t)
  pharmacology of, 308, 310, 310(t)
    clinical, 310–311
  therapeutic indications for, 309(t), 311
Neuromuscular blocking action, of nondepolarizing drugs, 310(t)
Nicotine, use of, by lactating women, 371–372, 372(t)
Nifedipine, clinical toxicology of, 202
  pharmacology of, *199,* 200, *200,* 201, *201*
    clinical, 201–202
  therapeutic indications for, 202
Nipride. See *Nitroprusside.*
Nitrate(s), organic, pharmacology of, 175(t), 183
Nitrate poisoning, in neonates, 342(t), 345